ANNALS OF THE NEW YORK ACADE

Volume 249

THYMUS FACTORS IN IMMUNITY

Edited by Herman Friedman

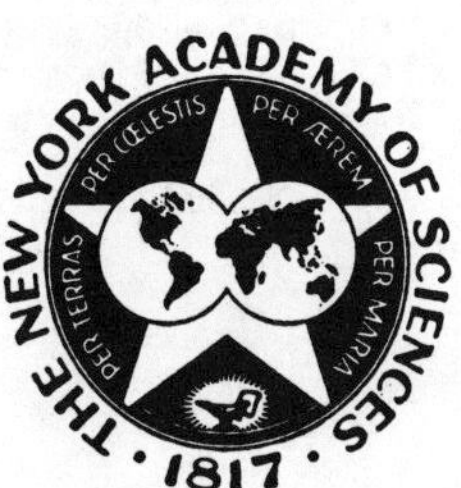

The New York Academy of Sciences
New York, New York
1975

Second printing December 1975

Library of Congress Cataloging in Publication Data

Main entry under title:

Thymus factors in immunity.

(Annals of the New York Academy of Sciences ; v. 249)
Papers presented at a conference held Apr. 3-5, 1974 by the New York Academy of Sciences.
1. Immune response--Congresses. 2. Thymus gland--Congresses. I. Friedman, Herman, 1931- ed. II. Series: New York Academy of Sciences. Annals ; v. 249.
Q11.N5 vol. 249 [QR186] 508'.1s [599'.02'9]
ISBN 0-89072-003-7 75-6939

PCP
Printed in the United States of America
ISBN 0-89072-003-7

ANNALS OF THE NEW YORK ACADEMY OF SCIENCES

Volume 249

February 28, 1975

THYMUS FACTORS IN IMMUNITY *

Editor
Herman Friedman

Conference Chairmen
Herman Friedman and Walter S. Ceglowski

CONTENTS

* This series of papers is the result of an international conference entitled Thymus Factors in Immunity, held by The New York Academy of Sciences on April 3–5, 1974.

Part IV. *In Vitro* Effects of Thymus Extracts and Products

Part V. *In Vivo* Effects of Thymus Extracts

Part VI. Role of Thymus Factors in Immunity: Perspectives

This monograph was aided by contributions from:

- CIBA-GEIGY
- WARNER-LAMBERT RESEARCH INSTITUTE
- WALLACE LABORATORIES
- SMITH, KLINE AND FRENCH LABORATORIES
- BURROUGHS-WELLCOME CO.
- UPJOHN CO.
- MERCK & CO.
- NATIONAL INSTITUTE OF ALLERGIES AND INFECTIOUS DISEASES
- SCHERING CORP.
- ENDO LABORATORIES

INTRODUCTORY REMARKS

Herman Friedman

Albert Einstein Medical Center
Philadelphia, Pennsylvania 19141

An extraordinary development of knowledge, concepts, interests and medical applications has occurred during the last two decades in the field of basic immunology. It is, for example, widely accepted that as late as the 1940's little was known concerning the cellular and molecular mechanisms involved in immunity. In contrast, it is now quite apparent even to the newcomer to immunology that this field is at the forefront of biomedical science. The increased interest and knowledge concerning the thymus gland has essentially paralleled the spectacular growth in the field of immunology itself. Although the thymus has been known as a lymphoid organ for many years, it has been only within the last decade and a half that the central role of the thymus in immunocompetence was again recognized and attempts made to understand the regulatory role of this important lymphoid organ. For example, diverse substances isolated from thymus extracts have been known for many years, and the existence of hormone-like factors, each with single or multiple biological activity, has been reported many times. For many years, however, studies concerning subcellular factors from the thymus gland were generally relegated to the sideline because of the extreme productivity and excitement engendered by the studies concerning cellular elements from the thymus, which influence the immune response mechanism.

It was only about 15 years ago that Jacques Miller first showed in the modern era that thymectomy of newborn mice impaired immune responsiveness to skin grafts. His studies were an outgrowth of the well known observations that thymectomy of leukemia-susceptible mice at birth interfered with the development of the leukemic process later in life. Such studies concerning leukemogenesis and thymectomy were thought unrelated to basic immunology per se. Once Miller showed the relationship between neonatal thymectomy and impairment of immunity, however, there was an almost explosive increase in studies concerning the role of the thymus in developmental immunology. The corollary studies by Robert Good and his associates concerning the role of the thymus as well as the bursa of Fabricius in immune responsiveness need not be restated here. The importance of the thymus in immunodeficiency diseases has been repeatedly discussed and, indeed, numerous earlier clinical studies had suggested that the thymus plays an important role in the immune defense mechanism. The dramatic findings that thymus and bone marrow cells collaborate synergistically, made by Claman and colleagues and then by Miller and Mitchell in the middle and late 1960's, pointed the way to the current investigations by numerous immunologists concerning interactions of different cell types in the immune response.

It seems reasonable to state that it was not until three or four years ago that the collaborative role between thymus and bone marrow cells appeared to investigators to be due not so much to a direct interaction among these cell types but to single or multiple factors released by thymus cells which influence bone marrow cells. These studies of factors released from T-cells after stimulation by antigen or other substances that can influence immune responsiveness (either enhancers or suppressors of antibody formation or cellular immunity) suggested that there may be a relationship between such studies and those by biochemists and endocrinologists concerning subcellular factors extracted from the thymus gland.

The purpose of this conference was to bring together in one place investigators from diverse areas of immunobiology and biochemistry who are making important contributions to the study of the mechanism and role of the thymus gland. Although much of the investigative work in immunobiology concerning the thymus and immunity has dealt with cellular elements, evidence has now become almost overwhelming that a thymus "hormone" or factor(s) may contribute to immune function and development of immunologic competence and/or maturation. Many cellular immunologists who are quite familiar with studies concerning soluble factors from T-lymphocytes, which are important in antibody formation and cell-mediated immunity, appear to be less familiar with the parallel yet similarly exciting studies from many biochemically orientated laboratories concerning factors that have been isolated from thymus glands and show activity in various biologic systems, including immunologic ones. Thus a major intention of this conference was to provide a forum for biologists, immunologists, and biochemists who are making important contributions to the study of thymus "hormones" and related areas of research.

As indicated in FIGURE 1, there is an obvious interrelationship between the studies concerning soluble factors evolving from thymocytes stimulated by antigen, which influence B-cells and the parallel studies by other investigators concerning the isolation of biologically active factors from the thymus of various animal species, including the cow. Thus, specific sessions for this Conference were planned, each chaired by world-renowned immunologists and immunochemists, for the presentation of specific papers by well-known scientists in the general area of the role of the thymus in immunity. The first session dealt with the general topic of Cellular Interactions and Thymus Functions in the Immune Response and was chaired by Dr. B. Waksman. Papers presented by Drs. Miller, Claman, Auerbach, Dutton, and Cudkowicz were concerned mainly with basic aspects of the role of the thymus and T-cells in immunity and how they regulate immune responsiveness.

The following session, chaired by Drs. H. Claman and G. Siskind dealt further with the general role of thymus factors in cellular and humoral immunity. Papers presented by Drs. Davies, Möller, Stutman, and Feldman, focused attention on the mechanisms involved in T- and B-cell interactions and the role of thymus factors in the effector stages of immune responses. The next session, chaired by Drs. W. Ceglowski and A. White, was concerned with the subject of preparation and characterization of thymic extracts. Investigators prominent in the area of thymus "hormones" and thymus-factor isolation presented descriptions of methods and procedures used for obtaining active preparations as well as of characteristics of calf thymus extracts and similar extracts from other sources. Information was presented characterizing these factors in terms of immunologic stimulation.

The next two sessions dealt with the effects of such thymus extracts, as well as thymus-cell products, on a variety of immune responses, both *in vivo* and *in vitro*. Papers were presented showing the variety of activities influenced by thymus cell factors, both in experimental animals and in man. Most noteworthy was the stimulation of human lymphocyte activity *in vitro* after treatment with thymic extracts. For example, human lymphocytes from individuals with immunodeficiency diseases recover their ability *in vitro* to perform a variety of normal "immune" functions after incubation with thymic factors. The mechanism whereby this occurs was discussed by a number of speakers.

The final session of the conference dealt with the "prospectus for the future" and the role of thymus factors in general immunity. Summation talks by a number of authorities in the field of immunology pointed to future applications of thymic "hormones" or factors in a wide variety of model systems

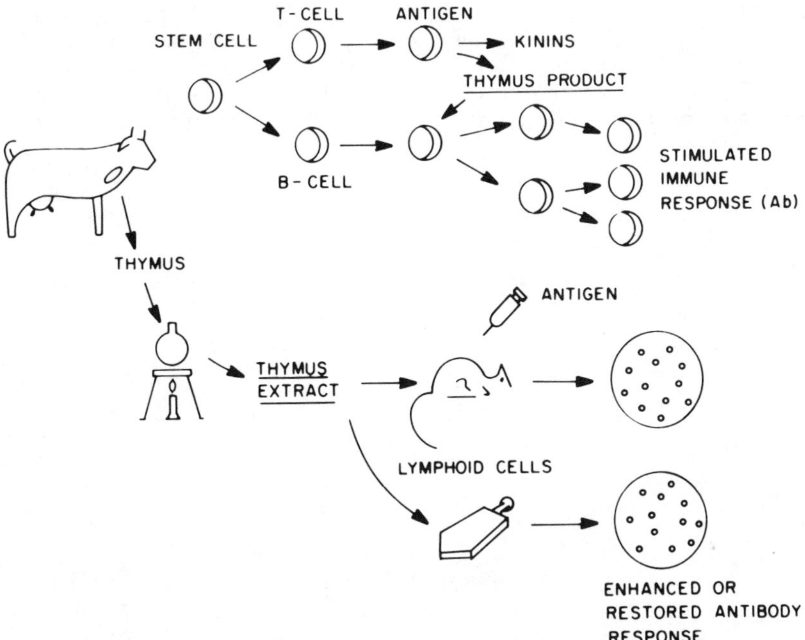

FIGURE 1. Schematic representation of model systems used to show immunological stimulatory activity of calf thymus extracts or factor(s) and possible relationship to T-cell products known to be important in cellular immunity and possibly as a helper factor(s) in humoral immunity.

and to the possibility that in the not-too-distant future such extracts and factors, as well as stimulation of thymus activity per se, will have an important place in the armamentarium of medicine.

Nearly all investigators who are actively engaged in studying some aspects of the role of soluble factors and subcellular extracts from thymus glands in immunity were present at the conference. A number of foreign immunologists and biochemists, including Drs. Bach, Davies, Globerson, Feldman, Feldmann, Mizutani, Möller, and Wecker were present. These investigators represented countries such as England, France, Japan, Israel, West Germany, Canada, and Australia, and lent a true international atmosphere to the conference. Last but not least Dr. A. White of California and Dr. J. Comsa of West Germany, among the first investigators in the area of thymic hormone factors from the calf in terms of immunologically active substances, were present as active participants. Dr. A. Goldstein of Texas, formally associated with Dr. White, provided invaluable assistance in the initial planning stages of the conference. All the participants who attended the evening banquet were very grateful to hear Dr. R. A. Good, from the Sloan-Kettering Institute, present his experiences and viewpoints, as well as perspectives, concerning the role of the thymus in immunobiology.

It is the expectation of those involved in organizing the conference, as well as the participants, that the proceedings of this conference, as well as proceedings of future conferences on the same subject, will bring to the attention of the immunology community not only the interesting and exciting data and experiments concernig the role of the thymus in immune responsiveness, but will also provide an impetus for further studies concerning the nature and significance of thymus extracts and products released by thymus cells involved in immune responses.

Part I. Cellular Interactions and Thymus Function in the Immune Response

T-CELL REGULATION OF IMMUNE RESPONSIVENESS *

J. F. A. P. Miller

The Walter and Eliza Hall Institute of Medical Research
Royal Melbourne Hospital
Victoria 3050 Australia

In 1961, data were available to show that mice thymectomized at birth were susceptible to infection, often died prematurely, had a diminished population of lymphocytes in blood and lymphoid tissues, and an impaired capacity to reject foreign skin grafts.[50] Defects in the ability of neonatally thymectomized mice to undertake cellular immune responses [51] and to produce antibody to some antigens [52] are now well established, and the origin, site of differentiation and fate of lymphocytes involved in immunity have been delineated. Hemopoietic stem cells (originating in the yolk sac, liver or marrow) migrate to the primary lymphoid organs, thymus and bursa, or bursa-equivalent, which in species other than birds may be the bone marrow itself. There the stem cells differentiate along lymphoid cell lines. Thymus-derived cells (T-cells †) populate the thymus-dependent areas of the lymphoid tissues and recirculate from blood to lymph. Nonthymus-derived cells (B-cells) colonize the thymus-independent areas of the secondary lymphoid organs, such as the follicles. As a result of interaction with antigen, T-cells differentiate to cells involved in cellular immunity and B-cells to antibody-producing cells.[56]

It is now evident that the thymus exerts a widespread influence, not only in the development of immune capacity, but also in the regulation of immune functions. Various factors are involved in the many activities of the thymus and of its cells, as is shown by the papers in this volume. In considering thymus factors in immunity, a distinction has to be made between those factors influencing the differentiation of the T-cell lineage (first section) and those factors produced by mature, antigen-activated T-cells which influence not only lymphoid cells but also other leucocytes and which play an essential role in regulating immune responsiveness (second and later sections).

* Publication number 1996 from The Walter and Eliza Hall Institute.

† Abbreviations used in this paper: ASC, *Ascaris suum;* B-cell, bone marrow-derived antibody-forming cell precursor; B_μ-cell, immediate precursor of IgM-secreting B-cells; B_γ-cell, immediate precursors of IgG-secreting B cells; cyclic AMP, adenosine 3′,5′-monophosphate; DNP, 2,4-dinitrophenyl; DNP-D-GL, DNP conjugate of a synthetic random copolymer of D-glutamic acid and D-lysine; DRC, donkey erythrocytes; Fla, flagellin of *Salmonella adelaïde,* FγG, fowl immunoglobulin G; Ig, immunoglobulin; KLH, keyhole limpet hemocyanin; MRC, mouse erythrocytes; MSH, *Maia squinada* hemocyanin; NIP, 4-hydroxy, 3-iodo, 5-nitrophenylacetyl; PFC, plaque-forming cells; poly A:U, polyadenylic-polyuridylic acid complex; SIII, type III polysaccharide from *Streptococcus pneumoniae;* T-cell, thymus-derived cell; (T,G)-A--L, poly-L(Tyr,Glu)-poly-D, L-Ala--poly-L-Lys.

Humoral Influences Regulating T-cell Development

In 1963, it was shown that the lymphoid tissues and immune capacities of neonatally thymectomized mice could in some cases be restored towards normal levels by inserting thymus tissue in a Millipore diffusion chamber, the pores of which prevented cell traffic into or out of the chamber.[65, 43] This raised the question as to whether the thymus might influence the differentiation of stem cells or prethymic cells by means of some thymus-specific humoral factor similar to inducers of differentiation acting on other cell lines of the hemopoietic system, e.g. erythropoietin. Recent work suggests that this is indeed the case.

We do not know how many differentiation steps there are between the uncommitted hemopoietic stem cell and the mature immunocompetent T-cell. By analogy with erythrocyte differentiation,[45] it may be that at least two types of differentiation processes are involved in the early history of the T-cell lineage. In the first, the stem cell becomes committed to the T-cell pathway and hence deprived of its other options (step 1, TABLE 1). Where and how this takes place is not known. It does seem, however, that it can occur in athymic mice (see below). The second step is likely to be initiated by a thymic humoral factor or thymic inducer acting on the committed prethymic cell and triggering its differentiation to the "immature" thymus cell (step 2, TABLE 1). This transition involves changes in surface phenotype characterized by the appearance of surface differentiation antigens coded by the sets of genes Thy-1 (θ), TL and Ly-1, Ly-2/3, Ly-5.[11] These changes can be induced *in vitro* within about two hours and do not therefore require cell division.[39] Inducible cells are present in athymic mice, clearly indicating that they have not been conditioned by the thymus or by a thymus humoral factor. Such cells should be identifiable by the presence on their surface of a receptor for the thymic inducer.

How specific is the thymus inducer responsible for step 2? Under normal, physiological conditions, the thymus itself must act as the inducer since normal mice have cells with the phenotypic characteristics of thymus cells (θ, TL and Ly antigens) and athymic mice have not. Under experimental conditions, however, not only can thymic extracts trigger step 2, but also other agents as cyclic AMP, poly A:U and endotoxin.[68] A specific thymus inducer should induce only differentiation of prethymic cells, in contrast to a nonspecific inducer, which might trigger differentiation not only of T-precursor cells but also of B or other precursor cells. It is necessary, therefore, to determine whether the inducer obtained from thymus extracts can or cannot induce the appearance of nonthymus-specific antigens (such as PC_1) on prethymic cells and whether it can or cannot provoke surface changes normally associated with T-cells on cells other than lymphoid cells, e.g. fibroblasts.

The majority of cells in the thymus have TL antigens (in TL^+ mice) and a high density of θ antigen.[69] These cells are cortisone-sensitive and not competent to initiate immune responses. A minority of thymus cells (10%) are cortisone-resistant and immunocompetent;[9] they have lost the TL antigens and have a much lower density of θ antigens ("low-θ cells"). They thus resemble mature peripheral T-cells in these respects. It is generally assumed that the high-θ, TL^+ cells are the immature, immunoincompetent, precursors of the low-θ, TL^- cells. Recently, however, the validity of this assumption has been questioned[69, 70] and a model proposed in which differentiation of prethymic cells can lead to one of two pathways, one of which is a direct transformation to a low-θ, TL$^-$ immunocompetent thymus cell, not involving prior transition through a high-θ, TL$^+$ cell. If this view can be substantiated, it becomes of extreme importance to determine whether agents like thymosin or thymin (which trigger the differentiation of high-θ, TL$^+$ cells) do indeed influence the differentiation pathway that leads to the generation of immunocompetent thymus cells: one must distinguish between surface phenomena and the acquisition of functional competence. Early reports on the immunocompetence of cells after thymosin treatment are not clear. In our laboratory, thymosin has not been effective *in vivo* in thymus-deprived mice.[72]

TABLE 1

HUMORAL FACTORS AND T-CELL DIFFERENTIATION

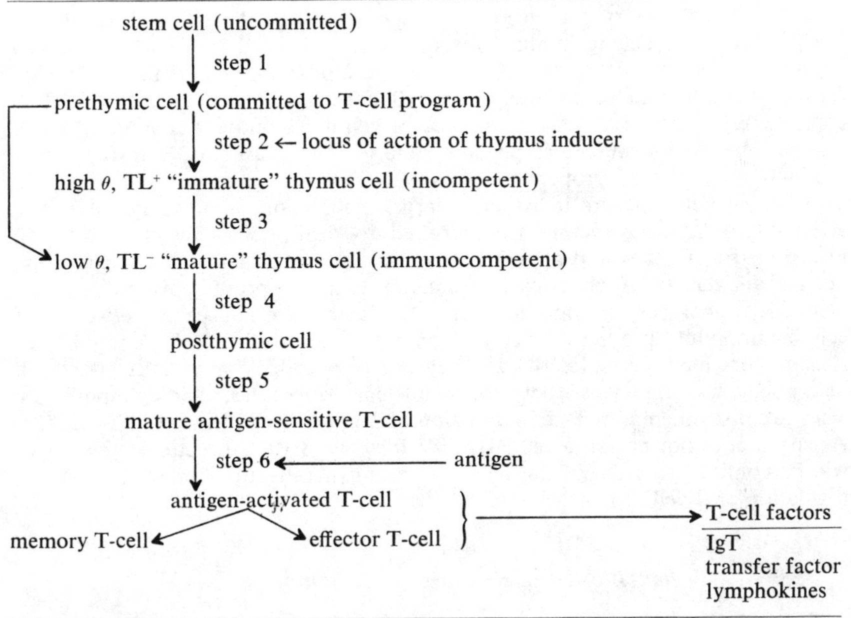

As regards postthymic cell differentiation, we do not know how many steps are involved. A thymus humoral factor has been implicated and said to activate "immature" postthymic cells into fully competent lymphocytes (step 4 and/or step 5).[66] Some investigators distinguish various stages of maturation of postthymic cells as T_1, T_2, T_3, T_4, etc., and others have claimed that collaboration occurs in some T-cell-mediated immune responses between T-cells of various postthymic maturation stages.[12] It is clear that much more data is required before the T-cell lineage can be mapped in a meaningful way.

T-cell Factors Regulating Immune Responsiveness

The mature antigen-sensitive T-lymphocyte can be influenced to differentiate further after antigenic stimulation. Just like the antigen-sensitive B-cell, the T-cell is capable of specific antigen recognition and, following antigen binding, of initiating immune responses.[5] The receptor that permits the B-cell to discriminate between various antigenic determinants has the same specificity as the secreted product (antibody) of the antigen-activated B-cell.[79] The nature of the analogous receptor on T-cells is the subject of much current debate. Some investigators[48] claim that it is an IgM-like molecule (known as IgT) cytophilic for macrophages. Other investigators have found it difficult to substantiate these claims,[77] and others[7] postulate the existence of receptors coded by a set of genes (Ir_1) different from those genes coding for immunoglobulin molecules. At the time of writing, it is still not clear whether IgT is secreted by antigen-activated T-cells and therefore whether it is one of the *T- and B-cell Collaboration in Antibody Responses*).

Among the factors produced by antigen-activated T-cells and regulating T-cell factors influencing immune responsiveness as listed in Table 1 (see also immune responsiveness are transfer factor and lymphokines (TABLE 1). Transfer factor is a low molecular weight (*ca.* 10,000 daltons) double stranded RNA complex acting essentially as an *initiator* of cellular immunity converting naive lymphocytes to an antigen-responsive state.[41] As a result of transfer factor production by a small proportion of natively sensitized specific T-lymphocytes, a cascading effect occurs in which a larger population of naive lymphocytes, activated by transfer factor, are recruited to deal more effectively with an infectious focus. It would appear that various transfer factors have specificity, not for antigen, but for a subset of antigen-sensitive (presumably T) lymphocytes. Lymphokines, in contrast to transfer factor, are nonspecific *effectors* of cellular immunity produced after antigen activation of T-cells.[42] A number of such factors have been described: they are responsible for various effects on macrophages, monocytes, polymorphonuclear leucocytes, and lymphocytes. They are instrumental in T-cell regulation of immune responsiveness (TABLE 2). As space does not permit a review of all these regulatory functions, this paper will be confined to a discussion of some recent investigations relevant to T-cell regulation of B-cell responsiveness.

T- and B-cell Collaboration in Antibody Responses

The finding that neonatal thymectomy impaired antibody responses to some antigens[52] was at first difficult to reconcile with the concept of a dual immune system. It was soon, however, shown that T-cells were required in order for B-cells to produce an optimal antibody response to certain types of antigens.[55, 13, 76] The concept of "T-dependent" and "T-independent" antigens therefore arose, and it became important to define the characteristic features which distinguished these two groups of antigens. T-independent antigens were found to have a structure characterized by repeating antigenic determinants. This was said to enable multivalent binding to the immunoglobulin receptors on the B-cell surface, a prerequisite for cell triggering.[21] T-dependent antigens lacked such physicochemical properties but were said to be able to activate T-cells (presumably after binding to antigen-recognition sites on the T-cells);

as a result, activated T-cells released special immunoglobulin molecules or IgT that were cytophilic for macrophages. The macrophage-carrying-IgT complexes were postulated to act as a matrix concentrating relevant antigenic determinants in a multivalent manner onto B-cell receptors.[19] There are several difficulties with such a hypothesis and, for convenience, they will be listed as follows.

First, T-independent antigens generally evoke only IgM antibody, not IgG, whether in the presence or absence of T-cells.[4] On the other hand, T-dependent antigens can generally produce some IgM response but no IgG in the absence of T-cells, whereas in their presence IgG responses occur. It would appear, therefore, that the assignment of an antigen to the T-dependent or T-independent class is not logical, since T-dependent antigens are in fact not strictly T-dependent insofar as the IgM response is concerned, whilst T-independent antigens are still unable to elicit an IgG response when T-cells are present. It would be more logical to distinguish those antigens that can activate T cells from those which cannot, and to ascribe the property of T-cell dependence, not

TABLE 2

T-CELL REGULATION OF IMMUNE RESPONSIVENESS

Cells Involved	Regulatory Role of T-Cells	References
T ⟶ T T ⟶ B	T-cells either promote or suppress function of other lymphocytes in both cellular and humoral immunity.	22, 53, 55, 58
T ⟶ macrophage	T-cells activate macrophages and enhance microbicidal activity.	46
T ⟶ mononuclear leucocytes T ⟶ polymorphonuclear leucocytes	T-cells produce factors which recruit inflammatory cells, e.g. in delayed hypersensitivity.	10
T ⟶ eosinophils T ⟶ basophils	T-cells help recruit eosinophils and basophils.	3, 16

to antigens, but to the type of antibody response. In fact the responses highly influenced by T-cells are high-affinity antibody production (e.g. secondary responses), IgE and IgG, whereas low-affinity antibody and IgM responses are marginally or not T-cell dependent (TABLE 3).

Second, the experimental systems that led to the formulation of the macrophage-IgT-antigen presentation hypothesis were set up entirely *in vitro*. This is unfortunate, because *in vitro* systems have thus far not been optimal in the induction of high-affinity antibodies and IgG antibodies, which are of major importance in the study of T-cell influence on B-cell responsiveness (TABLE 3). Only IgM antibody was assayed in such *in vitro* studies even though IgM antibody responses are the least T-cell dependent.

Third, it has been shown that allogeneic T- and B-cells fail to cooperate in contrast to syngeneic or semiallogeneic cells.[36] If the active T-cell product responsible for cooperation is an IgT molecule that has specificity for antigen and serves only to bind the antigen to macrophages, it becomes very difficult to understand why cooperation does not occur between allogeneic T- and B-cells.

Fourth, according to the macrophage-IgT-antigen presentation hypothesis, activated T-cells, by secreting specific immunoglobulin molecules cytophilic for macrophages, function essentially as antigen-concentrating devices to encourage effective binding of T-dependent antigens by B-lymphocytes. As a result, B-cells with lower antigen-binding potential would have their capacity to bind antigen increased and low-affinity antibody production should be enhanced. *In vivo,* however, the production of low-affinity antibody is the least T-cell dependent response: on the contrary, high-affinity antibody production is highly T-cell dependent (TABLE 3).

Fifth, perhaps the major difficulty with the macrophage-IgT-antigen presentation scheme is that of unequivocally demonstrating the release of IgT and its role in collaboration. Recent studies have shown that B-cell derived immunoglobulin can be carried not only by resting (G_0) T-cells [33, 34] but also by antigen-activated T-cells, in this case probably complexed with antigen.[32] Thus, T-cells activated to histocompatibility antigens had on their surface IgM antibody derived from B-cells contaminating the original thymus-cell suspension

TABLE 3

T-CELL-DEPENDENT HUMORAL ANTIBODY RESPONSES

Highly T-cell-dependent	Marginally or not T-cell-dependent
High-affinity antibody[24]	Low affinity antibody[24]
IgE[25]	IgM[57, 59]
IgG[57, 59]	

used to obtain activated T-cells. In addition, such activated T-cells also carried IgG antibody of which some, as determined by allotypic specificity, was derived from the irradiated host used to activate the thymus cells.[32] It is therefore clear that, in all experiments attempting to demonstrate a role for IgT, one must consider the possible existence of B-cell derived immunoglobulin.

Further reasons for not accepting the macrophage-IgT-antigen hypothesis of T- and B-cell collaboration will be pointed out in the next sections.

B-cell Responsiveness in the Absence of Appropriate Specific T-cells

Can B-cells be triggered to differentiate to antibody-forming cells (particularly to cells producing IgG antibody and high-affinity antibody) in the absence of a T-cell influence? At least four separate lines of evidence indicate that B-lymphocytes, in the absence of T-cells or of appropriate specific T-cells, not only can bind antigen (including so-called T-dependent antigens), but can also be influenced in a functional sense. These four lines of evidence are:

Antigen-Binding In Vitro

In vitro, B-lymphocytes, uncontaminated by T-cells (e.g. lymphoid cells from athymic nude mice) will bind antigen specifically, whether this be T-dependent or T-independent.[17] Evidently T-cells are not required for this binding.

Postantigen Transient Paralysis In Vivo

Specific transient unresponsiveness following short-term priming with antigen (about 24 hours) is demonstrable only on adoptive transfer[73] and appears to be a universal phenomenon since (1) it has been observed with particulate antigens such as erythrocytes and soluble antigens such as proteins; (2) it affects both T-cells and B-cells in humoral immune responses; (3) it affects both primed and unprimed B-cells; (4) it has been observed not only with humoral responses but also with T-cell mediated reactions (Sprent and Miller, data to be published); and (5) it has been observed with B-cells encountering T-dependent antigens in the absence of T-cells. The specific unresponsiveness exhibited by B-cells in the absence of T-cells was demonstrated in the following situations: athymic nu/nu mice, born from a fifth generation backcross of nu/+ mice to Balb/c, were given an intravenous injection of 10^9 sheep erythrocytes and 24 hours later cells from their spleens were transferred into irradiated BAB/14 mice together with sheep erythrocytes and T-cells from nu/+ donors. The direct and indirect plaque-forming cell responses to sheep erythrocytes were very low in contrast to those obtained in irradiated recipients of spleen cells of horse-erythrocyte-pretreated nu/nu mice.[61] B-cells must thus have been influenced by T-dependent antigens in the absence of T-cells.

IgG Expression on Cell Surface After T-cell-independent Encounter with T-dependent Antigen

It seems likely that the H-linked Ir-1 gene controls linked antigen recognition-dependent activation of T-cells.[7, 46] Both high- and low-responder mice have roughly the same number of antigen-binding B-cells. Following stimulation with antigen, both strains produce roughly the same amount of IgM antibody but only high-responders produce IgG antibody. Moreover, antigen-binding cells in high-responders increase to a much greater extent than they do in low-responders. After two challenges with antigen, however, antigen-binding cells in high- and low-responder mice have mainly IgG receptors even though low-responders fail to produce detectable amounts of IgG antibody.[30] It seems therefore that the switch from IgM to IgG precursor B-cells can be induced by antigen itself without the concomitant activity of appropriately activated specific T-cells.

Response of High-Affinity B-cells to Low *Doses of Hapten Carrier Conjugates in the Absence of Specific, Carrier-Primed T-cells*

Provided certain conditions of antigen dose and hapten density are fulfilled, B-lymphocytes can be triggered to produce IgG antibody (and even high-affinity antibody) in the absence of appropriate T-cells. The data of Klinman and Doughty[38] clearly show that, provided antigen dose is below a certain critical concentration, even memory B-cells can be triggered to produce high-affinity and IgG antibody in the absence of appropriate specific T-cells, and hence of any postulated IgT. These investigators treated spleen cell suspensions from immunized mice with anti-θ serum and complement before transferring the cells into nonimmune irradiated recipients. Fragments of spleens from irradiated mice were then explanted *in vitro,* stimulated with antigen and the amount of antibody released in the culture fluid measured. The anti-θ serum treatment reduced the degree of *in vitro* stimulation by hapten-homologous carrier complexes by 90%, but did not decrease at all the number of isolated precursor cells capable of being stimulated by *low* doses of hapten on heterologous carrier.

The experimental findings summarized in the four paragraphs above lead to the following conclusions: (1) B-lymphocytes, including precursors of IgG antibody-producers and high-affinity antibody-forming cells, can be stimulated by antigen in the absence of appropriate T-cells provided certain conditions of antigen dose are fulfilled; and (2) the effect of appropriately activated T-cells on B-cell responsiveness to antigen cannot therefore be a *sine qua non* for B-cell triggering, and, as a corollary, IgT, if it exists, cannot be an obligatory mediator of T- and B-cell collaboration. On the contrary, it would seem more logical to assume that the function of activated T-cells in B-cell responses is an immunoregulatory one.

Facilitation of B-cell Responses by Appropriately Activated T-cells

In *T- and B-cell Collaboration in Antibody Responses* it was reported that high-affinity antibody and IgG responses were highly T-cell dependent (TABLE 3). In the following section evidence was given that B-cells could produce such responses, but only if the antigen concentration was below a certain threshold. It is conceivable therefore that T-cells facilitate B-cell responses to antigen only if this exceeds a certain critical concentration effective presumably within the microenvironment of the B-cell. A number of experimental situations that are relevant to this possibility have been studied and are summarized below:

The antibody response to a hapten on an immunogenic carrier in mice previously exposed to the same hapten on a carrier that does not activate T-cells is negligible and there is no evidence of priming. Thus no IgG anti-DNP antibody could be detected in mice challenged with DNP.MSH one week after pretreatment with DNP.SIII, the carrier SIII being unable to activate T-cells.[60]

The antibody response to sheep erythrocytes of athymic nude mice given T-cells was markedly reduced if the mice had been pretreated one week before with the antigen given alone. Pretreatment with horse erythrocytes did not affect the anti-sheep response, indicating the specificity of the effect. It was also shown that the lymphoid cell population of sheep erythrocyte-pretreated nude mice was defective in its capacity to adoptively transfer IgG antibody responsiveness to sheep erythrocytes when injected together with T-cells in irradiated BAB/14 mice 1–3 weeks after pretreatment. In the one-host system, any IgM antibodies produced after the first injection with sheep erythrocytes, might well have inhibited B_{μ} cells from responding subsequently when sheep erythrocytes were given together with T-cells, but the adoptive transfer system established that B_γ cells must have been inhibited by the first contact with antigen in the absence of T-cells.[61]

The IgG antibody response of normal mice to a second challenge of a hapten on an immunogenic carrier when the first challenge was to the hapten on a nonimmunogenic carrier, such as autologous erythrocytes, is markedly reduced and often not detectable. Thus, for instance, a complete suppression of the indirect, but not the direct, antibody plaque-forming cell response to NIP conjugated to an immunogenic protein, FγG, was observed in mice pretreated with NIP-coated syngeneic erythrocytes. This occurred within 7 days, persisted for at least 2 months and was evident on adoptive transfer of spleen cells to irradiated mice. In this system, the possibility of a suppressive influence exerted by T-cells on anti-NIP antibody formation by B-cells was not supported by the fact that anti-θ-serum-pretreated NIP-tolerant spleen cells given to irradiated mice together with normal T-cells did not produce an anti-NIP

TABLE 4

PARALYSIS OF B_γ-CELLS BY NIP-CONJUGATED AUTOLOGOUS ERYTHROCYTES

CBA Cells Transferred	NIP PFC per Spleen at Day 7 in Irradiated CBA Mice Given NIP.FγG	
	Direct PFC	Indirect PFC
4×10^7 normal spleen cells *	11,000	27,000
4×10^7 spleen cells from NIP.MRC-pretreated mice *	4,100	0
4×10^7 spleen cells from NIP.MRC-pretreated mice depleted of T-cells by anti-θ serum + 10^7 cortisone-resistant thymus cells *	5,000	0
4×10^7 spleen cells from NIP.MRC-pretreated mice + 10^7 normal B-lymphocytes †	6,500	16,000

* Data from Reference 29.

† B-cells were separated from T-cells by cell electrophoresis of normal thoracic duct cells.

indirect plaque-forming cell response after challenge with NIP.FγG. On the other hand, the fact that the unresponsiveness could be reversed by supplementing with purified normal B-lymphocytes in the adoptive transfer system strongly suggests that the state of NIP tolerance was a stable property of the B-cell population (TABLE 4).[26, 28, 29] It is interesting to recall that syngeneic mouse erythrocytes persist for at least 2 to 3 months, and it is probable that there are no T-cells with reactivities directed towards the mouse's own erythrocytes. Thus, in the absence (or functional absence) of carrier-specific T-lymphocytes, the interaction of *excessive amounts* of persisting antigen with B_γ-lymphocytes must specifically suppress the potential of these cells to produce IgG antibody thus leading to a state of stable and specific B_γ-cell tolerance. These results are incompatible with the hypothesis that tolerance ensues when a complex made up of a postulated IgT and antigen reacts directly (not via macrophages) with the B-cell itself.[20]

Further experiments have shown that even in NIP-primed mice, the IgG anti-NIP response could be inhibited by treatment with NIP-coated syngeneic erythrocytes 10 days before secondary challenge with NIP.FγG.[29] Likewise with DNP.SIII, DNP-primed cells were much more susceptible to inhibition than unprimed DNP-sensitive cells.[60] In terms of antibody affinity, it has been shown that the production of high-affinity antibodies is more easily suppressed during tolerance induction than is the production of low-affinity antibodies,[71] and likewise IgG antibodies are more easily suppressed than IgM antibodies.[80] In keeping with these observations it is likely that B-cells with high intrinsic antigen-binding capacity will be more susceptible to receptor blockade *if antigen tends to persist* than B-cells with lower antigen-binding potential. This may be the reason why persistent, poorly degradable, antigens generally elicit only IgM responses and not IgG. On the other hand, degradable, nonpersistent, antigens elicit both IgM and IgG responses and it is the IgG response and the high-affinity antibody responses which are markedly diminished or abolished in the absence of T-cells, the IgM or low-affinity antibody responses being either unaffected or reduced significantly but not abolished. These observations would appear to link (1) antigen persistence, (2) susceptibility of potential IgG or high-affinity antibody producers to paralysis and (3) absence of a T-cell influence.[58]

Suppression of B-cell Responses by T-cells

Most studies have hitherto concentrated on defining a positive facilitating influence of T-cells on B-cell responsiveness to antigen. More recently, however, evidence, albeit indirect, has been presented by several groups [22] for a suppressive T-cell influence. Important observations worth citing are: (1) T-cell depleting procedures (such as thymectomy or treatment with antilymphocyte serum) have increased antibody production against so-called T-independent antigens.[37] (2) Conversely, addition of T-cells has sometimes caused a lowering in the antibody response.[2] (3) T-cells have been shown to play an active role in the phenomenon of allotype suppression.[31]

The possibility of a suppressor effect of T-cells on B-cell responsiveness in immunological tolerance became evident when it was found that cells from tolerant animals could, in some systems, be mixed with cells from normal animals and prevent these from responding adequately.[44, 23] Further evidence for the existence, in tolerant animals, of T-cells that exert an active suppressor effect on IgG antibody production has been obtained by our group.[6] Specific immunological tolerance was induced in CBA mice with a single injection of deaggregated FγG. The unresponsive state was stable on adoptive transfer and not reversed by pretreatment of tolerant cells with trypsin. Tolerant cells could suppress the IgG response of normal spleen cells or primed B-cells in an adoptive transfer system although the suppression was dose-dependent: low doses facilitating the response, higher doses suppressing it (Table 5). Incubation of the tolerant cell population with anti-θ serum and complement (Table 6), or with highly radioactive FγG (Table 7), under conditions known to abrogate T-cell facilitation, reversed the suppressor effect.

Much work has to be done before the mechanism of suppression by T cells can be understood. The following possibilities are being considered: (1) Two classes of T-cells exist, one facilitating immune responses, the other suppressing.

TABLE 5

HELPER AND SUPPRESSOR EFFECTS OF FγG-TOLERANT SPLEEN CELLS *

CBA Cells Transferred	Indirect PFC per Spleen at Day 7 in Irradiated CBA Mice Given FγG and DRC	
	Anti-FγG	Anti-DRC
10^7 normal spleen cells + 5×10^6 FγG-primed B-cells	10,270	8,990
10^8 normal spleen cells + 5×10^6 FγG-primed B-cells	56,000	38,750
5×10^6 FγG-primed B-cells	120	200
10^7 FγG-tolerant spleen cells + 5×10^6 FγG-primed B-cells	11,320	10,750
10^8 FγG-tolerant spleen cells + 5×10^6 FγG-primed B-cells	860	41,380

* Data from Reference 6.

The recent claim for an enhanced antibody response following passage of normal or primed spleen cells through columns of histamine-rabbit serum albumin-coated sepharose supports the idea that suppressor T-cells may be a distinct class of T-cells.[67] (2) Only one class of T-cells exists and suppressor activity results from excessive production of T-cell factors—the "supra-priming hypothesis." An overproduction of nonspecific lymphokines, either by too many T-cells or by hyperactive T-cell populations, may limit antigen availability to B-cells to such an extent that triggering is impaired or less antibody is produced. On the other hand, overproduction of a specific T-cell factor (IgT + antigen) may saturate Fc receptors on macrophages and allow direct interaction of IgT-antigen complexes with immunoglobulin receptors on B-cells.[20] Before

TABLE 6

θ-SENSITIVE SUPPRESSOR EFFECT OF FγG-TOLERANT SPLEEN CELLS *

CBA Cells Transferred	Indirect PFC per Spleen at Day 7 in Irradiated CBA Mice Given FγG and DRC	
	Anti-FγG	Anti-DRC
10^7 FγG-tolerant spleen cells	100	3,210
10^7 normal spleen cells	1,200	3,500
10^7 FγG-tolerant spleen cells + 10^7 normal spleen cells	30	6,020
10^7 anti-θ serum pretreated FγG-tolerant spleen cells + 10^7 normal spleen cells	4,650	7,390

* Data from Reference 6.

TABLE 7

ABROGATION OF SUPPRESSOR EFFECT OF FγG-TOLERANT SPLEEN CELLS BY ^{125}I-LABELED FγG *

CBA Cells Transferred	Indirect PFC per Spleen at Day 7 in Irradiated CBA Mice Given FγG and DRC	
	Anti-FγG	Anti-DRC
10^7 ^{127}I-FγG pretreated tolerant spleen cells	190	20,950
10^7 normal spleen cells	9,000	19,950
10^7 normal spleen cells + 10^7 ^{127}I-FγG pretreated tolerant spleen cells	720	59,760
10^7 normal spleen cells + 10^7 ^{125}I-FγG pretreated tolerant spleen cells	10,660	62,460

* Data from reference 6.

this can be envisaged as a mechanism, however, unequivocal demonstration of the production and export of T-cell immunoglobulin must be obtained *in vivo*.

If the supra-priming hypothesis is correct, one may predict that high doses of primed T-cells might suppress rather than facilitate B-cell responses [62] and that primed T-cells would reinforce the suppressor effect of tolerant T-cells. On the other hand, should primed T-cells abrogate the suppressor effect of tolerant T-cells, the possible existence of two distinct types of T-cells, one with facilitating and the other with suppressor activities, will have to be seriously considered.

Further clarification is required concerning the target of suppressor activity. In delayed hypersensitivity, it appears that T-cells, themselves, can suppress other T-cells.[81] In antibody formation, however, it is not known whether the suppressive effect is exerted directly on B-cells, via macrophages, or on other T-cells that would have facilitated the response of B-cells.

An understanding of the mechanism of T-cell suppression is urgently required as this phenomenon may play a role in immune homeostasis and self-surveillance against autoantigens.

Evidence for a Nonspecific Influence of T-cells on B-cell Responsiveness

There is much evidence to suggest that the influence by which T-cells modify B-cell responsiveness to antigen is nonspecific with respect to the antigenic determinants that activate T- and B-cells in the system used. The evidence for a nonspecific influence of activated T-cells modifying B-cell responsiveness *in vivo* has been obtained in systems in which a large number of T-cells were activated to an irrelevant antigen. Two such systems have been reported: (1) the "allogeneic effect," [1, 35] and (2) the "primed B-cell effect." [54]

As an example of the allogeneic effect, recent work on the response to NIP-coated erythrocytes may be given. NIP-coated F_1 or parental mouse erythrocytes do not give a detectable anti-NIP antibody response when given in one injection to normal mice. A substantial anti-NIP response was, however, obtained in F_1 mice if parental spleen cells were given at the same time as the

NIP-coated erythrocytes (TABLE 8). The primary anti-NIP antibody response produced under these conditions presumably resulted from the stimulation of the T-cells in the parental spleen cell population to the foreign histocompatibility antigens of the F_1 hosts with subsequent release of nonspecific factors capable of triggering NIP-sensitive B-cells.[27] The observed effect is consistent with a mechanism of T- and B-cell collaboration via nonspecific factors released from H-2 activated T-cells and acting in conjunction with antigen bound to immunoglobulin determinants on B-cells. It is difficult to explain these data in the basis of a specific IgT acting as collaborative factor.

Several other experimental systems allow the same conclusion. Thus, parental nonresponder $H2^{kk}$ cells transferred to nonresponder $H2^{kq}F_1$ mice enabled a primary IgG anti-(T, G)-A- -L antibody response after a single challenge.[63] Likewise, allogeneic cell transfer has overcome the requirement for carrier-specific T-cells in enabling a primary IgG response to antigens such as DNP-D-GL, which otherwise is not only poorly immunogenic but also tolerogenic to B_γ cells.[64]

It has been said that the allogeneic effect is too artificial to give a true insight into the physiological mechanisms of T- and B-cell cooperation. There are, however, other situations *in vivo* in which T-cells activated to irrelevant antigens can influence the responsiveness of B-cells to T-dependent antigens. For example, irradiated mice receiving KLH-primed T-cells (depleted of B-cells by passage through an anti-immunoglobulin column) and DNP.Fla-primed B-cells (depleted of T-cells by anti-θ serum treatment) produce a good IgG anti-DNP response to a challenge of DNP.KLH but little response to a challenge of KLH given together with DNP.FγG. If, however, the irradiated mice received, in addition, a *small number* of KLH-primed B-cells, their response to DNP.FγG was markedly enhanced when the antigen KLH was also given (TABLE 9). This so called "primed B-cell effect" suggests that KLH-primed B-cells can, presumably after binding KLH, activate KLH-primed T-cells more effectively than can KLH given without primed B-cells. It also suggests that T-cells, activated to KLH in this way, can influence the responsiveness of DNP-sensitive B-cells when DNP is conjugated to the irrelevant carrier FγG. The T-cell influence in this system cannot therefore be a specific one. Somewhat similar observations have been made in another *in vivo* system in which cells primed to DNP-ASC produced IgE anti-DNP responses upon challenge with DNP.KLH plus ASC.[25] The *in vivo* response to hapten and carrier on separate

TABLE 8

ALLOGENEIC CELL DEPENDENCE OF PRIMARY RESPONSE TO NIP.MRC *

Parental (CBA) Spleen Cells Given	Days Between Cell Transfer and Challenge with 2×10^9 NIP.MRC	NIP PFC per Spleen in Unirradiated (CBA × C57BL)F_1 Recipients	
		Direct PFC	Indirect PFC
none	—	0	0
5×10^7	same day	4000	16,000
5×10^7	2 days	0	5,400

* Data from Reference 27.

molecules may be explained not only by the inherently strong immunogenicity of the carrier proteins employed, but also by an enhancing effect of ASC-primed B-cells on the activation of ASC-primed T-cells in the presence of ASC.

In summary, it may be said that B-cells can bind antigen via their immunoglobulin determinants in the absence of any T-cell influence. Recent experimental evidence indicates that B-cells with high antigen-binding capacity (i.e. those B-cells that have the potential to produce high-affinity antibody in particular, or IgG antibody in general) are readily paralyzed in the absence of T-cells. Conversely, B-cells with lower antigen-binding capacity (such as cells producing low-affinity antibody in particular and IgM antibody in general) are not as easily paralyzed by antigen in the presence or in the absence of T-cells, possibly because antigen can readily dissociate from their receptors. T-cells are activated by antigen generally only if such antigen is presented on some surface such as the cell membrane of a macrophage.[78] It may be, however,

Table 9

Effect of Primed B-cells on T-cell Activation *In Vivo*

CBA Cells Transferred *	Antigen Challenge	Indirect DNP PFC per Spleen at Day 7 in Irradiated CBA Mice
5×10^6 KLH-primed T-cells + 5×10^6 DNP.Fla-primed B-cells	DNP.KLH	30,000
5×10^6 KLH-primed T-cells + 5×10^6 DNP.Fla-primed B-cells	DNP.FγG + KLH	4,000
5×10^6 KLH-primed T-cells + 5×10^6 DNP.Fla primed B-cells + 10^6 KLH-primed B-cells	DNP.FγG + KLH	25,000

* T-cells obtained by passing spleen cells through anti-immunoglobulin column; B-cells obtained by treating primed spleen cells with anti-θ serum and complement.

Unpublished data of Miller and Basten (1973). 8 mice per group.

that antigen bound to immunoglobulin determinants on B-cells is highly effective in activating T-cells. This may account both for the "primed B-cell effect" referred to above and for the phenomenon known as "original antigenic sin" in which the antibodies evoked by challenging with a structurally related antigen have a higher affinity for the first immunogen than for the second.[18] It may thus be assumed that under normal *in vivo* conditions, antigen bound to immunoglobulin determinants on B-cells recruits T-lymphocytes reactive to other determinants of the antigen. Possibly the T-cells recognize the B-cells bearing antigen-immunoglobulin complexes as foreign cells and are activated to produce nonspecific factors just as in cellular immunity. Among such factors are some which influence the mobility of phagocytic cells and the degradation of antigens by phagocytes.[10] This must lead to removal of antigen from the microenvironment of the B-cells and hence protect high affinity cells from paralysis. Among the products released by activated T-cells are presumably enzymes, such as proteases, which can activate components of the complement system.[14] Such components have been implicated in triggering of B-cells either by acting as an obligatory signal for cell transformation,[15] or by effecting release of antigen-antibody complexes bound to the B-cell membrane.[49] It is proposed, therefore, that T-cells modulate B-cell responsiveness by means of nonspecific factors and that T-cell immunoglobulin if it exists, does not play an obligatory role in B-cell triggering.

Implications

Experiments performed in the last 15 years have increased our knowledge of the physiology of the thymus and its relationship to the rest of the lymphoid system. The thymus is responsible for the construction of a pool of recirculating long-lived immunocompetent T-lymphocytes which, after antigen activation, have a major role in influencing immune responsiveness.

The discovery of the immunological function of the thymus has led to a better understanding of immunodeficiency diseases that afflict man. These can now be classified according to whether the T-cell system, the B-cell system or both are deficient. Replacement therapy (for instance implantation of thymus tissue or injection of a cell population containing stem cells) has been used with some success.[8] Measures that selectively deplete the T-cell population, for instance antilymphocyte serum, impair the capacity to reject grafts of foreign tissue and are being used in clinical medicine to prevent rejection of transplanted organs.[40]

By virtue of its capacity to recirculate, the T-cell is particularly well equipped for the task of seeking antigen and influencing the response of other lymphocytes and accessory cells. Support for such a role derives from the recent demonstration of rapid and complete recruitment of specific antigen-sensitive cells from the recirculating pool into regions where antigen has been deposited.[75, 74] This occurs during both cellular and humoral immunity. The ensuing interactions within lymphoid tissues between antigen-activated T-lymphocytes and effector cells—monocytes, macrophages, granulocytes or other lymphocytes—result in amplification and diversification of the immune response. This is manifest by simultaneous triggering of a wide range of host defence systems, constitutive as well as adaptive, including phagocytosis, microbicidal activity, the inflammatory response, kinin release and complement and coagulation cascades.

The T-cell/B-cell collaboration is the best characterized of the cellular interactions. There is compelling evidence for a crucial role of T-cells in determining the amount, class, and affinity of the antibody produced by B-cells in response to antigens. Indeed the switch from IgM to IgG production and the rise in affinity of the antibody produced, both seem to be under T-cell control (*T-cell and B-cell Collaboration in Antibody Responses*).

The knowledge that T-lymphocytes regulate the activities of other lymphocytes and leucocytes has wide practical implications in manipulation of the immune response:

Methods are available to augment the activities of T-lymphocytes. These include presentation of antigen in the appropriate form or by the appropriate route, the use of adjuvants such as the bacille Calmette-Guérin, or of the allogeneic effect. Such procedures, aimed at augmenting T-cell function, should enhance cellular immunity, microbicidal activity of macrophages and antibody production by B-cells. They may thus be beneficial in anergic states characterized by deficient T-cell functions, in various infectious diseases, such as leprosy, and in augmenting the efficacy of vaccinating procedures.

The suppressive effect of T-cells on B-cell responsiveness and on other T-cell activities (*Suppression of B-cell Responses by T-cells*) must be considered in the pathogenesis of autoimmune diseases. Further understanding of the mechanism of action of suppressor T-cells might conceivably lead to the control of some of these disorders.

The antibody response of B-lymphocytes can be turned off by antigenic determinants conjugated to materials (which can be synthesized) that are nondegradable, long-persisting and not T-cell activating (*Facilitation of B-cell Responses by Appropriately Activated T-cells*). This should provide a new approach to combat allergic disorders or complications (e.g. to penicillin) and possibly autoimmune diseases.

In some forms of cancer, where tumor cells have a distinct individual antigenicity of their own, the production of blocking factors may conceivably be diminished if the particular B-cells secreting enhancing antibody could be turned off by using one of the above methods.

A major unknown in all these systems is of course the identity of the various antigenic determinants concerned. Clearly, therefore, further detailed studies are required, not only in order to unravel precisely the many factors which activate or suppress T- or B-cell functions, but also to determine the chemical constitution of allergens, tumor-specific antigens, and other relevant cellular components. Such a knowledge may eventually allow precise immunological engineering and its application to clinical medicine.

References

1. Armerding, D. & D. H. Katz. 1974. J. Exp. Med. **140:** 19.
2. Baker, P. J., P. W. Stashak, D. F. Ambaugh, B. Prescott & R. Barth. 1970. J. Immunol. **105:** 1581.
3. Basten, A. & P. B. Beeson. 1970. J. Exp. Med. **131:** 1288.
4. Basten, A. & J. G. Howard. 1973. Contemp. Topics Imunobiol. **2:** 265.
5. Basten, A., J. F. A. P. Miller, N. L. Warner & J. Pye. 1971. Nature New Biol. **231:** 104.
6. Basten, A., J. F. A. P. Miller, J. Sprent & C. Cheers. 1974. J. Exp. Med. **140:** 199.
7. Benacerraf, B. 1974. Ann. Immunol. Inst. Pasteur **125C:** 143.
8. Bergsma, D. & R. A. Good, Eds. 1968. *In* The Immunological Deficiency Diseases of Man. Birth Defects Original Article Series. Vol. IV, No. 1. National Foundation. New York, N.Y.
9. Blomgren, H. & B. Andersson. 1970. Cell. Immunol. **1:** 545.
10. Bloom, B. R. & B. Bennett. 1970. Sem. Hematol. **7:** 215.
11. Boyse, E. A. & L. J. Old. 1969. Ann. Rev. Genet. **3:** 269.
12. Cantor, H. & R. Asofsky. 1972. J. Exp. Med. **135:** 764.
13. Claman, H. N. & E. A. Chaperon. 1969. Transplant. Rev. **1:** 92.
14. Cochrane, C. G. & H. J. Müller-Eberhard. 1968. J. Exp. Med. **127:** 371.
15. Dukor, P. & K-U. Hartmann. 1973. Cell. Immunol. **7:** 349.
16. Dvorak, H. F. & M. C. Mihm. 1972. J. Exp. Med. **135:** 235.
17. Dwyer, J. M., S. Mason, N. L. Warner & I. R. Mackay. 1971. Nature **234:** 252.
18. Eisen, H. N., J. R. Little, L. A. Steiner, E. S. Simms & W. Gray. 1969. Israel J. Med. Sci. **5:** 338.

19. FELDMANN, M. 1972. J. Exp. Med. **136:** 122.
20. FELDMANN, M. 1973. Nature New Biol. **242:** 82.
21. FELDMANN, M. & A. BASTEN. 1971. J. Exp. Med. **134:** 103.
22. GERSHON, R. K. 1974. Contemp. Topics Immunobiol. **3:** 1.
23. GERSHON, R. K. & K. KONDO. 1971. Immunology **18:** 723.
24. GERSHON, R. K. & W. E. PAUL. 1971. J. Immunol. **106:** 872.
25. HAMAOKA, T., D. H. KATZ & B. BENACERRAF. 1973. J. Exp. Med. **138:** 538.
26. HAMILTON, J. A. & J. F. A. P. MILLER. 1973. Eur. J. Immunol. **3:** 457.
27. HAMILTON, J. A. & J. F. A. P. MILLER. 1973. J. Exp. Med. **138:** 1009.
28. HAMILTON, J. A. & J. F. A. P. MILLER. 1974. Eur. J. Immunol. **4:** 261.
29. HAMILTON, J. A., J. F. A. P. MILLER & J. KETTMAN. 1974. Eur. J. Immunol. **4:** 268.
30. HÄMMERLING, G., T. MASUDA & H. O. MCDEVITT. 1973. J. Exp. Med. **137:** 1180.
31. HERZENBERG, L. A., E. B. JACOBSON, L. A. HERZENBERG & R. J. RIBLET. 1971. Ann. N.Y. Acad. Sci. **190:** 212.
32. HUDSON, L., J. SPRENT, J. F. A. P. MILLER & J. H. L. PLAYFAIR. 1974. Nature **251:** 60.
33. HUDSON, L., N. THANTREY, I. M. ROITT & L. N. PAYNE. 1974. Immunology. In press.
34. HUNT, S. & A. WILLIAMS. 1974. J. Exp. Med. **139:** 479.
35. KATZ, D. H. 1972. Transpl. Rev. **12:** 141.
36. KATZ, D. H., T. HAMAOKA, M. E. DORF & B. BENACERRAF. 1973. J. Exp. Med. **137:** 1405.
37. KERBEL, R. S. & D. EIDINGER. 1971. J. Immunol. **106:** 917.
38. KLINMAN, N. & R. A. DOUGHTY. 1973. J. Exp. Med. **138:** 473.
39. KOMURO, K. & E. A. BOYSE. 1973. J. Exp. Med. **138:** 479.
40. LANCE, E. M., P. B. MEDAWAR & R. N. TAUB. 1973. Advan. Immunol. **17:** 1.
41. LAWRENCE, H. S. 1974. Harvey Lectures. In press.
42. LAWRENCE, H. S. & M. LANDY, Eds. 1969. Mediators of Cellular Immunity. Academic Press. New York, N.Y.
43. LEVEY, R. H., N. TRAININ & L. W. LAW. 1963. J. Nat. Cancer Inst. **31:** 199.
44. MCCULLAGH, P. J. 1970. Australian J. Exp. Biol. Med. Sci. **48:** 369.
45. MCCULLOCH, E. A. 1970. *In* Regulation of Hematopoiesis. A. S. Gordon, Ed. Appleton-Century-Crofts. New York, N.Y.
46. MCDEVITT, H. O., K. B. BECHTOL, J. H. FREED, G. J. HÄMMERLING & P. LONAI. 1974. Ann. Immunol. Inst. Pasteur **125C:** 175.
47. MACKANESS, G. B. 1970. Sem. Hematol. **7:** 172.
48. MARCHALONIS, J. J. & R. E. CONE. 1973. Transpl. Rev. **14:** 3.
49. MILLER, G. W., P. H. SALUK & V. NUSSENZWEIG. 1973. J. Exp. Med. **138:** 495.
50. MILLER, J. F. A. P. 1961. Lancet **2:** 748.
51. MILLER, J. F. A. P. 1962. Ann. N.Y. Acad. Sci. **99:** 340.
52. MILLER, J. F. A. P. 1962. Proc. Roy. Soc. Series B. **156:** 410.
53. MILLER, J. F. A. P. 1972. Intern. Rev. Cytol. **33:** 77.
54. MILLER, J. F. A. P. & A. BASTEN. 1973. Unpublished results.
55. MILLER, J. F. A. P. & G. F. MITCHELL. 1969. Transplant. Rev. **1:** 3.
56. MILLER, J. F. A. P. & D. OSOBA. 1967. Physiol. Rev. **47:** 437.
57. MILLER, J. F. A. P., P. DUKOR, G. A. GRANT, N. R. ST. C. SINCLAIR & E. SACQUET. 1967. Clin. Exp. Immunol. **2:** 531.
58. MITCHELL, G. F. 1975. *In* The Lymphocyte: Structure and Function. J. J. Marchalonis, Ed. Dekker. New York, N.Y. In press.
59. MITCHELL, G. F., F. C. GRUMET & H. O. MCDEVITT. 1972. J. Exp. Med. **135:** 126.
60. MITCHELL, G. F., J. H. HUMPHREY & A. R. WILLIAMSON. 1972. Eur. J. Immunol. **2:** 460.
61. MITCHELL, G. F., L. LAFLEUR & K. ANDERSSON. 1974. Scand. J. Immunol. **3:** 39.
62. OKUMURA, K. & T. TADA. 1973. Nature New Biol. **245:** 181.

63. Ordal, J. C. & F. C. Grumet. 1972. J. Exp. Med. **136:** 1195.
64. Osborne, D. P., Jr. & D. H. Katz. 1973. J. Exp. Med. **137:** 991.
65. Osoba, D. & J. F. A. P. Miller. 1963. Nature. **199:** 633.
66. Rotter, V., A. Globerson, I. Nakamura & N. Trainin. 1973. J. Exp. Med. **138:** 130.
67. Shearer, G. M., K. L. Melman, Y. Weinstein & M. Sela. 1972. J. Exp. Med. **136:** 1302.
68. Scheid, M. P., M. K. Hoffmann, K. Komuro, U. Hämmerling, J. Abbott, E. A. Boyse, G. H. Cohen, J. A. Hooper, R. S. Schulof & A. C. Goldstein. 1973. J. Exp. Med. **138:** 1027.
69. Schlesinger, M. 1972. Progr. Allergy. **16:** 214.
70. Shortman, K. & H. Jackson. 1974. Cell. Immunol. **12:** 230.
71. Siskind, G. W. & B. Benacerraf. 1969. Advan. Immunol. **10:** 1.
72. Sprent, J. & J. F. A. P. Miller. 1970. *In* Annual Report of the Walter and Eliza Hall Institute of Medical Research, 74.
73. Sprent, J. & J. F. A. P. Miller. 1973. J .Exp. Med. **138:** 143.
74. Sprent, J. & J. F. A. P. Miller. 1974. J. Exp. Med. **139:** 1.
75. Sprent, J., J. F. A. P. Miller & G. F. Mitchell. 1971. Cell. Immunol. **2:** 171.
76. Taylor, R. B. 1969. Transplant. Rev. **1:** 114.
77. Vitetta, E. S. & J. W. Uhr. 1973. Transplant. Rev. **14:** 50.
78. Waldron, J. A., Jr., R. G. Hara & A. S. Rosenthal. 1973. J. Immunol. **111:** 58.
79. Warner, N. L. 1974. Advan. Immunol. **19:** 67.
80. Weber, G. & E. Kölsch. 1972. Eur. J. Immunol. **2:** 191.
81. Zembala, M. & G. L. Asherson. 1973. Nature **244:** 227.

"SIGNAL THEORY" IN CELLULAR IMMUNOLOGY: COLLABORATION BETWEEN T- AND B-LYMPHOCYTES IN THE IMMUNE RESPONSE

Henry N. Claman

Departments of Medicine and Microbiology
University of Colorado Medical Center
Denver, Colorado 80220

Two Universes of the Immune Response: Functional Separation

In the past, it has been useful to distinguish two universes of immune responses.[1] One used to be called *delayed hypersensitivity* because the reactions, such as the tuberculin skin test, were slow in time. When it was realized that these reactions were mediated by lymphocytes, investigators felt that this property was more essential to the characterization of the response than was the fact that it was slow in developing. Therefore, the term *cell-mediated immunity* (CMI) has replaced the older term, *delayed hypersensitivity*. Examples of immunologic phenomena in this area are the tuberculin-type skin tests to many microbial antigens, first-set allograft rejection, contact hypersensitivity, graft-versus-host (GvH) reactions, and perhaps resistance to viral infections and immune surveillance against malignancy.

The other universe is often called that of the *humoral antibody,* and consists of reactions mediated by immunoglobulin proteins containing various types of specific antibodies. Examples of these reactions include atopic diseases, such as allergic rhinitis and allergic asthma, antitoxic protection against certain bacterial diseases and some antiviral activity, some drug reactions, immune-complex disease such as systemic lupus erythematosus (SLE) and some autoimmune processes, e.g., autoimmune hemolytic anemia or erythroblastosis fetalis.

The functional separation of these two general universes was of considerable help in clarifying and distinguishing the mechanisms of various immunological phenomena.

Two Universes of the Immune Response: Anatomical Separation

About 1960, Glick and others[2,3] fortuitously discovered that, at least in the chicken, there was an anatomical separation of the two universes with regard to the primary lymphoid organs. Removing the bursa of Fabricius early in life led to severe impairment of the humoral antibody response, leaving CMI unimpaired. On the other hand, removal of the thymus early in life was followed by a failure of CMI to develop properly, but led to little deficiency in the humoral antibody-forming system. These experiments established the general concept that the thymus controlled the development and maintenance of the CMI system, and in the chicken, the bursa of Fabricius was responsible for the development of the immunoglobulin-producing system.

The picture was not so clear in the mouse. Miller[4] showed that although neonatal thymectomy did produce severe impairment of CMI (as it did in the chicken), it also caused impairment of the antibody response to antigens such as sheep erythrocytes (SRBC). It was interesting, however, that neonatally thymectomized mice had normal antibody responses to other antigens, e.g., pneumococcal polysaccharide.[5] Further confusion occurred with regard to the other limb of the immune response, the humoral antibody-forming system, because the controlling central organ of the chicken, the bursa of Fabricius, does not occur in mammals. What then, was the central lymphoid organ for the antibody system? At one time, it was thought to be the gut-associated lymphoid tissue (GALT) but this theory has since been modified.

Cooperation Between the Two Universes: T- and B-cells

In 1966[6] we reported our fortuitous findings that there was a synergism between thymus cells and bone marrow cells in the production of antibody to SRBC in the mouse. Neither cell population alone was very effective, but a mixture of the two produced far more antibody than could be accounted for by the sum of the antibody-forming ability of each population. We guessed that the antibody was made by cells derived from the bone marrow while the thymus cells served some auxiliary function of unknown mechanism. This guess was proved to be correct by Miller, Nossal and colleagues,[7] and the two groups of cells are now termed T-cells (for thymus-derived) and B-cells (for bone marrow-derived). The current consensus is that the origin of B-cells, and therefore the mammalian analogue of the bursa of Fabricius, is the bone marrow.

It was soon established that for a number of protein and other antigens, B-cells made the antibody while T-cells "helped" B-cells but did not themselves make antibody. This could account for the fact that while neonatally thymectomized mice had deficits in CMI, they also had deficits in antibody production to antigens such as SRBC because they could not provide "T-cell help." What about those antigens, e.g., pneumococcal polysaccharide, which produced normal antibody responses in thymus-deprived mice? It was found that there was a group of antigens that apparently could turn on B-cells without T-cell help. This group was consequently called the thymus-independent antigens and includes pneumococcal polysaccharide, dextran, levan, lipopolysaccharide (LPS) or bacterial endotoxin, polyvinylpyrrolidone (PVP), etc. These are polymeric antigens that have various unusual characteristics. They show T independence, an antibody response that is almost entirely IgM, little or no immunologic memory, and easy production of tolerance.

I have described elsewhere how Mitchison indicated that T-B-cell collaboration accounted for the puzzling phenomenon called the carrier effect.[8] The resultant model indicated that T-cells recognize foreign carriers and help B-cells make antibody to the attached hapten.

Signal Theory

If we concern ourselves with antibody production, the question now becomes: What is required to turn on a B-cell?

Because it is now fashionable to speak in terms of signals, the question should be put in the following form. What signals does a B-cell need to receive to be activated to start making antibody?

It seems to me that the original and incisive experiments in this area were reported by Dresser [9] in 1962 and I would dub him the original "two signal" man. He showed that mice given bovine gamma globulin (BGG) in adjuvant made antibody to BGG, but that similar mice first given soluble deaggregated BGG were later unable to respond to BGG in adjuvant. In other words, prior treatment with soluble BGG rendered a mouse tolerant to BGG in adjuvant. Dresser constructed a scheme which stated that for an antigen to be immunogenic, it also had to have "adjuvanticity" and that most antigens carried their own adjuvanticity with them. If the adjuvanticity was removed (as it appeared to be in the case of BGG by removing aggregates by ultracentrifugation) then the antigen in fact produced tolerance. In Aristotelian terms, the antigenic (specific) signal was necessary for antibody formation but not sufficient.

This work was done in the days when it was thought that only one lymphoid cell was required to produce antibody. Nevertheless, one can clearly see that it was recognized then that there were two signals involved.

I followed up Dresser's experiments to show that although soluble BGG would produce tolerance, soluble BGG given together with endotoxin (LPS) as a nonspecific adjuvant did not lead to tolerance. This apparently complete separation of the specific stimulus and the nonspecific stimulus led Talmage, Pearlman and me [10, 11] to draw a diagram of the situation (FIGURE 1). The concept of two signals—one to "tolerize" and two to induce antibody formation—has been ably expanded by Bretscher and Cohn.[12]

Today, we must think in terms of the three-cell model, namely, T-cells, B-cells and macrophages or accessory (A) cells.

B-cell Activation Without Thymic Help

This may be the simplest situation. In B-cells the receptor for antigen is apparently immunoglobulin (Ig), which is presumably a sample of the antibody the B-cell is programmed to manufacture when given the right signals. For some antigens (the so-called *T-independent antigens*) the right stimulus seems to be just antigen; i.e., the first signal alone. That is, presenting the B-cell with PVP or dextran leads to B-cell activation and antibody production. Upon further scrutiny, however, the situation is not quite so clear. First, these antigens are multivalent polymers of the same antigenic determinant, and the density of these antigenic determinants is crucial for B-cell activation. If the density is too low, (i.e., free haptenic antigen) the cell will not be turned on. Conversely, if there is too much antigen in the system, it will become tolerant. Therefore the first (specific) signal must be presented in the proper fashion. (Parenthetically, A-cells appear not to be required.)

Having satisfied the requirements for proper epitope presentation, is there then any need for a second nonspecific signal to turn on a B-cell to a T-independent antigen? The answer to this is not clear, but there is evidence that the second signal may be involved anyway. Moller [13] has argued that T-independent antigens are also B-cell mitogens, and that the function of the specific antigenic determinant is to "focus" the mitogen onto the relevant cells so that the mitogen can then turn on the proper B-cells to make antibody. In this case, therefore, even T-independent antigens carry both specific and nonspecific signals with them. A somewhat related point is that the deliberate addition of a nonspecific mitogenic signal, i.e., a mitogen for B-cells, can convert a tolerogenic specific signal to an immunogenic stimulus as shown by the BGG experiments mentioned above.[9, 11]

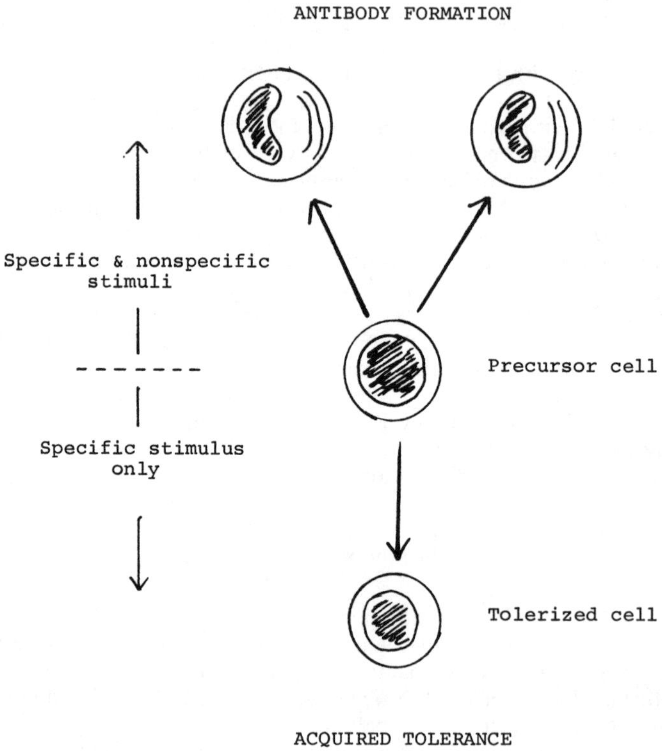

ANTIBODY FORMATION

Specific & nonspecific stimuli

Precursor cell

Specific stimulus only

Tolerized cell

ACQUIRED TOLERANCE

FIGURE 1. Schematic representation of the "two signal" model of Dresser, adapted from References 10 and 11.

B-cell Activation with Specific Thymic Help

The interpretation of the carrier effect in the context of thymus-marrow synergism stated that for thymus-dependent antigens B-cells would be activated to produce antihapten antibody if the hapten was presented on a carrier that could be recognized by T-cells. At first this "recognition" was felt to occur through a "focusing" of antigen by T-cells to form a matrix of hapten for presentation to B-cells. This is the "antigen-bridge" theory, which puts the T-cell in a rather passive role. It accounts for a number of experimental findings but suffers from the fact that it is statistically unlikely that an infrequent T-cell specific for the carrier would find itself so close to an infrequent B-cell specific for the hapten in question that the two could be connected via the antigen bridge.

It would be conceptually more comfortable if T-cells provided signals for B-cells via some diffusible substance that could affect B-cells at a (short) distance. A number of experiments by Feldmann[14] have indicated that T-cells and B-cells can interact *in vitro* across a cell impermeable membrane so that T-cell–B-cell contact is not required. Feldmann[15] also showed that antigen-activated specific T-cells do, in fact, release a specific factor (called IgT, which has the properties of monomeric IgM) that appears to require more antigen and a macrophage surface in order to activate B-cells. In this case, therefore, I interpret the data to mean that the antigen still gives the first (specific) signal to the B-cell but that adjuvanticity (the second signal) is provided by IgT and the macrophage surface. This kind of T-cell factor has also been shown to be active *in vivo*.[16]

B-cell Activation with Nonspecific Thymus Help

The above findings indicate that activation of T-cells by specific carrier can provide help when the T-cell product is presented with the hapten-carrier to the B-cell. Recently, however, there has been abundant evidence that T-cells can provide help for B-cells if they are activated by agents unrelated to the antigen that the B-cell will recognize. This can take at least two forms. In one, T-cells activated to carrier A can produce a factor that, with antigen C, can induce B-cells to make anti-C. A related situation (the allogenic effect) is one in which T-cells can be activated by a GvH reaction to provide second signals that, together with antigen C, can induce B-cells to make anti-C.[17] In these respects, the factors may be called "nonspecific" with regard to the B-cell and its antigen, although it should be quite clear that the T-cells themselves must be capable of responding to the antigenic or GvH stimulus in the first place. A second variation is that nonspecific T-cell mitogens, such as concanavalin A, can provide soluble factors that will, with antigen, provide help for B-cells.[18, 19] In this case, presumably, a very large proportion of the available T-cell population can be activated, rather than a small clone reacting to a specific antigenic or allogenic stimulus.

B-cell Activation for Thymus-Dependent Antigens Without Any Thymic Help: the Final Indignity

Lastly, it appears that even with a "thymus-dependent" antigen such as SRBC, you can get two signals *without T-cells at all!* In this case, the specific antigenic signal (SRBC) is given together with the nonspecific signal in the form of lipopolysaccharide (LPS), a potent B-cell mitogen. The combination leads to specific B-cell triggering with the formation of anti-SRBC antibodies.[20]

These various mechanisms are outlined in TABLE 1.

Final Comments

This brief analysis may "help" to tie up some of the many new ideas and the extraordinary amount of data that have been recently gathered bearing on the question of how B-cells are triggered into antibody formation. There are many points that were not covered, such as patching and capping, cyclic AMP and cyclic GMP, details of T- and B-cell tolerance and other timely subjects. I did not discuss at all how (or if) the two signals interact with each other, or where they act, on the membrane or inside the cell, because I don't know. Doubtless, the answers will be forthcoming soon.

TABLE 1

METHODS OF TRIGGERING B-CELLS TO PRODUCE ANTIBODY TO ANTIGEN A

Antigen	Signal 1	Signal 2
thymus-independent	AgA	Ag as mitogen?
thymus-dependent	(1) AgA	specific T-cell help from T-cells activated by antigen A
	(2) AgA	nonspecific T-cell help from T-cells activated by another antigen
	(3) AgA	B-cell mitogen acting without T-cells

References

1. GOOD, R. A. Disorders of the Immune System. 1971. *In* Immunobiology. R. A. Good & D. W. Fisher, Eds. : 3–17. Sinaner Associates. Stamford, Conn.
2. GLICK, B., T. S. CHANG & R. G. JAAP. 1956. The Bursa of Fabricius and Antibody Production. Poultry Sci. **35:** 224.
3. WARNER, N. L., A. SZENBERG & F. M. BURNET. 1962. The Immunological Role of Different Lymphoid Organs in the Chicken. I. Dissociation of Immunological Responsiveness. Australian J. Exp. Biol. Med. Sci. **40:** 373.
4. MILLER, J. F. A. P. & D. OSOBA. 1967. Current Concepts of the Immunological Function of the Thymus. Physiol. Rev. **47:** 437–520.
5. HUMPHREY, J. H., D. M. V. PARROTT & J. EAST. 1964. Studies on Globulin and Antibody Production in Mice Thymectomized at Birth. Immunology **7:** 419.
6. CLAMAN, H. N., E. A. CHAPERON & R. F. TRIPLETT. 1966. Thymus-Marrow Cell Combination—Synergism in Antibody Production. Proc. Soc. Exp. Biol. Med. **122:** 1167.
7. NOSSAL, G. J. V., A. CUNNINGHAM, G. F. MITCHELL & J. F. A. P. MILLER. 1968. Cell-to-Cell Interaction in the Immune Response. III. Chromosomal Marker Analysis of Single Antibody-Forming Cells in Reconstituted, Irradiated or Thymectomized Mice. J. Exp. Med. **128:** 839–854.
8. CLAMAN, H. N. & D. E. MOSIER. 1972. Cell-Cell Interactions in Antibody Production. Progr. Allergy. **16:** 40–80.
9. DRESSER, D. W. 1962. Specific Inhibition of Antibody Production. II. Paralysis Induced in Adult Mice by Small Quantities of Protein Antigen. Immunology **5:** 378–388.

10. Talmage, D. W. & D. S. Pearlman. 1963. The Antibody Response: A Model Based on Antagonistic Actions of Antigen. J. Theoret. Biol. **5:** 321–339.
11. Claman, H. N. 1963. Tolerance to a Protein Antigen in Adult Mice and the Effect of Nonspecific Factors. J. Immunol. **91:** 833.
12. Bretscher, P. & M. Cohn. 1970. A Theory of Self-Nonself Discrimination. Science **169:** 1042–1049.
13. Coutinho, A. & G. Moller. 1973. Mitogenic Properties of the Thymus-independent Antigen Pneumococcal Polysaccharide SIII. Eur. J. Immunol. **3:** 608.
14. Feldmann, M. & A. Basten. 1972. Specific Collaboration Between T and B lymphocytes Across a Cell-impermeable Membrane. Nature New Biol. **237:** 13–15.
15. Feldmann, M., R. E. Cone & J. J. Marchalonis. 1973. Cell Interactions in the Immune Response *In Vitro.* VI Mediated by T Cell Surface Monomeric IgM. Cell. Immunol. **9:** 1–11.
16. Taussig, M. J. 1974. T Cell Factor which can Replace T Cells *In Vivo.* Nature **248:** 234–6.
17. Katz, D. H., W. Paul, E. A. Goidl & B. Benaceraff. 1971. Carrier Functions in Antihapten Antibody Responses. III Stimulation of Antibody Synthesis and Facilitation of Hapten Specific Secondary Antibody Responses by Graft Versus Host Reactions. J. Exp. Med. **133:** 169–186.
18. Dulton, R. W., R. Falkoff, J. A. Hurst, M. Hoffman, J. W. Kappler, J. R. Keltmann, J. F. Lesley & D. Vann. 1971. *In* Progress in Immunology. : 355. B. Amos, Ed. Academic Press. New York, N.Y.
19. Gorczynski, R. M., R. G. Miller & R. A. Phillips. 1973. Reconstitution of T Cell-Depleted Spleen Cell Population by Factors Derived from T Cells. I. Conditions for the Production of Active T Cell Supernatants. J. Immunol. **110:** 968–983.
20. Jones, J. M. & P. D. Kind. 1972. Enhancing Effect of Bacterial Endotoxins on Bone Marrow Cells in the Immune Response to SRBC. J. Immunol. **108:** 1453–5.

ONTOGENY OF THYMUS CELL FUNCTION *

A. Chakravarty, L. Kubai, Y. Sidky, and R. Auerbach

Department of Zoology
University of Wisconsin
Madison, Wisconsin 53706

In our laboratory we have been studying the differentiation of the mouse embryonic thymus both in terms of the ontogeny of thymic lymphocytes and in terms of the functional capacity of these cells in both humoral and cellular immune systems. For our studies we have primarily employed *in vitro* procedures and have used tissue culture both to obtain differentiation of thymic lymphocytes from early embryonic thymus rudiments, and, subsequently, to assess immunocompetence of such *in vitro*-derived cells.

Our experiments have used two test systems: one for assessment of cellular immunity, the other for detection of humoral immune function. For cellular immunity we have used the *in vitro* graft-versus-host (GvH) reaction, described originally by Auerbach and Globerson [1,2] and recently modified to permit quantitative assessment of immunocompetence.[3] In this reaction, cells to be assessed for immunocompetence are added to neonatal semiallogeneic spleen explants where they can induce splenomegaly; this splenomegaly is detected by the increase in incorporation of isotope-labeled amino acids into the test explants. Both the onset of spleen-fragment enlargement and the degree of enlargement can be used to characterize the relative immunocompetence of various cell suspensions.[3] The *in vitro* GvH reaction has, for example, been used to show that thymus cells from adult mice are only about 10% as active as spleen cells, but that a 10–20-fold increase in activity occurs when thymus cells from corticosteroid-treated animals are used. Similarly, we have been able to show that aliquots of thymus cell suspension treated with anti-TL serum are as effective as control serum treated aliquots in spite of the 90% cytotoxicity of the anti-T1 serum.[4]

In our studies of humoral immunity we have restricted our investigations to the study of the response to sheep red blood cells (SRBC). For most of these studies we have employed the Click modification of the Mishell-Dutton cell suspension culture system;[5] the organ culture methods developed by Globerson and Auerbach [1,6] were employed for some ancillary studies. For both procedures assessment of immunological response was measured by enumeration of direct (19S) plaque-forming cells (PFC), using the Cunningham-Szenberg liquid monolayer assay.[7]

The Primitive Thymus Stem Cell

As background information for the studies of thymus stem-cell differentiation we determined the onset of immunocompetence as measured by the *in vitro*

* Supported by Grant GB 36767 from the National Science Foundation and Grant CA 13548 from the National Cancer Institute.

gvh reaction. In confirmation of earlier *in vivo* studies,[8,9] we found that neonatal thymus cells were as effective as were adult thymus cells.[10] (TABLE 1). We were unable to obtain positive responses with any embryonic thymus cells, however, suggesting that a considerable time period was required following the appearance of thymic small lymphocytes at day 16 of embryonic life before immunocompetence could be exerted as measured by our assay.

TABLE 1

ABILITY OF SEMIALLOGENEIC EMBRYONIC, NEWBORN OR ADULT THYMUS CELLS TO INDUCE SPLENOMEGALY (GRAFT-VERSUS-HOST REACTION) *In Vitro*

Source of Thymus Cells	Number of Cells	Number of Experiments	Number of Cultures	Spleen Index
adult	1.0×10^6	24	145	1.25 *
newborn	1.0×10^6	28	212	1.25 *
19–day embryo	1.0×10^6	4	41	1.01
18–day embryo	1.0×10^6	10	107	0.99
17–day embryo	1.0×10^6	5	47	1.12
16–day embryo	1.0×10^6	5	38	0.99
13–day embryo, after 7 days in organ culture	1.0×10^6	1	4	1.45 *
adult	0.2×10^6			(1.00) †
newborn	0.2×10^6			(0.97) †
13–day embryo, after 7 days in organ culture	0.2×10^6	5	20	1.22 *
13–day embryo, 850 R x-ray, then 7 days *in vitro*	0.2×10^6	7	27	1.33 *
13–day nu/nu embryo, 7 days *in vitro*	0.2×10^6	3	4	1.29 ‡
13–day embryo, 1–3 days in hydrocortisone, 4–6 days further culture	0.2×10^6	5	18	1.18 ‡

* Highly significant; see Auerbach and Shalaby (1973) for validation and experimental detail.

† From previous experiments.

‡ $.05 > p < .10$.

In Vitro *Maturation*

Some time ago work from our laboratory showed that the thymus rudiment isolated from 12–13 day embryos, is capable of becoming lymphoid when grown *in vitro* for 6–7 days[11,12] demonstrating that the thymus rudiment at the time of explanation must have contained a stem-cell population capable of differentiating into morphologically normal thymus lymphocytes. The yet earlier history of that stem-cell population (i.e. yolk-sac-derived) suggested by the work of Moore and Owen[13] and Owen and Richter,[14] need not concern us within the context of the studies we are reporting. To examine the functional capacity of tissue-culture-derived thymus lymphocytes, thymus rudiments from 13-day C57BL/6 embryos were cultured for one week, and lymphocytes from such cultures were then assayed for their ability to induce spleen enlargement in BDF_1 neonatal spleen explants. The experiments showed that not only are *in vitro*-derived thymus lymphocytes immunocompetent, but their effectiveness is equivalent to that of the cortisone-resistant thymus cell; i.e. splenomegaly could be induced by as few as 5×10^4 cells (TABLE 1). This finding suggests that the primitive thymus stem cells present in 13-day rudiments are capable of exhaustive differentiation in the absence of bone-marrow-derived precursor cells to yield a population of lymphocytes enriched for effector activity for cell-mediated immunity.

Radiation Sensitivity

To examine the radiation sensitivity of the thymus stem cell, thymus rudiments from 13-day embryos were irradiated with x-rays ranging from 250 R to 1000 R and then cultured for a 6–7 day period.[15] Irradiation had a profound effect on growth of the rudiment, as seen by the fact that the overall size of the explants as well as the total number of lymphocytes was drastically reduced at the higher doses. For example, whereas thymus rudiments *in vitro* yield about 5×10^4 to 10^5 lymphocytes,[16] rudiments irradiated with 1000 R give rise to only about 10^4 cells. Interestingly, however, histological examination showed that the differentiation of lymphocytes appeared normal; i.e. although the explants were smaller, their histiotypic development was not severely altered. Indeed, it appeared that the most pronounced radiation effect was seen in the mesenchymal tissue suggesting that stem-cell proliferation, rather than differentiation, was dependent on the induction effects known to be operative in thymus development.[17]

To assess the immunocompetence of thymic lymphocytes obtained following x-irradiation, 13- or 14-day rudiments were irradiated with 850 R and subsequently cultured for 6–7 days. After this time cell suspensions were prepared and assayed in the *in vitro* GvH reaction assay. As can be seen from TABLE 1, irradiated thymus explants yielded lymphocytes capable of causing a gvh reaction.

Sensitivity to Corticosteroids

Relatively low concentrations of some corticosteroids can inhibit the *in vitro* lymphoid differentiation of the 13-day embryonic mouse thymus.[18] Corticosterone was the most effective of the steroids studied, and thymus lymphoid differentiation remained arrested as long as the culture medium contained as little as 0.6 μg/ml. After careful washing and further culturing for 4–6 days, thymus rudiments developed lymphocytes that were normal in appearance and the cultures were essentially indistinguishable from untreated control cultures.[18]

Thymus lymphoid cells obtained from corticosterone treated rudiments have now been tested in the *in vitro* GvH reaction assay. As can be seen from TABLE 1, these lymphocytes are capable of inducing splenomegaly *in vitro*, indicating that they are capable of acting as effector cells in cell-mediated immunity.

It had previously been noticed that corticosterone treatment causes a disappearance of basophilic cells in the thymus rudiment, yet it is the basophilic cells that have been considered to be the stem cells for thymus lymphocytes.[13] We must therefore entertain the suggestion that the basophilic cells are not the sole stem cells within the thymus rudiment. It may well be, however, that corticosterone treatment leads to cytochemical alterations within the stem cells resulting in their inability to absorb basophilic dyes.

Thymocytes from Nude Embryos

Although mice homozygous for the nude gene are thymusless from birth, it had previously been reported that thymus rudiments do indeed appear during embryogeny, but that these fail to complete their migration into the thoracic cavity.[19] To examine the nature of thymus stem cells in nu/nu mice, 13-day embryos from crosses of nu/+ × nu/+ (Balb/C) were dissected to obtain thymus rudiments and skin fragments. Since at the time of dissection it was not possible to distinguish nu/nu embryos from normal ones (nu/+ or +/+) each embryo was separately handled. Thymus rudiments from each embryo were grown in organ culture, while several fragments of skin from each embryo were grafted into the anterior eye chamber of adult Balb/C mice. After one week in culture, thymuses were either fixed for histological examination or prepared as a cell suspension to be tested for GvH competence. Eye-chamber grafts were recovered after two weeks and scored for the presence of hair.

When skin fragments from normal embryos are grown in the anterior eye chamber, they readily produce hair;[20] nude skin grafts, however, fail to do so. Thus eye-graft assessment permitted the distinction of nu/nu embryonic thymus from normal thymus. Admittedly, this distinction could only be made after the experimental studies of thymus cultures was completed, and for this reason each pair of thymuses had to be handled separately throughout, limiting the number of lymphocytes that could be tested in any single GvH assay. Histological examination of nu/nu thymus cultures revealed that lymphopoiesis in such cultures was normal; there was no visible distinction between cultures derived from nu/nu embryos and those from their littermates. Furthermore, nu/nu lymphocytes gave positive spleen indexes and the mean spleen index of nu/nu lymphocytes was not distinguishable from the index of littermate controls (Table 1).

Kindred has recently reported that thymuses grafted into nu/nu animals become populated with cells from the nu/nu host.[21] Similarly, studies carried out with thymus extracts indicate that bone marrow cells from nu/nu mice can become θ-positive T-cells.[22] Our work suggests that not only are there presumptive T-cells in nu/nu mice, but there are embryonic thymus stem cells, and that these cells can be detected in the thymus itself.

Thymus Helper Cell Function

Although many studies have described interactions between T- and B-cells in the immune response to SRBC, thymus cells themselves have not been able to act synergistically when assayed directly. Thus virtually all studies involving T-B collaboration have employed the use of an intermediate irradiated host, previously injected with thymus cells and usually with antigen. This thymus "education" or "activation" has been an obligatory event in yielding functional thymus-derived cells.

To obtain thymus-cell helper function without cell passage, thymus cells were incubated for 24 hours with 5 μg concanavalin-A,[23] as suggested by studies of Anderson *et al.*[24] and Sjöberg *et al.*[25] To test for helper-cell activity, thymus cells were then washed and 3×10^6 cells were combined with 5×10^6 spleen cells obtained from adult, irradiated, thymectomized animals previously injected with bone marrow cells (B spleen cells). After 4 days of culture in the presence of SRBC the cultures were examined for presence of PFC. The results (FIGURE 1) clearly indicate that the pretreatment of thymus cells with concanavalin A permits them to act as helper cells in the immune response to SRBC. The specificity of action of concanavalin A was suggested by the fact that con-A-treated bone marrow cells failed to enhance the immune response.

Against this background information about adult thymus cells, we next examined the ontogeny of thymus helper-cell activity.[23, 26, 27] We found that even thymus lymphocytes obtained from 16-day embryos were capable of collaborating in the response to SRBC following 24 hours of incubation in medium containing con-A. Moreover, although the activity of 16-day embryonic thymus cells appeared lower on a per cell basis, the capacity of embryonic thymus cells obtained from 18-day embryos was virtually identical with that of adult thymus cells (FIGURE 2). Since, moreover, the 16-day embryonic thymus has a lymphocyte population in which only a small proportion of cells

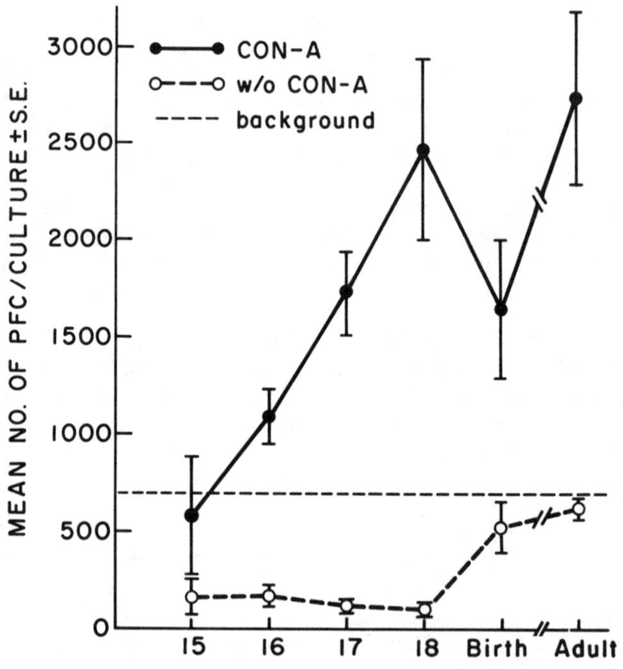

FIGURE 1. Functional ontogeny of T-cells.

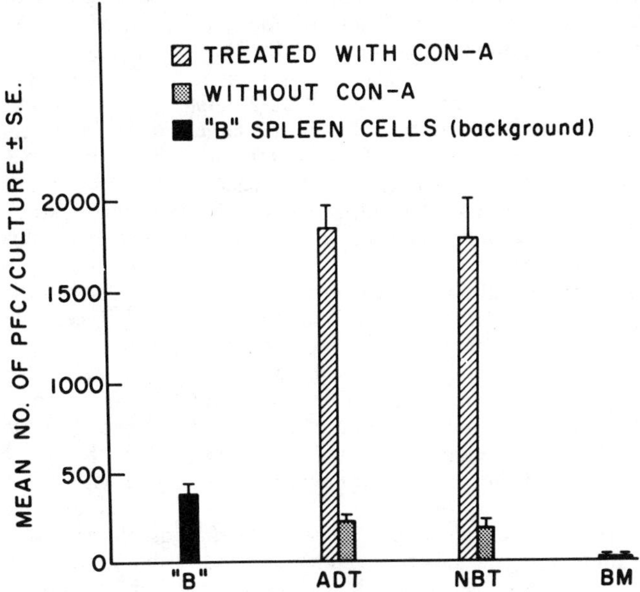

FIGURE 2. *In vitro* collaboration.

are small lymphocytes,[16, 28] our findings suggest that as soon as thymic small lymphocytes appear they have the ability to collaborate in the response to SRBC provided they are activated by con-A *in vitro*.

In an effort to determine the mechanism of con-A action on thymus cell activity, the θ and H-2 antigenicity of thymus cells before and after con-A treatment was determined.[23, 26, 27] The results indicate that con-A treatment is accompanied by a decrease in θ and an increase in H-2 surface antigens, a change generally considered indicative of thymus cell maturation;[29-31] moreover, this shift in antigen levels of thymocytes by con-A treatment is achieved equally in both embryonic and adult thymus cell populations.

In contrast to our findings of con-A-induced maturation of helper cell function, we found that con-A treatment of embryonic thymus cells did not alter the ontogeny of immunocompetence as measured in the gvh reaction. Thus, there appears here to be a real dissociation between the maturation of helper cell activity and of GvH reactivity of thymus cells. Such a dissociation had previously been suggested by Feldman *et al.*[32]

GENERAL COMMENTS

Our *in vitro* studies of embryonic thymus rudiments seem to define a thymus stem cell that is somewhat different from the thymus precursor cell residing in the bone marrow of adult animals. Clearly, it is radiation resistant; it need not be Giemsa-positive; and it is not destroyed by corticosteroid treatment. Moreover, the presence of a thymus stem cell in nude embryos needs to be recognized.

We have found that concanavalin-A activation of thymus cells can lead to functional helper cells without influencing the maturation of the effector cells for cell-mediated immunity as measured by the gvh reaction. This should serve as a caution that any single scheme for thymus cell maturation may not accurately reflect the complex series of differentiative events leading to the production of immunocompetent cells. At the same time, since concanavalin-A can cause detectable maturational shifts in H-2 and θ antigenicity of embryonic cells without concomitantly causing them to become immunocompetent in the gvh assay, it is clear that the shift in surface antigenicity associated with maturation is not the only signal of functionality of developing thymus lymphoid cell populations.

The ontogeny of immune competence appears to coincide with the morphological appearance of lymphocytes, at least to the extent that such lymphocytes can be activated to function as helper cells in the immune response to SRBC. Moreover, the demonstration that even before thymus cells make their appearance, there may be immunocompetence of liver cells [33–35] and even of yolk-sac cells [36] indicates that the differentiation of immunocompetence is achieved early in development, concomitant for cellular immunity with the appearance of blood-borne cells, and for humoral immunity no later than with the appearance of thymus lymphocytes.

One of us has argued elsewhere [37, 38] that this finding places new constraints on current immunological theories of tolerance and on the machinery by which an embryo can learn epigenetically to recognize self as different from non-self; for many of the antigens against which the embryo must not respond do not arise until long after the immune system itself has achieved competence. The concept of allosteric stem-cell tolerance [37, 38] attempts to explain tolerance as the result of an immune-type response leading to the production of blocking factors.

Finally, an earlier analogy drawn between the ontogeny of thymus cells and the ontogeny of germ cells may be recalled in the light of several newer findings about the thymus stem cell.[40] The fact that the thymus stem cell is alkaline phosphatase positive [41] brings to mind the studies on presumptive germ cells which have relied so heavily on just that property of these cells.[42] The radiation-resistance of the primordial germ cells has long been in sharp contrast to the radiation sensitivity of later stages in the development of the functional germ cells; a similar pattern is now seen for the thymus, where the stem cell, in contrast to the mature thymocytes, is also highly radiation-resistant. Perhaps the most striking parallel, however, resides in the complex cell surface changes that accompany activation, as measured by altered antigenicity and functionality following mitogenic stimulation.

References

1. Globerson, A. & R. Auerbach. 1965. Primary immune reactions in organ cultures. Science **149:** 991–993.
2. Auerbach, R. & A. Globerson. 1966. *In vitro* induction of the graft versus host reaction. Exp. Cell Res. **42:** 31–41.
3. Auerbach, R. & M.-R. Shalaby. 1973. Graft-versus-host reaction in tissue culture. J. Exp. Med. **138:** 1506–1520.
4. Doell, R. & R. Auerbach. Unpublished observations.

5. Click, R. E., L. Benck & B. J. Alter. 1972. Immune response *in vitro*. I. Culture conditions for antibody synthesis. Cell. Immunol. **3:** 264–276.
6. Globerson, A. & R. Auerbach. 1966. Primary antibody response in organ cultures. J. Exp. Med. **124:** 1001–1016.
7. Cunningham, J. A. & A. Szenberg. 1968. Further improvement in the plaque technique for detecting single antibody forming cells. J. Immunol. **14:** 599–600.
8. Cohen, M. W., G. J. Thorbecke, G. M. Hochwald & E. B. Jacobson. 1963. Induction of a graft-versus-host reaction in newborn mice by injection of newborn or adult homologous thymus cells. Proc. Soc. Exp. Biol. Med. **114:** 242–244.
9. Umiel, T. & R. Auerbach. 1973. Studies on the development of immunity: The graft-versus-host reaction. Pathobiol. Ann. **7:** 27–45.
10. Chakravarty, A., L. Kubai, C. Landahl, J. Roethle, M.-R. Shalaby & R. Auerbach. 1973. Studies on the development of immunity in the mouse. Phylogenic and Ontogenic Study of the Immune Response and its Contribution to the Immunological Theory. : 269–278. INSERM Coll. Soc. Franc. d'Immunol.
11. Ball, W. D. & R. Auerbach. 1960. *In vitro* formation of lymphocytes from embryonic thymus. Exp. Cell Res. **20:** 245–247.
12. Auerbach, R. 1961. Experimental analysis of the origin of cell types in the development of the mouse thymus. Develop. Biol. **3:** 336–354.
13. Moore, M. A. S. & J. J. T. Owen. 1967. Experimental studies on the development of the thymus. J. Exp. Med. **126:** 715–725.
14. Owen, J. J. T. & M. A. Ritter. 1969. Tissue interaction in the development of thymus lymphocytes. J. Exp. Med. **129:** 431–437.
15. Kubai, L. & R. Auerbach. 1973. Radiation resistant thymic stem cells. Proc. Soc. Exp. Biol. Med. **142:** 554–559.
16. Auerbach, R. 1964. Experimental analysis of mouse thymus and spleen morphogenesis. *In* The Thymus in Immunobiology. R. A. Good & A. Gabrielsen, Eds. : 95–113. Harper and Row.
17. Auerbach, R. 1960. Morphogenetic interactions in the development of the mouse thymus gland. Develop. Biol. **2:** 271–284.
18. Sidky, Y. 1968. Effect of steroids on thymus lymphoid development *in vitro*. Anat. Rec. **161:** 187–191.
19. Wortis, H. H., S. Nehlsen & J. J. Owen. 1971. Abnormal development of the thymus in "nude" mice. J. Exp. Med. **134:** 681–692.
20. Auerbach, R. 1954. Analysis of the developmental effects of a lethal mutation in the house mouse. J. Exp. Zool. **127:** 305–330.
21. Kindred, B. 1975. Am. Zool. In press.
22. Boyse, E. A., G. H. Cohen, J. A. Hooper, R. S. Schulof & A. L. Goldstein. 1973. Differentiation of T cells induced by preparations from thymus and by non thymic agents. The determined state of the precursor cell. J. Exp. Med. **138:** 1027–1032.
23. Chakravarty, A. 1974. Functional ontogeny of thymus cells. (Abstr.) Fed. Proc. **33:** 735.
24. Andersson, J., G. Möller & O. Sjöberg. 1972. Selective induction of DNA synthesis in T and B lymphocytes. Cell. Immunol. **4:** 381–393.
25. Barth, R. F. & O. Singla. 1973. Differential effects of concanavalin-A on T-helper dependent and independent antibody responses. Cell. Immunol. **9:** 96–103.
26. Chakravarty, A. 1975. Ph.D. Dissertation. University of Wisconsin. Madison, Wisc.
27. Chakravarty, A. 1975. In preparation.
28. Ball, W. D. 1963. A quantitative assessment of mouse thymus differentiation. Exp. Cell Res. **31:** 82–88.

29. OWEN, J. J. T. & M. C. RAFF. 1970. Studies on the differentiation of thymus-derived lymphocytes. J. Exp. Med. **132:** 1216–1232.
30. OWEN, J. J. T. 1972. The origin and development of lymphocytes populations. *In* Ontogeny of acquired Immunity. Ciba Found. Symp. R. Porter & J. Knight, Eds. : 35–64. Elsevier. Amsterdam, The Netherlands.
31. RAFF, M. C. 1971. T and B lymphocytes in mice studied by using antisera against surface antigenic markers. Am. J. Pathol. **65:** 467.
32. SEGAL, S., I. R. COHEN & M. FELDMAN. 1972. Thymus-derived lymphocytes: Humoral and cellular reactions distinguished by hydrocortisone. Science **175:** 1126–1128.
33. UMIEL, T., A. GLOBERSON & R. AUERBACH. 1968. Role of the thymus in the development of immunocompetence of embryonic liver cells *in vitro*. Proc. Soc. Exp. Biol. Med. **129:** 598–600.
34. UMIEL, T. 1971. Thymus-influenced maturation of embryonic liver cells. Transplantation **11:** 531–535.
35. UMIEL, T. 1973. Requirements for development of immunocompetence of embryonic liver cells: The graft-versus-host response. Differentiation **1:** 295.
36. HOFMAN, F. & A. GLOBERSON. 1973. Graft-versus-host response induced *in vitro* by mouse yolk sac cells. Eur. J. Immunol. **3:** 179–181.
37. AUERBACH, R. 1974. Development of immunity and the concept of stem cell tolerance. Am. Zool. In press.
38. AUERBACH, R. 1974. Towards a developmental theory of immunity: Ontogeny of immunocompetence and the concept of allosteric tolerance. *In* Cellular Selection and Regulation in the Immune Response. G. Edelman, Ed. : 59–70. Raven Press. New York, N.Y. In press.
39. AUERBACH, R. & J. ROETHLE. 1974. Tolerance to heterologous erythrocytes. Science **183:** 332–334.
40. AUERBACH, R. 1970. Toward a developmental theory of antibody formation: The Germinal Theory of immunity. *In* Developmental Aspects of Antibody Formation and Structure. J. Sterzl & I. Riha, Eds. : 23–33. Academic Press. New York, N.Y.
41. RUUSKANEN, O. & K. KOUVALAINEN. 1974. Differentiation of thymus and thymocytes. A study in foetal guinea-pigs using alkaline phosphatase as a label of thymocytes. Immunology. **26:** 187–195.

MITOGENS AND T-CELL HETEROGENEITY *

Richard W. Dutton

Department of Biology
University of California, San Diego
La Jolla, California 92037

Numerous plant lectins have been shown to bind to receptors on the surface of lymphoid cells, and in some cases these cells may be triggered into new patterns of activity. These activities may involve proliferation, the production of various lymphocyte mediators, or the development of new functions whose mechanisms are not understood.

We have studied the effect of concanavalin A (Con-A) on the *in vitro* immune response of mouse spleen cell suspensions in some detail.[1, 2] The results may be summarized as follows.

Con-A added to spleen cell suspensions from normal mice stimulates thymidine incorporation and inhibits the primary and secondary IgM response to sheep (SRBC) or burro (BRBC) erythrocytes or the anti-trinitrophenyl (TNP) response to TNP-SRBC. The optimal concentration of Con-A for both these effects is 2 μg/ml.

If the addition of Con-A is delayed for 24 hours after the initiation of the culture, inhibition is no longer observed. In fact, the addition at 24 hours frequently causes stimulation of the immune response. The inhibitory effects of Con-A are also abolished by treatment with goat anti-mouse brain antisera followed by complement, or by x-irradiation. The latter effect can be most easily demonstrated by the addition of control or irradiated spleen cells from normal mice to spleen cells from athymic nu/nu mice. The Con-A-induced inhibitory activity is missing from the spleens of adult thymectomized irradiated bone marrow restored (AT×BM) and nu/nu mice.

In the absence of inhibitory effects, it can be demonstrated that Con-A (again at 2 μg/ml) will induce a stimulatory effect on the immune response to heterologous erythrocytes. The cell mediating the stimulatory effect is present after treatment with goat anti-mouse brain and complement, is present in AT×BM mice, and persists in the spleens of adult thymectomized mice long after thymectomy.[3] It is present in lymph node cells but virtually absent from thymus. It is not present in the spleens of nu/nu mice. These observations are summarized in TABLE 1. We have also shown that spleen cell suspensions preincubated with Con-A for 24 hours will inhibit the humoral response of fresh syngeneic spleen cells in the absence of Con-A.[1] Rich and Pierce [4] have shown that culture supernatants from Con-A-treated spleens contain an inhibitory factor that is not cytotoxic but that will suppress the response of untreated spleen cells to foreign erythrocytes.

It is important to realize that all that can be measured in these experiments are *activities* and these activities represent the *net effect* resulting from the

* This work was supported by United States Public Health Service Grant AI08795 and American Cancer Society Grant IM-1G. R. W. Dutton was supported by a Career Development Award from the American Cancer Society, PRA-73.

TABLE 1

SUMMARY OF THE PROPERTIES OF INHIBITORY AND STIMULATORY ACTIVITIES

Present In:	Inhibitory Activity	Stimulatory Activity
normal spleen	yes	yes
antiserum-treated * spleen	no	yes
normal lymph node	yes	yes
AT×BM	no	yes
adult thymectomized spleen (25 wks)	? † maybe	yes
nude spleen	no	no
normal spleen preincubated for 24 hrs	no	yes
sensitive to irradiation	yes	no ‡

* In the original studies [1] the antiserum used was goat anti-mouse brain. This completely eliminated carrier specific "helper" activity and Con A-induced inhibitory activity, but had no apparent effect on the Con-A stimulatory activity. More recently studies with a rabbit anti-mouse brain serum (unpublished) show that treatment with this antiserum does cause some reduction in Con A-induced stimulatory activity.

† When Con-A is added (at zero time) to spleen cell cultures taken from mice at various times after adult thymectomy, a gradual shift from inhibition to stimulation is observed.[3] This may be the consequence of changes in the level in both inhibitory and stimulatory cells and it is not possible from this data to calculate a half life of the disappearance of the separate activities.

‡ Irradiation of normal spleen cell cultures shifts the balance from inhibition to stimulation. The inhibitory activity is very radiosensitive whereas the stimulatory activity appears to be only slightly affected.[2] It has not been possible to determine the true radiosensitivity of the separate activities.

balance of the inhibitory and stimulatory effects that may be present. To illustrate this, when unirradiated cells are added to the spleens of nude mice, Con-A increases the response when small numbers of normal spleen cells are added, but inhibits when larger numbers are added (up to 10^6 cells/ml). If the normal spleen cells are treated with varying doses of irradiation it can be seen that the inhibitory effects are very radiosensitive whereas the stimulatory effects are only moderately affected. The result is that the addition of large numbers of irradiated cells (2×10^6) now produces much greater stimulatory effects in the presence of Con-A.[2]

Since stimulatory activity is absent from the spleens of nu/nu mice, it seems reasonable to conclude that both inhibitory and stimulatory activities are mediated by T-cells. The essential question that arises from these studies is whether we are dealing with the Con-A-induced activities of a single T-cell or two separate T-cells.

The properties listed in TABLE 1 suggest that there may be two separate cells, but it is still possible that we are dealing with a quantitative distinction—inhibition could merely be the consequence of too much stimulation. All the properties or treatments that distinguished the two effects could be argued to be the result of a reduction in numbers of a single effective cell type from the inhibitory range to the stimulatory range (irradiation, anti-mouse brain sera, adult thymectomy, etc.). Three arguments, however, strongly suggest that we are dealing with two cell responses. First, there is no concentration of unirradiated spleen cells that will give as much stimulation to nude spleen cell suspensions (stimulator negative, inhibitor negative) in the presence of Con-A, as will the optimal concentration of irradiated normal spleen.[2] Second, phytohemagglutinin (PHA), which is known to stimulate only a subpopulation of peripheral T-cells,[5] will only induce inhibition. There is no concentration of cells or PHA that will induce stimulation.[2] Third, Rich and Pierce[4] have shown that a soluble factor responsible for the inhibitory effects of Con-A will only inhibit the response. Lower concentrations of the inhibitor do not stimulate the response.

Recently we have obtained an additional piece of information concerning the appearance of the stimulatory cell during development. This information is illustrated by the results presented in TABLE 2. Spleen cell suspensions from normal mice of various ages were irradiated and assayed for stimulatory activity. Two $\times 10^6$ irradiated cells from mice of various ages were added to aliquots of a pool of spleen cells from nu/nu mice containing 2×10^6 cells. Con-A was added at 2 μg/ml. It can be seen that no stimulatory activity could be measured in spleens from mice less than five weeks old. These results could be explained by a late development of the stimulatory activity in young mice or by the presence of an excess of inhibitory activity that was effective after irradiation (1000 R). The latter explanation, however, would seem to be unlikely. The response of spleen cells from young mice are very small, and inhibition with Con-A is hard to measure (TABLE 3).

In fact, the addition of Con-A at zero time causes even a slight stimulation; when added at 24 hours it causes a substantial increase in the response. This argues against the presence of excessive inhibitory activity in young mice and suggests that the inhibitory activity (or cell) is also slow to appear after birth.

Although there is no evidence either for or against equating the cell(s) mediating inhibitory or stimulatory activity with the cell that responds to Con-A by proliferation, it is of interest to note that this activity also develops progressively over the first seven weeks after birth.[6]

TABLE 2

DEVELOPMENT OF CON-A-INDUCED STIMULATORY ACTIVITY IN THE SPLEENS OF YOUNG BDF_1 (C57BL/6 $\times$ DBA2) MICE *

Con-A	—	+	+	+	+	+	+
Irradiated spleen BDF_1	—	—	New-born	1 wk	2 wks	5 wks	8 wks
Response (PFC/culture)	0	0	0	0	0	10	68
	0	0	0	0	0	14	28
	0	0	0	0	0	24	82
	1	0	0	0	0	4	96
	0	0	0	1	0	9	74

* All cultures contained 2×10^6 spleen cells from nu/nu mice. BRBC (3×10^6/culture) were added at t=zero, and the response was assayed at day 4. Con-A, where present, was at 2 μg/ml. The irradiated cells received 1000 R.

TABLE 3

RESPONSES OF YOUNG MICE *

	2 wks	5 wks	8 wks
No addition	35	60	555
Con-A at 0 hrs	50	165	465
Con-A at 24 hrs	410	735	3200

* 5×10^6 spleen cells from BDF_1 mice of various ages were incubated in 1 ml of medium. SRBC were added at t=zero. Con-A was added at the times indicated at a final concentration of 2 μg/ml. The PFC/culture were assayed at day 4.

References

1. DUTTON, R. W. 1972. Inhibitory and stimulatory effects of concanavalin A on the response of mouse spleen cell suspensions to antigen. I. Characterization of the inhibitory cell activity. J. Exp. Med. **136**(6): 1445–1460.
2. DUTTON, R. W. 1973. Inhibitory and stimulatory effects of concanavalin A on the response of mouse spleen cell suspensions to antigen. II. Evidence for separate stimulatory and inhibitory cells. J. Exp. Med. **138**(6): 1496–1505.
3. KAPPLER, J. W., P. C. HUNTER, D. JACOBS & E. LORD. 1974. Functional heterogeneity among the T-derived lymphocytes of the mouse. I. Analysis by adult thymectomy. J. Immunol. **113:** 27.
4. RICH, R. R. & C. W. PIERCE. 1974. Biological expressions of lymphocyte activation. III. Suppression of plaque-forming cell responses *in vitro* by supernatant fluids from concanavalin A-activated spleen cell cultures. J. Immunol. **112:** 136.
5. STOBO, J. D. 1972. Phytohemagglutinin and concanavalin A: probes for murine "T" cell activation and differentiation. Transplant. Rev. **11:** 60–86.
6. MOSIER, D. E. 1974. Ontogeny of mouse lymphocyte function. I. Paradoxical elevation of reactivity to allogeneic cells and phytohemagglutinin in BALB/c fetal thymocytes. J. Immunol. **112**(1): 305–310.

IN VITRO INDUCTION OF THYMUS-DERIVED CELL-MEDIATED CYTOTOXICITY TO TRINITROPHENOL-MODIFIED SYNGENEIC LYMPHOCYTE SURFACE PROTEINS

Gene M. Shearer

Immunology Branch
National Cancer Institute
Bethesda, Maryland 20014

Introduction

Thymus-derived lymphocytes appear to play an active rôle in many aspects of immunity. These include: (1) helper cell [1–4] and suppressor or regulator cell [5–7] functions for modulation of antibody production; (2) delayed hypersensitivity; [8] (3) graft-versus-host (GvH) reactions; [9] (4) mixed lymphocyte reactions; [10, 11] and (5) cell-mediated cytotoxicity.[12–20] In the mouse, the evidence that the induction and effector phases of specific cell-mediated cytotoxicity involve thymus-derived cells has been provided by studies demonstrating that both of these phases are sensitive to anti-θ antiserum and complement [12, 17–20] and that *in vitro* induction of cell-mediated cytotoxicity can be generated by thymus-derived thoracic duct lymphocytes [14] and by cortisone-resistant thymocytes.[15, 16]

Murine cell mediated cytotoxic reactions have been demonstrated against alloantigens, usually involving differences at the major histocompatibility complex between responding lymphocytes and stimulating cells.[12–20] Cytotoxic reactions against either modified or unmodified "self-antigens" have been more difficult to demonstrate. Mouse spleen cells cultured *in vitro* with syngeneic fibroblasts were capable of syngeneic GvH reactions when injected into syngeneic neonates,[21] and mixed lymphocyte reactivity between syngeneic cells of certain mouse strains have been demonstrated.[11, 22] A few examples of cell-mediated cytotoxicity directed against unmodified [23, 24] and modified [25] syngeneic tumor cell antigens have been reported. The present study shows that trinitrophenol (TNP) modification of mouse spleen cells resulted in the formation of new antigenic regions on the modified cells. *In vitro* culture of unmodified, syngeneic, thymus-derived lymphocytes with TNP-modified spleen cells resulted in the generation of cytotoxic effector cells that were not TNP-specific but were directed primarily against modified cell-surface proteins. The specificity observed between TNP-modified "immunogen" and target cells suggested that the proteins modified by TNP were controlled by genes within distinct regions of the major (H-2) histocompatibility complex.

Materials and Methods

Spleen cells from normal, young, adult mice were cultured *in vitro* with unmodified or TNP-modified syngeneic or congenic spleen cells by a modification [26] of the Mishell-Dutton technique.[27] Five days later, the effector cells generated in culture were harvested and incubated with ^{51}Cr-labeled unmodified or TNP-modified syngeneic or congenic spleen target cells. The percentage of specific lysis was determined after a four-hour incubation of effector and target cells by the method described by Canty and Wunderlich.[26] Spontaneous release of ^{51}Cr by spleen cell targets in the presence of unsensitized spleen cells was 15–30%. Nevertheless, significant specific lysis was obtained after subtraction of the relatively high spontaneous ^{51}Cr release characteristic of spleen cell targets. These results have been verified using TNP-modified tumor target cells (which give lower spontaneous lysis, 5–15%) with the appropriate H-2 types.

Spleen and tumor cells were modified with TNP by incubation of the cells with 10 mM 2,4,6-trinitrobenzene sulfonic acid at pH 7.3 for 10 minutes at 37° C. The cells were then washed twice in Hank's balanced salt solution containing 10% fetal bovine serum.

Results and Discussion

The cytotoxic results obtained using unmodified and TNP-modified syngeneic as well as congenic target cells are summarized in TABLE 1. Trinitrophenol modification of the target cells was necessary but not sufficient to obtain lysis of target cells. Unmodified B10.A spleen targets were not significantly lysed, whereas 28.6% lysis was obtained when the same target cells were modified with TNP (first two lines of TABLE 1). In order to determine whether the cytotoxicity was specific for the TNP moiety, B10.A effector spleen cells that had been sensitized *in vitro* with TNP-modified syngeneic spleen cells were assayed with modified spleen targets from the B10.D2, B10.BR and C57BL/10 congenic lines. These mouse strains differ at distinct regions of the major histocompatibility complex (MHC) as discussed elsewhere.[28] Designations of the K, Ir, Ss-Slp, and D regions of the MHC for the four strains studied are

TABLE 1

In Vitro INDUCTION OF CYTOTOXICITY OF B10.A SPLEEN CELLS TO TNP-MODIFIED SYNGENEIC SPLEEN CELLS ASSAYED WITH UNMODIFIED AND TNP-MODIFIED SYNGENEIC AND CONGENIC SPLEEN TARGET CELLS *

Target Cells	% Specific Lysis ± S.E.	MHC †			
		K	Ir	Ss-Slp	D
B10.A	2.7 ± 2.6	K	K	D	D
B10.A-TNP	28.6 ± 3.3	K	K	D	D
B10.D2	4.1 ± 2.5	D	D	D	D
B10.D2-TNP	6.3 ± 2.3	D	D	D	D
B10.A-TNP	23.2 ± 1.1	K	K	D	D
B10.BR-TNP	14.1 ± 2.1	K	K	K	K
B10.A-TNP	37.3 ± 1.6	K	K	D	D
B10-TNP	6.9 ± 1.1	B	B	B	B

* Effector:target cell ratio=8:1.

† MHC: Major histocompatibility complex.

TABLE 2

SUMMARY OF EXPERIMENTS INDICATING THAT THE PHENOMENON IS DUE TO T-CELL-MEDIATED CYTOTOXICITY

Parameter Tested in the Induction or Effector Phase	% Specific Lysis ± S.E.	
	Experimental	Positive Control
1. lymphocyte-dependent antibody is not detected in the culture media	0	37.3 ± 1.6
2. TNP-lysine does not block the effector phase	20.0 ± 2.2	23.2 ± 1.1
3. spleen cells from althymic nude donors do not generate effector cells	−0.9 ± 0.4	13.8 ± 2.1
4. effector cells are sensitive to rabbit anti-mouse brain serum	−0.2 ± 1.0	17.0 ± 1.5
5. effector cells can be generated by cortisone-resistant thymocytes	10.0 ± 1.1	10.4 ± 2.2

shown on the right side of the table. Specific lysis did not occur when either modified B10.D2 or C57BL/10 spleen cells were used as targets (compare lines 2 and 7 with lines 4 and 8, respectively). Significant cytotoxicity (14.1 ± 2.1%) was obtained, however, when TNP-modified B10.BR spleen cells targets were used, although it was not as great as in the case of target cells syngeneic with the TNP-modified "immunogen" and responding cell population (compare line 5 with 6). Thus, the cytotoxicity was not specific for TNP exclusively, but was primarily directed against modified syngeneic cell-surface proteins, which may or may not have included the TNP moiety as an integral part of the recognition unit. Were TNP the only requirement for recognition and cytolysis, B10.D2 (B10 is an exceptional strain as shown below) modified spleen cells should have been as effective targets as modified B10.A spleen cells when B10.A responding cells were sensitized against TNP-modified syngeneic spleen cells. Since these congenic mouse strains differ only at the major histocompatibility complex (H-2), the results suggest that the cellular proteins modified by TNP so as to be immunogenic to syngeneic lymphocytes were controlled by genes within distinct regions of the MHC. One or more of these genes would appear to be located within the K, Ir portion of the MHC, since some cross-reactivity was observed between TNP-modified B10.A and B10.BR spleen cells when cells for these two strains were used as "immunogen" and targets, respectively.

A number of criteria were used to demonstrate that the phenomenon was attributed to thymus-derived cell mediated cytotoxicity against modified lymphocyte proteins and that it was not due to lymphocyte-dependent antibody.[29] These include (see TABLE 2): (1) lack of detectable lymphocyte-dependent antibody in the culture media; (2) failure of TNP-lysine to block the effector phase of cytolysis under conditions identical to those that block lysis due to lymphocyte-dependent antibody; (3) failure of spleen cells from athymic nude donors to generate effector cells;[15] (4) sensitivity of effector cells to rabbit anti-mouse brain serum and complement;[19, 29, 30] and (5) generation of effector cells *in vitro* using cortisone-resistant thymocytes.[15, 16] Thus, both the effector and induction phases of cytotoxicity to TNP-modified syngeneic B10.A spleen cells are thymus-dependent, and the response can be generated exclusively from a population of cortisone-resistant thymocytes.

The ability of various congenic and noncongenic inbred mouse strains to generate *in vitro* cell-mediated cytotoxicity to TNP-modified syngeneic spleen cells when assayed with modified syngeneic targets was also controlled by genes within the major histocompatibility complex (TABLE 3). Of the C57BL/10 congenic strains tested, B10.A, B10.D2, and B10.BR were "responders," whereas C57BL/10 was a "nonresponder." The (B10 × B10.A)F_1 hybrid was a high responder, suggesting that the gene(s) controlling this phenomenon is dominant.[31]

The SJL/J and DBA/1 inbred strains were also found to be responder and nonresponders, respectively. However, in contrast to the (B10 × B10.A)F_1 mice, (SJL × DBA/1)F_1 mice were nonresponders. The apparent recessive nature of responsiveness in this case is similar to the "recessive" immune re-

TABLE 3

STRAIN DISTRIBUTION OF INDUCTION OF CELL-MEDIATED CYTOTOXICITY TO TNP-MODIFIED SYNGENEIC SPLEEN CELLS *In Vitro* *

Mouse Strain	% Specific Lysis ± S.E.	H-2 Type
B10.A	37.3 ± 1.6	a
B10	1.8 ± 1.8	b
(B10 × B10.A)F_1	32.9 ± 1.4	a/b
B10.D2	34.4 ± 1.0	d
B10.BR	37.1 ± 2.7	k
SJL/J	34.5 ± 1.7	s
DBA/1	6.0 ± 2.5	q
(DBA/1 × SJL/J)F_1	3.9 ±	s/q
NZB	2.6 ±	d
NZW	0.0 ±	z

* Effector:target cell ratio=8:1.

sponse gene controlling antibody production to TNP on a mouse serum albumin carrier.[32] This raised the possibility that a portion of the specificity of cytolysis in the SJL/J strain was directed against TNP exclusively. In fact, some cytotoxic cross-reactivity was observed when the effector cells from cultures in which SJL/J spleen cells were sensitized with TNP-modified syngeneic spleen cells were assayed with H-2-unrelated modified target cells (data not shown).

Both young adult NZB and NZW mice were nonresponders to modified syngeneic spleen cells. Older animals of these strains that exhibit autoimmune disorders[33] have not yet been tested.

The cellular and molecular bases for unresponsiveness in the C57BL/10 and DBA/1 strains are currently under investigation. Since the effector cells are of thymic origin, one might speculate that the phenomenon is controlled by a classical immune response (Ir) gene involving a defect in the responding population of thymus-derived cells.[31] Unlike most other known Ir genes, however, a cellular component of this model is contributed by the "immunogen" itself. Therefore, a defect could reside in the H-2-linked control of the synthesis of a cell-surface protein on C57BL/10 spleen cells, which cannot be conformationally altered by TNP so as to be immunogenic in the B10 congenic strains. Were this to be the site of the defect (not necessarily the only defect), (B10 × B10.A)F_1 responder cells should respond to TNP-modified F_1 or B10.A spleen cells, but not to TNP-modified B10 cells. Furthermore, the use of modified B10 spleen cells as targets should fail to detect F_1 cytotoxic effector cells even when immunized against modified F_1 or B10.A spleen cells. Both of these predictions were verified (data not shown). Thus, at least one genetic defect involves the failure of B10 cells to be modified in such a way as to be immunogenic to responding cells.

It remains to be established whether the H-2-linked genetic parameters associated with this phenomenon map in the same region of the MHC as classical Ir genes,[34, 35] and whether this model serves any significant role in natural immunobiology. The possibility is raised that these lymphocyte surface proteins modified by TNP and controlled by genes within the MHC represent the so-called Ir gene products.

Acknowledgments

I wish to gratefully acknowledge the skilled technical assistance of Carol Garbarino. I thank Dr. Pierre Henkart for testing culture media for lymphocyte-dependent antibody, Drs. Barry S. Handwerger and Ronald S. Schwartz for providing rabbit anti-mouse brain serum, and Marilyn Schoenfelder for typing the manuscript.

[NOTE ADDED IN PROOF: More recent studies indicate that C57Bl/10 spleen cells can be modified by TNP so as to be immunogenic to syngeneic-responding lymphocytes. Studies are in progress to elucidate possible differences in the immunogenicity of modified B10 spleen cells as a function of the degree of TNP-lation.]

References

1. CLAMAN, H. N., E. A. CHAPERON & R. F. TRIPLETT. 1966. Immunocompetence of transferred thymus-marrow cell combinations. J. Immunol. **97:** 828–832.
2. MILLER, J. F. A. P. & G. F. MITCHELL. 1968. Cell to cell interaction in the immune response. I. Hemolysin-forming cells in neonatally thynectomized mice reconstituted with thymus or thoracic duct lymphocytes. J. Exp. Med. **128:** 801–820.
3. MITCHISON, N. A. 1971. The carrier effect in the secondary response to hapten-protein conjugates. II. Cellular cooperation. Eur. J. Immunol. **1:** 18–27.
4. KUNIN, S., G. M. SHEARER, S. SEGAL, A. GLOBERSON & M. FELDMAN. 1971. A bicellular mechanism in the immune response to chemically defined antigens. III. Interactions of thymus and bone marrow-derived cells. Cell. Immunol. **2:** 229–238.
5. GERSHON, R. K., P. COHEN, R. HENCIN & S. A. LIEBHABER. 1972. Suppressor T cells. J. Immunol. **108:** 586–590.
6. SHEARER, G. M., K. L. MELMON, Y. WEINSTEIN & M. SELA. 1972. Regulation of antibody response by cells expressing histamine receptors. J. Exp. Med. **136:** 1302–1307.
7. SHEARER, G. M., Y. WEINSTEIN & K. L. MELMON. 1974. Enhancement of im-

mune response potential of mouse lymphoid cells fractionated over histamine columns. J. Immunol. **113:**.
8. Lawrence, H. S. & M. Landy. 1969. *In* the Mediators of Cellular Immunity. : 71. Academic Press. New York, N.Y.
9. Cantor, H. & R. Asofsky. 1972. Synergy among lymphoid cells mediating the graft-versus-host response. III. Evidence for interaction between two types of thymus-derived cells. J. Exp. Med. **135:** 764–779.
10. Howe, M. L., A. L. Goldstein & J. R. Battisto. 1970. Isogeneic lymphocyte interaction: Recognition of self antigens by cells of the neonatal thymus. Proc. Nat. Acad. Sci. U.S. **67:** 613–619.
11. Von Boehmer, H. & W. J. Byrd. 1972. Responsiveness of thymus cells to syngeneic and allogeneic lymphoid cells. Nature New Biol. **235:** 50–52.
12. Cerottini, J. C., A. A. Nordin & K. T. Brunner. 1970. *In vitro* cytotoxic activity of thymus cells sensitized to alloantigens. Nature **227:** 72–73.
13. Wagner, H. 1971. Cell-mediated immune response *in vitro:* Independent differentiation of thymocytes into cytotoxic lymphocytes. Eur. J. Immunol. **1:** 498–499.
14. Sprent, J. & J. F. A. P. Miller. 1972. Interaction of thymus lymphocytes with histoincompatible cells. III. Immunological characteristics of recirculating lymphocytes derived from activated thymus cells. Cell. Immunol. **3:** 213–230.
15. Wagner, H. 1972. The correlation between the proliferative and the cytotoxic responses of mouse lymphocytes to allogeneic cells *in vitro.* J. Immunol. **109:** 630–637.
16. Wagner, H., A. W. Harris & M. Feldman. 1972. Cell-mediated immune respones *in vitro:* II. The role of thymus and thymus-derived lymphocytes. Cell. Immunol. **4:** 39–50.
17. Cerottini, S. C., A. A. Nordin & K. T. Brunner. 1970. Specific *in vitro* cytotoxicity of thymus-derived lymphocytes sensitized to alloantigens. Nature **228:** 1308–1309.
18. Goldstein, P., H. Wigzell, H. Blomgren & E. Suedmyr. 1972. Cells mediating specific *in vitro* cytotoxicity. II. Probable autonomy of thymus-processed lymphocytes (T cells) for the killing of allogeneic target cells. J. Exp. Med. **135:** 890–906.
19. Goldstein, P., V. Schirrmacher, B. Rubin & H. Wigzell. 1973. Cytotoxic immune cells with specificity for defined soluble antigens. II. Chasing the killing cells. Cell. Immunol. **9:** 211–225.
20. MacDonald, H. R., R. A. Phillips & R. G. Miller. 1973. Allograft immunity in the mouse. II. Physical studies of the development of cytotoxic effector cells from their immediate progenitors. J. Immunol. **111:** 575–789.
21. Cohen, I. R., A. Globerson & M. Feldman. 1971. Autosensitization *in vitro.* J. Exp. Med. **133:** 834–845.
22. Von Boehmer, H. & P. B. Adams. 1973. Syngeneic mixed lymphocyte reaction between thymocytes and peripheral lymphoid cells in mice: Strain specificity and nature of the target cell. J. Immunol. **110:** 376–383.
23. Wagner, H. & M. Rollinghoff. 1973. Cell-mediated immunity *in vitro* against syngeneic mouse plasma tumor cells. Nature New Biol. **241:** 53–54.
24. Lundak, R. L. & D. L. Raidt. 1973. Cellular immune response against tumor cells. I. *In vitro* immunization of allogeneic and syngeneic mouse spleen cell suspensions against DBA mastocytoma cells. Cell. Immunol. **9:** 60–66.
25. Martin, W. J., J. R. Wunderlich, F. Fletcher & J. K. Inman. 1971. Enhanced immunogenicity of chemically-coated syngeneic tumor cells. Proc. Nat. Acad. Sci. U.S. **68:** 469–472.
26. Canty, T. G. & J. R. Wunderlich. 1970. Quantitative *in vitro* assay of cytotoxic cellular immunity. J. Nat. Cancer Inst. **45:** 761–772.
27. Mishell, R. I. & R. W. Dutton. 1967. Immunization of disocciated spleen cell cultures from normal mice. J. Exp. Med. **126:** 423–442.
28. Bach, F. H., M. B. Widmer, M. L. Bach & J. Klein. 1972. Serologically defined

and lymphocyte-defined components of the major histocompatibility complex in the mouse. J. Exp. Med. **136:** 1430–1444.

29. BRITTON, S., H. PERLMAN & P. PERLMANN. 1973. Thymus-dependent and thymus-independent effector functions of mouse lymphoid cells. Comparison of cytotoxicity and primary antibody formation *in vitro*. Cell. Immunol. **8:** 420–434.
30. GOLUB, E. S. 1971. Brain-associated θ antigen: Reactivity of rabbit anti-mouse brain with mouse lymphoid cells. Cell. Immunol. **2:** 353–361.
31. MCDEVITT, H. O. & B. BENACERRAF. 1969. Genetic control of specific immune responses. Advan. Immunol. **11:** 31–74.
32. RATHBUN, W. E. & W. H. HILDEMANN. 1970. Genetic control of the antibody response to simple haptens in congenic strains of mice. J. Immunol. **105:** 98–107.
33. HOWIE, J. B. & B. J. HELYER. 1968. The immunology and pathology of NZB mice. Advan. Immunol. **9:** 215–266.
34. LIEBERMAN, R., W. E. PAUL, W. HUMPHREY, JR. & J. H. STIMPFLING. 1972. H-2 linked immune response (Ir) genes. Independent loci for Ir-IgG and Ir-IgA genes. J. Exp. Med. **136:** 1231–1240.
35. MCDEVITT, H. O., B. D. DEAK, D. C. SHREFFLER, J. KLEIN, J. H. STIMFLING & G. D. SNELL. 1972. Genetic control of the immune response. Mapping of the Ir-l locus. J. Exp. Med. **135:** 1259–1278.

IDENTIFICATION OF θ-BEARING T-CELLS DERIVED FROM BONE MARROW CELLS TREATED WITH THYMIC FACTOR *

H. C. Miller and W. J. Esselman

Departments of Microbiology and Public Health, and Surgery
Michigan State University
East Lansing, Michigan 48824

A glycolipid, isolated from mouse thymus and brain tissue, is capable of inhibiting the cytotoxicity of anti-BAθ † antiserum.[1] The BAθ antigen, which was extracted into lipid solvents, was found in the upper-aqueous phase of Folch partitions and was characterized as a G_{D1b} ganglioside. Observations of other investigators are consistent with this claim. Earlier work of Reif and Allen[2] revealed that θC3HeB/Fc isoantigen of thymus could not be dialyzed and could not be recovered in active form after treatment with lipid solvents. Recently Vitetta *et al.*[3] presented evidence that the θC3H and BAθ antigens of mice were glycolipid in nature. The antigenic activity specified by AKR anti-θC3H antiserum was also found to cochromatograph with a ganglioside (G_{M1}) that lacks one of the sialic acid residues found on the BAθ antigen.[4]

Incubation of mouse bone marrow cells with thymic factor obtained from bovine thymus tissue results in development of cells with T lymphocyte markers (i.e., θ, azathioprine sensitivity, allograft responsiveness and rosette formation)[5] as well as functional helper T-cells, which induce B-cells to become antibody-forming cells.[6]

We now report the detection of BAθ and θC3H bearing cells in various density gradient fractions of mouse bone marrow following treatment of the cells with thymic factor. Differences in cell glycolipids are compared for purified marrow cells before and after TF treatment.

Materials and Methods

Mice

CBA/J female mice, 3 to 5 months old, were used as donors of bone marrow cells.

* Supported in part by grants from the National Cancer Institute (CA-13396), from the Kidney Foundation of Michigan (ORD 12164), and from National Institutes of Health GRS (RR-0565606).

† Abbreviations: BAθ, brain-associated θ antigen; TF, thymic factor; TF-marrow cells, thymic factor-treated marrow cells; SDS, sodium dodecylsulfate; BSA, bovine serum albumin; Gal, galactosyl; Glc, glucosyl; GalNAc, *N*-acetylgalactosyl; NANA, *N*-acetylneuraminyl; cer, ceramide (2-*N*-acylsphingosine); G_{M3}, NANA-Gal-Glc-Cer; G_{M2}, GalNAc-Gal(NANA)-Glc-Cer; G_{M1}, Gal-GalNAc-Gal(NANA)-Glc-Cer; G_{D1a}, Gal(NANA)-GalNAc-Gal(NANA)-Glc-Cer; G_{D1b}, Gal-GalNAc-Gal(NANA-NANA)-Glc-Cer; G_{T1}, Gal(NANA)-GalNAc-Gal(NANA-NANA)-Glc-Cer.

Cell Suspensions

Bone marrow cells, harvested from the long bone of 12-week-old female mice, were suspended in Eagle's medium. Nucleated, viable cells were counted and washed by centrifugation.

Density Gradient Separation

The cells were subjected to equilibrium centrifugation in a discontinuous gradient of bovine serum albumin (BSA) as previously described.[7,8] Cell fractions were collected from the interphases, beginning at the top, between 17 and 19% BSA. The fractions were diluted in Ca- and Mg-free phosphate-buffered (pH 7.2) saline (PBS), washed once by centrifugation, and resuspended in PBS.

Thymic Factor

Thymic factor (TF), fraction 3, prepared from calf thymus according to Goldstein *et al.*[9] was a generous gift of Dr. Allyn Rule (School of Medicine, Tufts University, Medford, Massachusetts). TF was stored in lyophilized form at −20° C until needed.

Antiserum, Complement, and Cytotoxic Tests

Brains of CBA/J mice were removed, homogenized, and injected into Dutch Belt rabbits for production of anti-BAθ antiserum according to the protocol used by Golub.[10] The cytotoxic titer of the antiserum used for all experiments reported herein was 1:128. This antiserum and normal rabbit serum (C) were absorbed with CBA/J mouse erythrocytes, liver and agarose. Anti-θC3H antisera were produced in AKR/J female mice by injection of CBA thymocytes intraperitoneally according to the method of Reif and Allen.[11] The cytotoxic titer of the pooled antisera was 1:64. Either 0.05 ml of absorbed rabbit anti-CBA brain antiserum diluted 1:10 or AKR anti-θC3H diluted 1:4 was added to 0.1 ml of cells at a density of 2×10^7/ml; 0.05 ml of absorbed C was added next and incubated 1 hour at 37° C. Cytotoxicity was determined by trypan blue exclusion.

Radiolabeling of Cells

Bone marrow cells collected from layers 2 (21% BSA) and 3 (23% BSA) were combined (2.5×10^7 cells) and were incubated simultaneously with 50 μg/ml thymic factor, 25 μCi D-[1-^{14}C]galactose (45 mCi/mmole, New England Nuclear, Boston, Massachusetts) and 150 μCi L-[4,5-^{3}H]leucine (30 Ci/mmole, New England Nuclear). The incubation was performed in Hank's balanced salt solution for 2 hours at 37° C in a CO_2 incubator. An equal number of control cells (2.5×10^7) were incubated with the same amounts of radioactive precursors. At the end of the incubation the cells were washed 3 times and the pellets were prepared as described below.

Lipid Extraction and Separation

Cell pellets were extracted with 3 ml of chloroform-methanol 2:1 (v/v) and the extract was subjected to a Folch partition as described previously.[12] The ganglioside-rich Folch upper phase was fractionated by thin-layer chromatography on 0.25 mm Silica Gel G plates (Analtech, Inc., Wilmington, Delaware). The plates were developed with chloroform-methanol-2,5 N ammonium hydroxide 60:40:9 (v/v/v). Radioactivity was determined by scanning of the plates with a Berthold Radio Scanner (Varian Instruments, Palo Alto, California). Radioactivity was also determined by elution of the ganglioside bands as described previously.[1] Because of the small amounts of gangliosides obtained from the cell pellets, cold carrier mouse-brain gangliosides were added to the lipid extract before thin-layer chromatography.

Protein Fractionation

Radioactivity of the lipid-free protein residues was determined by removing an aliquot of the protein after dissolution in 1% SDS, 2% 2-mercaptoethanol, 50 mM tris buffer, pH 7.4. The protein solution was heated at 60° C for 30 minutes, sonicated briefly and subjected to electrophoresis on 1% SDS polyacrylamide gels.[13]

Results

Density distributions of nucleated marrow cells following equilibrium centrifugation in discontinuous gradients of BSA are presented in Table 1. The numbers of cells obtained for each fraction were reproducible. Although the majority of the cells was found in the higher density fractions not presented here, pilot studies suggested these were not pertinent to the experiments described below.

Table 1

Density Distribution Profile of Nucleated Cells of Mouse Bone Marrow 2.5×10^8 Cells were Layered on the Top of the Gradient

Fraction Number	BSA Concentration	Nucleated Cells * $\times 10^6$
1	19	1.3
2	21	1.8
3	23	3.2
4	25	13.2
5	27	23.4
6	29	49.3

* Mean of three individual separation runs.

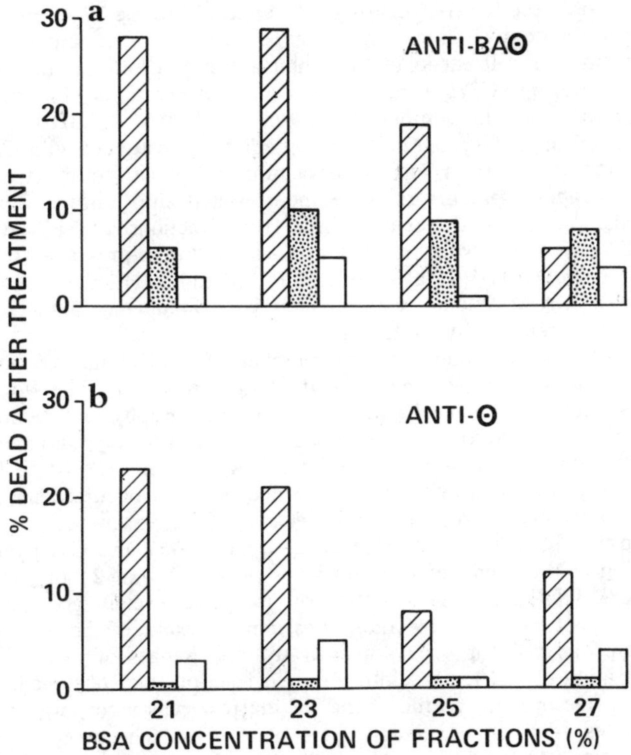

FIGURE 1. Anti-θ-sensitive T-cells derived from density gradient fractionation of bone marrow cells; (a) shows results of fractions of marrow cells treated with rabbit anti-mouse brain antibodies in the presence of complement following treatment with thymic factor (striped area); in absence of pretreatment with thymic factor (stippled areas); and cells treated with thymic factor followed by incubation with complement only (open areas); (b) represents exactly the same design with AKR anti-CBA thymus antiserum treatment of the fractions. Percent killing was determined by trypan blue exclusion.

Bone marrow cells from the various density gradient fractions were incubated with TF for one hour. Presence of BAθ or θC3H on TF-treated marrow cells was detected by treatment of aliquots from each BSA fraction with rabbit anti-BAθ or AKR anti-θC3H antisera and complement. In addition, control-cell suspensions from each fraction were either not exposed to TF, exposed to TF and complement only, or exposed to TF only. Results of this experiment are presented in FIGURE 1. The plots are normalized by first subtracting controls for each fraction in which the cytotoxicity due to complement treatment alone was measured. Although not presented here, background values for these ranged from 1–2% killing only. Numbers of BAθ-bearing cells (FIGURE 1a) which appear following TF treatment are highest in the low density fractions, i.e., 21 and 23% BSA concentration. Only 9% of the cells in the 25% BSA fraction were above respective controls, i.e., those exposed to TF and complement only. No detectable BAθ-bearing cells appeared in the 27% BSA fraction. Cell killing in the controls that were not exposed to TF treatment was presumably due to antistem-cell effects of the rabbit anti-mouse brain antiserum.[14]

The cells bearing θC3H were found in all BSA fractions (FIGURE 1b). It should be noted that, in comparison to cells with BAθ, θC3H-bearing cells were also found in fraction 5 (27% BSA) following treatment with TF.

In an attempt to further specify the action of thymic factor on bone marrow cells, metabolic precursors were incorporated into differentiating bone marrow cells. Bone marrow cells isolated from fractions 2 (21% BSA) and 3 (23% BSA) were incubated at 37° C for 2 hours in the presence of 50 μg/ml thymic factor, 25 μCi [1-^{14}C]galactose and 150 μCi [4,5-^{3}H]leucine as described in MATERIALS AND METHODS. Control cells were incubated in the same way except for the absence of thymic factor.

The TF marrow cells and an equal number of control marrow cells were treated with chloroform-methanol to extract lipid material. The Folch upper phase lipids were fractionated by thin-layer chromatography and monitored for ^{14}C radioactivity (FIGURE 2). Significant [^{14}C]galactose radioactivity was incorporated into the glycolipids of TF marrow cells in contrast to low level incorporation into control cells. Maximal incorporation occurred in glycolipid (G_{M1}) which we have proposed to be θC3H antigen.[4] Smaller amounts of [^{14}C]galactose were incorporated into G_{D1a}, G_{D1b} (BAθ) and G_{T1} gangliosides. Incorporation at the origin of the thin layer plate (FIGURE 2) may be due to free galactose, UDP-galactose or very large molecular weight glycolipids. The presence of small water-soluble molecules can be excluded because the lipid extracts were dialyzed for 4 days against several changes of distilled water.[12] No incorporation of [^{3}H]leucine into the lipid fractions was observed.

The lipid-free protein residue of the TF marrow cells incorporated approximately 3 times as much [^{3}H]leucine as control cells. The protein residue in both cases demonstrated little or no incorporated [^{14}C]galactose. Preliminary evidence obtained by electrophoretic separation of the protein residue on 9% SDS polyacrylamide gels of TF marrow cells indicated that there was no selective increase in the polypeptide profile. Thus, it appeared that there was a general increase in protein biosynthesis with TF treatment.

DISCUSSION

Precursors of T-cells are found in lower density regions of BSA discontinuous density gradients. This observation confirms the recent report of Komuro and Boyse[15] in which they used mouse marrow, spleen or fetal liver that had been subjected to BSA density gradient separation followed by exposure to "thymic extract." A unique aspect of the observations reported in FIGURE 1 is that cells bearing θC3H antigen are found in the 27% BSA fraction whereas BAθ-bearing cells were not detected here. The most obvious interpretation of this finding is that at least two populations of cells with the different θ antigens arise after TF treatment. Perhaps some of the cells may have BAθ, some θC3H and others could conceivably have both. Studies are presently under way to resolve this matter as well as to correlate these topical differences with the various aspects of T-cell helper function. Although the results reported in FIGURE 1 represent one set of observations for pooled fractions of marrow cells, we have repeated these density gradient separations and θ determinations three times with almost identical results.

When radioactive precursors were incubated with marrow cells and thymic factor, a significant increase in incorporation was observed. [^{14}C]galactose was incorporated more rapidly into G_{M1} ganglioside (θC3H antigen) thus pos-

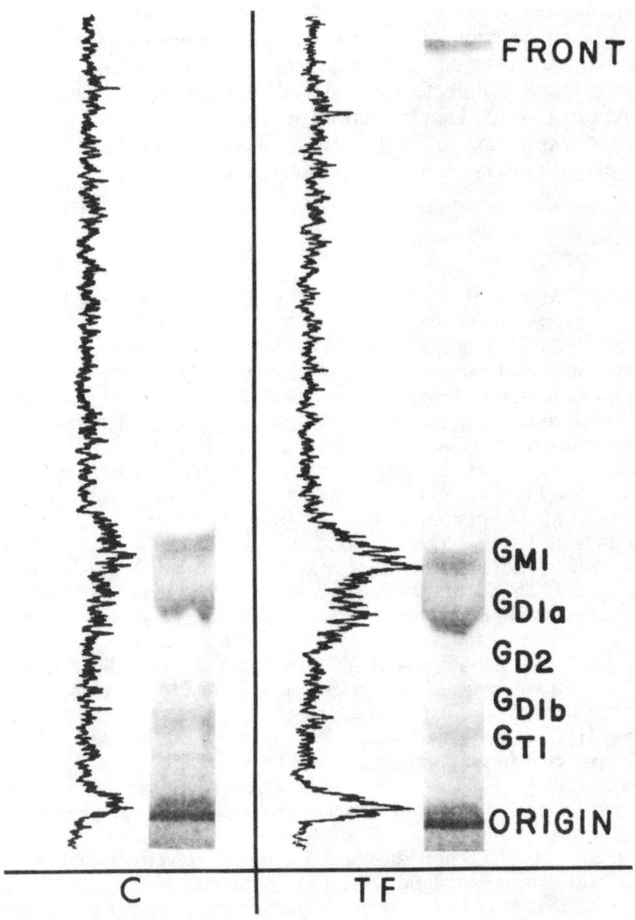

FIGURE 2. Effect of thymic factor on incorporation of [^{14}C]galactose into bone marrow cell glycolipids. C, Folch upper phase gangliosides isolated from marrow cells incubated with [1-^{14}C]galactose and [3,4-^{3}H] leucine; TF, Folch upper phase gangliosides isolated from marrow cells incubated with thymic factor, [1-^{14}C]galactose and [3,4-^{3}H] leucine. The thin layer plate was developed as described in MATERIALS AND METHODS. The radioactive scan shown to the left of each thin layer chromatogram is for ^{14}C and no ^{3}H activity was observed. Cold carrier mouse-brain gangliosides were added to the small amounts of lipids obtained from the cell extracts.

sibly accounting for the appearance of this antigen on TF treated marrow cells. [^{3}H]leucine incorporation into cell proteins was also stimulated, thus indicating that the general biosynthetic processes of the cells was elevated in TF marrow cells. This finding is in accord with the finding of Komuro and Boyse [16] that the appearance of T-cell specific antigens (TL and θ [Thy 1]) on thymic-extract-treated spleen cells depends on protein biosynthesis. The action of TF on marrow cells was rapid since the appearance of specific surface antigens occurred within a one-hour period.

Whether incorporation of [^{3}H]leucine and [^{14}C]galactose is due only to the action of thymic factor on specific precursor cells remains to be determined by the use of pure thymic factor and cells containing a higher population of specific precursor cells. Determination of further details of lymphocyte differentiation and expression of cell surface changes and their correlation with functional cell-cell interaction are in progress.

References

1. Esselman, W. J. & H. C. Miller. 1974. Brain and thymus lipid inhibition of antibrain-associated θ-cytotoxicity. J. Exp. Med. **139:** 445.
2. Reif, A. E. & J. M. Allen. 1964. The AKR thymic antigen and its distribution in leukemias and nervous tissues. J. Exp. Med. **120:** 413.
3. Vitetta, E. S., E. A. Boyse & J. W. Uhr. 1973. Isolation and characterization of a molecular complex containing Thy-1 antigen from the surface of murine thymocytes and T cells. Eur. J. Immunol. **3:** 446.
4. Esselman, W. J. & H. C. Miller. 1974. The ganglioside nature of θ antigens. Abstr. Fed. Proc. **33:** 771.
5. Bach, J.-F., M. Dardenne, A. L. Goldstein, A. Guha & A. White. 1971. Appearance of T-cell markers in bone marrow rosette-forming cells after incubation with thymosin, a thymic hormone. Proc. Nat. Acad. Sci. U.S. **68:** 2734.
6. Miller, H. C., S. K. Schmiege & A. Rule. 1973. Production of functional T cells after treatment of bone marrow with thymic factor. J. Immunol. **111:** 1005.
7. Dicke, K. A., G. Tridente & D. W. van Bekkum. 1969. The selective elimination of immunologically competent cells from bone marow and lymphocyte cell mixtures. Transplantation **8:** 422.
8. Miller, H. C. & G. Cudkowicz. 1971. Density gradient separation of marrow cells restricted for antibody class. Science **171:** 913.
9. Goldstein, A. L., F. D. Slater & A. White. 1966. Preparation, assay, and partial purification of a thymic lymphocytopoietic factor (thymosin). Proc. Nat. Acad. Sci. U.S. **56:** 1010.
10. Golub, E. S. 1971. Brain-associated θ antigen: Reactivity of rabbit anti-mouse brain with mouse lymphoid cells. Cell. Immunol. **2:** 353.
11. Reif, A. E. & J. M. Allen. 1966. Mouse thymic isoantigens. Nature **209:** 521.
12. Esselman, W. J., R. A. Laine & C. C. Sweeley. 1972. Isolation and characterization of glycosphingolipids. Methods Enzymol. **28:** 140.
13. Fairbanks, G., T. L. Steck & D. F. H. Wallach. 1971. Electrophoretic analysis of the major polypeptides of the human erythrocyte membrane. Biochemistry **10:** 2606.
14. Golub, E. S. 1972. Brain-associated stem cell antigen: An antigen shared by brain and hemopoietic stem cells. J. Exp. Med. **136:** 369.
15. Komuro, K. & E. A. Boyse. 1973. Induction of T lymphocytes from precursor cells *in vitro* by a product of the thymus. J. Exp. Med. **138:** 479.
16. Komuro, K. & E. A. Boyse. 1973. *In vitro* demonstration of thymic hormone in the mouse by conversion of precursor cells into lymphocytes. Lancet **1:** 740.

THYMIC HORMONES?

A. J. S. Davies

Chester Beatty Research Institute, Institute of Cancer Research London SW3 6JB, England

The notion that the thymus produces a hormone is attractive. It could be that the putative factor has an influence on cells outside the thymus that reflects the differentiational influence it has on cells within the organ. Alternatively, the effect of the hormone on cells outside the organ could be very different from whatever humoral factors may cause differentiation within the thymus. But, however appealing is the idea of a thymic hormone, and whatever the rewards for its translation into a properly characteriezd reality, the evidence adduced so far has not been received with universal acclaim.

I intend to illustrate here, by brief consideration of a series of experiments done over a number of years, that it is all too easy to get inconclusive results from procedures designed to explore the possibility of a thymic hormonal influence. Such results in biological experimentation are often meaningless and are rarely talked about for this reason. As will be seen, however, one result was positive, and it has certainly helped me to retain interest in the problem.

The test system adopted has in most instances been a thymectomized irradiated adult mouse injected after irradiation with 5×10^6 syngeneic bone-marrow cells.[1] For convenience, I shall call these animals "deprived mice." Others, I am led to believe, have termed them, pejoratively, B mice. I have selected only the major experiments we performed—many others, all inconclusive, were carried out on various extracts of thymuses. In all instances the aim was to replace the thymic function by means of an extract or serum humoral factor of thymic origin.

First, I was much impressed in 1965 by the results of de Somer and his colleagues,[2] who had shown that a simple extract of an incubated calf thymus restored immunological responsiveness to neonatally thymectomized mice. I made a similar extract which was injected into thymectomized irradiated bone-marrow-injected mice 30 days after their construction. All the injected mice died promptly. Realizing my ineptitude I then obtained, by the kindness of de Somer, a sample of his effective (and nonlethal) extract and in a large series of experiments was unable in any way to influence the peripheral blood lymphocyte levels or immunological responses of our test mice. Clearly we must have been using the wrong amount of extract and the wrong test system.

Next, in conjunction with Dr. N. R. St C. Sinclair, a much more determined attempt was made on the problem in 1966. A saline extract was made of thymuses from mice that had received 850 R followed by an injection of syngeneic bone marrow 17, 18, or 19 days previously. We knew from other studies that at this time the thymus was of maximal importance in relation to recovery of immunological responsiveness. These extracts were injected into thymectomized mice that had 17, 18, or 19 days previously been irradiated with either 850 R or 600 R. All the 850 R mice and half the 600 R animals were injected with syngeneic bone-marrow subsequent to irradiation. The extracts were injected on three consecutive days in such a manner that each recipient on a particular day received the "saline equivalent" of a thymus harvested from a donor animal that was at the same time after irradiation as the recipient. The impeccable logic of the experiment need not be spelled out here. Thirty-five days after irradiation all mice were injected IP with 5×10^8 sheep red blood cells, and titrations of the hemolytic and hemagglutinating antibodies were made on days 7, 14, and 25 after the first injection and 7 and 21 days after the second injection. There were eight mice in each group, and controls were injected with normal thymus extract or nothing. The adoption of recipients given 600 R $\pm$ bone marrow was to explore the possibility that 850 R was such a high radiation dose as to leave too few residual cells upon which our putative hormone could have its impact. 600 R we felt might give our experiments a better chance.

The results were a complete failure in that the only statistically significant result was that mice injected with thymic extract showed depressed antibody responses 21 days after the second injection of sheep red blood cells. There was no difference between irradiated and nonirradiated thymus as a source of 'hormone.' This result did not inspire us with confidence and I do not intend further to analyse the reasons for failure except to say that our multitude of assumptions piled one on top of another had clearly produced a poor experiment. I deeply suspect that such things happen in other laboratories but rarely see any concrete evidence that this is so.

A third attempt on the problem was made in the summer of 1967 when we were joined for a few months by Dr. Alicja Ryzewska. Her wish was to repeat some of the experiments with Millipore chamber encapsulated thymus grafts, which were at that time all the rage. As before, our test system was to be thymectomized, irradiated adult mice injected with bone marrow after irradiation. Later I was to learn that such mice had about 10% of the usual number of 'T'-cells and that these cells were distributed round the body in blood, spleen and lymph nodes in the same manner as in normal mice. We elected also to use as positive control mice animals implanted with thymus grafts under the kidney capsule. The experiment also included many variants designed to illustrate the specificity of the effect of a thymus in the Millipore chamber. Experimenters always travel hopefully, especially when they are on short-term fellowships.

Groups of 20 mice were implanted each with empty Millipore chambers or chambers containing either a single neonatal thymus lobe, or ½ a neonatal spleen or 15×10^6 thymocytes or an adult lymph node or ½ a neonatal spleen + a neonatal thymus lobe or an epithelial thymic graft (obtained by prior depletion of a thymus in a Millipore chamber *in vivo*). In some mice two chambers each containing a single thymus lobe were implanted. All grafts were chromosomally marked vis-a-vis their host. All grafts had in addition to the chromosome marker a minor histocompatibility difference the influence of which can probably be ignored. All animals were subjected to examination of their blood at 35 and 80 days after irradiation and implantation of the various "grafts." Particular attention was paid to lymphocyte numbers. Some mice at day 36 were injected with 5×10^8 sheep red blood cells IP and their sera were titrated for agglutinating antibodies 3, 5, 7, and 14 days later. At 21 days a second injection of sheep red blood cells was made and the titration sequence was repeated. At the end of the experiment all animals were bled again, the peripheral blood lymphocyte counts were determined and detailed histopathological examinations were made. In addition, we performed cytological analysis on the spleens of some of the thymus grafted mice two days after the second injection of sheep red blood cells. We knew from previous experience that at this time about 50% of the cells in division were T-cells brought into division by the stimulation with antigen. These experiments occupied nearly three competent research workers for all or a proportion of their time for over three months. In fiscal terms the experiment probably cost nearly £3,000 and would certainly have cost much more if contracted out to a commercial concern. A much less expensive experiment could have given the same (negative) result. The mistake I made was to assume that what had been so confidently stated in the literature about the efficacy of restoration of immunological responsiveness by encapsulated thymus grafts would hold in our own experimental system.

We learned that about 30% of Millipore chambers leaked, because there were living cells *inside* some empty chambers fifty days after their implantation in the peritoneal cavity. (We were using circular lucite rings with membrane glued to either end of the ring rather than envelope type chambers). Also two such chambers tended to cause sufficiently pronounced inflammatory changes as to be evident (just) in an elevated peripheral blood granulocyte count. Although minor restoration of immunological responsiveness was discovered particularly after a second injection of sheep red blood cells in mice receiving a loaded as opposed to an empty chamber the thymic nature of the load seemed to be irrelevant (i.e. ½ spleen was as good as a single encapsulated thymus graft). In no instance did the immunological responsiveness of chamber-engrafted mice approach nearer than 3% of the responsiveness of mice given a naked graft under the kidney capsule. No thymus-graft-derived cells were observed in the spleens of mice receiving the encapsulated thymus although there were plenty in those mice given nonencapsulated grafts under the kidney capsule. The histopathological findings were similarly uninspiring.

Dr. Myra Small came to our laboratory in 1972, there having been some five years during which work on thymic hormones had proved unpopular. In the intervening years there had been developed many methods other than strictly immunological for detecting and quantitating lymphoid cell populations. Dr. Small, who derived from Professor Nathan Trainin's laboratory, came with fully-fledged thymus extracts that had previously been shown to have effects in systems which were not particularly suitable for analysis of the nature of the target cell(s) of these thymic extracts. Her efforts in my laboratory were manifold and heroic. I shall here briefly outline a few of them.

There has been much talk recently of T1- and T2-cells by which, it seems, is implied that thymus-derived cell populations differ in the length of time they have been out of the organ of their origin, T1 being the more recently emerged. There is some confusion here. A variety of experiments performed with thymocytes as a putative source of T1-cells have also been described. My bias is to refer to T-cells as extra-thymic lymphocytes of thymic origin. It has also been suggested that thymic hormones have an effect on T-cells outside the thymus.[3] It is quite easily possible to show in mice that have been thymectomized (as adults), irradiated, injected with bone marrow and implanted with a chromosomally marked thymus graft that cells of thymic graft origin will respond to antigenic stimulus.[1] Further it can be inferred that in addition to providing a population of its own cells the graft acts as a "staging-house" in which cells from the bone-marrow are "processed" into 'T'-cells.[4] If these inferences are correct, there is a temporal difference between the T-cells that derived from the stem cells native to the graft and those that derived (later) in the graft from stem cells from the bone marrow. If these musings are true, it might be possible to drive T1-cells by means of antigenic stimulus to T2-cells. If the bulk of T1-cells have the marker of the bone-marrow graft whereas the bulk of T2-cells have the marker of the thymus graft the antigen-induced drive might be perceptible by cytological analysis. If one now supposes that the T1 → T2 conversion is in some way thymus dependent, then injection of a putative thymus hormone might alter the numbers of cells of a particular chromosomal phenotype responding by mitosis after an injection of antigen—i.e. in the instance under discussion, the proportion of native thymus graft cells would fall as the T2 cell population became enriched by erstwhile T1 cells having the bone-marrow marker. Without going into details of the results suffice it to say that on three separate occasions no such effect was observed.

Dr. Small showed that when CBA spleen cells were injected into irradiated (CBA × C57BL)F_1 mice a fatal graft-versus-host reaction ensued. She also found, five days after injection, that the dividing population in the spleen of the recipient was 100% donor cells and, furthermore, she showed by using appropriately constructed donor chimeras that the mitosing cells were entirely 'T' cells. Having established this, Dr. Small went on to show that if she injected mixtures of CBA/H.*T6T6* and CBA/H cells (i.e. chromosomally distinct but otherwise entirely comparable populations of cells) that she could record proportions of cells in division which reflected exactly her expectations made on the basis of cell counts. Using this system, Dr. Small went on to incubate one of the injected cell populations with extract of mouse thymuses in order to determine whether she could in any way affect the behavior of the incubated cells. (i.e. would the proportion in which the 'T'-cells were found participating in a graft-versus-host reaction be altered by incubation with extract.) No alterations were perceptible.

On several occasions Dr. Small had found that injections of mouse-thymus extract had improved the capacity to respond to PHA *in vitro* of the spleens of thymectomized irradiated bone-marrow injected mice. It seemed possible that this effect was real and it was thought that in the culture system adopted only T-cells were brought into division. Accordingly, Dr. Small set out to attempt to identify the target cells which seemed to have been affected by her extracts. The method was to make CBA mouse chimeras by a sequence of thymectomy, irradiation and syngeneic bone-marrow injection. CBA/H.*T6T6* thymus grafts were then implanted under the kidney capsule of each recipient and left intact for 30 days, at which time they were surgically removed. On previous occasions it has been found that 90% of the T-cells of such animals have the T6T6 chromosome marker. Specifically the T-cell populations in the bone-marrow are so marked.

Dr. Small took bone marrow from such chimeras and injected it into thymectomized, irradiated (CBA/H.*T6T6* × CBA/H)F_1 mice. Thirty days later she injected the thymus extract and four days later removed the spleens and placed them in tissue culture with PHA. She performed a cytological analysis in order to determine whether the spleens from thymus extract injected as opposed to noninjected mice had a higher proportion of T6T6 cells. The answer was no, but that there was a slight excess of CBA/H cells in the cultures from the extract injected mice. If anything, this elaborate and difficult experiment, which Dr. Small carried out with great skill, indicated that non-T-cells had been slightly encouraged to respond to PHA by injection of thymus extract.

Overall, however, Dr. Small was disappointed that none of the experiments she carried out in my laboratory had given clear-cut results. All were based on the mitotic performance of (largely T) lymphocytes and it may be that this particular behavioral attribute cannot directly be affected by thymus extracts.

Another approach was directed toward the capacity of mouse lymphocytes to form more or less fragile associations *in vitro* with heterologous erythrocytes, a phenomenon which has come to occupy the hours of many scientists in recent years. Jean-François Bach [5] and his colleagues have found that in normal mice this rosetting capacity is inhibitable *in vitro* to a large extent by azathioprine and have suggested on good evidence that many of the "spontaneous" spleen RFC (rosette forming cells) in the mouse are 'T'-cells. In accord with this hypothesis is the finding that RFC whose rosetting facility is highly azathrioprine-sensitive are rare in the spleens of neonatally thymectomized or nude or thymectomized, irradiated and bone-marrow injected mice.[6] Paradoxically, they are also apparently rare in the spleens of adult thymectomized mice,[7] which are probably not very deficient in T-cells as judged by their immunological performances. Whatever the explanation, it seems that various thymus extracts can *in vitro* or after injection *in vivo* restore the azathioprine sensitivity of the spleen cells of adult thymectomized mice in relation to the formation of rosettes with sheep red blood cells *in vitro*.[8, 9] There is no dispute over the facts here—the interpretation is, however, more troublesome.

More important perhaps is the demonstration by Bach and his associates that the serum of normal mice, but not of thymectomized mice, contains a restorative factor that is similar in its action to thymus extracts.[8, 9] It is with this serum factor that we are here concerned.

The relevant experiments are simple. Normal CBA/H mice had implanted under their kidney capsules eight entire thymus lobes that had previously been taken from 1–3 day-old CBA/H.*T6T6* mice. These implantations were performed by Dr. E. Leuchars, who placed two lobes at the pole of each of the two kidneys of each recipient. Some control mice were grafted with neonatal kidneys in the same situations. Other mice were left ungrafted but served as age-matched controls. As will be seen in the experimental results, the grafts were later removed from some of the mice. Sera were evaluated for their capacity to restore azathioprine sensitivity in relation to the rosette forming cell capacity to the spleen cells of adult thymectomized mice *in vitro*. These animals from which the test spleens derived had been thymectomized not less than a week before they were killed. The serum evaluations were performed by Dr. Mireille Dardenne [7] on coded serum samples as described elsewhere.

The results are shown in TABLE 1. In all instances the thymus-grafted mice had a higher titer of serum factor than did the normal mice. In some instances these differences are statistically significant. In one instance, however, (at 56 days) some of the control kidney-grafted mice also had higher serum titers than did normal mice.

The experiments were designed only to see whether from the serum of a mouse its thymic mass can be determined. The answer is yes, but there may be other organs whose mass or activity is unusual that can interfere with the specificity of the assay.

In writing this paper I felt that I would make myself responsible for the opinions expressed as the results are largely though not entirely inconclusive. None of the work could, however, have been accomplished without the active collaboration of those working in the thymic hormone field. I am grateful to them for their friendship and open-mindedness. I remain undecided as to whether there exist true thymus-specific hormones or whether the thymus liberates a message quantitatively different from the messages that other similarly mitotically active organs may emit.

It is a well known fable that there is a crock of gold at the end of the rainbow. Many spades have been blunted in an attempt to dig it up. It is most important that people should keep trying however many failures there seem to be. There is a powerful imaginative appeal in doing so. The production of a specific hormone by the thymus sometimes seems to me rather like a crock of gold at the end of an immunological rainbow.

TABLE 1

MEAN SERUM TITERS OF "THYMIC FACTOR" IN MICE THAT HAVE RECEIVED EIGHT THYMUS GRAFTS AT VARIOUS EARLIER TIMES *

Time after Grafting	Normal	Thymus Grafted	Kidney Grafted
7	5.8	8.8	5.0
14	5.8	6.4	7.8
16		3.8 +	
21	6.2	7.0	5.4
33	6.0	7.0	5.2
56	6.8	10.6	9.2
		9.8	
139	6.0 (n=2)	9.0 (n=2)	5.5 (n=3)
		8.1 − (n=3)	

* See text. Control mice received kidney grafts or nothing. + indicates that the thymus graft had been removed 2 days previously. − indicates that the thymus graft had been removed 105 days previously. (n=5, neg. log 2)

References

1. DAVIES, A. J. S., E. LEUCHARS, V. WALLIS & P. C. KOLLER. 1966. Transplantation **4:** 438.
2. DE SOMER, P., P. DENYS, JR. & R. LEYTEN. 1963. Life Sci. **11:** 810.
3. DAVIES, A. J. S. 1969. Transplant. Rev. **1:** 43.
4. DOENHOFF, M. J., A. J. S. DAVIES, E. LEUCHARS & V. WALLIS. 1970. Proc. Roy. Soc. Series B **176:** 69.
5. BACH, J. F. 1973. Contemporary Topics in Immunobiology. Vol. **2:** Chapter 12. Plenum Publishing Corporation. New York, N.Y.
6. BACH, J. F. & M. DARDENNE. 1972. Cell. Immunol. **3:** 11.
7. BACH, J. F., M. DARDENNE & A. J. S. DAVIES. 1971. Nature **231:** 110.
8. DARDENNE, M. & J. F. BACH. 1973. Immunology **25:** 343.
9. BACH, J. F. & M. DARDENNE. 1973. Immunology **25:** 353.

Discussion of the Paper

Dr. J. F. A. P. Miller: In the last experiment, Dr. Davies, did you look at the effect of grafting other lymphoid tissues?

Dr. A. J. S. Davies: Yes, but fetal lymph nodes are very small for implantation.

Dr. Josephson: Was the thymic hormone of which you spoke derived from Hassel's corpuscle or from the basothelial element of the lymphatic tissues?

Dr. A. J. S. Davies: Unfortunately the experiments that were carried out were not designed with that particular point in mind. I can not give any satisfactory answer.

FACTORS INFLUENCING ACTIVATION OF B-CELLS IN IMMUNITY *

Göran Möller † and Antonio Coutinho

Division of Immunobiology
Karolinska Institutet, Wallenberglaboratory
104 05 Stockholm 50, Sweden

Bone marrow-derived (B) lymphocytes are equipped with surface bound immunoglobulin (Ig) receptor molecules. The properties of these receptors (class, specificity and affinity) are similar to those of the antibodies produced by the cells after antigenic stimulation.[15] It is generally accepted that the first event in antigen triggering of B-lymphocytes is the binding of antigenic determinants by the Ig receptors. All the different hypotheses advanced to explain B-cell triggering share one basic assumption; namely, that the Ig receptors are directly responsible for cell activation and deliver the initial triggering signal to the cell. However, the postulated signal generated by the combination between the Ig receptor and the antigen is often insufficient for B-cell activation and the same antigen-Ig receptor interaction can also result in paralysis. Thus, it is well known that antigen-sensitive B-cells do not become activated after binding thymus-dependent (TD) antigens without the participation of several "helper mechanisms" and that they never become activated after binding haptens.

Several hypotheses have been put forward to explain these findings. One of these postulates that B-cells can never be triggered without helper mechanisms, the main helper mechanism being T-cells, which work by carrying or releasing "associative antibodies." [1] In terms of this concept, thymus-independent (TI) antigens do not exist and, furthermore, an interaction between the Ig receptors and the antigen in the absence of T-cells, always results in paralysis. This is the most extensively worked out two signal theory, which ascribes a dominant role to T-cells in the induction of immune responses. All the other two signal hypotheses are similar in design and differ mainly in the nature of the postulated second signal (specific, specific and nonspecific, nonspecific), and furthermore, they do not clearly propose a mechanism for tolerance induction.

The main difficulty with these models is explaining how B-cells can be activated by nonspecific ligands (mitogens—see below) and consequently this type of induction has been termed "abnormal." Furthermore, the increasing evidence for the existence of truly thymus-independent immune responses cannot be accounted for.

Another set of hypotheses does not postulate two signals for activation.

* The experimental work reported was supported by grants from the Swedish Cancer Society, the Swedish Medical Research Council, the Wallenberg Foundation, and the Jeansson Foundation.

† No attempts have been made to review the literature relevant to the topic. Instead references are given to review articles and only when judged necessary to technical publications.

Instead it is suggested that B-cell triggering is dependent on the "pattern" of antigenic presentation to the cell surface receptors. Macromolecules with repeated epitopes would trigger B-cells directly, because they would be capable of cross-linking the specific Ig receptors. Molecules with a nonrepeated structure could only activate B-cells if presented to the latter in a "locally concentrated" form. All hypotheses of this type are variants of the "antigen concentration" [8, 9, 14] model, and all suggest that T-cells are active in triggering, because they concentrate the TD antigen, either directly, or via the macrophage surface, even though it is known that T-cells bind less antigen and with lower stability than B-cells. The actual triggering signal would always be delivered by the Ig receptors when they have been aggregated or cross-linked to a sufficient extent.

It is not the purpose of the present article to discuss the different hypotheses in detail. Rather, we want to analyze their common denominator; i.e., the dogma that the Ig receptors are always directly responsible for triggering at some stage. We shall not discuss the fact that the immunoglobulin receptors on B-lymphocytes are competent to interact with the antigenic determinants, but we want to analyze the subsequent step leading to triggering, with particular emphasis on the question of whether the triggering signal is delivered by the Ig receptor or whether immunocyte triggering is caused by a signal that is not related to the immunoglobulin receptor. Therefore, it is important to distinguish antigen binding from the triggering event. We will focus the discussion on the induction of primary IgM responses.

Evidence That Ig Receptors Cause Triggering of B-lymphocytes

Although it is generally accepted that the Ig receptors are responsible for triggering, the available evidence is weak. The well established findings that removal of cells having a certain Ig class or a certain specificity (by the use of specific antibodies, antigen coated columns, or highly radioactive antigens) results in the failure of the population to synthesize the class or specificity of antibody involved are not at all informative. It is obvious that removal of cells having the capacity to produce antibodies with certain characteristics also eliminates antibody synthesis of this type, irrespective of the mechanism of triggering. Unfortunately, deletion experiments of this type have been misinterpreted in many contexts, and have been used as arguments for (or against) a certain mechanism of activation.

Another type of argument for the direct participation of Ig receptors in B-cell triggering is based on the findings that certain anti-Ig sera are competent to induce DNA synthesis in blood lymphocytes from certain species.[12] So far, these findings are restricted to rabbit and guinea-pig lymphocytes, whereas lymphocytes from humans and mice are not activated at all or to a very small extent. Furthermore, the cells activated in rabbit blood (80–90% of which are Ig positive) are not characterized with regard to B or T origin nor have any functional properties (e.g. induction of Ig synthesis) been analyzed. It is important to point out that in the mouse system anti-Ig sera do not trigger B-lymphocytes even though the Ig receptors are cross-linked and capping occurs.

It seems reasonable to conclude that the available experimental evidence does not critically support the concept that B-cells can be triggered after an interaction between the specific Ig receptor and the antigenic determinants present on immunogenic thymus-dependent molecules.

How Specific is Triggering?

It follows from all the hypotheses ascribing the triggering event to an interaction between Ig receptor and antigen that activation of B-cells necessarily exhibits specificity for the antigen. It is of interest, therefore, that B-cell activation has been achieved in a completely nonspecific way in several experimental systems. The first and most extensively studied system makes use of B-cell mitogens. A variety of substances of microbiological, plant, or synthetic origin have the ability to induce Ig synthesis in B-cells, although there is no complementarity between the mitogen and the combining site of the Ig receptors.[16] Since TD antigens or haptens cannot by themselves trigger the corresponding B-cells, but mitogens can whether or not the Ig receptor has reacted with the antigen, it is clear that the triggering signal in this case is not delivered by the Ig receptor, but is nonspecific. Attempts have been made to explain mitogen triggering in terms of a two-signal concept by assuming that the Ig receptors of the activated cells have reacted with cross-reacting antigens in the culture medium or with autologous cells and that the mitogen delivers the second (nonspecific) signal. This is unlikely for several reasons. First, triggering can be achieved in serum-free medium and is not influenced by the addition of free hapten. Thus, cells that have combined with corresponding antigens are triggered to the same extent as cells that have not reacted with antigen. Secondly, if the cross-reacting antigens are present on autologous cells, the two-signal hypothesis postulates that this would lead to paralysis and therefore, that such cells could not be induced.[1] As a rescue operation, it was postulated that the affinity for the cross-reacting autologous antigens was too low for paralysis to occur.[18] However, if this is so, it follows that it is easier to activate cells than to paralyze them, although the virtue of the two-signal concept was precisely to make paralysis the first and easiest event.

It seems unescapable to us that mitogen activation is caused by one nonspecific signal that is unrelated to the Ig receptor. There are other examples of nonspecific triggering. Thus, there is a large body of evidence that specific or mitogen-activated T-cells can serve as helper cells in the induction of immune responses to unrelated antigens.[16] Furthermore, products from T-cells have the same capacity and seem to act as nonspecific B-cell mitogens (see, e.g. references 3 & 11). Although most studies of this type have been performed *in vitro,* it seems established that analogous phenomena work *in vivo.* The first example was the "original antigenic sin," but there is now much evidence that B-cells can be activated *in vivo* by a nonspecific signal[7] (the allogeneic effect, conversion of nonresponder mice to responders and increases of background PFC in the absence of antigen both *in vivo* and *in vitro* by graft-versus-host reactions, etc.). These studies only show that one signal can be nonspecific, and they are therefore compatible with a two-signal model for triggering (but not with a one specific signal concept) and only the finding that the T-cell factor can act as a nonspecific B-cell mitogen argues against both of the mentioned hypotheses.

Mitogens and Thymus-independent Antigens

The mitogen experiments show that B-cells are immunocompetent and can be activated into high-rate antibody producing cells by a nonspecific signal. There is no reason to separate B-cells involved in the IgM response to TI antigens from those activated by TD antigens. This follows from work with B-cell mitogens, which are able to interact directly with Ig positive cells, in the absence of any helper cells, and trigger them into polyclonal antibody synthesis also detectable against TD antigens. The fact that this activation is polyclonal shows that activation may proceed independently of specific combining sites on the cell surface. A strong argument for this point is the demonstration that B-cells of a certain specificity can be activated by nonspecific mitogens, even when the specific Ig combining sites were occupied by a free specific ligand (hapten). These findings raise an important question: is nonspecific triggering caused by mitogens restricted to induction of polyclonal antibody synthesis, or can it operate physiologically for the induction of specific immune responses? One way to study this question was to analyze the specificity of triggering achieved by immunogenic molecules that are known to be capable of directly activating specific immune responses in B-cells (thymus-independent antigens).

It is well established that TI antigens do not require the participation of helper cells, such as T-cells or macrophages, for the induction of immune responses, and therefore, they can directly induce B-cells to divide and differentiate into high-rate antibody producing cells. According to hypotheses explaining B-cell activation via specific receptors, this property of TI molecules is due to their polymeric structure, which allows a stable multipoint binding to the cell surface and induces cross-linking of the surface Ig receptors, postulated to be essential for cell activation. *Therefore, only antigen specific cells should be activated by these molecules, since only these would display the relevant Ig receptors to be redistributed or cross-linked.*

It is now well established that TI antigens at higher concentrations induce polyclonal antibody synthesis in B-cells, suggesting that most, if not all, mature B-cells, possessing different Ig specificities, had been triggered.[2] Thus, TI molecules have the intrinsic property to activate B-cells directly. This cannot be mediated by the antigenic determinants of the TI antigens, since B-cells of a variety of different specificities were activated. It follows that the B-cells were not triggered via the surface Ig receptors. These findings show that B-cells may be activated by other mechanisms than the combination of the antigen with the specific receptor, and suggest a common explanation for thymus-independent immunocyte triggering based on B-cell mitogenic properties of the antigenic molecules.

Specific Triggering

Since the TI antigens possess both antigenic determinants and mitogenic properties it seemed plausible that the interaction between the immunoglobulin receptors and antigenic determinants on these molecules resulted in a preferential binding of mitogen molecules to the cells, which would be triggered by the mitogenic properties of the TI antigens. Therefore, the immune response to these antigens would be thymus-independent, because the helper function of

T-cells would not be needed. Thymus-dependent antigens on the other hand, which lack mitogenic properties, could only combine with the immunoglobulin receptors, but by themselves not deliver the necessary triggering signal. This signal would be delivered by the activated T-cells, but would also lack immunological specificity. It is obviously necessary to explain how a nonspecific triggering signal can give rise to a specific immune response. The proposed scheme is outlined in essence in FIGURE 1. It is suggested that the role of the immunoglobulin receptor is only to act as a passive focusing device causing the binding of the antigen molecule to the surface of the cells. (It should be pointed out that we base our concept of triggering on the findings with mitogens that cells are activated by the *quantity not the quality* of the triggering signal. This is a concept that appears to be shared by proponents of most theories of lymphocyte activation). In a low concentration of TI antigens, only specific antigen-reactive B-cells would be competent to bind a sufficient number of the mitogen molecules to become triggered. Other cells having different immunoglobulin receptors (nonspecific cells) would not bind the necessary concentration of mitogen molecules to become activated. At a high concentration of antigen the nonspecific cells would also interact with a sufficient number of TI antigen molecules to become triggered into immunoglobulin synthesis and then they

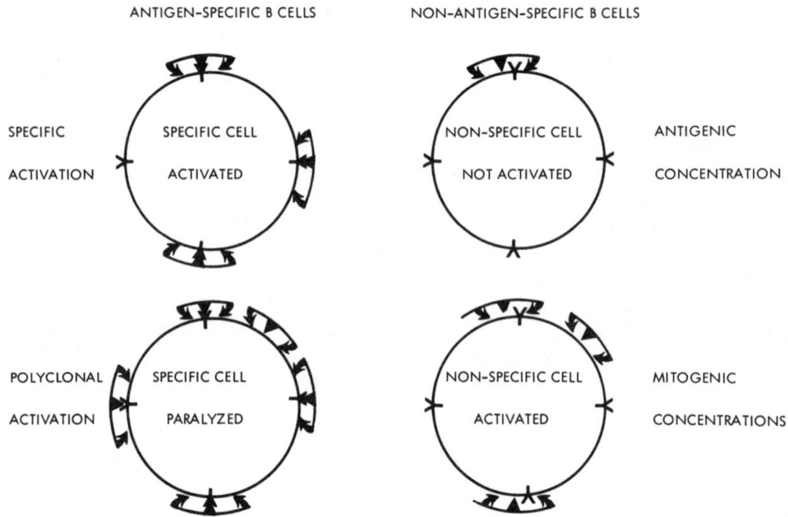

FIGURE 1. Schematic outline of the proposed hypothesis demonstrating the focusing function of specific Ig receptors. At low (antigenic) concentrations of TI antigens (⟲▼⟳) which display both antigenic determinants (▼) and mitogenic properties (↘), the specific Ig receptors on antigen-sensitive cells will preferentially concentrate the mitogenic molecules on their surface. Therefore, the threshold level of mitogen molecules required for triggering will only be reached on the membrane of these specific cells. Consequently the response will be detected as antigen-specific and thymus-independent. High (mitogenic) concentrations of the same molecules will bind nonspecifically to all B-cells and will induce polyclonal responses, but at the same time they will reach the paralytic threshold on antigen-specific cells, which always bind an additional amount of molecules by the presence of specific Ig receptors.

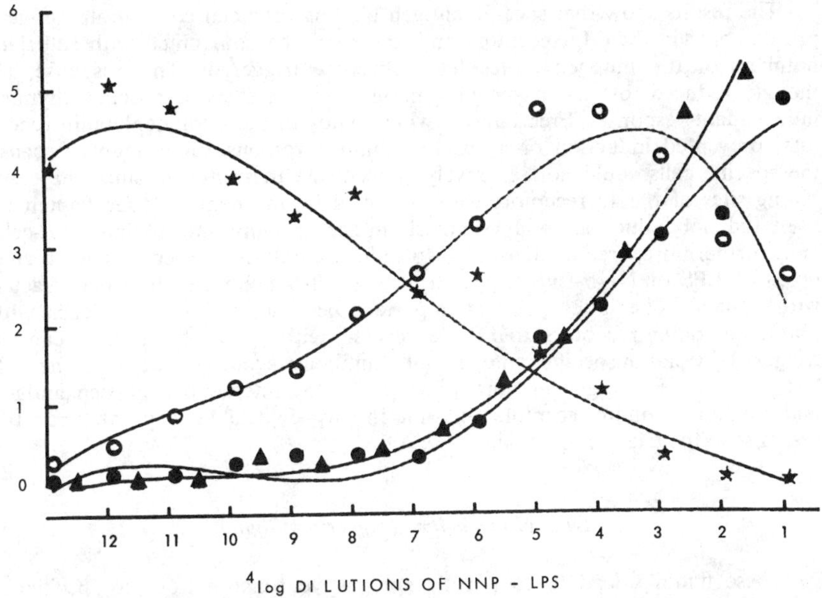

FIGURE 2. Results of one experiment testing the hypothesis outlined in FIGURE 1. Normal mouse spleen cells were cultured in the presence of different concentrations of NNP-LPS in serum-free medium. After two days, the responses induced in these culture were measured. Activation of DNA synthesis, as well as induction of antibody production against an irrelevant antigen (SRC), was determined. In addition, high and low affinity antibody synthesis against the specific hapten NNP was measured. Background values in unstimulated cultures were subtracted from each experimental group, and the net responses were plotted in a Hewlett-Packard 9820A calculator, using a program for least square fit.

▲———▲ C.P.M./culture (Y:0 to 84,000)
●———● anti-SRC PFC/culture (Y:0 to 300)
★———★ high avidity anti-NNP PFC/culture (Y:0 to 1,500)
○———○ low avidity anti-NNP PFC/culture (Y:0 to 6,000)

will express the immunoglobulin for which they are genetically coded. However, in this case also, the specific antigen-binding cells would bind a much higher number of TI molecules and they would be specifically turned off from responding, because superoptimal doses of mitogen molecules always turn off the response.

This hypothesis was tested experimentally, and the results were in agreement with the proposal. In these experiments the hapten NNP was coupled to the mitogen LPS. At low doses of this hapten-mitogen conjugate a specific antihapten response was obtained, which was thymus-independent. At higher doses polyclonal activation occured, but the specific NNP-response disappeared (FIGURE 2). When free hapten in the form of NNP-cap was added to the cultures, the specific immune response to NNP at lower doses of NNP-LPS was abolished. However, at conjugate doses inducing polyclonal activation, the NNP-reactive cells responded in the same manner as all other cells, even in the presence of free hapten.

The results show that specific antigen binding cells can concentrate antigen, presumably via their Ig receptors and, therefore, be confronted with sufficient numbers of the mitogen molecules to become triggered. This response, although induced by a nonspecific mitogen, appears as a specific thymus-independent response. Free hapten, which binds to the immunoglobulin receptors, prevented induction of a specific immune response, presumably because the specific cells could not selectively concentrate the mitogen, since the combining sites of the Ig receptors were occupied by the hapten. Free hapten by itself did not induce antibody synthesis in the specific antigen-binding B-cells and, furthermore, free hapten failed to induce paralysis in B-cells, since higher doses of LPS or NNP-LPS triggered also the B-lymphocytes that had reacted with hapten. The latter point is important because it shows that cells with immunoglobulin receptors that have reacted with a specific antigen can be triggered by a nonspecific mitogen into antibody synthesis, whether the cell has reacted with antigen or not, showing that the interaction between antigen and immunoglobulin receptors did not in any detectable way influence the response to the triggering signal.

One Nonspecific Triggering Signal

These findings lead us to postulate a passive function for the specific Ig receptors on the immunocompetent B-cells, which are not directly involved in delivering the triggering signal to the cells. They would act only as passive focusing devices for mitogenic molecules. This hypothesis has as yet only received experimental support for the induction primary IgM responses to thymus-independent antigens, and implies that no signal is generated from the combination of the specific site on the surface Ig molecule with the antigenic determinants present on the immunogenic molecules. Since the antigen-sensitive B-cells can specifically bind mitogenic molecules (thymus-independent antigens) by recognizing their antigenic determinants, the specific cells will become triggered at immunogenic (low) concentrations of these substances on the membrane, whereas nonspecific cells will not, because they lack the additional, specific binding of the mitogen molecules. By increasing the concentrations of these substances, the nonspecific binding to nonspecific cells will allow triggering concentrations to be reached on every mitogen-sensitive B-cell, and the response will be polyclonal. However, the relevant triggering signal is the same in both situations, and is generated exclusively by the mitogenic properties of these molecules.

The distinctive features of this hypothesis are the following two postulates: (1) only one signal is required for triggering, and (2) this signal is nonspecific and delivered to the cell by surface structures other than the combining sites of specific Ig receptor. However, the mitogen receptors need not be identical for different mitogens. Furthermore, the cells become activated only when a sufficient number of these receptors have interacted with any of the inducing molecules.

Cross-Linking of Ig Receptors

This proposal is not a semantic variation of previous hypotheses, such as those suggesting that antigen presentation in a certain "pattern" capable of inducing cross-linking of Ig receptors would cause triggering.[5] The cross-linking concept has been used in several hypotheses of B-cell activation to explain both thymus-independent and thymus-dependent immunocyte triggering. Although we do not think that cross-linking is an absolute or necessary requirement for triggering, it may play an accessory role also in cell activation by nonspecific mechanisms.

When cross-linking of Ig receptors is considered to be the triggering signal, it is usually assumed that cell activation results from an extensive alteration of the membrane mobility.[6] It has not been specified how restriction in mobility of "peripheral" membrane proteins could interfere with the mobility of the lipid components of the plasma membrane, a proposal which seems unlikely,[13] or how restricted mobility could lead to cell activation.

As mentioned above, cross-linking of surface Ig receptors by anti-Ig sera does not lead to cell-activation. Therefore, it is unlikely that B-cell triggering is caused by a cross-linking of Ig receptors as such. It could be argued that triggering occurs only if cross-linking of Ig receptors is superimposed on some specific signal generated at the Ig combining site, and that the cell is activated only by an antigen-induced cross-linking. However, it is well known that highly hapten-substituted TD proteins, even of very high molecular weight, which should cause extensive Ig cross-linking, do not induce B-cell activation, whereas in contrast, even the low hapten substitution of thymus-independent antigens (B-cell mitogens) leads to direct B-cell activation, specific at low concentrations, but polyclonal at high concentrations. Thus, it has been shown that the anti-DNP response to DNP_{1800}-KLH (1 epitope/555 MW) is entirely thymus-dependent, whereas $DNP_{0.7}$-POL (1 epitope/57.000 MW) was thymus-independent.[4] We also carried out analogous experiments using haptens coupled to proteins or to insoluble particles (Sepharose®) but it was not possible to trigger an immune response, in spite of the fact that multipoint binding would be expected to occur and that certain antigen concentrations would be expected to lead to receptor redistribution and receptor cross-linking.

Furthermore, when antigen-induced redistribution of Ig surface receptors was studied in specific antigen-binding cells, it was possible to show "capping" of these receptors only with antigen concentrations[10] that were paralytogenic. This is not surprising in view of the findings that cross-linking of other surface receptors, which are known to be involved in triggering (Con-A receptors), does not correlate with cell activation. Thus, Con-A cross-links surface receptors in both T- and B-cells, although only T-cells are activated, and furthermore, activating and nonactivating Con-A concentrations cross-link to the same extent.

On the other hand, the importance of the focusing function of the Ig receptors can be explained by the very high affinity of the interaction between the antigen and the combining sites of the Ig receptor on the specific cell, which is probably several orders of magnitude higher than that of the interaction between the nonspecific receptor and the complementary structures on the mitogenic molecules. It is probably advantageous that the affinity of the latter reaction is low, because this prevents dangerous or nonsense activation of B-cell clones. Therefore, efficient interaction between ligands and such low affinity receptors can only be achieved by multipoint binding of polymeric structures in high concentrations in the medium (commonly termed mitogenic activation) or else by stabilizing the binding by high affinity receptors directed against the antigenic determinants on the same molecule (commonly called TI antigenic activation). This may explain the requirement for polymeric structures of B-cell mitogens and TI antigens, as well as the fact that for a given substance the MW requirements for TI antigenicity are less restricted than for polyclonal mitogenicity.

All these observations suggest that cross-linking of *some,* but *not every* surface structure on B-cells *may* lead to cell activation. It seems likely that the Ig receptors do not belong to the relevant sites, which can trigger the cell after cross-linking. If activation is achieved by cross-linking of "integral" membrane proteins, the relevant signal is still nonspecific, since the specific surface receptors are not directly involved. However, if cross-linking is not the relevant signal, even when nonspecific receptors are involved, and is only an accessory mechanism for stabilizing a weak binding, it should be predicted that small, nonpolymeric molecules which have a high affinity for the nonspecific receptors would be capable of cell activation, overcoming the requirement for multipoint binding. This is actually the case, since hydrophilic molecules of about 10 residues of substituted pentose (MW 2,000) are among the best B-cell mitogens known.[17] If an intensive alteration of the membrane structure is required for triggering, this can obviously be achieved by small molecules, interacting at a restricted site on the membrane and, therefore, extensive modification of the membrane is not required, excluding cross-linking as a necessary initial step in activation. Whether the interaction of these small molecules at a limited site on the membrane structure is sufficient for triggering or whether a signal generated at several single receptors is necessary to induce B-cells is still unknown and requires further investigation.

Thymus-dependent Responses

The present "one nonspecific signal" concept for B-cell activation can be easily extended to thymus-dependent immune responses. In this case, the immunogenic molecules, lacking mitogenic properties, are not competent to activate B-cells directly and, therefore, require the help of other cell types for the induction of immune responses. Ig surface receptors would in this case focus nonspecific triggering signals provided by other cells or products of other cells onto the specific B-cells by bringing them in close contact via antigen bridging. Some important points need to be stressed in this context. (1) The helper cell activity can be "bypassed" by providing the specific cells with nonspecific triggering signals (see below), such as B-cell mitogens (LPS, POL and SIII). (2) The "physiological" T-cell-mediated help has been shown to be nonspecific in a number of independent systems. (3) Monovalent antigenic molecules, such as haptens, which seem to be bound perfectly well by both B- and T-cells, are not competent to induce immune responses, suggesting that some bridging mechanism is likely to be involved.

Much attention has been focused on nonspecific T-cell factors in connection with the mechanism of cell cooperation. These products can be shown to be differentogens for B-cells, in the sense that B-cells, exposed to the factors in the absence of the antigen, develop polyclonally into high-rate antibody producing cells both *in vitro* and *in vivo.* However, two important points should be kept in mind, both arguing for a requirement for cell-to-cell contact in cooperation: (1) T-cells have been shown to be entirely substituted by these factors only when *in vitro* responses to red blood cells are measured, and there are claims that it is impossible to substitute nonspecific T-cell factors for T-cells in the responses to antigens that are more thymus-dependent (proteins), which completely lack any B-cell activating capacity, in contrast to red cells. (2) The *in vivo* allogeneic effect (but not the allogeneic effect *in vitro*) requires that the B-cells must belong to the target cell population. These two points suggest a need for a close cell-to-cell contact, possibly involving interaction between the two different plasma cell membranes. If this is the case, histocompatibility may be a necessary requirement for cell cooperation to occur, both between T- and B-cells, and between macrophages and T-cells. However, it is also possible that the requirement for very close T-B cell-to-cell contact is due to a need for high concentrations of the nonspecific T-cell factors during physiological conditions.

There are several reasons why it is unlikely that antigen presentation is involved in this interaction. (1) The Ig receptors do not seem to generate the triggering signal. (2) Cooperation should be theoretically expected to operate between two B-cells or between B-cells and macrophages (in the absence of T-cells), which could mutually stabilize the binding, or build a matrix of antigenic determinants for each other. There are some reasons why two B-cells could not cooperate, but few why macrophages and B-cells could not, but the main point (the Ig receptor is not responsible for activation) is not part of any of these arguments.

Although several studies have shown that soluble T-cell factors act nonspecifically, it has also been claimed that they are effective because they contain specific T-cell released Ig.[5] Recently, it has been shown that macrophage supernatants can enhance the primary immune response to TD antigens, and it was suggested that macrophages released a protein that provided the second triggering signal.[19] We have confirmed that macrophages in culture release a factor which: (1) acts synergistically with SRC in the induction of a primary immune response, (2) can replace the macrophages in the induction of primary anti-SRC responses, and (3) is a B-cell mitogen that activates DNA synthesis and polyclonal antibody synthesis in nonsensitized cells (FIGURES 3, 4, 5).

Although the macrophage supernatant behaved as a B-cell mitogen, it could still be argued that Ig was responsible for the effect. Therefore, studies were done to see whether other cell types could release factors competent to act in a similar way. It was found that mouse embryo fibroblasts (syngeneic or allogeneic) could replace macrophages in the induction of a primary anti-SRC response (FIGURE 6). Furthermore, supernatants from fibroblast cultures acted like macrophage supernatants and worked synergistically with SRC in the induction of primary immune responses in serum-free medium, and replaced macrophages in the induction of a primary immune response to SRC (FIGURES 7, 8). Finally, the fibroblast supernatant acted as a B-cell mitogen (FIGURE 9).

Taken together, the findings suggest that macrophages and fibroblasts secrete B-cell mitogens behaving as well-characterized B-cell mitogens, such as LPS. Since also fibroblasts secrete these factors it can be excluded that Ig is responsible for the effect. It is likely that the need of macrophages in primary responses to TD antigens is due to the fact that they release B-cell mitogens, which provide the triggering signal.

Synergism Between Antigens and Mitogens

One type of experimental finding has been used as an argument for a role of the Ig receptor in B-cell activation, namely the well-documented fact that

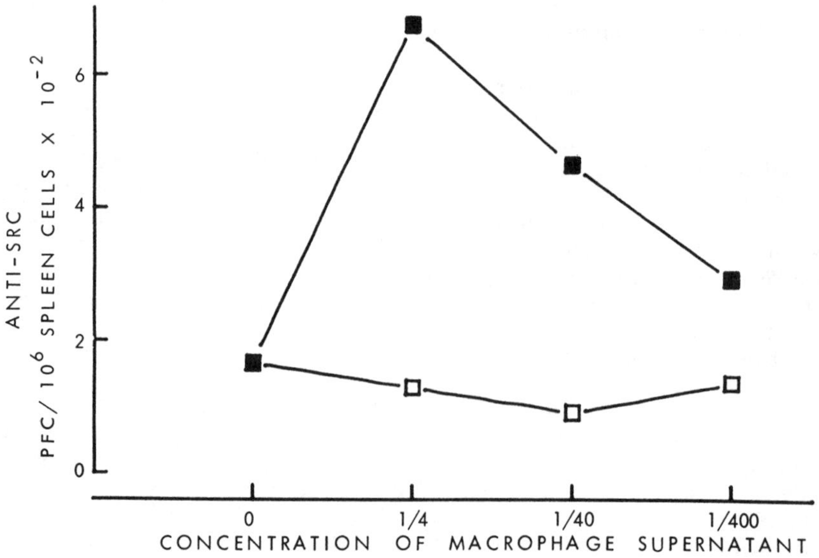

FIGURE 3. Immune response to SRC in normal A × C57L spleen cells in serum-free medium after addition of supernatants from a two-day culture of A × C57L macrophages (□——□) or after addition of supernatants and SRC (■——■). The plaque assay was carried out on day 4.

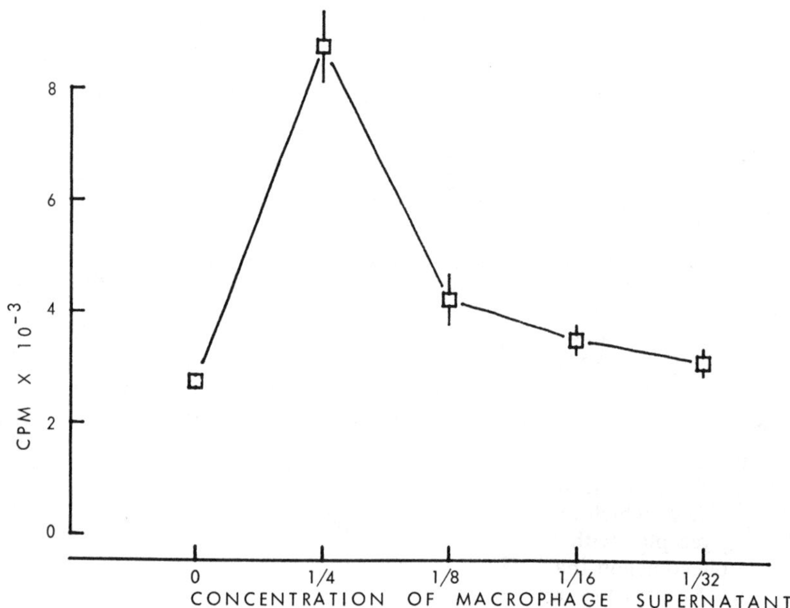

FIGURE 4. Ability of macrophage supernatants to induce DNA synthesis in syngeneic lymphocytes in serum-free medium. The macrophages were cultivated for two days in serum-free medium, the supernatant removed and added to A × C57L lymphocytes. Thymidine incorporation was determined between day 2 and 3.

B-cell mitogens and red-cell antigens can work synergistically during the induction of immune responses. Thus, the simultaneous stimulation of a lymphocyte by antigen and mitogen results in an increased response, as compared to the responses induced by either alone. These findings argue against most two-signal concepts of B-cell activation, as well as against one-signal theories, whether the signal is specific or nonspecific. In the two-signal hypothesis of Cohn each signal is *qualitatively* different from the other, and *each signal alone is incapable of induction.* Since *both* signals are *necessary,* there is no possibility for a synergistic action between them. Actually synergy is compatible only with a hypothesis that requires two signals (one of which is specific—Ig receptor—and the other nonspecific), and where the two signals cannot be qualitatively

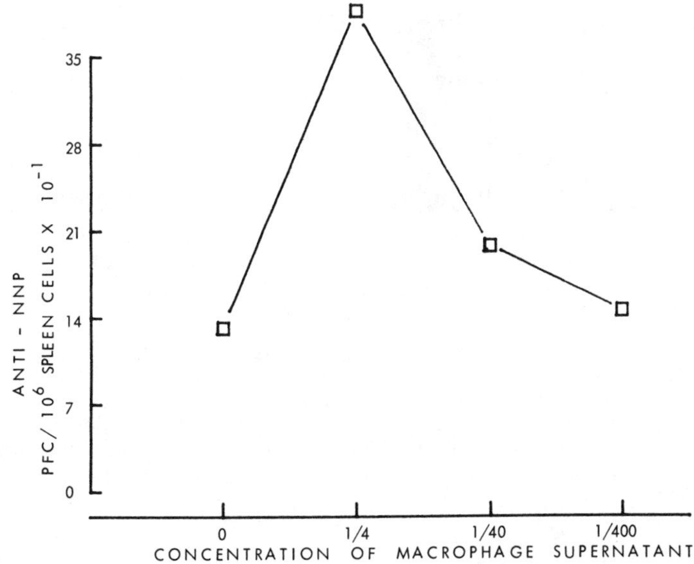

FIGURE 5. Ability of macrophage supernatants to induce polyclonal activation of antibody synthesis. Experimental conditions were as in FIGURE 4, but the response was determined by measuring the number of PFC against NNP-SRC, utilizing a high epitope density in order to allow detection of polyclonal antibody synthesis.

distinguished by the responding cells. For several reasons, which will shortly be discussed below, it appears to us that the phenomenon is caused by trivial events, none of which involves the generation of any signal by the combination of the Ig receptor with the antigen. First, we want to point out that synergy is not a phenomenon that can be reproduced with all different antigens and/or mitogens. Synergy has been reported to occur *in vitro* between red-cell antigens and LPS, PPD or T-cell replacing factor (TRF), both in FCS supplemented cultures and in serum-free media. A weak synergy between haptens and hapten-substituted proteins and LPS in FCS supplemented cultures has been reported,[18] but no specific or insignificant synergism could be found by us in serum-free cultures between a range of LPS concentrations and the haptens NNP, FITC,

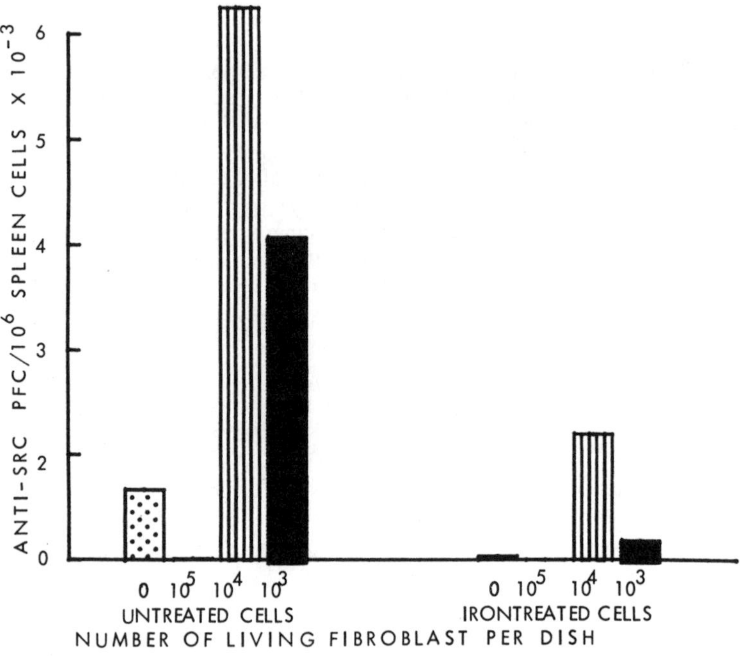

FIGURE 6. Induction of a primary immune response to SRC in petri dishes containing the indicated numbers of living syngeneic fibroblasts. Spleen cells from untreated A × C57L mice were added to the petri dishes directly or after treatment with iron powder to remove adherent cells. The antigen (SRC) was present in all dishes and the response determined at day 4. Controls (which are not shown) were carried in the absence of SRC. In this case there was virtually no response to SRC in any culture at day 4.

or the same haptens coupled to various degrees onto HSA or HGG, whether the protein was soluble or aggregated (FIGURE 10). Finally, there was no synergy between LPS and a 1000-fold different concentrations of FITC coupled to Sepharose beads used in a 1000-fold range of concentrations. However, if the Sepharose particles were not removed they caused PFC (FIGURE 11). This was due to release of absorbed anti-FITC antibodies from the particles in the PFC assay. This phenomenon was only observed in the presence of LPS or FCS, which stimulate polyclonal antibody synthesis. Analogous experiments with FITC-HGG using different epitope densities and protein concentrations coupled to Sepharose were equally negative (FIGURE 12). In contrast FITC-LPS on Sepharose induced a primary anti-FITC response (FIGURE 12). As will be mentioned below, there is also evidence that synergy requires helper cells (macrophages and T-cells) and thus may not reflect a basic phenomenon of B-cell triggering.

FIGURE 8. Synergy between fibroblast supernatants and SRC in the induction of a primary immune response to SRC.

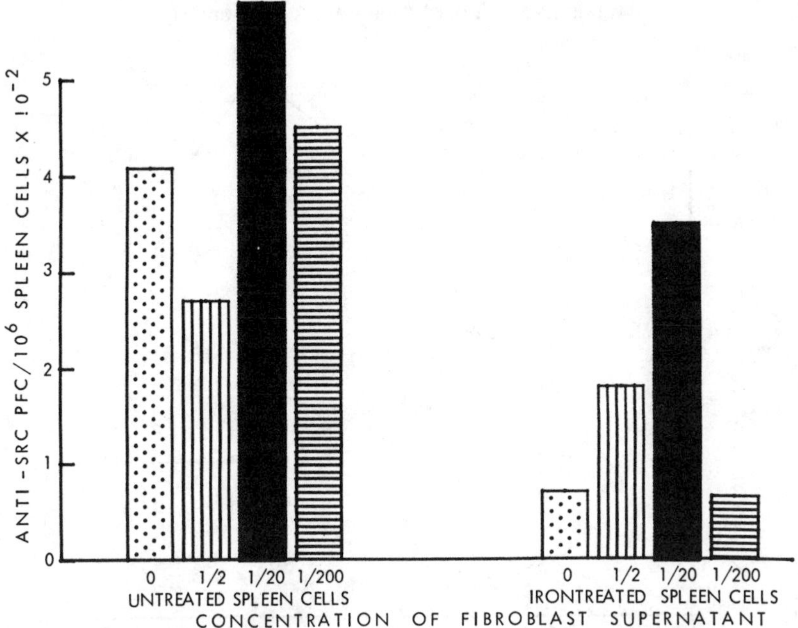

FIGURE 7. Fibroblast supernatants can replace macrophages. Untreated A × C57L spleen cells were cultivated alone or in the presence of various dilutions of fibroblast supernatants. SRC were added to all cultures. In one group the lymphocytes were untreated, in the other treated with iron particles to remove adherent cells. The response was determined at day 4.

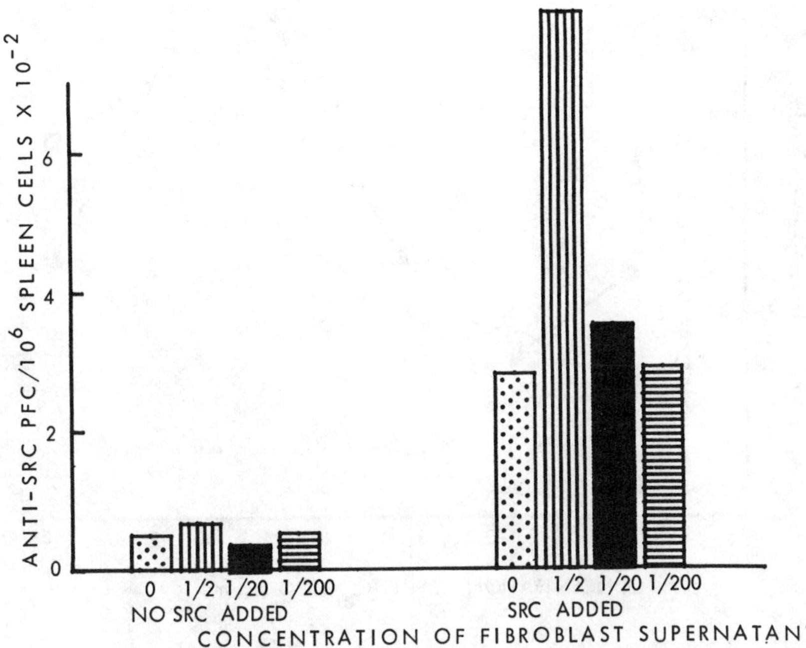

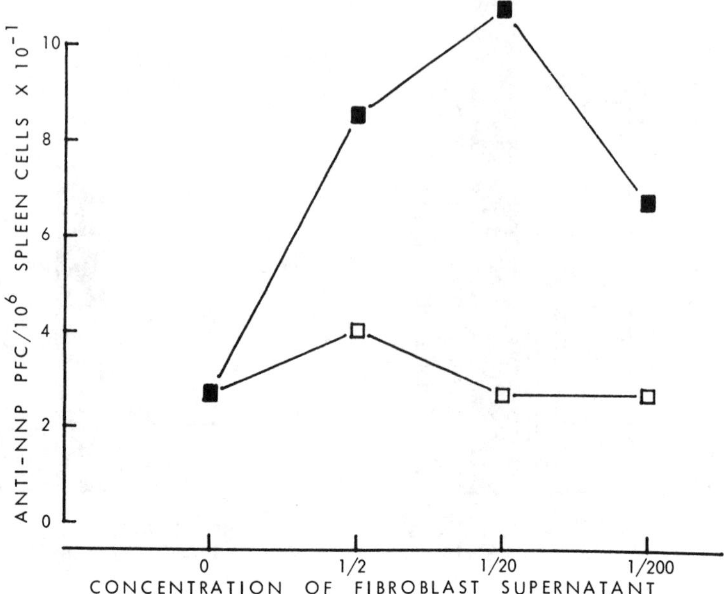

FIGURE 9. Polyclonal induction of antibody synthesis by fibroblast supernatants. Lymphocytes were cultured in normal medium (□——□) or in medium containing the indicated concentrations of macrophage supernatants (■——■). At day two the PFC against NNP-SRC was determined.

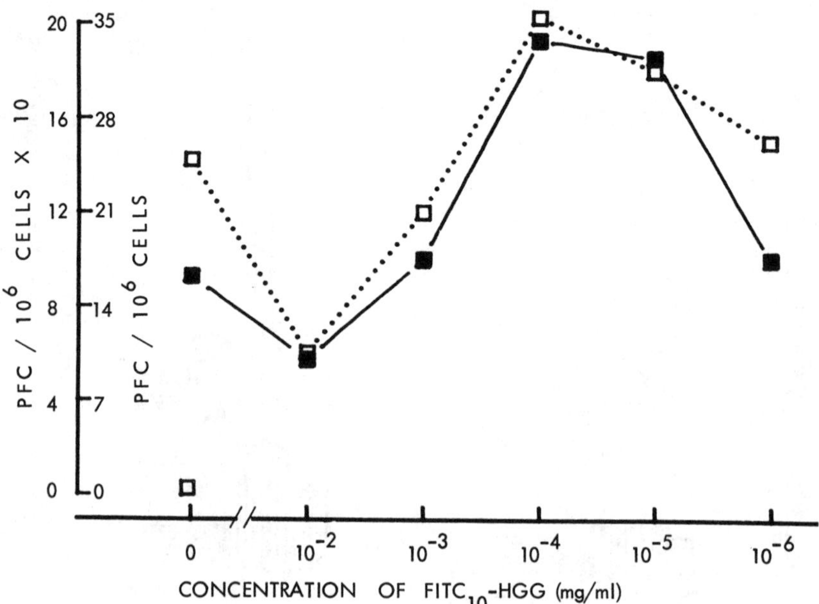

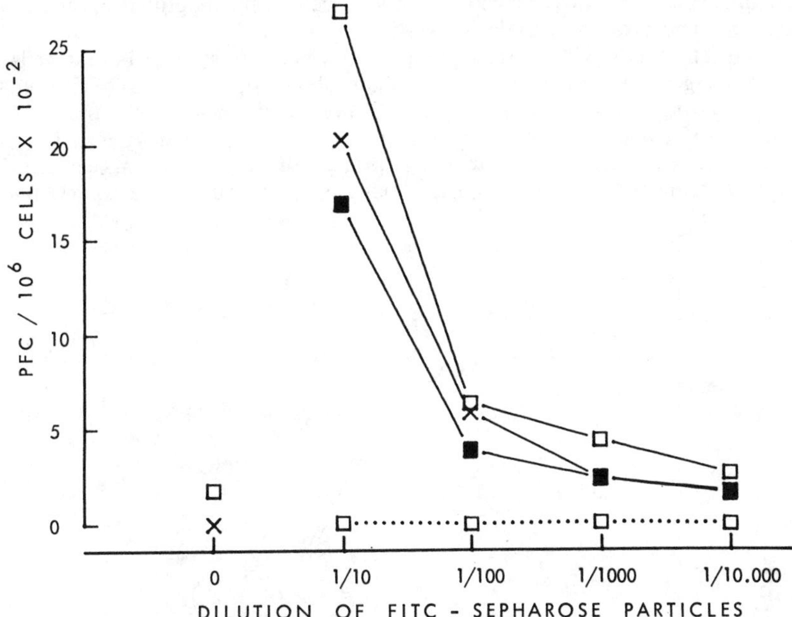

FIGURE 11. Attempts to detect synergy between different preparations of FITC-Sepharose and 100 μg LPS in serum-free spleen cell cultures assayed at day 4. The cultures were treated with LPS plus FITC-Sepharose 1 (■), 2 (□) or 3 (×). In addition, the various FITC-Sepharose particles were added to cultures alone (□- - -□) or they were treated with LPS alone (□) or left untreated (×). The Sepharose particles were *not* removed prior to assay.

Here is a summary of some trivial explanations of synergy.

The antigen contains a mitogen. This has been clearly shown with SRC (A. Coutinho, to be published). Thus, concentrated soluble extracts from SRC are strong B-cell mitogens capable of inducing polyclonal antibody synthesis. Therefore, synergy between SRC and B-cell mitogens may be another example of synergy between two B-cell mitogens in suboptimal concentrations. Lymphocytes specific for SRC would bind the antigen preferentially and therefore be confronted with a higher concentration of the mitogen present on SRC than nonspecific cells. Synergy between mitogen and SRC is more evident with weak B-cell mitogens (such as those present in fetal calf serum or in supernatants from activated T-cells (TRF)) than with strong mitogens (LPS). In

---

FIGURE 10. Response to FITC after the addition of various concentrations of $FITC_{(10)}$-HGG to normal lymphocyte cultures in the presence of 100 microg/ml of LPS (□- - - -□). The same cells were also tested against SRC (■——■). Controls (□) indicate the response in cultures given neither LPS nor $FITC_{(10)}$-HGG. Cultures treated only with the hapten-protein conjugate were also negative. The response was determined at day 4. The left scale refers to FITC PFC, the right to SRC.

the latter case, the most striking synergy is seen with suboptimal concentrations of LPS, in accordance with this suggestion.

Synergy occurs via accessory cells. It has been shown that both T-cells and macrophages are needed for full expression of synergy, whereas B-cell mitogens are fully active in the absence of any of these helper cells. Therefore, synergy may often be due to effects of antigen on helper cells. (1) Antigen and mitogen may be concentrated on macrophage surfaces. If so, specific antigen-sensitive cells reacting with the macrophage-bound antigen will at the same time be

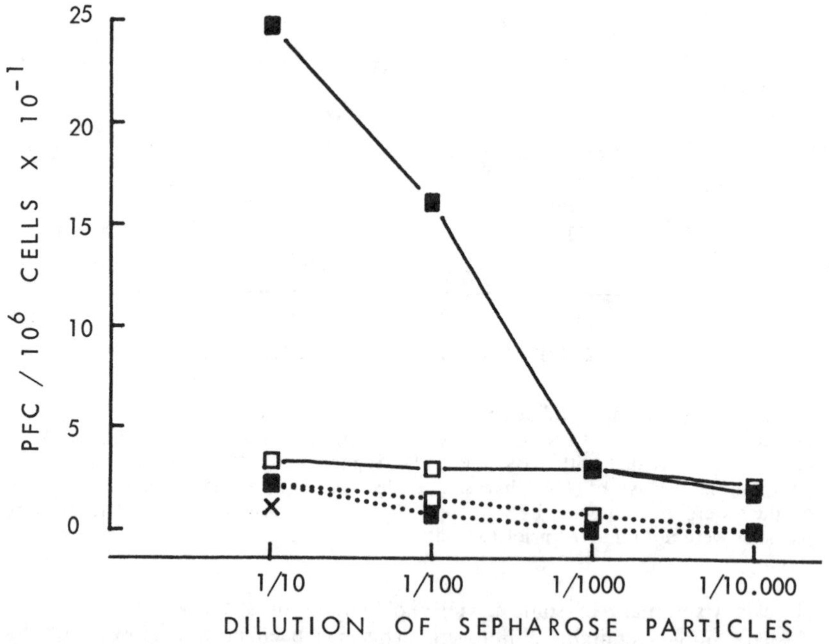

FIGURE 12. Ability of $FITC_{10}$-LPS and $FITC_{10}$-HGG to induce a primary anti-FITC response in spleen cells cultured in serum-free medium for 4 days. The $FITC_{10}$-LPS treated cultures were tested against FITC (■——■) and against SRC (■- - -■). Also the $FITC_{10}$-HGG cultures were tested against FITC (□——□) and SRC (□- - -□). The background response against FITC in untreated cultures is also indicated (×). The Sepharose particles were removed by sedimentation prior to assay.

exposed to higher mitogen concentrations. (2) Mitogen may activate macrophages. It has been shown that LPS activates macrophages in various ways. One effect may be to stimulate the release of soluble factors acting as B-cell mitogens or increasing cell survival in culture. These factors may be preferentially concentrated on antigen-binding B-cells, because antigen may bridge macrophages (having cytophilic antibody) and specific B-cells, thus establishing a situation analogous to the T-B cell collaboration. (3) Mitogens may work in synergy with B-cell mitogens released by activated T-cells. Since T-cells help the expression of synergy and since antigen may directly activate T-cells, it is possible that the released T-cell factors and B-cell mitogens work together in triggering B-cells, as postulated for T-B cells collaboration *in vivo*. No experiments so far have been performed in pure populations of B-cells and it was even found that removal of adherent cells from normal spleen populations completely abolishes synergism antigen-mitogen.

Antigen bound to specific B cells could amplify mitogenic effects on these cells by several mechanisms. (1) The mitogen and the antigen could bind each other. Many B-cell mitogens bind readily to antigens, such as SRC, and actually this binding constitutes the method for detecting anti-LPS PFC. It has already been shown that LPS coated to SRC makes this antigen TI most likely because antigen-sensitive B-cells binding the SRC via the Ig receptor will be exposed to LPS and triggered mitogenically. Obviously, this mechanism applies to any mitogen-antigen complex, and the result will always be a preferential activation of antigen-binding cells, though without generation of any specific signal. (2) Antigen could redistribute cell-surface components on the antigen-sensitive cells and cause an exposition of mitogen receptors or modify the turnover of these structures. In essence, such a cell could bind more mitogen and therefore be selectively triggered by the mitogen. (3) Antigen could stabilize the binding of the mitogen to the cell. Since most B-cell mitogens appear to bind weakly to the B-cell surface, it seems possible that antigen bound to a specific B-cell may cause a more efficient binding of the mitogen by sterically preventing the mitogen from dissociating from the cell. (4) Antigen may displace normal serum suppressor from the cell surface. It has been adequately demonstrated that normal sera of different origins contain serum suppressors that markedly inhibit B-cell activation. These suppressors bind to B-cells and suppress their ability to become triggered. It is possible that antigen bound to Ig receptors may displace these serum suppressors from the B-cell surface. Such cells would then be much more readily accessible to activation by B-cell mitogens. This hypothesis is confirmed by experimental findings, showing that the synergism SRC-LPS is increased 10-fold when very low concentrations of mouse serum is added to the cultures (W. W. Bullock, unpublished).

Many of the listed possibilities are likely to occur and a few have been demonstrated in direct experiments. Most of the possibilities are individually adequate to explain synergy, but it is not unlikely that several mechanisms operate at the same time. However, before these trivial explanations can be ruled out, it does not appear fruitful to base concepts of immunocyte activation of synergy between mitogen and antigen.

Summary

The hypotheses so far advanced for B-cell activation by antigen are based on the assumption that the interaction between antigen and the Ig receptors delivers at least the initial triggering signal. There are few, if any, experimental findings to support this assumption. On the contrary, a variety of findings indicate that the Ig receptors do not deliver any signal to the cells, whereas activation can be regularly achieved without participation of Ig receptors. The available evidence forces us to suggest that antigen-induced B-cell triggering is always caused by one nonspecific signal, which is delivered to the cells by surface structures, which are not the Ig receptors. For distinctive features of this hypothesis see *One Nonspecific Triggering Signal.* Various competing hypotheses for B-cell activation have been analyzed, but none of them appears to satisfy the experimental findings.

Acknowledgments

The technical assistance of Miss Susanne Bergstedt, Miss Yrsa Avellan, and Miss Lena Lundin is gratefully acknowledged.

References

1. COHN, M. 1973. Conference Evaluation and Commentary. *In* Genetic control of Immune Responsiveness. H. O. McDevitt & M. Landy, Eds. Academic Press. New York, N.Y.
2. COUTINHO, A. & G. B. MÖLLER. 1973. Cell mitogenic properties of thymus-independent antigens. Nature New Biol. **245:** 12.
3. DUTTON, R. W., R. FALKOFF, J. A. HIRST, M. HOFFMANN, J. W. KAPPLER, J. R. KETTMAN, J. F. LESLEY & D. VANN. 1971. Is there evidence for a non-antigen specific diffusable chemical mediator from the thymus-derived cell in the initiation of the immune response? *In* Progress in Immunology. B. Amos, Ed. Academic Press. New York, N.Y.
4. FELDMAN, M. 1972. Induction of immunity and tolerance *in vitro* by hapten protein conjugates. I. The relationship between the degree of hapten conjugation and the immunogenicity of dinitrophenylated polymerized flagellin. J. Exp. Med. **135:** 735.
5. FELDMAN, M. & G. J. V. NOSSAL. 1972. Tolerance, enhancement and the regulation of interactions between T cells, B cells and macrophages. Transplant. Rev. **12:** 3.
6. GREAVES, M. & G. JANOSSY. 1972. Elicitation of selective T and B lymphocyte responses by cell surface ligands. Transplant. Rev. **11:** 87.
7. KATZ, D. & B. BENACERRAF. 1972. The regulatory influence of activated T cells on B cell responses to antigen. Adv. Immunol. **15:** 2.
8. MITCHISON, A. 1971. Cell cooperation in the immune response: the hypothesis of an antigen presentation mechanism. Immunopathology **6:** 52.
9. MÖLLER, G. 1970. Immunocyte triggering. Cell. Immunol. **1:** 573.
10. RAFF, M. C., S. DEPETRIS & M. FELDMAN. 1973. Monospecificity of bone marrow-derived lymphocytes. J. Exp. Med **137:** 1024.
11. SCHIMPL, A. & E. WECKER. 1972. Replacement of T cell function by a T cell product. Nature New Biol. **237:** 15.
12. SELL, S. 1970. Development of restrictions in the expression of immunoglobulin specificities by lymphoid cells. Transplant. Rev. **5:** 19.
13. SINGER, S. J. & G. L. NICOLSON. 1972. The fluid mosaic model of the structure of cell membranes. Science **175:** 720.
14. TAYLOR, R. & G. M. IVERSEN. 1971. Hapten-competition and the nature of cell cooperation in the antibody response. Proc. Roy. Soc. Series B. **176:** 393.
15. Transplantation Reviews. 1970. Antigen-binding lymphocyte receptors. **5:**.
16. Transplantation Reviews. 1972. Lymphocyte activation by mitogens. **11:**.
17. VOGT, W., H. RUEHL, B. WAGNER & T. DIAMANTSTEIN. 1973. Stimulation of DNA synthesis in mouse lymphoid cells by polyanyons *in vitro.* II. Relationship between adjuvant activity and stimulation of DNA synthesis by polyanions. Eur. J. Immunol. **3:** 493.
18. WATSON, J., E. TRENKNER & M. COHN. 1973. The use of bacterial lipopolysaccharides to show that two signals are required for the induction of antibody synthesis. J. Exp. Med. **138:** 699.

19. Schrader, J. W. 1973. Mechanism of activation of the bone-marrow-derived lymphocyte. III. A distinction between a macrophage-produced triggering signal and the amplifying effect on triggered B lymphocytes of allogeneic interaction. J. Exp. Med. **138:** 1466.

Discussion of the Paper

Dr. H. Claman: We will entertain questions for Dr. Möller. What is the affinity of those cells activated nonspecifically by a hapten?

Dr. G. Möller: As far as we can determine, low affinity antibodies dominate. If one prepares a hapten inhibition curve, one finds the same number of high affinity antibody as when one treats specifically.

Dr. H. Claman: Is the actual distribution affinity the same in both of these populations?

Dr. G. Möller: We can select the affinity we test for by varying the density on the target cell.

Dr. A. J. S. Davies: Is your hypothesis related only to serum-free tissue culture circumstances?

Dr. G. Möller: We have already published data with pneumococcal polysaccharide that show high doses induced polyclonal inactivation, a time-independent specific immune response. Dextran can interfere.

Dr. A. J. S. Davies: It seems quite clear that dextran in particular leads to the production of very many plaque-forming cells *in vivo* but it is our finding that no mitosis occurs.

Dr. G. Möller: That is why I wish to do away with the term mitogen, since we are actually dealing with activation. There are certain activators which don't act on the same cell population.

Dr. D. Talmadge (*University of Colorado School of Medicine, Denver, Colo.*): If antibody only acts to focus antigen, than it is clear enough that a thymus-independent antigen is its own trigger. For thymus dependent antigens one must have T-cells and macrophages. Therefore, isn't the question "how does it work?" First, we have the necessity for a bridge in very close contact between T- and B-cells. I believe this is due to Ig binding on the B- and T-cells. Macrophages may be important, especially if coated with cytophillic antibodies which bind the antigen. B-cells may be involved in the macrophage release of many mitogenic factors. This again probably requires close cell contact. The two important cells for triggering B-cells are T-cells and macrophages; both of these release very potent mitogens. This could be explained by the bridging mechanism.

Dr. B. Waksman: Dr. Möller, I would like to ask a naive question: Low doses of sheep red blood cells in the intact animal are good stimuli for specific anti-SRBC antibody production; if in that context LPS has no effect on T-cells, why is it a good adjuvant if administered simultaneously but separately? In your model how does LPS act as an adjuvant for the sheep red blood cell response?

Dr. G. Möller: If you agree that the sheep red blood cell induces a true thymus-independent response, then you do not need macrophages and T-cells. If you separate B- and T-cells in culture, you need macrophages. My feeling is that LPS binds or activates macrophages. Thus we stimulate a macrophage mitogen.

DR. B. WAKSMAN: Thus you feel that the action of LPS *in vivo* is by way of macrophages and antigen handling?

DR. G. MÖLLER: B-cells could be involved also.

DR. B. WAKSMAN: But you really do not need macrophages because according to your model sheep red blood cells carry their own B-cell mitogenicity.

DR. G. MÖLLER: Remember that B-cell mitogens act synergistically, thus these mitogens can enhance immune responses. This could occur also with SRBC but perhaps not with protein antigens. It is interesting that one gets a thousand to ten thousand fold synergism with SRBC, but less with protein antigens.

DR. H. FRIEDMAN: I am not quite sure if your model applies to IgG production. As far as T-dependency is concerned, one must realize that IgG production is far more dependent than IgM.

DR. G. MÖLLER: Yes, I implied that different mitogens act on different subpopulations. Our guess for the moment is that mitogens like PPD, PVP, etc., as well as T-cell and macrophage factors, are specifically designed to act on the IgG subpopulation, whether it existed there from the beginning or occurred by a "switch" on mechanism. LPS would have no effect on this population. The effect of LPS on IgG memory cells to SRBC is compared to the IgM. Again my guess is that different mitogens act on different cells.

HUMORAL THYMIC FACTORS INFLUENCING POSTTHYMIC CELLS *

Osias Stutman

Memorial Sloan-Kettering Cancer Center
New York, New York 10021

The concept of a humoral function for the thymus developed largely from ablation-replacement experiments in mice in which thymus grafts restored the immune vigor depleted by neonatal thymectomy, but the immunocompetent cells produced by such a procedure were mainly of the host type.[1] These results were interpreted as the consequence of either traffic of host cells to and from the thymus graft [2] and/or to the effect of thymic humoral factor(s) acting at a distance on the host cells.[1, 3] Although both interpretations were, and still are, not mutually exclusive, the quantitative contribution of each component to lymphoid maturation under physiological conditions is unknown. The humoral theory gained strength from experiments showing the restorative activity of thymus grafts enclosed within diffusion chambers (DC) that precluded the passage of large number of cells [4, 5] and even with truly cell-impermeable DC.[6] In such experiments the restorative effects were obtained only when the DC contained thymus and not with other lymphoid or endocrine tissues.[6] The isolation of different factors extracted from thymic tissue that could mimic some of the thymic functions in mice strengthened the humoral theory.[7, 8] However, the isolation and purification of such humoral factors has proven a difficult task. For at least for one of these factors, the demonstration of biological effects *in vivo* has produced both positive [9] and negative results [10–12] using the same product and comparable techniques and procedures.

During our analysis of the restoration of immune functions in neonatally thymectomized mice, especially when using thymus in DC, we observed that the animals became refractory when such treatment was delayed for 30 to 60 days after neonatal thymectomy.[13] We then used 45-day old neonatally thymectomized animals and studied the effect of various cell supplements in augmenting the capacity of thymus grafts or thymus enclosed in DC to restore immune functions.[14, 15] We found that lymphoid and hematopoietic cells from adult or newborn animals acted synergistically with thymus in DC in the restoration.[14] Embryonic hematopoietic cells cooperated effectively only with thymus grafts and not with thymic tissue enclosed within DC.[15] It was concluded from these studies that adult and newborn tissues contained cells that had already received some thymic influence to become a postthymic population sensitive to the humoral activity of the thymus. Embryonic tissues contained cells that still required thymic influence, through traffic into the organ, to become sensitive to the humoral activity of the thymus.[16] These two types of cells were termed postthymic and prethymic, respectively.[13–16] Our studies with the postthymic cells clearly indicated that the actual content of immunocompetent cells was not a component of the cooperation of cells and thymus in

* Supported by United States Public Health Grants CA-08748, CA-15988 and American Cancer Society PR-71.

DC since newborn spleen, which is practically devoid of competent lymphocytes, was as effective as adult spleen in such cooperative restoration.[14–16] These results suggested that the postthymic pool may be composed of both immunoincompetent and competent thymus-dependent lymphoid cells. In the present experiments we will show that we can indeed isolate a population of postthymic cells that are not immunologically competent and that may act as precursor in the periphery for the development of competent T-cells. Our previous experiments[13] as well as studies of the traffic patterns of hematopoietic stem cells originating from embryos, newborn, or adult mice[17, 18] showed that the postthymic cell pool is incapable of self-renewal in absence of the thymus and that the pool is replenished by migration of prethymic cells to the thymus and by further export of those cells to the peripheral lymphoid tissues.[19]

It is also apparent that the target cells for the action of at least one of the thymic extracts[20] and of a thymic factor obtained from serum[21, 22] are indeed cells that have received thymic influence and may be equated with what we call postthymic immunoincompetent cells. It is most probable that the *in vitro* effects produced by such thymus extracts and measured as changes in surface properties or as expression of T-cell antigenic markers[23–26] may be the result of direct action on such postthymic cells. On the other hand, the intrathymic step of differentiation by which immigrant precursors of hematopoietic origin differentiate into thymocytes may be detected by some of the *in vitro* tests since an antigenic marker for intrathymic thymocytes (TL) that is absent in extrathymic lymphocytes can be expressed in such cells after incubation with thymic extracts.[24–26] However, further analysis of such interesting *in vitro* experiments is needed before the site of action of the thymic products is defined.

Our present results indicate that: (1) the extrathymic pool of postthymic cells in the periphery is composed of at least two subsets of cells, one which is immunologically incompetent and another which has the characteristics of a competent T-lymphocyte; (2) the immunoincompetent postthymic cells have peculiar physical and functional characteristics different from the mature immunologically competent T-lymphocyte (see TABLE 7 for summary of differences); (3) relatively pure populations of immunoincompetent postthymic cells can generate immunocompetent lymphocytes that have T-cell characteristics and such differentiation seems to be influenced by humoral thymic products; and (4) the immunoincompetent postthymic cell may be a precursor of the competent postthymic cell, indicating that further maturation takes place in the peripheral lymphoid tissues.

MATERIALS AND METHODS

Mice of C3Hf, CBA/H, CBA/HT6T6 and C57BL/6 strains were used in the experiments. The origin of these strains and the animal care conditions have been described in previous publications.[14, 15, 17]

Techniques for neonatal thymectomy, thoracic duct cannulation, preparation of cell suspensions and cell injections have been also described.[14, 15] Analysis of metaphases for chromosome characterization using CBA/HT6T6 cells were done as previously described.[17] Diffusion chambers (DC) using lucite rings and Millipore filters of either 0.22 or 0.10 μ mean pore size were prepared as in a previous publication.[6] Such filters have been shown to be impermeable to the passage of cells.[6] The chambers were implanted intraperitoneally (IP) and unless otherwise stated in the text, contained one lobe from the thymus of a newborn C3Hf or CBA/HT6T6 mouse. Graft-versus-host (GvH) assays were performed as in previous publications[14, 15] by injection of 10×10^6 test C3Hf spleen cells into (C3Hf $\times$ C57BL/6)F1 hybrids and determining spleen indices 8 days after IP cell injection. A positive GvH assay was considered to exist when the spleen index obtained from comparing animals injected with syngeneic F1 cells versus animals injected with the test cells was 1.30 or higher. (For calculation of spleen indices see references 6, 14, 15.) *In vitro* responses to phytohemagglutinin were measured as described previously.[17] Other techniques and procedures will be described and referenced in the text.

Experimental Design

The basic experimental system used consisted of the treatment of 50-day old neonatally thymectomized C3Hf mice by IP implantation of thymus enclosed in DC (in some experiments free thymus grafts were used) in association with variable IP doses of dispersed cells (usually 20×10^6 cells) from different newborn or adult syngeneic donors. The cells were obtained mainly from adult spleen or marrow and from newborn hemopoietic liver or spleen. The cells in some experiments were derived from animals treated *in vivo* (either adult thymectomy or short treatments with antilymphocyte serum) or submitted to different *in vitro* treatments designed for the selective elimination of cells (i.e., by lysis with anti-Thy.1.2 antiserum and complement) or by different separation procedures. Such procedures will be discussed in the text. Thirty days after these treatments, the spleens from such animals and controls (treated with thymus in DC alone or with cells alone) were tested for their GvH capacity. Restoration of GvH capacity by these procedures begins at 7–10 days after treatment. The results are expressed as the number of animals giving positive GvH reactions (i.e., immunologically restored) per total number of animals treated. Animals that were either incompletely thymectomized or showed defective diffusion chambers were excluded from the experiments. The incidence of such technical failures in the experiments described in the present paper was 11%.

Since all the animals were injected with the same number of viable nucleated cells (20×10^6) and the anti-Thy.1.2 treatment eliminated equally well the functional postthymic population in each of those tissues regardless of the actual proportion of cells lysed, it is apparent that the functional postthymic cell capable of cooperation with thymus in DC represents a minority of 1% or less of the total population in such tissues. The functional cooperative capacity also does not correlate with the content of immunocompetent postthymic cells, since of the four tissues studied the only one with significant numbers of competent postthymic cells is the adult spleen.

Results and Discussion

Effect of Anti-Thy.1.2 (θ) Treatment on Cooperative Restoration

Table 1 shows the effects of pretreatment *in vitro* of the different cell types (adult marrow or spleen and newborn liver or spleen) with anti-Thy.1.2 anti-

TABLE 1

EFFECT OF ANTI-THY.1.2 TREATMENT ON RESTORATION OF GvH REACTIONS IN 50-DAY OLD NEONATALLY THYMECTOMIZED C3HF MICE BY SYNGENEIC LYMPHOID OR HEMOPOIETIC CELLS IN ASSOCIATION WITH THYMUS GRAFTS IN DIFFUSION CHAMBERS

Treatment *	Restoration of GvH Capacity † Controls	Anti-Thy.1.2
adult bone marrow	6/12 (50%)	2/20 (10%)
adult spleen	9/16 (56%)	2/19 (10%)
newborn liver	13/23 (56%)	3/30 (10%)
newborn spleen	8/16 (50%)	1/20 (5%)

* Graft and cells were implanted intraperitoneally. Diffusion chambers made with filters of 0.10 μ pore size, containing one thymus lobe from newborn C3Hf donors. The cell dosage was 20×10^6 viable nucleated cells. The cells were incubated *in vitro* (see text) with normal AKR serum or with AKR anti-Try.1.2 serum and rabbit complement. The dilution of antiserum used was 1:16, capable of 95–100% lysis of C3Hf thymocytes.

† Restoration of GvH reactivity was measured in spleen cells 30 days after treatment, and tested in (C3Hf×C57BL/6)F1 hybrids (see text). Restoration with thymus in diffusion chamber alone was 1/20 (5%). Results expressed as number of animals with normal GvH responses (spleen indices of 1.30 or more) per total number of mice treated.

body and complement (C) on the capacity of these cells to cooperate with thymus in DC in the restoration of GvH reactivity in 50-day old neonatally thymectomized C3Hf mice. The control cells from adult or newborn origin in association with thymus in DC produced restoration of GvH activity in 50 to 56% of the treated animals at the cell dose used, and these results are comparable to those obtained with normal cells in our previous experiments.[14, 15] As was shown in our previous experiments, thymus in DC alone produced restoration in only 5% (1 of 20 animals) and the cells alone (not included in the table) were totally ineffective. The controls were incubated for 45 minutes with normal AKR serum and rabbit C whereas the experimental cells were incubated with anti-Thy.1.2 antibody produced in AKR mice plus C. (For details on preparation, purification, and cytotoxic capacities of the anti-Thy.1.2 antibody see reference 27.) TABLE 1 also shows that when the same adult or newborn cells are treated with anti-Thy.1.2 antibody and C, thus lysing the Thy.1.2 positive cells, the cooperative effect of these cells with thymus in DC was completely abolished and restoration of GvH capacity ranged from 5 to 10%, comparable to the effects of thymus in DC alone. These results indicate that the postthymic population capable of cooperative restoration of immune function when associated with thymus in DC is eliminated by pretreatment *in vitro* with anti-Thy.1.2 (θ-C3H) antibody and C. In contrast with the uniform effect of anti-Thy.1.2 on the restorative capacities of the different cell types, the actual proportion of cells lysed by the treatment was quite different since the percent lysis of adult marrow was 1 (0–5 range), adult spleen 34 (25–42), newborn liver 1 (0–5) and newborn spleen 5 (1–10).

Effect of Adult Thymectomy on Cooperative Restoration

TABLE 2 shows that when the donors of marrow or spleen cells were thymectomized as adults (at 35 days of age), the capacity of such cells to cooperate with thymus in DC in the restoration of GvH capacity in 50-day old neonatally thymectomized C3Hf mice declined progressively with time after the operation. Sixty days after adult thymectomy, the marrow and spleen were practically ineffective in cooperation (lines 7 and 11, TABLE 2). Even large numbers of marrow cells from adult thymectomized animals obtained 60 days after the operation were totally ineffective (line 8, TABLE 2). This effect of adult thymectomy becomes apparent in marrow approximately at 40 days after the operation (line 5, TABLE 2), and similar results have been obtained with spleen cells from adult thymectomized donors (not included in the table—unpublished observations). Thus, it is apparent that the functional postthymic population capable of the cooperative effect with thymus in DC is sensitive to adult thymectomy and decreases within 40 to 60 days after such operation. Its thymus dependency is also evidenced by the fact that such a population can not be replaced in the absence of a thymus. These early effects of adult thymectomy contrast with the time required for decay of the immunocompetent postthymic cells in mice (usually 6 months or more).[28] On the other hand, the timing of this decay correlates well with the results obtained with thymus

TABLE 2

EFFECT OF ADULT THYMECTOMY ON THE CAPACITY OF BONE MARROW OR SPLEEN CELLS TO RESTORE GvH REACTIONS IN 50-DAY OLD NEONATALLY THYMECTOMIZED SYNGENEIC C3HF MICE WHEN ASSOCIATED WITH A THYMUS IN DIFFUSION CHAMBER

Treatment of Cell Donor *	Type of Cell	Time After Adult Tx (Days)	Thymus in DC †	Restoration of GvH Capacity ‡
sham tx	marrow	60	yes	6/12 (50%)
sham tx	marrow	60	no	0/12
tx	marrow	15	yes	5/10 (50%)
tx	marrow	30	yes	4/10 (40%)
tx	marrow	40	yes	3/12 (25%)
tx	marrow	50	yes	2/13 (15%)
tx	marrow	60	yes	1/10 (10%)
tx	marrow	60 §	yes	2/10 (20%)
sham tx	spleen	60	yes	7/12 (58%)
sham tx	spleen	60	no	1/10 (10%)
tx	spleen	60	yes	2/10 (20%)
none	none	—	yes	1/20 (5%)

* Adult thymectomy (tx) or sham-tx was performed at 35 days of age. Cell dosage was 20×10^6 marrow cells and 10×10^6 spleen cells injected intraperitoneally.

† Thymus from newborn syngeneic mice in diffusion chambers (DC) prepared with 0.22 μ pore size filters and implanted intraperitoneally.

‡ Spleen cells from the treated animals were tested 30 days after treatment. For description of GvH assay, see text.

§ Cell dosage was 250×10^6 marrow cells injected ip.

in DC implanted at different times in neonatally thymectomized animals: in such experiments the mice became refractory to the restorative effect of thymus in DC at approximately 40 days after neonatal thymectomy.[13]

Effect of Antilymphocyte Serum (ALS) on Cooperative Restoration

TABLE 3 shows the effect of a single dose of rabbit anti-mouse lymphocyte serum on the capacity of adult marrow or spleen cells to cooperate with thymus in DC in the restoration of GvH reactivity in 50-day old neonatally thymectomized C3Hf mice. (For details on the preparation and administration of ALS see reference 29.) It is clear that ALS treatment had no effect on such cooperative capacity. On the other hand, it abolished completely the capacity of 50×10^6 spleen cells to restore adoptively the GvH capacity in the thymectomized animals (line 12, TABLE 3). Adoptive restoration is mediated by the immunocompetent cells present in the inoculum, is dependent only on the donor cells, and does not require the presence of the thymus.[28] These results show that: (1) the postthymic cell capable of cooperation with thymus in DC is insensitive to short-term ALS treatment, indicating that it is probably a nonrecirculating tissue-fixed cell; and (2) adoptive restoration mediated by immunocompetent postthymic cells on the contrary, is completely abolished by ALS treatment.

TABLE 3

EFFECT OF ANTILYMPHOCYTE SERUM (ALS) ON THE CAPACITY OF BONE MARROW OR SPLEEN CELLS TO RESTORE GvH REACTIONS IN 50-DAY OLD NEONATALLY THYMECTOMIZED SYNGENEIC C3HF MICE IN ASSOCIATION WITH THYMUS IN DIFFUSION CHAMBERS

Treatment of Cell Donor *	Cell Type	Cell Dose $\times 10^6$	Thymus in DC †	Restoration of GvH Capacity ‡
nothing	marrow	20	yes	6/10 (60%)
NRS	marrow	20	yes	7/12 (60%)
ALS	marrow	20	yes	6/12 (50%)
NRS	marrow	20	no	0/12
ALS	marrow	20	no	0/10
NRS	spleen	10	yes	6/10 (60%)
ALS	spleen	10	yes	7/12 (60%)
NRS	spleen	10	no	0/10
ALS	spleen	10	no	1/10 (10%)
NRS	spleen	50	no	6/12 (50%)
ALS	spleen	50	no	0/13
none	none	—	yes	0/13

* Cell donors were injected IP with 0.5 ml of either normal rabbit serum (NRS) or rabbit anti-mouse lymphocyte serum (ALS) at 60 days of age and the cells were obtained 48 hours later.

† On thymic lobe from newborn C3HF mice with DC made with filters of 0.22 μ mean pore size. "No" indicates empty chamber implanted ip.

‡ Number of mice with positive GvH per total mice treated, 30 days after treatment.

TABLE 4

EFFECT OF FRACTIONATION OF NEWBORN OR ADULT SPLEEN CELLS IN BOVINE SERUM ALBUMIN (BSA) GRADIENTS ON CAPACITY TO COOPERATE WITH THYMUS IN DIFFUSION CHAMBERS TO RESTORE GvH REACTIONS IN 50-DAY OLD NEONATALLY THYMECTOMIZED C3HF MICE

Cell Type	BSA Fraction *	Cell numbers $\times 10^6$	Thymus in DC †	Restoration of GvH Capacity †
adult spleen	A+B	50	no	0/22
adult spleen	A+B	25	no	0/17
adult spleen	C+D	25	no	8/10 (80%)
adult spleen	A+B	25	yes	7/12 (60%)
adult spleen	A+B	15	yes	6/12 (50%)
newborn spleen	A+B	25	no	0/19
newborn spleen	A+B	25	yes	6/10 (60%)
newborn spleen	A+B	15	yes	5/10 (50%)
newborn spleen	A+B	10	yes	6/12 (50%)
newborn spleen	C+D	50	no	1/10 (10%)
newborn spleen	C+D	50	yes	2/12 (17%)

* Bands from BSA gradients: A (10–23% BSA), B (23–26), C (26–29) and D (29–35) as described in reference 30.

† For details on thymus in DC and GvH assays see footnotes in previous tables.

Effect of BSA Gradient Fractionation on Cooperative Restoration

The previous results as well as our previously published work [14, 15] strongly supported the idea that the immune restoration in the present experimental model was mediated by the action of humoral thymic factors (i.e., thymus within DC) on a population of cells within the cell inoculum that we termed postthymic cells. Our results also indicated that such a population may not be necessarily immunocompetent and that it was apparently postthymic since it had Thy.1 antigens on its surface (see TABLE 1), that it was short-lived and thymus-dependent for its renewal (TABLE 2), and that it was apparently not recirculating as suggested by its resistance to ALS treatment (TABLE 3). Since, as mentioned previously, newborn spleen was as effective as adult spleen in the cooperative restoration,[14] it seemed the appropriate source to characterize the immunoincompetent postthymic cell.

TABLE 4 shows some of such attempts using BSA gradients. The gradients, using BSA (Pentex Biochemical, Kankakee, Ill.) were prepared as described in reference 30 and centrifuged at 4° C in a 39SW rotor at 13,500 rpm in a Beckman L-2 ultracentrifuge for 30 minutes. The average distribution of cells in each layer was quite comparable for newborn or adult spleen: layer A 10–15%, B layer 40–45%, C layer 35–40% (newborn spleen usually 16–20% with a proportionate increase in layers B and D) and D layer 5–10%. The number of cells seeded per run was usually 5×10^8. TABLE 4 shows that: (1) the A + B layers of both adult and newborn spleen when given alone do not produce any restoration of GvH capacity (lines 1, 2 and 6, TABLE 4); (2) layers C + D from adult spleen can produce adoptive restoration in the absence of thymus in DC (line 3, TABLE 4) whereas C + D layers from newborn spleen are totally ineffective even at a higher dose (line 10, TABLE 3); (3) C + D layers from newborn spleen did not show significant cooperative restoration when associated with thymus in DC (line 11, TABLE 4), these results indicating that the postthymic cell capable of cooperation was not within the layers containing the dense cells; (4) all the cooperative activity, both in the adult and the newborn spleen, was detected in the A + B layers; i.e., the layers containing the less dense cells. The results are pooled for both layers since no important differences were observed between A and B.

The next series of experiments were designed to determine if the cells in layers A + B of the newborn spleen had Thy.1.2 antigens on their surface. TABLE 5 shows these results. As was observed in TABLE 1, pretreatment of the unfractioned newborn spleen cells with anti-Thy.1.2 and C abolished the cooperative capacity of such cells, when associated with thymus in DC, to restore GVH activity in 50-day old neonatally thymectomized mice. Similarly, treatment of the A + B layers with anti-Thy.1.2 and C completely abolished the cooperative efficiency of such cells. The actual percent of cells lysed in these

TABLE 5

EFFECT OF ANTI-THY.1 ANTIBODY AND C ON THE CAPACITY OF A+B LAYERS FROM BSA GRADIENTS OF NEWBORN SPLEEN TO COOPERATE WITH THYMUS IN DC FOR THE RESTORATION OF GVH CAPACITY IN 50-DAY OLD NEONATALLY THYMECTOMIZED C3HF MICE

Cell Fraction *	Pretreatment †	Restoration of GvH Reactivity †
whole (newborn spleen)	control	6/10 (60%)
whole (newborn spleen)	anti-Thy.1.2	0/12
A+B (newborn spleen)	control	6/12 (50%)
A+B (newborn spleen)	anti-Thy.1.2	1/20 (5%)

* For details on cell fractions see TABLE 4 and text. The animals were injected with 20×10^6 viable whole spleen cells or 10×10^6 viable cells from fraction A+B.

† For details on thymus in DC and GvH assays see footnotes in previous tables.

experiments was 6% (4–11%) in the unfractioned cells and 1% (0–5%) in the A + B layer. Again these results indicate that it is actually a small proportion of postthymic cells which have the functional capacity for cooperation with thymus in DC.

Additional studies on these cell fractions (Stutman, unpublished observations) can be summarized as follows: fractions A + B from adult spleen have a high background of spontaneous [^{3}H]thymidine incorporation, have a poor response to phytohemagglutinin (PHA), have no response in mixed leukocyte cultures, are incapable of producing GvH reactions, and are found to lodge mainly in the spleen when they are labeled with ^{51}Cr and injected intravenously and the organ distribution measured 4 to 24 hours after cell injection. The A + B cells from newborn spleen have practically the same characteristics as those from adult spleen. The spleen-seeking characteristics of these cells fit well with the ALS data presented in TABLE 3, which suggested that the cells capable of cooperation were insensitive to ALS treatment and probably nonrecirculating.

Effect of Tritiated Thymidine Suicide on Cooperative Restoration

The high background incorporation of [^{3}H]thymidine by the A + B layer suggested a rapidly dividing population. In these experiments, whole newborn spleen or A + B layers from newborn spleen were incubated for 24 hours with 10 μc per ml/10^6 cells of [^{3}H]thymidine of high specific activity (18 c/mmole). Control cells were incubated either in absence of [^{3}H]thymidine, with [^{3}H]-thymidine of low specific activity, nonradioactive thymidine or [^{3}H]water (Scwartz Bio Research, Orangeburg, N.Y.). Restoration of GvH capacity when 20×10^6 cells were used in association with thymus in DC was: 4/8 (50%) for the animals injected with whole spleen controls; 3/4 for the animals injected with A + B layer control and 0/7 and 0/6 respectively for the animals injected with the cells treated with "hot" [^{3}H]thymidine.

These observations strengthen the view that the restoration of GvH by these cells is mediated by precursor cells and not by contamination with immunocompetent cells, since such cells are not affected by incubation with high doses of [^{3}H]thymidine, results which corroborate previous experiments in the rat.[31]

Isolation of Immunoincompetent Postthymic Cells by Velocity Sedimentation

Attempts to separate the immunoincompetent postthymic cells by velocity sedimentation at unit gravity [32] will be described.

Velocity sedimentation at unit gravity was performed as described in reference 32 with minor modifications (a siliconized glass funnel was used instead of a plastic one). When adult spleen was fractioned we observed the following: (1) the fraction that migrated at 3.0 to 4.0 mm/hr (mean 3.7 mm/hr) was enriched for Thy.1-positive cells (76–88% Thy.1-positive versus 31–36% for the unfractioned spleen) and contained the immunocompetent postthymic cells (those which had good response to PHA and mixed leukocyte cultures and were capable of restoring adoptively the thymectomized animals); (2) the fraction that migrated at 5.0 to 7.0 mm/hr (mean 5.9 mm/hr) contained the postthymic cells capable of cooperation with thymus in DC (this fraction had 12–20% Thy.1-positive cells, showed no response to PHA, no response in mixed leukocyte cultures and could not restore the thymectomized animals when administered alone at dosages ranging from 20 to 100×10^6 cells, i.e., there was no capacity for adoptive restoration); (3) the 5.0 to 7.0 mm/hr fraction could restore 7 of 10 mice (70%) when 10×10^6 cells were injected IP in association with thymus in DC in 50-day old neonatally thymectomized mice, and this effect could be abolished by pretreatment *in vitro* with anti-Thy.1.2 and C; (4) fractionation of newborn spleen showed again that the main component of cells capable of cooperative restoration of GvH capacity when associated with thymus in DC was located in the fraction that migrated at 5.0–7.0 mm/hr (mean 5.8 mm/hr); however, restoration was also observed in the 4.0–5.0 mm/hr fraction, which was not the case with adult spleen: the 5.0–7.0 mm/hr fraction restored 6 of 8 mice at 10×10^6 cell-dosage when associated with thymus in DC whereas the 4.0–5.0 mm/hr fraction restored 3 of 8 animals (thymus in DC alone restored only 1 of 8 treated animals whereas the cells alone or associated with an empty chamber were negative in 7 and 8 instances respectively); and (5) the 3.0 to 4.0 mm/hr fraction of newborn spleen was slightly enriched for Thy.1 cells (22–28% Thy.1-positive versus 5–14% for the unfractioned spleen) and showed some degree of PHA reactivity and mixed leukocyte reactivity, although at dosages ranging from 20 to 50 × 10^6 cells it could not produce adoptive restoration of thymectomized hosts. A more detailed description of these studies will be published elsewhere.

In summary, by velocity sedimentation at unit gravity (which separates cells by volume) two distinct cell populations could be isolated from spleen: one with a mean migration of 5.9 mm/hr, which is immunoincompetent but can cooperate with thymus in DC in restoring GvH reactivity in 50-day old neonatally thymectomized mice (immunoincompetent postthymic cell) and another fraction with a mean migration of 3.7 mm/hr, which is immunologically competent and enriched for Thy.1-positive cells and can produce adoptive restoration of thymectomized animals (immunocompetent postthymic cell).

When ^{51}Cr-labeled cells from such fractions (obtained from adult spleen) were injected into normal syngeneic mice, it was observed that the 5.9 mm/hr fraction migrated mainly to spleen whereas the 3.7 mm/hr fraction migrated mainly to lymph nodes. For details on ^{51}Cr-labeling and migration studies see references 33 and 34.

The cells separated by velocity sedimentation that showed cooperative activity with thymus in DC were also tested for other surface determinants: (1) treatment *in vitro* with anti-TL and C had no cytotoxic nor functional effect; (2) treatment with polyvalent rabbit anti-mouse Ig antiserum and C had minimal cytotoxic effects (5–12% lysis) and no functional effects on cooperative efficiency. For details on TL see references 24–26, and for details on anti-Ig see reference 27.

It should be mentioned that the sedimentation values for other cell types are well established and could be used as comparison: erythrocytes, 2.0 mm/hr, granulocytes two peaks at 4.3 mm/hr and 5.9 mm/hr, 19S plaque-forming cells 4.7 mm/hr, 7S plaque-forming cells 4.4 mm/hr, cells required for initiation of an *in vivo* response to sheep red cells 3.0 mm/hr, and hemopoietic stem cells (CFU) 4.2 and 3.7 mm/hr.[35-37]

A summary of our experiments, which are still in progress, indicates that the immunoincompetent postthymic precursor cell, which has a sedimentation velocity of 5.8 to 6.1 mm/hr, can be isolated from adult spleen, newborn spleen, adult bone marrow, and embryonic hemopoietic liver at ages ranging from day 14 to birth. Such cells could not be obtained from embryonic liver of younger embryos. The tissue distribution of such cells agrees with our previous functional studies.[14, 15]

Effect of Adherence to Plastic or Nylon Wool on Cooperative Restoration

When newborn spleen cells were cultivated in plastic culture flasks for 6 hours and the nonadherent cells recovered and used in the model system, only a slight decrease in effectiveness was observed (i.e., 6 of 10 mice restored for the nonincubated cells and 5 of 10 for the nonadherent cells).

However, when the newborn spleen cells were passed through nylon wool columns (prepared using nylon wool obtained from Fenwal Laboratories, Morton Grove, Ill. in 10cc plastic syringes and the cells were incubated within the column for 30 minutes as described in reference 34) the cooperative capacity was completely abolished. The results showed that when such cells were simply passed through the column the capacity to produce restoration of GvH when associated with thymus in DC was 5 of 10 (50%) whereas the cells incubated within the column did not restore GvH in any of 12 treated mice. In these experiments 20×10^6 viable cells were injected IP and the results should be compared with those in TABLE 1, which used unmodified newborn spleen cells. Similar results were obtained by the incubation of bone marrow cells within the nylon wool columns (Stutman, unpublished).

These results indicate that the population of immunoincompetent postthymic cells adheres to nylon wool, a property not shared by the immunocompetent postthymic cells.

Direct Evidence That Immunoincompetent Postthymic Cells are Precursors for Immunocompetent T-lymphocytes

To demonstrate in a direct way that the cells purified by BSA gradient fractionation or velocity sedimentation were indeed postthymic precursors for the immunocompetent postthymic lymphocytes in the periphery, advantage was taken of the availability of congenic strains of mice, which differ only on a pair of autosomal chromosomes readily detected in metaphase.[7, 17, 18] The model in this experiment consisted of 50-day old neonatally thymectomized CBA/H mice grafted ip with either an empty chamber or a chamber containing a CBA/HT6 thymus (these mice are obtained by mating CBA/H with CBA/HT6T6 and have only one marker T6 chromosome) and also injected ip with purified immunoincompetent postthymic cells obtained from newborn CBA/HT6T6 spleen (20×10^6 cells from either BSA gradients or velocity sedimentation). Thirty days after such treatment the spleens or thoracic duct lymphocytes (from 12-hour drainages) were tested for their capacity to respond *in vitro* to PHA or in mixed leukocyte reactions (MLR) to allogeneic C57BL/6 cells. Chromosome analysis of the responding cells was performed after 48 and 72 hours in culture, respectively and scored as percent T6T6 metaphases per total metaphases scored. For details on chromosome preparation, PHA responses and MLR reactivity see references.[17, 19, 38] The results of such experiments are presented in TABLE 6.

It is apparent that: (1) both fractionation procedures give comparable results; (2) the fractioned cells alone or in association with an empty DC produce only minimal numbers of dividing cells in spleen, and no dividing cells with the T6T6 marker can be detected in thoracic duct lymph (lines 1, 3 and 5, TABLE 6); (3) when such fractioned cells are associated with a thymus in DC, a high number of dividing cells can be detected responding to PHA or in MLR that have the T6T6 marker of the immunoincompetent precursor: 68 to 74% of the cells responding in spleen to PHA are derived from the T6T6 inoculum (lines 2 and 6, TABLE 6) and 73% of the cells in spleen responding in MLR have the T6T6 marker; (4) the responses in thoracic duct show that practically all the cells responding to PHA are derived from the injected T6T6 precursors, and a high percentage of the cells responding in MLR are of such origin; and (5) additional controls, not included in the table, indicated that in unstimulated cultures of spleen or thoracic duct the percent of cells with the T6T6 marker was 17% in spleen and 1% in thoracic duct

TABLE 6

EFFECT OF PURIFIED IMMUNOINCOMPETENT POSTTHYMIC CELLS FROM NEWBORN CBA/HT6T6 SPLEEN ON COOPERATIVE RESTORATION OF *In Vitro* RESPONSES TO PHA AND MIXED-LEUKOCYTE REACTIONS WHEN ASSOCIATED WITH THYMUS IN DC

Experimental Model *	Response †	Percent T6T6 Metaphases ‡ Spleen	Thoracic Duct
A+B bands plus empty DC	PHA	9 (266)	0 (320)
A+B bands plus thymus in DC	PHA	74 (395)	96 (420)
A+B bands alone	MLR	5 (232)	0 (333)
A+B bands plus thymus in DC	MLR	73 (350)	89 (320)
5.0–7.0 mm/hr fraction	PHA	5 (288)	0 (350)
5.0–7.0 mm/hr fraction plus thymus in DC	PHA	68 (345)	98 (420)

* The A+B bands from BSA gradients or the 5.0–7.0 mm/hr fraction from velocity sedimentation (see text for description) were prepared from newborn CBA/HT6T6 spleen. Twenty million cells were injected ip either alone, in association with an empty DC implanted ip, or with a DC containing a CBA/HT6 newborn thymus. The hosts were 50-day old neonatally thymectomized CBA/H mice. The responses in lymph nodes or thoracic duct cells (obtained from 12-hour drainages) were measured 30 days after treatment.

† PHA responses measured 48 hours after culture and MLR responses measured 72-hour cultures. For procedures see references 17 and 38.

‡ Metaphases with the T6T6 marker are expressed as percent of the total. The actual number of metaphases scored is in parentheses. The results are pooled from 3 animals per point.

for those animals treated with cells and thymus in DC and 5% in spleen and 0% in thoracic duct for those treated with cells alone.

In summary: immunoincompetent nonrecirculating postthymic cells, purified to a reasonable degree by physical methods, become recirculating and capable of producing mitotic responses to PHA and allogeneic cells within 30 days after injection into syngeneic thymectomized hosts, provided that a thymus in a DC in also included.

Such "maturation" requires time, since the first cells with T6T6 markers in thoracic duct (or in lymph nodes) start to appear 5 to 7 days after treatment provided that a thymus in a DC or a free thymus graft is also included (Stutman, unpublished observations).

Summary of the Physical and Functional Characteristics of the Immunoincompetent Postthymic Cell

The postthymic immunoincompetent precursor cells have the following characteristics (summarized in TABLE 7): (1) in the adult they are present mainly in marrow and spleen (in newborn or late embryos they are present in hemopoietic liver and spleen); (2) after intravenous injection of ^{51}Cr-labeled cells they show preferential migration to spleen; (3) they are not recirculating cells and cannot be detected in thoracic duct; (4) they are immunoincompetent and thus by themselves cannot produce adoptive restoration of immune functions in thymectomized hosts; (5) they are depleted within 30–60 days after adult thymectomy; (6) they are resistant to short-term treatments with antilymphocyte serum; (7) they are a rapidly dividing population than can commit [^{3}H]thymidine suicide; (8) in BSA gradients, they appear in the less dense fractions; (9) by velocity sedimentation, they appear to be large cells with a sedimentation velocity of 5.5 to 6.1 mm/hr; (10) they adhere to nylon wool; and (11) they have Thy.1 (θ) antigen on their surface and no detectable amounts of TL antigen or immunoglobulins. It is also apparent that the listed properties are significantly different from those of the immunocompetent postthymic cell or T-lymphocyte in the periphery. The experiments with the T6T6 chromosome markers also indicate that, as part of a maturation step, such immunocompetent postthymic cells can acquire new characteristics such as recirculation capacity, lymph-node seeking traffic patterns and the capacity to respond mitotically to such stimuli as PHA or allogeneic cells. Those results also indicate that this maturation step appears to be dependent on the thymus and probably mediated by its humoral action (i.e., thymus in DC).

The exact correlation of this subpopulation of postthymic cells with other subpopulations that interact synergistically with competent T-cells in the generation of GvH reactions [39] or other reactions [40] deserves further study. Our own preliminary results indicate that the purified immunoincompetent postthymic population may contain cells that are sensitive to antigen and can be driven by antigen alone (in the absence of thymus) to differentiate into

Table 7

Characterization of Two Subpopulations of Postthymic Cells in Mouse Tissues

Biological Characteristics *	Immunoincompetent	Immunocompetent
tissue distribution (adult)	spleen, marrow	lymphoid tissues
(newborn)	spleen, liver	—
traffic patterns	spleen-seeking	lymph-node seeking
recirculation (presence in TD)	no	yes
capacity of adoptive restoration of thymectomized animals	no	yes
effect of adult thymectomy	depletion (30–60 days)	none (within 60 days
effect of short term ALS treatment	none	depletion
[^{3}H]thymidine suicide	yes	no, usually.
BSA gradients	A-B layers	C-D layers
flotation velocity (adult spleen)	5.9 mm/hr	3.7 mm/hr
(adult marrow)	5.4 mm/hr	3.6 mm/hr
(newborn spleen)	5.8 mm/hr	?
adherence to plastic	yes, partial	no
adherence to nylon wool	yes	no
surface antigens: Thy.1	yes	yes
TL	no	no
Ig	no	no

* See text for details. TD: thoracic duct. BSA gradients: A-B layers (10–26%); C-D layers (26–35% BSA).

competent T-lymphocytes. These experiments, still in progress, indicate that 50-day old neonatally thymectomized mice injected only with immunoincompetent postthymic cells and subsequently immunized with heavily irradiated xenogeneic rat cells, can specifically destroy the appropriate rat cells *in vitro* (Stutman, unpublished). It is obvious that these experiments have to be expanded and correlated with the known facts about generation of killer T-lymphocytes.[41]

The semantic argument on whether the presently described population of precursor postthymic cells is a T_1,[40] T_2 being the competent T-lymphocyte, or a T_0-cell,[42] or equated with any other sub-set of T-cells may be settled by performing comparative studies.

Similarly, the relevance of the present experiments describing a noncompetent postthymic cell that acts as precursor for the competent T-lymphocyte in the periphery, with the attempts to define the target cells for the action of thymic extracts or hormones,[22] will be evaluated through further work.

The fact that the immunoincompetent postthymic precursor cell is present in newborn and embryonic tissues as early as two days after appearance of the thymus,[15, 18] suggests that the predetermined state of the T-cell precursor [25, 26] may be still a thymus-dependent event mediated perhaps through traffic. Thus, the *in vitro* effects of thymus extracts may be expressed mainly on postthymic cells. Experiments using pure prethymic cells such as yolk sac or embryonic liver of less than 14 days [18] may resolve this question.

In his original description of the absence of the thymus in a child who died at eight days of age of "convulsions," Harington indicated that

> the nature and uses of the thymus gland still lie in so much obscurity (that) . . . by collation and placing on record this and similar examples, we may hereafter succeed in discovering the physiology of an apparatus apparently of great importance to foetal and infantile organizations.[43]

It is apparent from the present conference that although we have apparently overcome the stage of "collation and placing on record" our understanding of thymic physiology is still incomplete and fragmentary.

References

1. Dalmasso, A. P., C. Martinez, K. Sjodin & R. A. Good. 1963. Studies on the role of the thymus in immunobiology. Reconstitution of immunologic capacity in mice thymectomized at birth. J. Exp. Med. **118:** 1089–1109.
2. Ford, C. E. & H. S. Micklem. 1963. The thymus and lymph-nodes in radiation chimeras. Lancet **1:** 359–362.
3. Osoba, D. & J. F. A. P. Miller. 1963. Evidence for a humoral thymus factor responsible for the maturation of immunological faculty. Nature **199:** 633–654.
4. Law, L. W., N. Trainin, R. H. Levey & W. F. Barth. 1963. Humoral thymic factor on mice: Further evidence. Science **143:** 1049–1051.
5. Osoba, D. 1965. The effects of thymus and other lymphoid organs enclosed in millipore diffusion chambers on neonatally thymectomized mice. J. Exp. Med. **122:** 633–650.
6. Stutman, O., E. J. Yunis & R. A. Good. 1969. Carcinogen-induced tumors of the thymus. III. Restoration of neonatally thymectomized mice with thymomas in cell-impermeable chambers. J. Nat. Cancer Inst. **43:** 499–508.
7. Goldstein, A. L., F. D. Slater & A. White. 1966. Preparation, assay and par-

tial purification of a thymic lymphocytopoietic factor (thymosin). Proc. Nat. Acad. Sci. U.S. **56:** 1010–1017.

8. Trainin, N. & M. Linker-Israeli. 1967. Restoration of immunologic reactivity of thymectomized mice by calf thymus extracts. Cancer Res. **27:** 309–313.
9. Goldstein, A. L., Y. Asanuma, J. R. Battisto, M. A. Hardy, J. Quint & A. White. 1970. Influence of thymosin on cell-mediated and humoral immune responses in normal and in immunologically deficient mice. J. Immunol. **104:** 359–366.
10. Kruger, J., A. L. Goldstein & B. H. Waksman. 1970. Immunologic and anatomic consequences of calf thymosin injection in rats. Cell. Immunol. **1:** 51–61.
11. Lance, E. M., S. Cooper Gillette, A. L. Goldstein, A. White & M. M. Zatz. 1973. On the mode of action of thymosin. Cell. Immunol. **6:** 123–131.
12. Stutman, O. & R. A. Good. 1973. Thymus hormones. *In* Contemporary Topics in Immunobiology. A. J. S. Davies & R. L. Carter, Eds. Vol. **2:** 299–319. Plenum Press. New York, N.Y.
13. Stutman, O., E. J. Yunis & R. A. Good. 1969. Carcinogen-induced tumors of the thymus. IV. Humoral influences of normal thymus and functional thymomas and influence of post-thymectomy period in restoration. J. Exp. Med. **130:** 809–819.
14. Stutman, O., E. J. Yunis & R. A. Good. 1970. Studies in thymus function. I. Cooperative effect of thymic function and lymphohemopoietic cells in restoration of neonatally thymectomized mice. J. Exp. Med. **132:** 583–600.
15. Stutman, O., E. J. Yunis & R. A. Good. 1970. Studies on thymus function. II. Cooperative effect of newborn and embryonic hemopoietic liver cells with thymus function. J. Exp. Med. **132:** 601–612.
16. Stutman, O., E. J. Yunis & R. A. Good. 1969. Thymus: an essential factor in lymphoid repopulation. Transplant. Proc. **1:** 614–615.
17. Stutman, O. 1970. Hemopoietic origin of cells responding to phytohemagglutinin in mouse lymph nodes. *In* Proceedings of the 5th Leukocyte Culture Conference. J. E. Harris, Ed. 671–681. Academic Press. New York, N.Y.
18. Stutman, O. & R. A. Good. 1971. Immunocompetence of embryonic hemopoietic cells after traffic to thymus. Transplant. Proc. **3:** 923–925.
19. Stutman, O. 1972. Traffic of cells and development of immunity. *In* Membranes and viruses in Immunopathology. S. B. Day & R. A. Good, Eds. **:** 437–450. Academic Press. New York, N.Y.
20. Lonai, P., B. Mogilner, V. Rotter & N. Trainin. 1973. Studies on the effect of a thymic humoral factor on differentiation of thymus-derived lymphocytes. Eur. J. Immunol. **3:** 21–26.
21. Bach, J. F. & M. Dardenne. 1973. Studies on thymus products. II. Demonstration and characterization of a circulating thymic hormone. Immunology **25:** 353–366.
22. Bach, J. F. 1973. Target cell of thymic hormone. Lancet **II:** 1320.
23. Bach, J. F., M. Dardenne, A. L. Goldstein, A. Guha & A. White. 1971. Appearance of T-cell markers in bone marrow rosette forming cells after incubation with thymosin, a thymic hormone. Proc. Nat. Acad. Sci. U.S. **68:** 2734–2738.
24. Komuro, K. & E. A. Boyse. 1973. *In-vitro* demonstration of thymic hormone in the mouse by conversion of precursor cells into lymphocytes. Lancet **1:** 740–743.
25. Komuro, K. & E. A. Boyse. 1973. Induction of T lymphocytes from precursor cells *in vitro* by a product of the thymus. J. Exp. Med. **138:** 479–482.
26. Scheid, M. P., M. K. Hoffmann, K. Komuro, U. Hammerling, J. Abbot, E. A. Boyse, G. H. Cohen, J. A. Hooper, R. S. Schulof & A. L. Goldstein. 1973. Differentiation of T cells induced by preparations from thymus and by nonthymic agents. J. Exp. Med. **138:** 1027–1032.

27. STUTMAN, O. 1972. Lymphocyte subpopulation in NZB mice: deficit of thymus dependent lymphocytes. J. Immunol. **109:** 602–611.
28. STUTMAN, O., E. J. YUNIS & R. A. GOOD. 1972. Studies on thymus function. III. Duration of thymic function. J. Exp. Med. **135:** 339–356.
29. STUTMAN, O. 1972. Immunologic studies on resistance to oncogenic agents in mice. Nat. Cancer Inst. Monograph **35:** 107–115.
30. KONDA, S., E. STOCKERT & R. T. SMITH. 1973. Immunologic properties of mouse thymus cells: Membrane antigen patterns. Cell. Immunol. **7:** 275–289.
31. MCGREGOR, D. D. 1969. Effect of tritiated thymidine and 5-bromodeoxyuridine on development of immunologically competent lymphocytes. Immunology **16:** 83–90.
32. MILLER, R. G. & R. A. PHILLIPS. 1969. Separation of cells by velocity sedimentation. J. Cell. Physiol. **73:** 191–202.
33. ZATZ, M. M. & E. M. LANCE. 1970. The distribution of chromium 51-labelled lymphoid cells in the mouse: a survey of naatomical compartment. Cell. Immunol. **1:** 3–17.
34. STUTMAN, O. 1973. Lymphocyte sequestration: its role in tumor immunity. Transplant. Proc. **5:** 707–710.
35. PHILLIPS, R. A. & R. G. MILLER. 1970. Antibody-producing cells: analysis and purification by velocity sedimentation. Cell Tissue Kinet. **3:** 263–274.
36. MILLER, R. G. & R. A. PHILLIPS. 1970. Sedimentation analysis of the cells in mice required to initiate an *in vivo* immune response to sheep erythrocytes. Proc. Soc. Exp. Biol. Med. **135:** 63–67.
37. WORTON, R. G., E. A. MCCULLOCH & J. E. TILL. 1969. Physical separation of hemopoietic stem cells differing in their capacity for self-renewal. J. Exp. Med. **130:** 91–103.
38. TAKIGUCHI, T., W. H. ADLER & R. T. SMITH. 1971. Cellular recognition in vitro by mouse lymphocytes: effects of neonatal thymectomy and thymus graft restoration on alloantigen and PHA stimulation of whole and gradient-separated sub-populations of spleen cells. J. Exp. Med. **133:** 63–80.
39. CANTOR, H. & R. ASOFSKY. 1970. Synergy among lymphoid cells mediating the graft-versus-host reactions produced by BALB/C lymphoid cells of different anatomic origin. J. Exp. Med. **131:** 235–246.
40. RAFF, M. C. & H. CANTOR. 1971. Subpopulations of thymus cells and thymus-derived lymphocytes. *In* Progress in Immunology. B. Amos, Ed. : 83–94. Academic Press, New York, N.Y.
41. MILLER, J. F. A. P., A. BASTEN, J. SPRENT & C. CHEERS. 1971. Interaction between lymphocytes in immune responses. Cell. Immunol. **2:** 469–495.
42. BACH, J. F. & M. DARDENNE. 1973. Antigen recognition by T lymphocytes. III. Evidence for two populations of thymus-dependent rosette-forming cells in spleen and lymph nodes. Cell. Immunol. **6:** 394–406.
43. HARINGTON, H. 1828–1829. Absence of the thymus gland (Letter to the Editor). London Med. Gazette **3:** 314.

DISCUSSION OF THE PAPER

DR. A. GOLDSTEIN: I would like to make a comment on some of the data dealing with a negative experiment with thymosin in nude mice. We have initiated experiments ourselves in nude mice; there are also several other similar studies that are presently in progress around the country. In contrast to Dr. Stutman's data, we have found effects of thymosin in the systems we have looked at. We have not been able to totally reconstitute the nude mouse, but we certainly have data to indicate that there is an effect. I feel strongly that if a thymus preparation does not work, it is called thymosin and, of course, if it works it is called something else in some other laboratory. I wish to comment that the particular fraction mentioned by Dr. Stutman was not delivered by me personally and I have been told privately by Dr. Stutman that he received it from someone else.

DR. O. STUTMAN: What is the point of your statement Dr. Goldstein?

DR. A. GOLDSTEIN: The point is simply that in our hands we do have evidence that thymosin fraction-5 does do something in the nude mouse.

DR. J. F. A. P. MILLER: Isn't it true that you must be dealing with two different phenomena, because according to the literature thymosin is supposed to induce TL positive cells to appear but both your T1 and T2 tests were negative.

DR. STUTMAN: The TL studies are very important. In leukemia, transformation occurs for TL antigens. Cells may have the T-antigen for only very limited periods of time. Thus the fact that these cells are T1 negative indicates that we are dealing with an extrathymic event.

CELLULAR INTERACTIONS CONTROLLING THE IMMUNE REACTIVITY OF T-LYMPHOCYTES *

Irun R. Cohen and Michael Feldman

Department of Cell Biology
The Weizmann Institute of Science
Rehovot, Israel

Cell interactions were first shown to determine developmental processes in embryogenesis and, in fact, the analysis of such interactions constituted the "golden age" of experimental embryology.[1] Thus, the first manifestation of histogenesis in the early embryo, the differentiation of the neural tissue, results from an interaction between the endomesoderm and the ectoderm, the latter responding to a developmental signal emitted by the endomesodermal cells. The newly formed neural tissue in turn originates signals that trigger other cells to further developmental processes. Thus, the eye cup formed from a lateral extension of the embryonic brain signals the differentiation of the lens, the latter evokes the differentiation of the cornea, etc.

Most of the developmental systems that were shown to be based on cell interactions were confined to the early stages of embryogenesis. In our studies on the differentiation of thymus-derived (T) lymphocytes we found that developmental processes that take place constantly in the adult organism are also based on cell interactions. Furthermore, regulation of the extent of differentiation of specific effector T-lymphocytes in response to antigenic stimuli is also subject to control mechanisms based on cell interactions.[2–4]

The sequence of developmental processes of thymus-derived lymphocytes could be classified into two distinct stages. The first stage constitutes the appearance of lymphocytes in the thymus capable of recognizing antigenic signals. Such lymphocytes leave the thymus and colonize the spleen and lymph nodes. The second developmental stage involves the response of T-lymphocytes to antigenic signals, which can take place in a number of distinct ways. Thus, when a given cell-bound antigen triggers T-lymphocytes capable of recognizing the antigen, killer cells develop capable of specifically lysing target cells possessing the same surface antigens that triggered their development.

Studies carried out in our laboratory indicated that both these stages, i.e. the differentiation of T-cells within the thymus and their differentiation in response to antigen, are regulated by cell interactions.[2–4]

In Vitro *Induction of T-cell Properties by Thymus Reticulum Cells*

The initial development of immunocompetent T-lymphocytes takes place within the thymus from precursors of exogenous origin. Hemopoietic tissues, such as bone marrow, give rise to precursor cells that migrate to the thymus

* This work was supported by a grant from the Talisman Foundation, New York, N.Y. and by Contract NCI-G-72-3890 from the National Institutes of Health, Bethesda, Md.

and differentiate there to lymphocytes, characterized by reactivity to lectins and by their capacity to recognize and respond to antigenic stimuli. Such precursor cells appear to establish within the thymus cell-to-cell contact with thymus reticulum cells. It therefore appeared that cellular interactions between the thymus reticulum and precursor cells originating in the bone marrow may trigger the developmental processes that result in the manifestation of immune reactivity by thymic lymphocytes.

To test this interaction we prepared monolayer cultures of rat thymus reticulum cells and studied their effects on populations of lymphocytes depleted of differentiated T-lymphocytes. B mice were prepared by subjecting hybrid (C3H/eb × C57BL/6)F_1 mice to thymectomy, lethal x-irradiation, and injection of bone marrow. Spleen cells from such animals and from normal control

TABLE 1

EFFECTS OF THYMUS RETICULUM CELLS ON SPLEEN CELLS FROM THYMUS-DEPRIVED B MICE; REACTIVITY TO CON-A AND ABILITY TO TRIGGER A SYNGENEIC LYMPH NODE RESPONSE

Mouse Spleen Cells *	Rat Monolayer Cells	Con-A Reactivity Index †	Lymph Node Index ‡
normal	fibroblasts	1.63	6.7 ± 1
normal	thymus reticulum	not done	6.4 ± 1
B	fibroblasts	0.87	2.7 ± 1
B	thymus reticulum	1.59	6.7 ± 2

* Spleen cells from normal or thymus-deprived B mice were incubated for 24 hours with rat monolayers of fibroblasts or thymus reticulum cells.

† The spleen cells were removed from the monolayers and cultured for 48 hours with or without con-A (10 μg/ml). DNA synthesis was measured by the uptake of [^{3}H]thymidine and the con-A reactivity index was expressed as the ratio of cpm of con-A treated to control cultures.

‡ Sensitization of the mouse spleen cells against rat antigens was tested by injecting the cells into the right foot pads of syngeneic mice and measuring the lymph node index 6 days later. The lymph node index was computed as the mean ratio of the weight of the right lymph node to that of the control left lymph node ± standard deviation.

donors were incubated for 24 hours with thymus reticulum monolayers then collected and tested for the acquisition of two properties of competent T-lymphocytes: reactivity to Concanavalin A (con-A) and immune reactivity to cell-surface antigens.

Lymphocyte transformation stimulated by con-A was measured by assaying DNA synthesis reflected in uptake of tritiated thymidine after 48 hours of culture with the lectin. TABLE 1 shows the results [2] expressed as the ratio of thymidine uptake of con-A treated, to that of untreated lymphocytes. The ratio produced by spleen cells from normal mice incubated with rat fibroblasts was 1.63. In contrast, spleen cells from B mice incubated with fibroblasts could not respond to con-A and demonstrated a ratio of 0.87. Incubation of spleen cells from the B animals with cultures of thymus reticulum cells, however, conferred reactivity to con-A (ratio = 1.59). Hence, rat thymus reticulum cells appear to be able to render mouse spleen cells competent to respond to stimulation with con A.[2]

In previous studies we found that thymus-deprived (T) lymphocytes can be sensitized *in vitro* against cell-surface antigens. This sensitization can be induced against foreign cells,[5–7] or against cells obtained from syngeneic animals to produce autosensitization.[8–10] The sensitized state of the lymphocytes is easily detected by injecting them into the foot pads of syngeneic recipient animals.[3] Enlargement of draining popliteal lymph nodes indicates that the injected lymphocytes were sensitized. Specific cytotoxic lymphocytes were shown to develop within these enlarged lymph nodes. The ability to undergo sensitization *in vitro* and stimulate a lymph node response *in vivo* was found to be a function of T-lymphocytes.[3]

We used this system to test whether incubation with reticulum cells *in vitro* could induce immunocompetence of lymphocytes from thymus-deprived B mice.[2] Spleen cells from control or B mice were cultured on, and tested for sensitization against, monolayers of rat fibroblasts or thymus reticulum cells after 24 hours of incubation. The lymph node assay in syngeneic mice was used to measure the degree of sensitization against the rat cells. The results [2] are shown in Table 1. Spleen cells from normal mice produced the same lymph node index (about 6.5) whether they were sensitized against rat fibroblasts or reticulum cells. Hence, both cell types appear to be equally immunogenic for normal lymphocytes. In contrast, spleen cells from thymus-deprived B mice sensitized against fibroblasts manifested a markedly decreased ability to stimulate a lymph node response (index = 2.7). Incubation with reticulum cells, however, restored the response completely (index = 6.7). These results indicate that reticulum cells induced in spleen cells from thymus-deprived mice the capacity to become sensitized against rat antigens and stimulate a lymph node response in syngeneic recipient mice.

Previous studies of this laboratory indicated that the specificity of cell mediated immune reaction is based on a state of diversity among T-cells.[11–13] This was derived from experiments in which fibroblast monolayers of various histocompatibility phenotypes were used as cellular immunoadsorbents. Normal unsensitized lymphocytes were incubated on the monolayers for 30–120 minutes; the nonadherent lymphocytes were separated from those that adhered to the fibroblasts and were transferred for sensitization to fresh fibroblasts. The nonadherent lymphocytes were found to have a markedly reduced capacity to become sensitized to fibroblasts genetically identical to the immunoadsorbent fibroblasts although they retained the capacity to react against genetically nonrelated fibroblasts.[11]

The diversity thus found among T-lymphocytes with regard to receptors for cell-surface antigens was previously assumed to originate in the thymus. The prevailing theories for the lymphocyte diversity have been based on mechanisms involving active lymphocyte proliferation. The high rate of lymphocyte proliferation taking place within the fetal and neonatal thymus seemed therefore to support the assumption of the thymic origin of T-cell diversity. Yet, we obtained immune reactivity within 24 hours of interaction of precursor lymphocytes with thymus reticulum cells, a period that allows a few, if any, cell cycles. If the reactivity we measured is indeed specific (i.e. is based on a stage of diversity among T-cells) then diversity must have existed *prior* to the interaction of the lymphocytes with the thymus reticulum. The conclusion from this would be that immunologically incompetent precursor T-cells that acquire immunocompetence within the thymus do possess the capacity to synthesize specific receptors *prior* to their interaction with the reticulum cells. The thymus reticulum thus induces the capacity to respond to antigenic signals. The precursor T-cells, however, appear to be already diverse with regard to their potential ability to recognize antigens even before they differentiate within the thymus.

It is generally accepted that bone marrow stem cells give rise to both antibody-producing B-lymphocytes and to T-lymphocytes. One could have postulated that the two lymphocyte populations arise from the same pool of precursors. Accordingly, cells that randomly migrate to the thymus will acquire T-cell properties, whereas those reaching the spleen will differentiate to B-cells. It appears, however, that if diversity exists before the cells reach the thymus, then the precursors of T-cells and those of B-cells must constitute two distinct populations already in the bone marrow. This is because the receptors for antigens of B cells are immunoglobulins whereas the T-cell receptor in our system does not possess properties of a known immunoglobulin.[15]

Interactions Between T-lymphocytes and the Differentiation of Effector Cells

The differentiation of T-lymphocytes was shown to involve interaction between the thymus reticulum and precursor cells. T-lymphocytes may undergo further maturation after leaving the thymus due to a hormone-like substance secreted by the thymus.[16] The lymphocytes are now at a stage in which they can fully react to antigenic stimuli. Do such reactions involve cell interactions between T-lymphocytes? Experiments designed to assay for such interactions consisted of sensitizing T-lymphocytes *in vitro* on monolayers of syngeneic or allogeneic fibroblasts, and then assaying their effects *in vivo* following inoculation into the foot pads of animals syngeneic to the lymphocytes.[13, 17] The result was that sensitized lymphocytes caused enlargement of the draining lymph nodes. These lymph nodes were found to contain effector cells that caused specific lysis of target cells syngeneic to the sensitizing ones.

The lymphocytes that populated the enlarged lymph nodes and manifested effector activity could have derived from one or both of two sources. They could be the clonal progeny of the lymphocytes that were sensitized *in vitro*. Alternatively, they might be cells that were recruited from the recipient lymphocyte population and acquired effector properties following interaction with the sensitized lymphocytes. To differentiate between these two possibilities, experiments were done in which either the injected lymphocytes or the host rat were irradiated to inhibit cell replication.[3]

The result was that lymph node enlargement following sensitization of Lewis rat thymus lymphocytes on allogeneic BN, or xenogeneic C3H mouse fibroblasts was not prevented by irradiating (1000 R) the *in vitro* sensitized lymphocytes. On the other hand, irradiating the recipient (600 R) prevented lymph node enlargement and the appearance of cytotoxic effector cells. Hence, the effector lymphocytes in the enlarged lymph nodes are recipient cells that seem to have differentiated following a signal emitted by the *in vitro* sensitized T-lymphocytes. Whether or not this signal involves a cell to cell contact, or whether an extracellular substance is emitted from the sensitized lymphocytes remains an open question. The fact that the reaction is local tends to suggest a cell to cell interaction, although no direct evidence for this is as yet available.

To explore the nature of the recruiting and recruited cells, a mouse allogeneic system was investigated. The C57BL 3LL Lewis lung carcinoma was used.[18] Allografts of the 3LL tumor give lethal takes in C3H allogeneic recipients. We tested whether normal C3H thymus lymphocytes sensitized *in vitro* against alloantigens of C57BL will protect C3H recipients against the progressive growth of the C57BL 3LL tumor. C3H thymocytes were cultured *in vitro* on C57BL fibroblasts. The sensitized C3H lymphocytes were separated from the sensitizing fibroblasts and injected into the foot pads of syngeneic C3H mice. An enlarged lymph node response was obtained and allografts of the 3LL tumor were rejected by the C3H recipients (TABLE 2). This resistance cannot be attributed to the possible immunizing effect of C57BL fibroblasts that were carried over with the lymphocytes, since the injection of 10^4 C57BL fibroblasts did not induce resistance to the 3LL carcinoma in the C3H recipients. Experiments were then made to test whether the effector cells are the clonal

TABLE 2

RECRUITMENT OF T-LYMPHOCYTES IN THE REJECTION OF A TUMOR ALLOGRAFT

C3H Thymocytes *	C3H Recipients	% Mice Developing 3LL Tumors
1. anti-C57BL	normal	10 †
2. anti-C57BL, irradiated (2000 R)	normal	10 †
3. anti-C57BL	irradiated (600 R)	90
4. anti-C57BL	B mice	90
5. anti-C57BL spleen cells of B-mice	normal	100
6. unsensitized + C57BL fibroblasts (10^4)	normal	90

* C3H thymus or spleen cells from B mice were sensitized for 18 hours *in vitro* in the absence of serum against fibroblasts of C57BL origin. The sensitized lymphocytes (10^7) were then injected into the right foot pads of C3H recipients. These foot pads were injected 5 days later with 10^6 tumor cells.

† $P < 0.005$ compared to Group 6.

progeny of the sensitized lymphocytes or whether they are cells recruited from the recipient's lymphocyte population. It was found that lymphocytes which had been exposed to 2000 R following *in vitro* sensitization elicited resistance to the tumor allografts. On the other hand, when sensitized lymphocytes were injected to animals exposed previously to 600 R, resistance was not conferred. Hence, the effector cells were not the clonal descendants of the sensitized lymphocytes but were recruited by them within the lymph nodes of the recipient mouse. B mice were then used either as donors or as recipients to study the origin of participating lymphocytes. In neither case was resistance obtained. Hence, both the recruitor and recruited lymphocytes were thymus-derived lymphocytes. Thus, T-T interaction determined the production of T effector cells.

Do the interacting T-cells, the recruitors and the recruited, constitute distinct populations of T-cells? When the adherent population of T-lymphocytes, i.e. the subpopulation that recognizes the specific antigens of the fibroblast monolayer, is sensitized *in vitro* for 5 days it differentiates *in vitro* to specific effectors.[5, 6] Had the adherent population represented predominantly the "recruitors" of the previous experiments, this would have suggested that at least *in vitro,* the "recruitors" can themselves differentiate to effectors. An alternative interpretation could be that the "adherent" cells contained two distinct types of antigen specific cells, the antigen-recognizing and the potential effector cells. Following the sensitization of the antigen-recognizing cell, the potential effector is signalled in culture to develop to a killer. In fact, a bicellular interaction between antigen-sensitive and potential effectors in the *in-vitro* system of sensitization leading to the production of specific killers was demonstrated previously in our laboratory.[19] Furthermore, it appears that, although the antigen-sensitive and the effector cell recognize the same antigenic specificity, the receptors for cell surface antigens of the two cells behave differently. Recognition by the antigen-sensitive cell can be blocked by soluble factors (antigens) whereas the recognition of the effector cell cannot. This may support, although certainly does not prove, the possibility of two distinct T-cell populations.

Be the nature of the interacting cells as it may, the type of cell cooperation just described seems to control the extent of the immune reaction. It is based on signals that trigger the production of specific effectors, thus representing a system of cell interactions augmenting cell-mediated immune responses.

Suppressor T-cells Control the Differentiation of Effector Lymphocytes

The question of whether the differentiation of effector T-cells is controlled also by lymphocytes that exert a suppressive, as distinct from an augmenting effect, was studied in experiments using lymphocytes from tumor-bearing mice.[4] Spleen cells from C57BL mice bearing the 3LL lung carcinoma were investigated. When tested *in vitro,* such spleen cells were found to have a strong cytotoxic effect on the tumor target cells. Pretreatment of such cell populations with anti-θ serum plus complement abolished the cytotoxic activity. Hence, mice bearing the syngeneic 3LL tumor develop immune effector T-cells. To test the effect of these lymphocytes on tumor growth *in vivo,* tumor cells were mixed with spleen cells from either normal or tumor-bearing mice and the mixed cell population was inoculated into the foot pads of C57BL mice. The result was that the rate of growth and incidence of tumor metastases in mice that received immune spleen cells was greater than in those inoculated with normal spleen cells (TABLE 3). To test the nature of the immune cells that caused enhancement of tumor growth, anti-θ serum was applied prior to cell inoculation. The removal of θ-positive cells diminished the enhancing effect. In fact, even spleen cell populations from normal donors had an enhancing effect, relative to the growth of tumors when no spleen cells were inoculated. This relative enhancement by normal lymphocytes was also inhibited by anti-θ serum.

T-lymphocytes from tumor-bearing mice could enhance the growth of tumors by either of two mechanisms: (1) such lymphocytes could by themselves directly stimulate the growth of tumor cells, or (2) they could suppress mechanisms of the recipient mice that might otherwise inhibit tumor growth.

To distinguish between these possibilities, recipient mice were irradiated with either 450 R or 750 R and assayed for the effects of immune spleen cells

TABLE 3

T-LYMPHOCYTES FROM TUMOR-BEARING OR NORMAL MICE ENHANCE THE INCIDENCE OF 3LL TUMORS IN RECIPIENT MICE *

Origin of Donor Spleen Cells	Incidence of Tumors at Day 14 (%) — Treatment of Spleen Cells with Serum + Complement: Normal Serum	Anti-θ Serum
tumor-bearing mice	100	70
normal mice	30	0

* 5×10^4 3LL tumor cells were mixed with 5×10^6 C57BL spleen cells from tumor-bearing or normal mice and injected into the right foot pads of C57BL mice irradiated with 450 R one day earlier.

on tumor growth. We found that spleen cells from tumor-bearing mice markedly enhanced the growth of tumors in recipients irradiated with 450 R. Recipients irradiated with 750 R, however, demonstrated an equally rapid growth of tumor cells, regardless of whether or not they were injected with lymphocytes from normal or tumor-bearing mice (TABLE 4).

Hence, T-lymphocytes from tumor bearing mice appeared to facilitate tumor growth by suppressing a radiosensitive antitumor mechanism in the recipient mice.[4]

It thus appears that the control of host resistance to tumor growth is mediated by suppressor T-cells that may suppress the differentiation of specific effector cells. When the latter are suppressed, tumor growth is enhanced. What, then, is the nature of the suppressor T-lymphocyte compared to the effector T-lymphocyte? One possibility is that the two populations of T-lymphocytes differ in their life span. To test this we thymectomized adult mice. One would expect short-lived T-lymphocytes to gradually decrease in number following thymectomy. If the suppressor T-cells are short-lived cells, then the growth of the 3LL tumor in adult thymectomized animals should show a reduced rate compared to normal intact animals. In the absence of suppres-

TABLE 4

EFFECT ON TUMOR DEVELOPMENT OF SPLEEN CELLS FROM NORMAL OR TUMOR-BEARING MICE IN IRRADIATED RECIPIENT MICE *

Origin of Donor Spleen Cells	Incidence of Tumors at 14 Days (%) — Irradiated Recipients: 450 R	750 R
tumor-bearing mice	100	100
normal mice	20	100

* 2.5×10^6 C57BL spleen cells were mixed with 5×10^4 3LL tumor cells and injected into the right foot pads of C57BL mice which had been irradiated one day earlier.

sors, the effectors will exert a stronger effect and decrease tumor growth. Alternatively, if the effectors are short-lived cells, enhanced growth would be expected following adult thymectomy. As seen in TABLE 5 adult thymectomy resulted in a significant reduction of tumor metastases; therefore, resistance to tumor growth seems to be regulated by short-lived T-cells that act on effector cells. If, as seems likely, the effectors are also thymus-derived, then a cellular interaction between suppressor T- and effector T-cells seems to control tumor growth.

Suppressor T-cells were recently claimed to regulate antibody production. Furthermore, with regard to thymus-independent antigens (i.e. polyvinyl pyrrolidone—PVP), suppressor T-cells were found to be short-lived cells, since adult thymectomy resulted in an increased antibody production to such antigens.[20, 21] In the cases of thymus-independent antigens, it is most probable that the suppressor T-cells act on B-lymphocytes. The same T-B suppressing interaction appears to operate in some cases of tolerance to thymus-dependent antigens.[22] In our system, however, we seem to be dealing with suppressor T-cells that

TABLE 5

EFFECT OF ADULT THYMECTOMY ON THE NUMBER OF LUNG METASTASES *

Time Between Thymectomy and Tumor Challenge	Mean No. of Lung Metastases per Mouse ± S.E. †		P value
	Control	Thymectomized	
2 weeks	23.0 ± 3.9	9.6 ± 2.3	< 0.01
5 weeks	42.7 ± 9.9	20.5 ± 4.6	< 0.05
24 weeks	18.9 ± 3.3	6.8 ± 1.6	< 0.005

* Normal 6-week-old mice were thymectomized and inoculated subcutaneously with 0.5×10^6 3LL tumor cells after various time intervals. The number of lung metastases was scored three weeks after tumor challenge.

† S.E.—Standard error.

act, in all probability, on effector T-cells. Whether or not this interaction involves cell to cell contact, or whether it is mediated by cell products is still an open question. So is the question of whether the T-lymphocytes of tumor bearing mice that mediate cytotoxicity *in vitro* constitute a population distinct from that which mediates suppression *in vivo*.

Thus, two types of cell interaction between T-lymphocytes seem to control the differentiation of effector cells: T-lymphocytes can signal the formation of effector T-cells; T-lymphocytes can also suppress the formation of effectors. What is the relation between subpopulations of T-cells interacting in the control of cell mediated immunity, and those recently described with regard to other properties of T-cells? Thus, spleen-seeking and lymph-node-seeking T lymphocytes were described as manifesting different properties.[23] Whereas both are reactive to con-A, only the lymph-node-seeking population seems to be equally reactive to phytohemagglutinin (PHA). The latter seems to have a higher density of θ antigen, and seems to represent the recirculating component of T-cells. Since such T-lymphocytes might represent the short-lived cells, one may seek among them the suppressor T-cells that control the differentiation of effector cells. This gains further support from preliminary observations claiming that the precursors of the effector cells respond to con-A but not to PHA.[23] It is clear that the precise nature of interacting T-cells invites further analysis. In conclusion: differentiation of T-cells capable of responding to cell-surface antigens and the extent of differentiation of T-effectors in response to antigenic stimuli, depends upon processes of cell interaction. The *in vitro* induction of T-cell properties in spleen cells of **B** mice by thymus reticulum indicates that the precursors of T-cells are a diverse population with regard to their cell receptors for antigen, prior to their interaction with thymus tissue. The extent of production of specific T-effector is controlled by two types of T-cells: one that signals the production of effectors, the other that suppresses it. Hence, the functional differentiation of the T-lymphocyte immune system is regulated by a number of cellular interactions. These interactions, analogous to some of those observed during histogenesis in the embryo, demonstrate that cellular control of differentiation is probably a general phenomenon occurring throughout the life time of the organism.

References

1. WEISS, P. 1939. Principles of Development. Henry Holt & Co. New York, N.Y.
2. WEKERLE, H., I. R. COHEN & M. FELDMAN. 1973. Thymus reticulum cell cultures confer T cell properties on spleen cells from thymus deprived animals. Eur. J. Immunol. **3:** 745–748.
3. COHEN, I. R. 1973. The recruitment of specific effector lymphocytes by antigen reactive lymphocytes in cell mediated autosensitization and allosensitization reactions. Cell. Immunol. **8:** 209–220.
4. TREVES, A. J., C. CARNAUD, N. TRAININ, M. FELDMAN & I. R. COHEN. 1974. Enhancing T lymphocytes from tumor bearing mice suppress host resistance to a syngeneic tumor. Eur. J. Immunol. In press.
5. GINSBURG, H. 1968. Graft-versus-host reaction in tissue culture. I. Lysis of monolayers of embryo mouse cells from strains differing in the H-2 histocompatibility locus by rat lymphocytes sensitized *in vitro*. Immunology **14:** 621–635.
6. BERKE, G., W. AX, H. GINSBURG & M. FELDMAN. 1969. Graft reaction in tissue culture. II. Quantification of the lytic action on mouse fibroblasts by rat lymphocytes sensitized on mouse embryo monolayers. Immunology **16:** 643–657.
7. COHEN, I. R., A. GLOBERSON & M. FELDMAN. 1971. Rejection of tumor allograft by mouse spleen cells sensitized in vitro. J. Exp. Med. **133:** 821–833.
8. COHEN, I. R., A. GLOBERSON & M. FELDMAN. 1971. Autosensitization *in vitro*. J. Exp. Med. **133:** 834–845.
9. COHEN, I. R. & H. WEKERLE. 1972. Autosensitization of lymphocytes against thymus reticulum cells. Science **176:** 1324–1325.
10. COHEN, I. R. & H. WEKERLE. 1973. Regulation of autosensitization. The immune activation and specific inhibition of self-recognizing T lymphocytes. J. Exp. Med. **137:** 224–238.
11. WEKERLE, H., P. LONAI & M. FELDMAN. 1972. Fractionation of antigen reactive cells on a cellular immunoadsorbent: Factors determining recognition of antigens by cells. Proc. Nat. Acad. Sci. U.S. **69:** 1620–1624.
12. ALTMAN, A., I. R. COHEN & M. FELDMAN. 1973. Normal T cell receptors for alloantigens. Cell. Immunol. **7:** 134–142.
13. LONAI, P., A. ELIRAZ, H. WEKERLE & M. FELDMAN. 1973. Depletion of specific graft-versus-host reactivity following adsorption of nonsensitized lymphocytes on allogeneic fibroblasts. Transplantation **15:** 368–374.

14. BURNET, M. 1969. Cellular Immunology. : 367. Melbourne University Press. Melbourne, Australia.
15. WEKERLE, H. & M. FELDMAN. 1973. Diversity of T cells recognizing transplantation antigens: Mechanism of antigen recognition. Transplant. Proc. **1:** 133–135.
16. ROTTER, V., A. GLOBERSON, I. NAKAMURA & N. TRAININ. 1973. Studies on characterization of the lymphoid target cell for activity of a thymus humoral factor. J. Exp. Med. **138:** 130–142.
17. TREVES, A. J. & I. R. COHEN. 1974. Recruitment of effector T lymphocytes against a tumor allograft by T lymphocytes sensitized *in vitro*. J. Nat. Cancer Inst. **51:** 1919–1925.
18. COHEN, I. R. & A. J. TREVES. 1974. Recruitment of effector lymphocytes in autosensitization and transplantation reactions. *In* Lymphocyte Recognition and Effector Mechanisms : 633–638. K. Lindahl-Kiessling & D. Osoba, Eds. Academic Press. New York, N.Y.
19. LONAI, P. & M. FELDMAN. 1970. Cooperation of lymphoid cells in an in vitro graft reaction system. The role of the thymus cells. Transplantation **10:** 372–381.
20. KERBEL, R. S. & D. EIDINGER. 1971. Variable effects of anti-lymphocyte serum on humoral antibody formation: Role of thymus dependency of antigen. J. Immunol. **106:** 917–926.
21. KERBEL, R. S. & D. EIDINGER. 1972. Enhanced immune responsiveness to a thymus-independent antigen early after adult thymectomy: Evidence for short-lived inhibitory thymus-derived cells. Eur. J. Immunol. **2:** 114–118.
22. ZAN-BAR, I., D. NACHTIGAL & M. FELDMAN. 1974. Mechanisms in immune tolerance: I. A specific block of immunological memory in HSA tolerant mice. Cell. Immunol. **10:** 19–30.
23. STOBO, J. D. & E. W. PAUL. 1973. Functional heterogeneity of murine lymphoid cells. III. Differential responsiveness of T cells to phytohemagglutinin and con A as a probe for T cell subsets. J. Immunol. **110:** 362–375.

DISCUSSION OF THE PAPER

DR. N. TALAL: To go back to the blocking experiments, you told us that it was not an autoantibody for the reasons that it does not react with the target cell. Does it contain antigenic fragments, or might it be a thymic hormonal factor?

DR. M. FELDMAN: No, had it been a thymic humoral factor, then it would not show blocking. In all probability these are soluble antigens which are being shed off normally. I personally believe that under normal conditions antigens are being shed continuously from the cell membranes; these block receptors for "self."

THE ROLE OF THE THYMUS IN SPONTANEOUS AUTOIMMUNE THYROIDITIS *

Noel R. Rose

Department of Immunology and Microbiology
Wayne State University School of Medicine
Detroit, Michigan 48201

There is a significant body of evidence linking thymic dysfunction with autoimmunity in animals and man. For instance, in myasthenia gravis thymomas are found in about 15% of cases. A certain proportion of patients with Hashimoto's disease and systemic lupus erythematosus seem to have thymic enlargement, atrophic thymuses, or thymic germinal centers.[15, 18, 19] Alarcon-Segovia *et al.*[1] reported two cases in which systemic lupus erythematosis developed after thymectomy.

NZB mice present the best studied examples of spontaneously occurring autoimmunity in animals. These mice develop Coombs-positive hemolytic anemia at three to nine months of age. When NZB mice are crossed with NZW mice, the F_1 hybrids (B/W) often develop positive LE cell tests similar to those seen in human systemic lupus erythematosus, as well as lupus-like nephritis. Quite early in the study of these animals, Burnet and Holmes[5] suggested that the presence of germinal centers in the thymic medulla of NZB mice indicated that some thymic dysfunction is associated with the development of autoimmune disease. It was found that neonatal thymectomy of NZB mice led to earlier onset of autoimmune disease, characterized by anemia and the premature appearance of a direct Coombs test.[9] A naturally occurring thymocytotoxic antibody was detected in young NZB mice by Shirai and Mellors.[25] In experiments by Steinberg *et al.*,[28] when young B/W thymus was transplanted to neonatally thymectomized F_1 recipients, the accelerated development of antinuclear antibodies was prevented. Older B/W thymuses were ineffective. These results suggest some deficiency in the thymus of older B/W mice with respect to the induction or maintenance of tolerance.

NZB and B/W mice are not the only strains that develop autoimmunity following neonatal thymectomy. Yunis *et al.*[41] described the development of positive Coombs tests in neonatally thymectomized C_{57}Bl/Ks and A mice. Teague *et al.*[29] found that many A/Jax mice developed antideoxynucleoprotein antibodies spontaneously after 22 weeks of age. If thymus cells from young A/Jax mice were injected into older animals, the autoantibodies either disappeared or decreased in titer. The authors suggested that antibodies to nucleoprotein developed during aging due to failure of a thymic homeostatic function.

For several years we have been studying two examples of spontaneous autoimmune thyroiditis in animals. The obese strain (OS) of White Leghorn chickens was first described by VanTeinhoven and Cole.[31] They noticed that a few females of the closed flock of Cornell chickens spontaneously developed signs of hypothyroidism. When examined histologically, the thyroid glands

* These studies were supported in part by Public Health Service Research Grant CA02357 from the National Cancer Institute.

showed lymphocytic infiltration with formation of germinal centers. Extensive investigations by Witebsky *et al.*,[39, 17, 23] have established that the pathogenesis of this disease is autoimmune. Genetically, the incidence of disease is related to the major histocompatibility (B) locus of chickens.[24] Other controlling factors are also involved, however.

Cole *et al.*[7] and Wick *et al.*[37, 38] examined the effects of surgical bursectomy and thymectomy on thyroiditis of the OS chicken. Neonatal bursectomy reduced or entirely prevented the disease. Chicks reinjected with autologous bursa cells developed disease equivalent to that of untreated controls, although less antibody was detected in their sera.[20] Thymectomy in one experiment led to an increased severity and earlier onset of thyroiditis. In a second experiment, however, sham thymectomized controls showed no significant difference from neonatally thymectomized animals. Therefore, Welch and Kite and I [35] performed additional experiments to determine the effect of neonatal thymectomy on OS chickens. Two modifications of the earlier experimental protocols were introduced. First, the chickens were sacrificed at an earlier age (four weeks rather than seven weeks) in order that a significant increase in the severity of disease could be more reliably determined. Secondly, additional controls were included to study the possible effects of trauma to the thyroid gland during surgery. The thyroid pathology scores and results of thyroid antibody determinations by the tanned cell hemagglutination tests (HA) are shown in FIGURES 1a and 1b.

Neonatal thymectomy led to a significant increase in thyroid infiltration. The mean antibody titer was also raised. These effects were not due to trauma associated with surgical removal of the caudal thymus lobes adjacent to the thyroid. On the other hand, chickens from which all thymus tissue, except for the two most caudal lobes, was removed were similar to completely thymectomized animals.

The occurrence of spontaneous thyroiditis in older Buffalo strain (BUF) rats was first reported by Hajdu and Rona in 1969.[14] The feeding of methylcholanthrene increases the unique susceptibility of BUF rats to this genetically-determined disease.[11, 12] Its autoimmune nature was established by Silverman and Rose.[26] Like OS chickens, BUF rats developed thyroid autoantibodies as well as lymphocytic infiltrates of their thyroid glands. Experiments to determine the effects of adult and neonatal thymectomy on the incidence of spontaneous thyroiditis in BUF rats were undertaken in collaboration with Silverman.[27] The results are given in FIGURES 2a and b.

The incidence of disease in untreated BUF rats 16–20-weeks old was about 13%. This figure did not seem to be increased by sham thymectomy. Complete neonatal thymectomy sharply raised the incidence, however, whereas incomplete neonatal thymectomy had a moderate effect. Adult thymectomy performed at 21 days of age resulted in rats that did not differ from the untreated group. Further evidence of the role of the thymus in spontaneous autoimmune thyroiditis in the BUF rat is provided by the data in FIGURE 3. When the severity of thyroiditis was plotted against the amount of thyroid tissue found at autopsy, a negative correlation resulted. Of 10 rats with 65 mg of thymus remnants, all but three had moderate to severe disease, whereas only two of nine rats having more than 75 mg of thymus tissue had disease.

Burnet [5] first suggested that the thymus may exert an inhibitory function over aberrant clones of self-reacting lymphocytes that arise, perhaps, by somatic mutation. Allison *et al.*[3] have advanced the hypothesis that thymic-

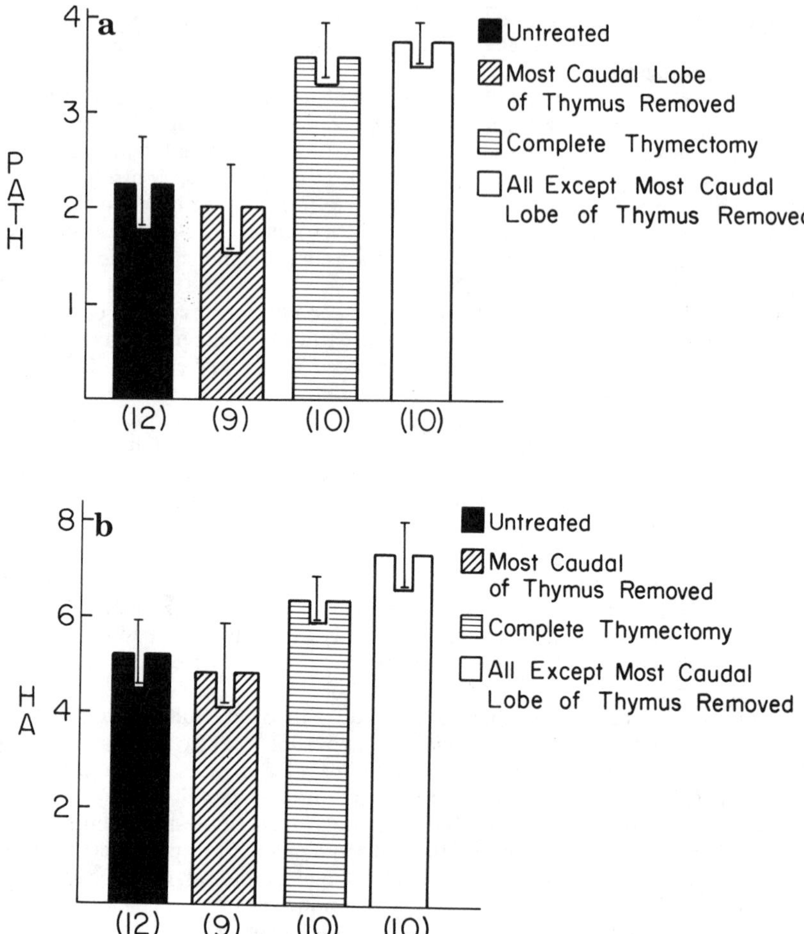

FIGURE 1. The effect of surgical thymectomy on the development of spontaneous autoimmune thyroiditis in OS chickens. Newly hatched OS chickens were divided into 4 groups. Group 1 was not treated. In group 2, the 2 most caudal thymus lobes adjacent to the thyroid were surgically removed. A complete thymectomy was carried out on the birds in group 3. In group 4 all of the thymus except the two most caudal lobes was excised. Following operation, the birds grew for 4½ weeks and were sacrificed. The thyroid histopathology scores (graded on the basis of 0 to 4+) are shown in FIGURE 1a, and the results of the tanned cell hemagglutination test with chicken thyroid extract (titer calculated as $\log_2$) are shown in FIGURE 1b. The figures in parenthesis indicate the number of animals in each group. The data are taken from P. C. Welch. 1972. *The role of the thymus and delayed hypersensitivity in spontaneous and experimental autoimmune thyroiditis in the chicken.* Ph.D. Dissertation, State University of New York at Buffalo.

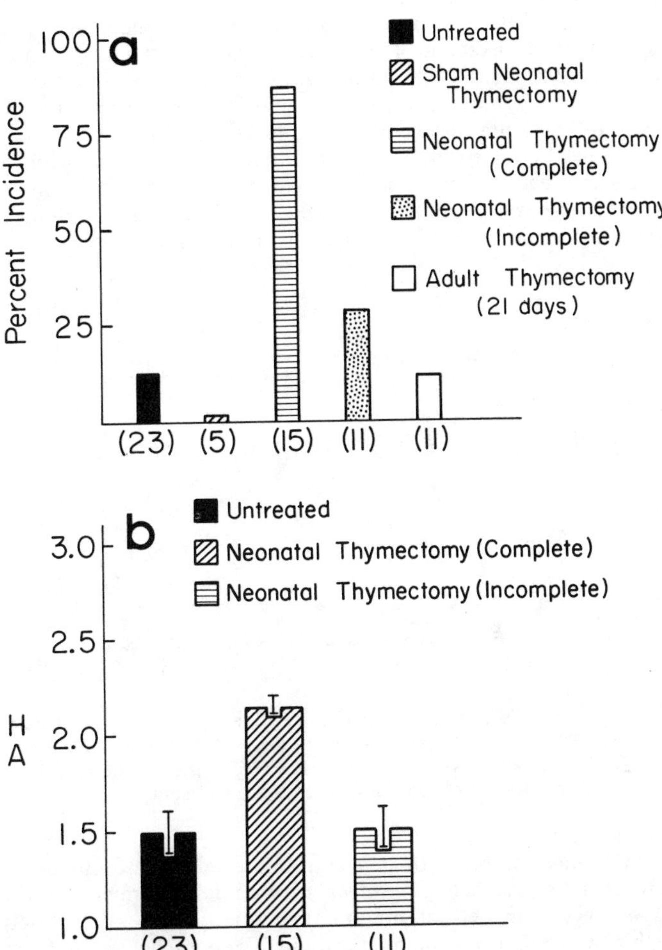

FIGURE 2. Effect of neonatal or adult thymectomy on spontaneous thyroiditis in BUF rats. Animals were surgically thymectomized or sham thymectomized at birth, or after 21 days, and were sacrificed at 14 to 16 weeks of age. By means of a "double blind" test, the animals were classified as positive or negative for thyroid histopathology, and the results given in Figure 2a. Tanned cell hemagglutinin tests were used to measure antibodies to rat thyroid extract, FIGURE 2b. The data are taken from D. A. Silverman. 1973. *Autoimmunity in Buffalo strain rats.* Ph.D. Dissertation, State University of New York at Buffalo.

derived (T) lymphocytes exert a double regulatory effect on autoimmunity. They suggested that T-cells are normally unresponsive to self-antigens and therefore do not cooperate with B-cells. The concept is similar to the one suggested by Clagett & Weigle [6] who found that T-cells are made more readily unresponsive than antibody-forming B-lymphocytes. Secondly, T-cells may exert a specific feedback control of autoantibody formation. As an example of this control, lymphoid cells from NZB mice transferred to F_1 recipients produced antibody against erythrocytes only if the suspensions were first treated with anti-θ serum and complement to destroy T-cells.[2]

Autoimmune thyroiditis induced by immunization with thyroglobulin of the same species is prevented by neonatal thymectomy of the chicken [16] and the rat.[4] The response to thyroglobulin seems to depend upon thymus-derived cells. We have recently found that lethally radiated mice reconstituted with

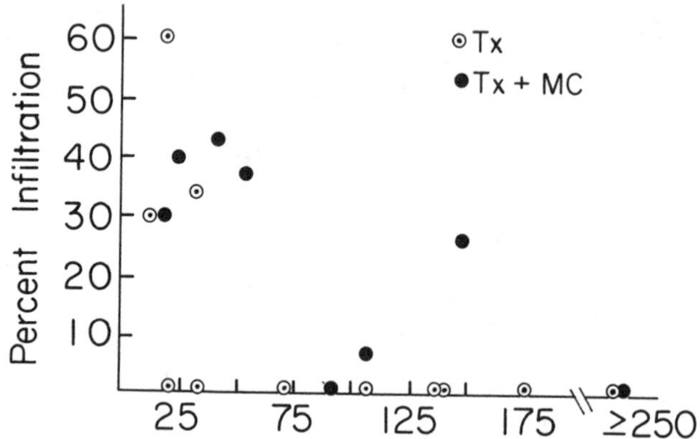

FIGURE 3. A comparison of the weight of residual thymus tissue in partially thymectomized BUF rats with the percent of the thyroid gland infiltrated by mononuclear cells. Tx=neonatally thymectomized; MC=fed methylcholanthrene. The numbers at the bottom of the figure represent thymus weight (mg).

syngeneic bone marrow cells (treated with anti-θ serum and complement) fail to respond to mouse thyroglobulin given with complete Freund adjuvant.[31]

The spontaneous models of autoimmune thyroiditis lend themselves to a study of the two proposed functions of the T-cell as helper and suppressor. In induced thyroiditis, thymectomy reduces the severity of disease because of the removal of helper T-cells. In the case of spontaneously developing disease, only small numbers of T-cells seem to be necessary to initiate the autoimmune response. The helper function of T-cells comes into play at the onset of immunocompetence. Removal of the thymus at birth, therefore, ablates only the inhibitory function of the thymus and is reflected in the increased incidence and severity of disease. Thymectomy of adults has relatively little effect on the course of the disease probably because T-cells have already migrated to the peripheral lymphoid tissues.

A genetic predisposition or irradiation is required to provide reactive populations of helper T- and B-cells unless deliberate immunization is performed. Neonatal thymectomy of normal White Leghorn chickens or of Lewis or

Fischer rats does not produce spontaneous thyroiditis. Penhale *et al.*[22] recently reported that Wistar rats subjected to repeated low doses of irradiation and to thymectomy develop typical autoimmune thyroiditis. Certain strains of mice also exhibit thyroiditis following early thymectomy, whereas other strains were refractory to the treatment.[21] In most animals, removal of the thymus by itself is insufficient to initiate an autoimmune response to the thyroid.

We recognize several alternative explanations for the augmenting effect of thymectomy on spontaneous autoimmune thyroiditis in the chicken and rat. Although a virus has not been connected with either of these conditions, it is possible that some infectious agent is involved.[42] If such were the case, one must imagine that thymectomy might increase susceptibility to the pathological effects while, in the chicken, bursectomy reduces it. An agent dependent upon bursa-derived or B-cells is a corollary requirement. Another explanation is that neonatal thymectomy allows greater proliferation of B-cells, perhaps by simply allowing more space in peripheral lymphoid organs. B-cell-mediated immunological responses would therefore be enhanced by thymectomy. Finally, it is possible that the thymus or thymus-derived lymphocytes suppress the autoimmune response to thyroglobulin. This conjecture receives support from recent investigations demonstrating a suppressor effect of the thymus or thymic factors in initiation of humoral antibody or cellular responses.[10, 14] Further investigations designed to demonstrate directly a possible suppressive effect of the thymus on the autoimmune response to thyroglobulin are presently underway in our laboratory.

A crucial question still to be resolved is whether the inhibitory action of the thymus on the development of autoimmunity is antigen-specific. Wick *et al.*[36] found that thymectomized OS chickens showed an increased incidence of autoantibodies to the liver and kidney. Some neonatally thymectomized BUF rats had weak antinuclear antibodies. There is no evidence that neonatal thymectomy results in wide-spread production of autoantibodies to many self-constituents, however, although such explanations have been put forth to explain the development of postthymectomy wasting disease.[8, 40] It seems likely that the production of one or more autoantibodies following thymectomy depends upon the particular autoimmune potential of the animal.

The ability of mice to respond to injections of mouse thyroglobulin is determined in a large measure by a principal gene linked to the major histocompatibility locus, H-2.[32] It has been localized at or near the previously described lr-la locus.[30] The ability to respond well to thyroglobulin can be transferred to irradiated, marrow-reconstituted recipients by thymus cells if taken from good responder donor mice. On the other hand, mice given the thymus of a poor responder strain responded poorly even after receiving marrow cells of a high responder strain.[32] In view of these observations and the studies described above, it is quite possible that genetic control determines the suppressor function of the thymus as well as its role of providing helper lymphocytes. We may eventually be able to separate these thymic functions and assign them to distinct cellular or humoral factors.

These results suggest the hypothesis that the development of autoantibodies may result from the failure of a normal, thymus-dependent regulatory mechanism designed to prevent the proliferation of autoimmune lymphocytes; that the ability of thymic control to cope with autoimmune potential may decrease during aging; and that the efficiency of thymic regulation is under genetic control.

Summary

In two models of genetically determined, spontaneous autoimmune thyroiditis, neonatal thymectomy increases the incidence and severity of disease. The simplest explanation is that the thymus, or thymus-derived cells, normally exert a suppressive effect on the autoimmune response to thyroglobulin in addition to the helper function that is necessary to initiate the autoimmune reaction.

References

1. Alarcon-Serovia, D., R. F. Galbraith, J. E. Maldonado & F. M. Howard. 1963. Systemic lupus erythematosis following thymectomy for myasthenia gravis. Lancet **1:** 662–665.
2. Allison, A. C. 1971. Unresponsiveness to self antigens. Lancet **ii:** 1401–1403.
3. Allison, A. C., A. M. Denman & R. D. Barnes. 1971. Cooperating and controlling functions of thymus-derived lymphocytes in relations to autoimmunity. Lancet **ii:** 135–140.
4. Busci, R. A. & H. R. Strausser. 1972. The effect of neonatal thymectomy on the induction of experimental autoimmune thyroiditis in the rat. Experientia **82:** 194–195.
5. Burnet, F. M. & M. C. Holmes. 1964. Thymic changes in the mouse strain NZB in relation to the autoimmune state. J. Pathol. Bacteriol. **88:** 229–241.
6. Clagett, J. A. & W. O. Weigle. 1974. Roles of T and B lymphocytes in the termination of unresponsiveness to autologous thyroglobulin in mice. J. Exp. Med. **139:** 643–660.
7. Cole, R. K., J. H. Kite & E. Witebsky. 1968. Hereditary autoimmune thyroiditis in the fowl. Science **160:** 1357–1358.
8. deVries, M. J., L. M. vanPutten, H. Balner & D. W. vanBekkum. 1964. Lesions suggerant une reactivite auto-immune chez des souris atteintes de la "runt disease" apres thymectomie neonatale. Rev. Fran. Etudes Clin. Biol. **9:** 381–397.
9. East, J., M. A. B. DeSousa, D. M. V. Parrott & H. Jaquet. 1967. Consequences of neonatal thymectomy in New Zealand black mice. Clin. Exp. Immunol. **2:** 203–215.
10. Gershon, R. K., P. Cohen, R. Hercen & S. A. Liebhaber. 1972. Suppressor T cells. J. Immunol. **108:** 586–590.
11. Glover, E. L. & M. D. Reuber. 1968. Chronic thyroiditis in Buffalo strain rats ingesting methylcholanthrene. Arch. Pathol. **86:** 542–544.
12. Glover, E. L., M. D. Reuber & E. F. Godfrey. 1969. Methylcholanthrene-induced thyroiditis susceptibility of Buffalo strain rats. Arch. Environ. Health **18:** 901–903.
13. Ha, T.-Y. & B. H. Waksman. 1973. Role of the thymus in tolerance X. Suppressor activity of antigen-stimulated rat thymocytes transferred to normal recipients. J. Immunol. **110:** 1290–1299.
14. Hajdu, A. & G. Rona. 1969. Spontaneous thyroiditis in laboratory rats. Experientia **25:** 1325–1327.
15. Irvine, W. J. 1970. The thymus in autoimmune disease. Proc. Roy. Soc. Med. **63:** 718–722.
16. Jankovic, B. D., M. Isoaneski, L. Popeskovic & K. Mitrovic. 1965. Experimental allergic thyroiditis (and parathyroiditis) in neonatally thymectomized chickens. Participation of the thymus in development of disease. Intern. Arch. Allergy Appl. Immunol. **26:** 18–33.
17. Kite, J. H., G. Wick, B. Twarog & E. Witebsky. 1969. Spontaneous thyroidi-

tis in an obese strain of chickens. II. Investigations on the development of the disease. J. Immunol. **103:** 1331–1341.

18. LARRSON, O. 1963. Thymoma and systemic lupus erythematosus in the same patient. Lancet **2:** 665–666.
19. MCKAY, I. E. & P. DEGAIT. 1963. Thymic "Germinal Center" and plasma cells in systemic lupus erythematosus. Lancet **2:** 667.
20. NILSSON, L.-A. & N. R. ROSE. 1972. Restoration of autoimmune thyroiditis in bursectomized-irradiated OS chickens by bursa cells. Immunology **22:** 13–23.
21. NISHIZUKA, Y., Y. TANAKA, T. SAKAKURA & A. KOJIMA. 1973. Murine thyroiditis induced by neonatal thymectomy. Experientia **29:** 1396–1398.
22. PENHALE, W. J., A. FARMER, R. P. MCKENNA & W. J. IRVINE. 1973. Spontaneous thyroiditis in thymectomized and irradiated Wistar rats. Clin. Exp. Immunol. **15:** 225–236.
23. ROSE, N. R., J. H. KITE, D. T. FLANAGAN & E. WITEBSKY. 1971. *In* Cellular interactions in the immune response. 2nd Intern. Convoc. Immunol., 1970. : 264–281. Karger. Basel, Switzerland.
24. ROSE, N. R., J. H. KITE, A. O. VLADUTIU, V. TOMAZIC & L. D. BACON. 1973. Genetic aspects of autoimmune thyroiditis. Intern. Arch. Allergy & Applied Immunol. **45:** 138–149.
25. SHIRAI, T. & R. C. MELLORS. 1971. Natural thymocytotoxic autoantibody and reactive antigen in NZB black and other mice. Proc. Nat. Acad. Sci. U.S. **68:** 1412–1415.
26. SILVERMAN, D. A. & N. R. ROSE. 1971. Autoimmunity in methylcholanthrene-induced and spontaneous thyroiditis in Buffalo strain rats. Proc. Soc. Exp. Biol. Med. **138:** 579–584.
27. SILVERMAN, D. A. & N. R. ROSE. 1974. Neonatal thymectomy increases the incidence of spontaneous and methylcholanthrene enhanced thyroiditis in rats. Science. **184:** 162.
28. STEINBERG, A. D., L. D. LAW & N. TALAL. 1970. The Role of NZB/NZW F_1 thymus in experimental tolerance and autoimmunity. Arthritis Rheumat. **13:** 369–377.
29. TEAGUE, P. O. & G. J. FRIOU. 1969. Antinuclear antibodies in mice. II. Transmission with spleen cells; inhibition with thymus or spleen cells. Immunology **17:** 665–675.
30. TOMAZIC, V., N. R. ROSE & D. C. SHREFFLER. 1974. Autoimmune murine thyroiditis. IV. Localization of genetic control of the immune response. J. Immunol. **112:** 965–969.
31. VANTIENHOVEN, A. & R. K. COLE. 1962. Endocrine disturbances in obese chickens. Anat. Rec. **142:** 111–122.
32. VLADUTIU, A. O. & N. R. ROSE. 1971. Autoimmune murine thyroiditis: Relation to histocompatibility (H-2) type. Science **174:** 1137–1139.
33. VLADUTIU, A. O. & N. R. ROSE. 1974. Cell transfer studies in murine thyroiditis. Fed. Proc. Am. Soc. Exp. Biol. **58:** 3433.
34. WEIGLE, W. O. 1971. Recent observations and concepts in immunological unresponsiveness and autoimmunity. Clin. Exp. Immunol. **9:** 437–447.
35. WELCH, P., N. R. ROSE & J. H. KITE. 1973. Neonatal thymectomy increases spontaneous autoimmune thyroiditis. J. Immunol. **110:** 575–577.
36. WICK, G. 1970. The effect of bursectomy, thymectomy, and x-irradiation in the incidence of precipitating liver and kidney autoantibodies in chicken of the obese strain (OS). Clin. Exp. Immunol. **7:** 187–199.
37. WICK, G., J. H. KITE & E. WITEBSKY. 1970. Spontaneous thyroiditis in the obese strain of chicken. IV. The effect of thymectomy and thymo-bursectomy on the development of the disease. J. Immunol. **104:** 54–62.
38. WICK, G., J. H. KITE, R. K. COLE & E. WITEBSKY. 1970. Spontaneous thyroiditis in the obese strain of chickens. III. The effect of bursectomy on the development of the disease. J. Immunol. **104:** 45–53.

39. WITEBSKY, E., J. H. KITE, G. WICK & R. K. COLE. 1969. Spontaneous thyroiditis in an obese strain of chickens. I. The demonstration of circulating autoantibodies. J. Immunol. **103:** 708–715.
40. YUNIS, E. J., R. HONG, M. A. GREIVE, C. MARTINEZ, E. A. CORNELIUS & R. A. GOOD. 1967. Post-thymectomy wasting associated with autoimmune phenomenon. J. Exp. Med. **125:** 945–966.
41. YUNIS, E. J., P. O. TEAGUE, O. STUTMAN & R. A. GOOD. 1969. Post-thymectomy autoimmune phenomena in mice. II. Morphologic observations. Lab. Invest. **20:** 46–61.
42. ZEIGEL, R. F., A. L. BARRON, J. H. KITE & E. WITEBSKY. 1970. Avian Diseases **14:** 617.

PART III. PREPARATION AND CHARACTERIZATION OF THYMIC EXTRACTS

PURIFICATION AND PROPERTIES OF BOVINE THYMOSIN *

John A. Hooper, Mildred C. McDaniel, Gary B. Thurman, Geraldine H. Cohen, Richard S. Schulof, and Allan L. Goldstein

Division of Biochemistry
University of Texas Medical Branch
Galveston, Texas 77550

INTRODUCTION

Major advances in our understanding of the role of the thymus gland and its endocrine secretions in the ontogenesis and homeostasis of the lymphoid system and in the mechanisms of immunological surveillance have been made in the past decade. The physiological consequences of experimental thymectomy in animals or the failure of the thymus to develop normally in man have demonstrated that this organ has an important influence on organ and tissue transplantation,[1, 2] the development of autoimmune diseases,[3, 4] tolerance,[5, 6] immunological deficiency states,[7, 8] and resistance to tumor induction by cells or oncogenic viruses.[9–12]

For the last ten years, beginning with studies initiated in the laboratory of Dr. Abraham White at the Albert Einstein College of Medicine, we have sought to identify biologically active thymic factors which could act in lieu of an intact thymus gland to reconstitute thymectomized animals or enhance immunological competence in normal animals. These studies resulted in the identification of a lymphopoietic factor in rat and mouse thymus extracts in 1965,[13] the preparation of a stable form of the biologically active fraction (thymosin) in 1966,[14] and its purification to homogeneity in 1972.[15]

In this paper we report a modified purification procedure that was designed to produce large amounts of purified thymosin. In collaboration with several laboratories we have also developed new bioassays and a variety of *in vivo* and *in vitro* systems designed to measure T-cell characteristics and function in man and other animals. A preliminary account of some of these studies has been given.[16]

MATERIALS AND METHODS

Thymus tissue, trimmed and quick frozen, was supplied by Insel and Cohen, Newark, N.J. Acetone, 99.5% was purchased in 55 gallon drums from Texas Solvents, Houston. Sephadexes® G-25 and G-50 were from Pharmacia, and microgranular DEAE cellulose (DE-32) was from H. Reeve Angel. A Buchler Polyprep 200 was used for preparative acrylamide gel electrophoresis. Ultrapure guanidinium chloride was purchased from Schwarz-Mann.

* These studies were supported by grants from the National Cancer Institute (CA 14108 and CA 15419) and the John Hartford Foundation, Inc.

Purification of Thymosin

Thymus tissue that had been thawed and trimmed free of adipose tissue was processed in batches of 5 kg. All operations were conducted at 4° C unless stated otherwise.

One kg of thymus tissue was homogenized in 3 liters of 0.15 M NaCl in a Waring blender for 3 minutes at top speed. Thirty ml of octyl alcohol were added to minimize foaming. The homogenate was centrifuged at 14,000 $\times g$ to sediment the nuclear material, and 2-liter portions of the supernatant were heated with stirring to 80° C in a boiling water bath. The voluminous precipitate of heat-denatured protein was removed by filtration through Miracloth. The clear yellow filtrate was cooled to 4° C and added slowly, with stirring, to 5 volumes of acetone at —10° C. The precipitate was collected on a large Buchner funnel, washed with several volumes of cold (—10° C) acetone, and dried in a dessicator under reduced pressure. The white powder obtained by this procedure was suspended in 10 volumes of 10 mM $NaPO_4$, pH 7.0, and was stirred at room temperature for one hour. A small amount of insoluble residue was removed by centrifugation at 15,000 $\times g$, and the sample was adjusted to a protein concentration of 25 mg/ml as determined by the Lowry procedure;[17] 33.3 ml of saturated ammonium sulfate solution adjusted to pH 7.0 with NH_4OH was added to each 100 ml of solution, and the solution was stirred for one hour. The precipitate was removed by centrifugation, and the supernatant was adjusted to pH 4.0 with 10% acetic acid. Solid ammonium sulfate (14.6 g/100 ml) was added, and the suspension was stirred for one hour. The precipitate was collected by centrifugation, dissolved in 10 mM Tris-Cl, pH 8.0 at a concentration of 10 mg/ml protein,[17] and subjected to ultrafiltration at room temperature in an Amicon DC-2 hollow fiber system (Concentration mode, HIDP10 membrane cartridge). The filtrate was collected at 4° C, concentrated by rotary evaporation under reduced pressure, and desalted on a 5 $\times$ 80 cm column of Sephadex G-25 (fine) equilibrated with deionized water. The protein peak which eluted in advance of the salt and nucleotide peak was pooled, concentrated by rotary evaporation, and dried by lyophilization. This material was stored dessicated at —20° C and was used routinely in many studies of thymosin biological activity, e.g. see Cohen *et al.*[27]

Further purification was achieved by column chromatography and preparative polyacrylamide gel electrophoresis. One gram of the lyophilized protein was dissolved in 100 ml of 50 mM Tris-Cl, 10 mM mercaptoethanol, pH 8.0, and the solution was percolated through a 2 $\times$ 40 cm column of DEAE cellulose (Whatman DE-32) equilibrated with the same buffer. After washing the column with one bed volume of starting buffer, the chromatogram was developed with a linear gradient formed by 800 ml of 10 mM mercaptoethanol in 50 mM Tris-Cl, pH 8.0, as the starting buffer and 800 ml 10 mM mercaptoethanol, 0.8 M NaCl in 50 mM Tris-Cl, pH 8.0, as the limit buffer. The thymosin-containing fractions were pooled and subjected to gel filtration on a 3.8 $\times$ 150 cm column of Sephadex G-50 (fine) equilibrated with 0.2 M KCl, 10 mM mercaptoethanol in 10 mM Tris-Cl, pH 8.0. The active fractions were desalted by gel filtration on G-25 and subjected to preparative polyacrylamide gel electrophoresis. This procedure utilized a 15% acrylamide gel (6 cm high) that had been preelectrophoresed with 5 mmoles of cysteine as a free radical scavenger.[18] The sample (150–200 mg) was electrophoresed at 100 mA using a standard pH 8.3 Tris-glycine buffer system,[19] and the first protein peak eluted from the bottom of the gel, which contains a single protein component, was designated as thymosin, fraction 8.

SDS-Polyacrylamide Gels

Gels containing 15% acrylamide and 1% bisacrylamide were prepared by the method of Swank and Munkries.[20] Other components and their final concentrations were 0.1% SDS (w/v), 0.075% TEMED (v/v), 0.1 M H_3PO_4, 8 M urea, and 0.07% ammonium persulfate (w/v). The gel solution was adjusted to pH 6.8 with Tris. The tray buffer was 0.1% SDS (w/v) in 0.1 M H_3PO_4 adjusted to pH 6.8 with Tris. A Hoefer vertical slab electrophoresis apparatus that formed gels 0.75 mm thick was used for these studies.

One mg protein samples were dissolved in 1 ml of 1% SDS, 8 M urea, 1% mercaptoethanol (v/v) and 10 mM H_3PO_4 adjusted to pH 6.8 with Tris. The samples were heated for 2 minutes in a boiling water bath and left at room temperature until used (1–2 hours). The solution was brought to 20% (w/v) with sucrose crystals. 2 μl of .05% bromphenol blue (w/v) were added to a 50 μl aliquot of the protein solution, and a 10 μl sample was layered on the gel surface underneath the tray buffer. Electrophoresis was toward the anode at 1 mA per sample well for 6 to 8 hours.

The gels were stained for 2 hours in a solution containing 1.25 g Coomassie Blue, 454 ml of 50% methanol, and 46 ml glacial acetic acid. Destaining was accomplished by dialyzing for 48 hours in a solution of 75 ml acetic acid, 250 ml methanol and 675 ml water using a Hoefer Slab Destainer.

The distance each protein migrated was measured to the nearest 0.5 mm and plotted against the log of the molecular weight.

Gel Filtration in Guanidinium Chloride

The gel filtration method of Fish *et al.*[21] was used to estimate the molecular weight of bovine thymosin. Sephadex G-50 (fine) equilibrated with 6 M guanidinium-Cl in 10 mM Tris-Cl, pH 7.5, was packed in a 1.5 × 80 cm column to a final bed volume of 141 ml.

Protein samples (10 mg) were dissolved in 0.5 ml of 6 M guanidinium-Cl in 10 mM Tris-Cl, pH 8.6, that had been saturated with nitrogen gas. The protein was reduced and carboxymethylated by a previously described procedure.[22] After carboxymethylation the reaction mixture was adjusted to pH 6.5 with 1.0 M HCl and diluted with 0.5 ml of column buffer that contained 0.6% blue dextran (w/v), 0.1% DNP-alanine (w/v) and 20% sucrose (w/v). A 200 μl aliquot of this solution was layered on the column, and the chromatogram was developed with 6 M guanidinium-Cl in 10 mM Tris, pH 7.5, at a flow rate of 4 ml/hr. Fractions of 2 ml per tube were collected, and absorbencies at 276 and 235 nm were determined.

Solute elution positions were defined as those tubes within the blue dextran (BD), protein (P), or DNP-alanine (DNP) peaks having maximum absorbancies at 276 or 235 nm. The distribution coefficient (K_D) of each protein was calculated by the following equation: [21]

$$K_D = \frac{Tube_P - Tube_{BD}}{Tube_{DNP} - Tube_{BD}}$$

A plot of the log molecular weight versus K_D was made with proteins of known molecular weight to calibrate the column. The molecular weight of thymosin was determined on the calibrated column.

Analytical Gels

Gels containing 15% acrylamide were run at both basic and acidic pH. The basic gel contained 15% acrylamide (w/v), 4.5% Tris (w/v), 0.029% TEMED (v/v), 0.15% bisacrylamide (w/v) and 0.07% ammonium persulfate (w/v) adjusted to a pH of 8.9 with 1 M HCl. Above the separating gel, a concentrating gel containing 2.5% acrylamide, 0.62% bisacrylamide, 0.713% Tris, 0.025% TEMED and .001% riboflavin, was photopolymerized; 1.8 ml of separating gel solution and 0.2 ml of concentrating gel solution were polymerized in 5 × 125 mm tubes. The tray buffer containing 25 mM Tris and 0.19 M glycine had a pH of 8.3. The protein sample (1–2 mg/ml) in 10% sucrose was layered onto the top of the gel. One ml of bromphenol blue was added to the upper buffer solution, and 2 mA per tube were applied until the dye front entered the separating gel whereupon the current was raised to 4 mA per tube. After electrophoresis, the gels were suspended in 20% trichloracetic acid (TCA) for 2 hours to fix the zones of protein and then stained for 2 hours in a fresh solution of Coomassie blue prepared from 1 volume of 1% Coomassie blue (in water) diluted to 20 volumes with 20% TCA. The gels were destained by dialysis in 10% TCA. Electrophoresis at pH 2.9 was performed by the method of Panyim and Chalkley.[23]

Assays for Thymosin Activity

Several *in vitro* bioassays used to measure thymosin activity are listed in TABLE 1. The rosette bioassay developed in collaboration with Bach and Dardenne[24] was used to measure thymosin activity during the purification procedure. A recently developed radioimmunoassay for thymosin was used to determine thymosin levels in the blood.

Rosette Assay[24]

Spleens from adult C57 black mice that had been thymectomized 14 days earlier were excised and homogenized with 2–3 ml of Hank's balanced salt solution in a glass homogenizer (teflon pestle). The homogenizer was rinsed twice with 2 ml of Hank's solution, and the rinses were combined with the original homogenate. The cells were poured through a double layer of nylon monofilament mesh (53 μ pore) and centrifuged at 200 × *g* for 7 minutes. The cells were resuspended in 20 ml of Hank's and centrifuged at 200 × *g*. The cells were suspended in 1.0 ml of Hank's solution for counting, and then they were diluted with Hank's to a concentration of 40×10^6 cells/ml.

Hank's solution in aliquots of 0.25 ml was placed in a series of 8 tubes. A 0.25 ml aliquot of an azathioprine solution (100 μg/ml in Hank's was added to the first tube and serially diluted (2-fold) in the remaining tubes to produce azathioprine concentrations of 50, 25, 12.5, 6.2, 3.1, etc. μg/ml. Two tubes containing only 0.25 ml Hank's served as incubated and unincubated controls. In a separate series of tubes, 0.125 ml of a thymosin or control protein solution was serially diluted with 0.125 ml of Hank's solution. To this series was added 0.125 ml of an azathioprine solution that would not inhibit rosette formation (20 μg/ml). One hundred μls of the spleen cell suspension were added to each tube. The cells were incubated for 90 minutes at 37° C in air. Immediately after the incubation, 12×10^6 sheep erythrocytes were added in 0.1 ml for a final volume of 0.45 ml, and the mixture was centrifuged at $200 \times g$ for 5 minutes. The cells were resuspended by gentle rotary agitation, and the number of rosettes present in duplicate fields of 6,000 cells were counted in a hemocytometer.

The parameter measured was the minimum amount of azathioprine that reduced the number of spontaneous rosette-forming cells by 50% in a given field. T-cell spontaneous rosette-forming cells (sRFC) are much more sensitive to azathioprine than are B-cell sRFC. Thus, the production of T-cells by thymosin treatment was indicated by a much lower concentration of azathioprine needed to reduce the number of sRFC by 50%.

Table 1

Bioassays for Thymosin

In Vitro	
Rosette (spontaneous, activated, and long-term)	
Cytotoxicity (expression of θ and TL)	
Mitogens (bone marrow conversion and amplification of T-cell responses)	
MLC ($T_1 \rightarrow T_2$ and amplification of T-cell responses)	
RIA (calf and human)	
Antibody formation	
In Vitro → In Vivo	In Vivo → In Vitro
GVH (bone marrow)	Mitogens
T- and B-cell cooperation	MLC
	Educated T-cells
In Vivo Animal Models	
Neonatally thymectomized mice	
Athymic "nude" mice	
Immunosuppressed mice (x-irradiation, ALS, steriods)	
NZB Mice (autoimmune disease)	
Normal mice	
Tumor-bearing mice	

Cytotoxicity Assay (θ and TL) [33]

This assay was developed by Komuro and Boyse [25] and is based on the principle that the presence of θ or TL antigen on a lymphoid cell surface may be used as a T-cell marker. The assay is derived from the finding by Boyse *et al.* that incubation of thymosin with a low-density, low-θ-bearing subpopulation of spleen or bone marrow cells from a θ-positive mouse strain (C_3H)

causes a quantitative increase in TL or θ antigen on responsive cell surfaces. To obtain thymosin-sensitive cells, a suspension of spleen or bone marrow cells was washed once in Medium 199, and the erythrocytes were removed by hypotonic shock. About 5×10^6 cells were suspended in 1 ml 35% bovine serum albumin (BSA, 300 milliOsmolar in medium 199) in a 5 ml Beckman cellulose nitrate tube. The cell suspension was overlayed with 1 ml each of 29%, 26%, 23% and 10% BSA (w/v) respectively, and the tube was centrifuged at 4° C in an SW50.1 rotor at 13,000 rpm for 30 minutes in a Beckman model L2-65B ultracentrifuge. Cells were collected at the four interfaces of the discontinuous gradient and were designated as A, B, C, or D from top to bottom, respectively. A or B cells were incubated with or without several concentrations of thymosin for two hours at 37° C. Nontoxic rabbit serum (complement) along with anti-θ C_3H or anti-TL mouse antiserum or rabbit anti-θ serum was added to the treated cells. After 45 minutes at 37° C trypan blue was added, and the proportion of dead cells containing trypan blue was determined in a hemocytometer. Controls included cells from congenic TL^- or C_3H θ-negative mice as well as complement-free and antiserum-free incubations. The inductive power of thymosin was calculated by subtracting the percentage of dead cells in the control tubes (no thymosin) from the percentage of dead cells after incubation with thymosin.

Graft-versus-Host (GvH) Assay [26]

Adult bone marrow cells were obtained from the femurs of CBA/J mice by aspiration with a syringe containing Medium 199 and 5% fetal calf serum. Cells were washed once and resuspended at the concentration of $5–10 \times 10^6$ cells/ml. Cells were incubated for 2 hours with varying concentrations of thymosin, control proteins, or with unsupplemented normal saline solution. The cells were washed, resuspended in Medium 199, counted and injected (usually 5×10^6 bone marrow cells per animal) intravenously into $B6AF_1/J$ hosts (4 per group) previously exposed to 800 R whole-body x-irradiation. The test animals were killed seven days later, and their spleens were weighed. The parameter measured was enlargement of the spleen due to the reaction of competent grafted T-cells. Normal bone marrow caused a minimal GvH reaction. Thymosin treatment of bone marrow increased the GvH response. The spleen index was calculated by dividing the spleen weight (mg) to body weight (g) ratio of the $B6AF_1/J$ mice that received allogeneic cells by the spleen weight to body weight ratio of mice that received the same number of similarly treated isogeneic cells. A spleen index greater than 1.3 was considered a positive GvH response.

Mixed Lymphocyte Culture (MLC) Assay

Methods for the MLC are presented elsewhere in this Annal.[27]

Radioimmunoassay for Thymosin [28]

The double antibody radioimmunoassay for bovine and human thymosin reported here was developed by Schulof *et al.*[28] Thymosin was iodinated by a modified chloramine-T method.[29] One mCi of carrier-free $Na^{131}I$ or $Na^{125}I$ was placed in a small disposable glass culture tube, and the pH was adjusted to 7.4 with 25 μl of 0.4 M phosphate buffer. Five μl of a 1 mg/ml thymosin solution was added, and the iodination reaction was initiated by rapid addition of 10 μl of freshly prepared 2.5 mg/ml chloramine-T in 10 mM phosphate buffer, pH 7.4. After 30 seconds the reaction was terminated by addition of 100 μl of a 2.5 mg/ml solution of $Na_2S_2O_5$ in 10 mM phosphate buffer, pH 7.4, and 50 μl of normal rabbit serum. The reaction mixture was immediately transferred to a 1 × 10 cm Sephadex G-50 column equilibrated with separated buffer (SB, 10 mM phosphate buffer, pH 7.4, 0.15 M NaCl, 0.1% bovine serum albumin, w/v, 0.1% sodium azide, w/v) in order to removed unreacted iodine from labeled thymosin. By this technique ^{131}I-labeled thymosin was prepared with a specific activity of 100–150 μCi/μg. ^{131}I-labeled thymosin behaved exactly like native thymosin on polyacrylamide gels and Sephadex G-50 columns.

Antisera to thymosin were prepared in adult female New Zealand White rabbits by two immunization procedures. Rabbits were immunized with 1 mg thymosin in 1 ml 0.15 M NaCl mixed with an equal volume of Freund's complete adjuvant. The first set of injections was administered in divided doses in the hind foot pads and in two subcutaneous sites. Subsequent injections were given in two subcutaneous sites.

One group of four rabbits was given 5 weekly injections. Another group was given 2 weekly injections followed by 3 monthly boosts. Animals were bled every 2 weeks from the marginal ear vein. Blood was allowed to clot at 5° C overnight, and serum from each animal was stored separately in small aliquots at −70° C. Goat anti-rabbit gamma globulin sera (GARGGS) were used for double antibody radioimmunoassay studies. Agar gel immunodiffusion tests were performed according to the method of Ouchterlony.[30]

Radioimmunoassays were carried out in disposable 12 × 75 mm glass culture tubes. Each tube contained (1) 0.5 ml of salt buffer (SB + 4% normal rabbit serum); (2) 100 μl of 10 mM EDTA in SB; (3) 100 μl of ^{131}I-labeled thymosin, which was diluted with SB to give 2500 cpm (0.1 ng); (4) 100 μl of standard solutions of unlabeled thymosin in SB; (5) 100 μl of antithymosin sera diluted in SB (antisera were used at a final dilution of 1:1000–1:5000, which bound 25–35% of labeled thymosin when no competing unlabeled hormone was present); and (6) 100 μl of thymectomized or normal guinea-pig serum. When assaying serum samples, 100 μl of appropriately diluted serum were used in (6), and 100 μl of SB were substituted in (4).

All assays were performed in duplicate and included control tubes without antisera (to test for coprecipitation) and standard tubes to determine total cpm added. After a 4 day incubation at 4° C, antibody-bound thymosin was precipitated by adding 100 μl of GARGGS and incubating for an additional 24 hours. The tubes were centrifuged for 30 minutes at 1300 × *g* in an International PR-2 refrigerated centrifuge. The supernatants were removed by suction, and the precipitates were counted in a Nuclear-Chicago Model 1185 gamma counter. The data were analyzed in the form of % labeled antigen bound by computing the mean and % standard error of each duplicate set on a Wang 720C Programmable Calculator.

Results and Discussion

The procedure used to isolate bovine thymosin is outlined in Figure 1. This procedure was designed to process large amounts of thymus tissue and to obtain the maximum yield of purified thymosin. Thus, the thymus tissue homogenate was centrifuged 3 liters at a time at 14,000 $\times g$ to sediment the large amount of chromatin that is characteristic of lymphoid tissue. A prior report[15] recommended a second centrifugation at 46,000 $\times g$ for two hours. This procedure is not practical in large-scale isolations and was omitted in these studies. Another effort-saving procedure was filtration of the hot suspension of heat-coagulated protein through Miracloth. This procedure produces a clear yellow filtrate that is readily cooled to 4° C. The acetone precipitation step precipitates all of the protein and a substantial quantity of nucleotide to give a dry powder that is equivalent to the previously reported fraction 3.[15]

The ammonium sulfate fractionation is designed to take advantage of the principles of isoelectric precipitation. Preliminary studies have revealed that thymosin is isoelectric at pH 4. Accordingly, the initial ammonium sulfate addition to 25% of saturation is performed at pH 7.0. This procedure removes a substantial amount of protein but no thymosin activity. After centrifugation, adjustment of the supernatant to pH 4 induces the appearance of a precipitate. An additional amount of protein is precipitated by raising the ammonium sulfate concentration to 50% of saturation. In this manner, 99% of the thymosin activity is recovered, and a substantial purification is achieved.

An ultrafiltration step has replaced the Sephadex G-150 procedure reported by Goldstein *et al.*[15] Early experiments showed that thymosin activity passed through Amicon UM-10 ultrafilters, which are impermeable to most proteins having a molecular weight larger than 15,000 daltons. Proteins with a molecular weight lower than 15,000 daltons permeate UM-10 filters with varying degrees of efficiency. The Amicon hollow fiber system with a PM-10 membrane cartridge was selected because of its high filtration rate (approximately 500 ml/hr.). Usually a 1000 ml protein solution from the preceding ammonium sulfate fractionation was concentrated to a volume of 100 ml. The colorless filtrate was collected in an Erlenmeyer flask packed in ice. The retentate was diluted with an equal volume of deionized water and concentrated to 100 ml or less. Thymosin activity was found only in the filtrate as measured by the rosette assay.

In our experience, ammonium sulfate fractionation, ultrafiltration and gel filtration on G-25 were essential for the complete removal of contaminating nucleotides. Upon desalting the ultrafiltrate on G-25, we always obtained a large protein peak followed by a peak of absorbance that contained both salts and nucleotides (data not shown). Protein determinations revealed that the nucleotide peak contained little protein. This fraction was cytotoxic in the rosette bioassay, and activity measurements were not possible. The lyophilized ultrafiltrate (thymosin fraction 5) was another fraction that could be stored until required for activity studies or further purification. On the basis of dry weight, this fraction is 99% protein and contains only a small amount of contaminating nucleotide. As shown in TABLE 2 this fraction is active *in vitro* in the rosette, cytotoxicity (expression of TL and Thy-1) and MLC assays as well as in several *in vivo* assays shown in TABLE 3. The activity seen is usually 2 to 100 times greater than thymosin, fraction 3, the acetone precipitate.

In an effort to standardize the ion-exchange column chromatographic procedure, the use of Ecteola-cellulose recommended by Goldstein *et al.*[15] was abandoned in favor of DEAE-cellulose chromatography as described in MATERIALS AND METHODS. In our hands this procedure yields a large "break-through" peak containing no thymosin activity as measured by the rosette bioassay (see FIGURE 1). Upon gradient elution, there are four to six peaks of absorbance

TABLE 2

In Vitro THYMOSIN ACTIVITY IN THE GVH, ROSETTE, CYTOTOXICITY AND MLC BIOASSAYS

	GVH *	Rosette †	Expression of TL or Thy-1 Antigen ‡	MLC §
Thymosin, fraction 3	2–10	10–30	N.T.**	N.T.
Thymosin, fraction 4	.5–5	10–20	N.T.	N.T.
Thymosin, fraction 5	.1–1	5–8	1–10	+
Thymosin, fraction 6	.01–.1	N.T.	N.T.	++
Thymosin, fraction 7	N.T.	.1–1.0	N.T.	+++
Thymosin, fraction 8	N.T.	4–6	.05–.1	+

* μg protein per 10×10^6 bone marrow cells. See reference 26.

† μg protein per 3×10^6 bone marrow cells.

‡ μg protein per 8×10^5 cells, performed by M. Scheid on a spleen cell subpopulation prepared as described in *Materials and Methods* (personal communication).

§ 8.0×10^5 thymocytes $+ 4.0 \times 10^5$ mitomycin treated spleen cells. (See also Cohen et al.[27]).

** N.T.=not tested.

at 276 nm, and the last peak eluted from the column is predominantly nucleotide as estimated from the ratio of absorbancies at 276 nm and 260 nm. This peak is also devoid of thymosin activity in the rosette bioassay. Thymosin activity was usually found in the two peaks of absorbance eluted prior to the nucleotide peak, but variations in the elution profile were observed until 10 mM mercaptoethanol was included in the chromatography buffers. As shown in TABLE 2

TABLE 3

THYMOSIN ACTIVITY IN MICE AS SHOWN BY A VARIETY OF ASSAYS THAT MEASURE LYMPHOCYTE FUNCTION

	Mice				
Fraction Tested	Nude *	Neonatal ThymX †	Adult ThymX ‡	Normal §	NZB **
Thymosin, fraction 5	+	+	+	+	+
Thymosin, fraction 6	+	+	+	N.T.	N.T.
Thymosin, fraction 8	+	N.T.	+	N.T.	N.T.

* Partial reconstitution of responses to the mitogens PHA and Con A. See reference 35.

† Enhancement of survival and reconstitution of responses to skin allografts. See references 38 and 39.

‡ Reconstitution of spontaneous rosette forming cell populations. See reference 24.

§ Enhanced responses to T- and B-cell mitogens (G. B. Thurman & A. L. Goldstein, unpublished observations).

** Reconstitution of suppressor cell populations (M. Dauphineé & N. Talal, this volume).

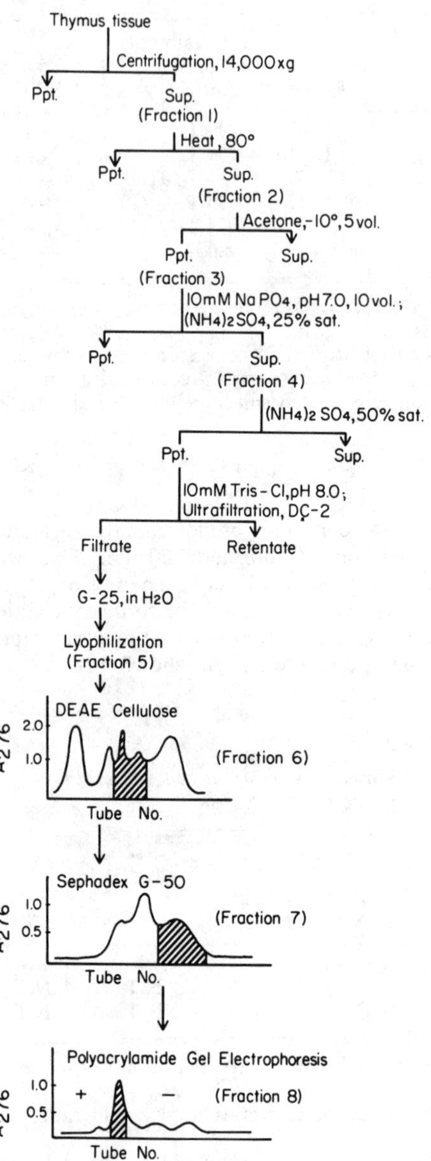

FIGURE 1. The purification of bovine thymosin.

the thymosin-containing fractions from DEAE cellulose are usually 10 times more active than the lyophilized ultrafiltrate (fraction 5) and are active *in vivo* in the nude and adult thymectomized mouse as measured by the increase in lymphocyte response to T-cell mitogens phytohemagglutinin (PHA-P) and concanavalin-A (Con-A) (TABLE 3, unpublished data).

A second separation on the basis of molecular size was accomplished by gel filtration on Sephadex G-50 as described in MATERIALS AND METHODS and illustrated in FIGURE 1. The thymosin-containing fractions from this procedure are highly active in the rosette and MLC assays as shown in TABLE 2.

The preparative polyacrylamide gel procedure yields a thymosin preparation (fraction 8) that appears to be completely free of nucleotide, carbohydrate and other nonprotein moieties. Unexpectedly, 4–6 μg of thymosin fraction 8 are required for the expression of activity in the rosette bioassay and in the MLC assay. In the nude mouse 2.5 μg/mouse/day for 3 days caused the development of small but significant responses to PHA-P and Con-A.[35] Fraction 8 thymosin was highly active in the cytotoxicity assay for the expression of TL or Thy-1 surface antigens (TABLE 2). These findings suggest that several assays should be used to measure the activity of thymic factors during their isolation. The data also indicate that an essential cofactor may have been removed by preparative electrophoresis or that the molecule was modified by this procedure. Pre-electrophoresis of the gel with cysteine was initiated as a precaution against modification by free radicals. This procedure has resulted in better yields of protein from the preparative electrophoresis, but biological activity was not always increased.

Thymosin purified by the procedure outlined in FIGURE 1 migrates as a single band on analytical polyacrylamide gels at pH 8.3 or pH 2.9 as shown in FIGURE 2. The preparation is free of nucleotide and contains no cyclic AMP as measured by the method of Gilman.[36]

Amino acid analyses were performed on 24, 48, and 72 hour acid hydrolysates of thymosin fraction 8. TABLE 4 shows the assumed number of residues per molecule based on these analyses. These data reveal that thymosin contains approximately 108 residues with a calculated molecular weight of 12,200. The molecule is rich in acidic residues and contains no unusual amino acids. The molecule contains only one tyrosyl residue and is negative in the Ehrlich reaction for tryptophan.[37] As a consequence, the molecule exhibits little ultraviolet absorption between 250 nm and 290 nm.

Estimates of molecular weight were performed on polyacrylamide gels that contained SDS. FIGURE 3 shows a slab gel on which the mobility of thymosin was compared to that of insulin, cytochrome C, lysozyme, myoglobin and ovalbumin. FIGURE 4 shows a graph of log molecular weight versus the migration distance in millimeters. These data indicate that bovine thymosin is approximately 12,000 in molecular weight.

Thymosin was reduced and carboxymethylated[22] and subjected to gel filtration on Sephadex G-50 equilibrated with 6 M guanidinium-Cl in 10 mM Tris-Cl, pH 7.5. The sample eluted as two peaks of absorbance at 235 nm. The gel filtration data for the proteins of known molecular weight and the thymosin preparation are shown in FIGURE 5 as a graph of the log molecular weight versus the distribution coefficient K_D. These data suggest that fraction 8 is composed of two polypeptide chains with molecular weights of 3,200 and 2,400. The data may be compatible with the data in FIGURE 4 if one assumes that native thymosin (MW 12,200) is composed of subunits. The occurrence of

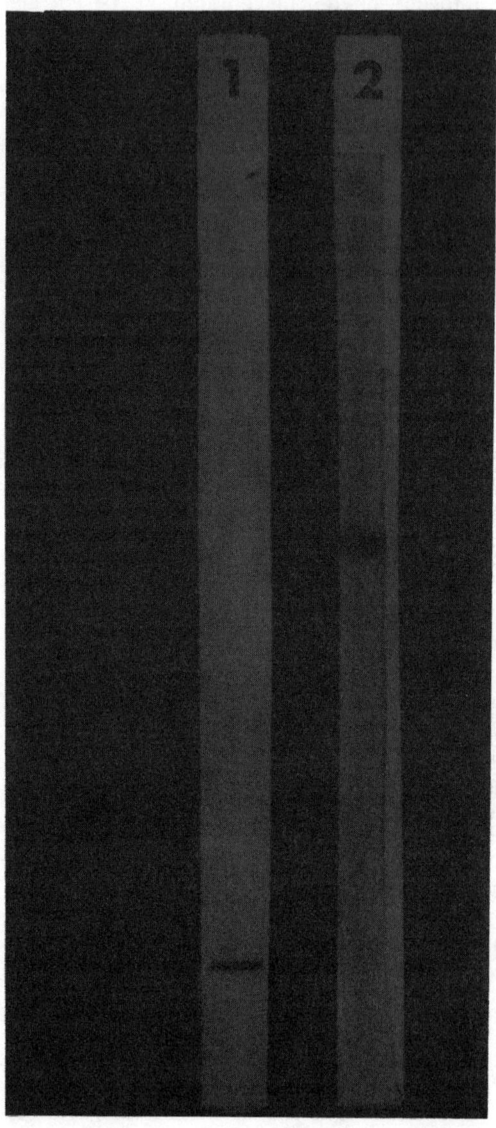

FIGURE 2. Acrylamide gels of thymosin at pH 8.3 (1) and pH 2.9 (2). Thymosin (100 μg) was applied to basic and acidic gels (5×125 mm) prepared as described in MATERIALS AND METHODS.

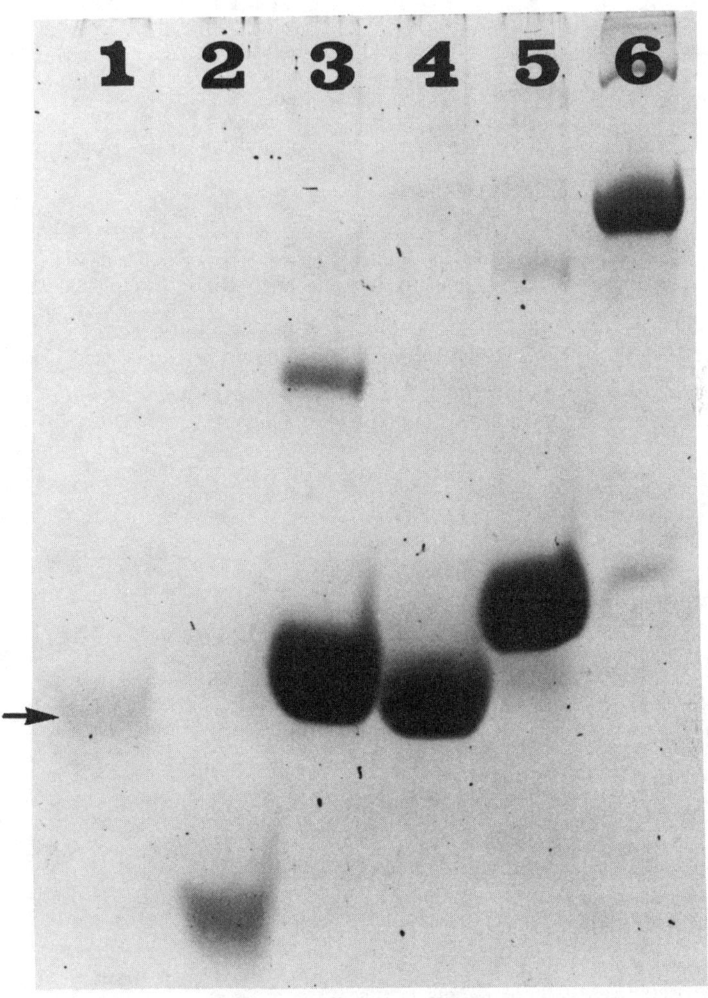
1
2
3
4
5
6

TABLE 4

AMINO ACID COMPOSITION OF BOVINE THYMOSIN *

Amino Acid	Residues/ Molecule	Amino Acid	Residues/ Molecule
lysine	4	alanine	7
histidine	1	cysteine ‡	1
arginine	2	valine	5
aspartic acid	22	methionine ‡	2
threonine †	4	isoleucine	3
serine †	5	leucine	6
glutamic acid	32	tyrosine	1
proline	5	phenylalanine	2
glycine	6		
		Total	108

* The data are presented as assumed numbers of residues per molecule. The molecular weight is approximately 12,200. A separate analysis for tryptophan was performed.[37]

† Extrapolated to zero time from 24, 48 and 72 hour hydrolysates.

‡ Determined as cysteic acid and methionine sulfone by performic acid oxidation.

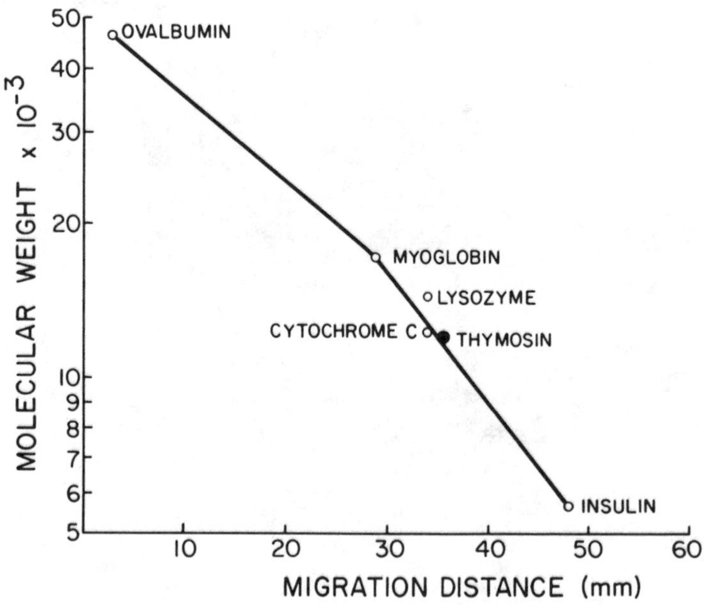

FIGURE 4. Data from the 15% polyacrylamide slab gel (0.75 mm thick) containing 0.1% SDS and 8 M urea (shown in FIGURE 3). The mobility in millimeters was plotted against the log molecular weight. These data indicate that thymosin has a molecular weight of 12,000.

single residues of histidine, cysteine, and tyrosine is shown in TABLE 4 indicates that the subunits are polypeptides of similar size but dissimilar sequence.

Several attempts to identify the amino terminal residue of bovine thymosin were unsuccessful. This is not surprising, since a molecule with the amino acid composition shown in TABLE 4 is very likely to have an amino terminal pyrrolidone-carboxylyl residue.

The modified purification procedure described in this paper has yielded sufficient quantities of fraction 5 thymosin to complete acute toxicity studies in

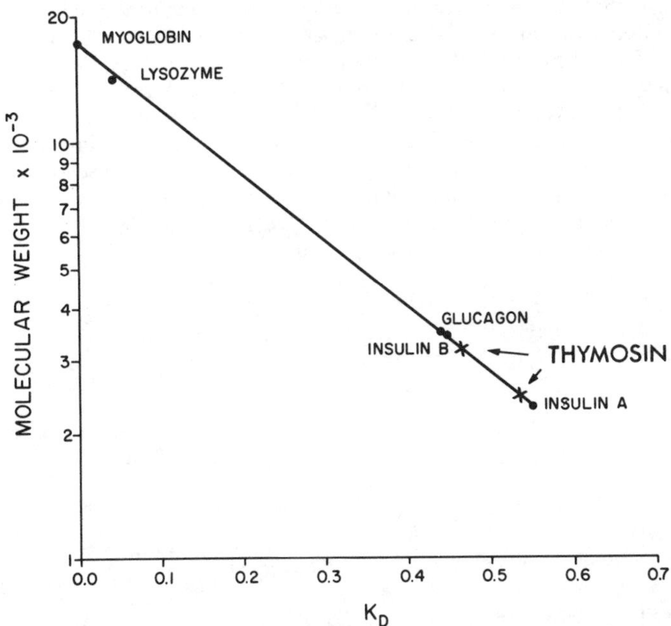

FIGURE 5. Determination of molecular weight by gel filtration on Sephadex G-50 equilibrated with 6 M guanidinium-Cl in 10 mM Tris-Cl, pH 7.5. Protein samples (200 μg) were reduced and carboxymethylated and run with standards of Blue Dextran-2000 and DNP-alanine. Using the tube number of maximum absorbance at 276 or 235 nm, a distribution coefficient, K_D, for each protein was calculated as described in MATERIALS AND METHODS. The graph of log molecular weight vs. K_D shows that thymosin eluted as two polypeptide chains with approximate molecular weights of 3200 and 2400.

mice and dogs. The results of these studies indicate a complete lack of toxicity of thymosin even at extremely high doses (1000 mg/kg/day for 14 days). There was no mortality, and all of the animals were healthy and normal appearing at the completion of the treatments. There were several interesting histological and immunological observations noted (unpublished data), which will be reported in detail elsewhere.

A sufficient quantity of pure thymosin is now available to complete the amino acid sequence determination. These studies are presently in progress.

Using the rosette assay[24] and a newly developed radioimmunoassay,[28] we found that thymosin circulates in the blood of a wide variety of mammals. The most compelling evidence that the thymosin-like activity indigenous to normal mouse serum is identical or closely related to thymosin extracted from thymus glands came from studies by Bach *et al.*[31] of serum thymosin activity in thymectomized mice injected with thymosin. Serum from thymectomized mice did not induce azathioprine sensitivity in rosette-forming cells *in vitro*. Injection of highly purified thymosin (prepared in our laboratory) into thymectomized mice restored serum thymosin activity so that it would transform rosette-forming cells *in vitro* into lymphocytes that were sensitive to azathioprine (or to antiheta or antilymphocyte serum). These data are shown in FIGURE 6. It should also be noted from FIGURE 6 that when purified thymosin was injected into thymectomized mice whose population of azathioprine-sensitive rosette-forming spleen cells had disappeared, a new population of rosette-forming cells sensitive to azathioprine appeared in the spleen within 24 hours after injection.

FIGURE 7 shows the effect of aging, immunodeficiency disease, and a neoplastic disease on circulating thymosin levels in man. These data compare thymosin biological activity measured by the rosette assay with thymosin immunological activity measured by radioimmunoassay. With the rosette assay,

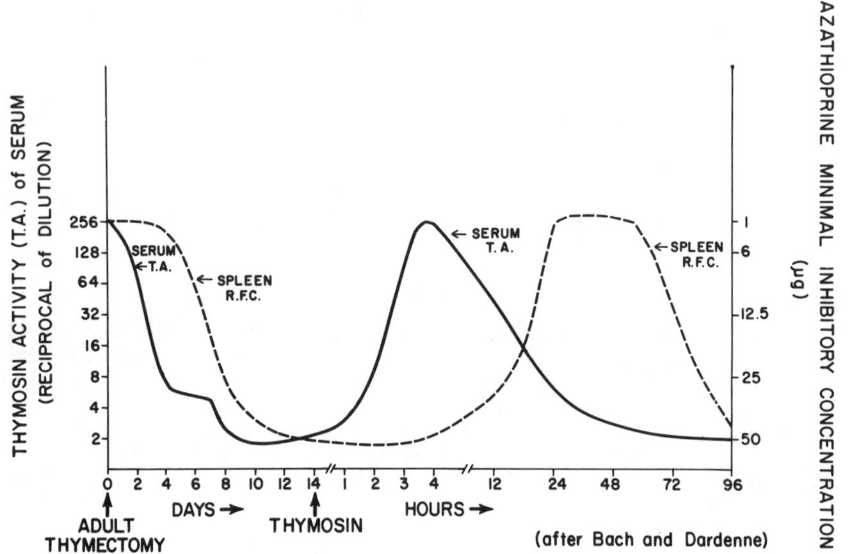

FIGURE 6. Effect of thymosin on thymus-dependent spontaneous rosette-forming cells (RFC) in the spleen. After adult thymectomy there was a rapid decrease in serum thymosin-like activity (serum TA) which was followed by a significant decrease in spleen RFC. Administration of a single intraperitoneal injection of thymosin resulted in a rapid rise in serum TA and within 24 hours, in the appearance of a new population of azathioprene-sensitive spleen cells. The reconstitution of RFC is transitory and is lost within 72 hours following a single injection of thymosin, suggesting the need for constant thymosin levels in the blood to maintain the population of spontaneous rosette-forming spleen cells.

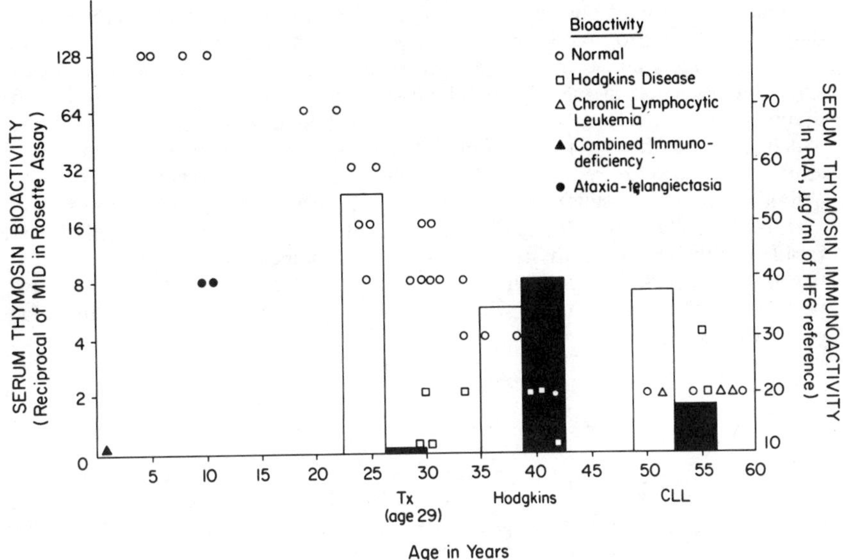

FIGURE 7. Effect of aging, immunodeficiency diseases, and cancer on circulating thymosin levels in man. These data compare thymosin biological activity measured by the rosette assay (serum thymosin bioactivity) with thymosin immunological activity measured by radioimmunoassay (serum thymosin immunoactivity). With the rosette assay, a significant decrease in serum thymosin with age was observed in normal individuals (○). The data also indicate that there are lower levels of thymosin activity in serum from younger patients with Hodgkin's disease (□), with sex-linked combined immune deficiency disease (▲), and with ataxia-telangiectasia (●). Preliminary data obtained by radioimmunoassay (RIA) are shown in bar graphs. The open bars indicate levels measured in normal individuals. Thymosin levels are decreased in patients thymectomized for myasthenia gravis (Tx) and in patients with chronic lymphocytic leukemia (CLL). In Hodgkin's disease, thymosin levels appear normal or slightly elevated by RIA in contrast to the rosette bioassay suggesting the existence of circulating thymosin molecules which are biologically inactive.

a significant decrease in serum thymosin activity in normal individuals with age was observed. The data also demonstrated that there were lower than average levels of thymosin activity in serum from younger patients with Hodgkin's disease, with sex-linked combined immune deficiency, and with ataxia-telangiectasia. Preliminary data obtained by radioimmunoassay are shown in the bar graphs. The open bars indicate levels measured in normal individuals. We observed a dramatic decrease in the serum thymosin level of a patient thymectomized for myesthenia gravis. We also observed low thymosin immunological activity in patients with chronic lymphocytic leukemia as compared to normal individuals of the same age group. In Hodgkin's disease, thymosin immunological activity appeared normal in contrast to the low biological activity demonstrated with the rosette bioassay. These data suggest that Hodgkin's patients may produce normal levels of a biologically inactive form of thymosin that has retained its antigenic characteristics as measured by radioimmunoassay.[32]

Our current working hypothesis of the mechanism of action of thymosin is diagrammed in FIGURE 8 and is discussed in more detail elsewhere in this volume.[27] Our studies suggest that thymosin acts on a cell that may not necessarily have resided in the thymus gland.[24, 26, 33, 34] The short time required for thymosin to convert a stem-cell population (thymosin-sensitive cell) into a T-cell suggests that thymosin probably derepresses or activates a cell that is already genetically programmed to differentiate into a T-cell. Thymosin-activated cells (T_1-cells) can, under the appropriate stimulus (antigens?), mature in the presence of additional thymosin into functional T-cells.[27] The rapidity with which the thymosin-sensitive cells appear in the spleen and leave the bone marrow (unpublished observations) after thymectomy suggests a possible reversion to a more primitive cell in the absence of the thymus gland or its secretions.

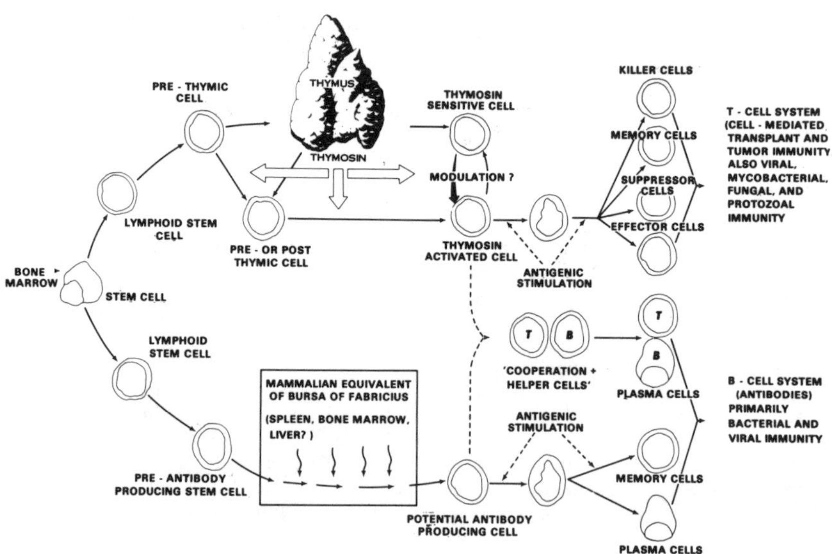

FIGURE 8. Maturation of the immune system under the influence of thymosin. Thymosin acts at key points in the development of T_1- and T_2-cells to cause primitive lymphoid T-cell populations to mature into immunologically competent cells.

SUMMARY

A modified purification procedure has been developed for bovine thymosin, and chemical characterization studies have been initiated. Amino acid analyses of acid hydrolysates reveal that thymosin fraction 8 contains approximately 108 residues of which half are aspartic and glutamic acid. The molecule contains one histidine, one cysteine, one tyrosine, and no tryptophan. Nucleotides are completely absent. From the composition and from electrophoretic studies using SDS-polyacrylamide gels, fraction 8 has an estimated molecular weight of 12,200. Preliminary studies suggest the presence of subunits.

Partially purified thymosin (fraction 5) contains several heat-stable acidic proteins with molecular weights that range from 1,200 to 14,000. It is not yet known whether all of the biological activity ascribed to thymosin fraction 5 resides within a single molecular species (fraction 8) or whether multiple thymic factors must act in concert to endow the host with its normal complement of immunity. The low specific activity of thymosin fraction 8 in some of the bioassays could reflect the removal of one or more active components that must be present for full expression of biological activity.

Other studies using a radioimmunoassay and a rosette bioassay indicate that thymosin is present in the blood of animals and man and that thymosin levels are altered in patients with known (or suspected) immunodeficiency disease and with age.

In vivo studies with thymosin, fraction 5, showed that a dose of 1000 mg/kg was not toxic or pathogenic to mice. As a result of successful progenicity, sterility, and toxicity studies our laboratory is now preparing to test thymosin in patients.

We report elsewhere in this volume (see Cohen *et al.*[27]) that thymosin acts on both stem cells (predetermined T-cells) and thymocytes (T_1-cells) to activate and/or derepress a cell that already has the capacity to function as a mature immunologically competent lymphocyte (T_2-cell).

Acknowledgments

We thank Dr. Abraham White and Mrs. Susan Haag of Syntex Research, Palo Alto, California, for performing some of the rosette assays shown in Table 2. We also thank Mr. Billy Jack Verret, Miss Barbara Simms, Mr. James Oliver and Mr. John McClure for their expert technical assistance.

[**Note Added in Proof:** Clinical trials with thymosin fraction 5 have now been initiated. Preliminary *in vitro* and *in vivo* studies show that thymosin can increase the number of peripheral blood T-cells of patients with a variety of primary and secondary immunodeficiency diseases and can partially reconstitute host immunological competence in ways similar to those seen in several animal models.[40, 41] Large-scale clinical trials are now in progress to determine the therapeutic potential of thymosin in patients having primary or secondary immunodeficiency diseases, cancer, or diseases related to aging.]

References

1. Miller, J. F. A. P. 1961. Lancet **2:** 748–749.
2. Martinez, D., J. Kersey, B. W. Papermaster & R. A. Good. 1962. Proc. Soc. Exp. Biol. Med. **111:** 41–43.
3. Burnet, F. M. 1962. Brit. Med. J. **2:** 807–811.
4. Goldstein, G. 1966. Lancet **2:** 1164–1167.
5. Isakovic, K., S. B. Smith & B. H. Waksman. 1965. Science **148:** 1333–1335.
6. Hess, M. W. 1968. Experimental Thymectomy. Possibilities and Limitations. Springer-Verlag. New York, N.Y.
7. Good, R. A., A. P. Dalmasso, C. Martinez, O. K. Archer, J. C. Pierce & B. W. Papermaster. 1962. J. Exp. Med. **116:** 773–795.
8. Bergsma, D., Ed. 1968. Immunologic Deficiency Diseases in Man. *In* Birth Defects Original Article Series. Vol. IV, No. 1. The National Foundation March of Dimes. New York, N.Y.

9. LAW, L. W. 1966. Cancer Res. **26:** 551–571.
10. MCENDY, D. P., C. BOON & J. FURTH. 1944. Cancer Res. **4:** 377–383.
11. FURTH, J. 1946. J. Gerontol. **1:** 46–52.
12. MILLER, J. F. A. P. 1967. The Thymus in Relation to Neoplasia. *In* Modern Trends in Pathology. T. Crawford, Ed. Vol. **2:** 140–175.
13. KLEIN, J. J., A. L. GOLDSTEIN & A. WHITE. 1965. Proc. Nat. Acad. Sci. U.S. **53:** 812–817.
14. GOLDSTEIN, A. L., F. D. SLATER & A. WHITE. 1966. Proc. Nat. Acad. Sci. U.S. **56:** 1010–1017.
15. GOLDSTEIN, A. L., A. GUHA, M. M. ZATZ, M. HARDY & A. WHITE. 1972. Proc. Proc. Nat. Acad. Sci. U.S. **69:** 1800–1803.
16. HOOPER, J. A., G. H. COHEN, R. S. SCHULOF, A. WHITE & A. L. GOLDSTEIN. 1973. Abstr. Fed. Proc. **32:** 489.
17. LOWRY, O. H., N. J. ROSENBROUGH, A. L. FARR & R. J. RANDALL. 1951. J. Biol. Chem. **193:** 265–275.
18. PETERSON, R. F. 1972. *In* Methods in Enzymology. C. H. W. Hirs and S. N. Timasheff, Eds. Vol. **25:** 178–182.
19. GABRIEL, O. 1971. *In* Methods in Enzymology. W. B. Jacoby, Ed. Vol. **22:** 565–578.
20. SWANK, R. T. & K. D. MUNKRIES. 1971. Anal. Biochem. **39:** 462–477.
21. FISH, W. W., K. G. MANN & C. TANFORD. 1969. J. Biol. Chem. **244:** 4989–4994.
22. DELANGE, R. J. 1970. J. Biol. Chem. **245:** 907–916.
23. PANYIM, S. & R. CHALKLEY. 1969. Arch. Biochem. Biophys. **130:** 337–346.
24. BACH, J. F., M. DARDENNE, A. L. GOLDSTEIN, A. GUHA & A. WHITE. 1970. Proc. Nat. Acad. Sci. U.S. **68:** 2734–2738.
25. KOMURO, K. & E. A. BOYSE. 1973. J. Exp. Med. **138:** 479–482.
26. GOLDSTEIN, A. L., A. GUHA, M. L. HOWE & A. WHITE. 1971. J. Immunol. **106:** 773–780.
27. COHEN, G. H., J. A. HOOPER & A. L. GOLDSTEIN. 1974. This volume.
28. SCHULOF, R. S., J. A. HOOPER, A. WHITE & A. L. GOLDSTEIN. 1973. Abstr. Fed. Proc. **32:** 962.
29. GREENWOOD, F. C. & W. M. HUNTER. 1963. Biochem. J. **89:** 114–123.
30. OUCHTERLONY, O. 1953. Acta Path. Microbiol. Scand. **32:** 231–240.
31. BACH, J. F., M. DARDENNE & J. C. SALEMEN. 1973. Clin. Exp. Immunol. **14:** 247–256.
32. GOLDSTEIN, A. L., G. H. COHEN, J. A. HOOPER, R. S. SCHULOF & A. WHITE. 1973. Fed. Proc. **33:** 2053–2056.
33. SCHEID, M. P., M. K. HOFFMAN, K. KOMURO, N. HAMMERLING, E. A. BOYSE, G. H. COHEN, J. A. HOOPER, R. S. SCHULOF & A. L. GOLDSTEIN. 1973. J. Exp. Med. **138:** 1027–1032.
34. LOWENBERG, B., H. T. M. NIEUVERKERK & D. VAN BEKKUM. 1972. Ann. Report of the Radiobiological Institute. 105–106. TNO. Rijswijk, The Netherlands.
35. THURMAN, G. B., B. B. SILVER, J. A. HOOPER, B. C. GIOVANELLA & A. L. GOLDSTEIN. 1973. *In* 1st International Workshop on Nude Mice. Gutar Fischer Verlag. Stuttgart, West Germany. In press.
36. GILMAN, A. G. 1970. Proc. Nat. Acad. Sci. U.S. **67:** 305–312.
37. REDDI, K. K. & E. KODICEK. 1953. Biochem. J. **53:** 286–294.
38. ASANUMA, Y., A. L. GOLDSTEIN & A. WHITE. 1970. Endocrinology **86:** 600–610.
39. GOLDSTEIN, A. L., Y. ASANUMA, J. R. BATTISTO, M. A. HARDY, J. QUINT & A. WHITE. 1970. J. Immunol. **104:** 359–366.
40. WARA, D. W., A. L. GOLDSTEIN, W. DOYLE & A. J. AMMANN. 1974. New Engl. J. of Med. In press.
41. GOLDSTEIN, A. L., D. W. WARA, A. J. AMMANN, H. SAKAI, N. S. HARRIS, G. B. THURMAN, J. A. HOOPER, G. H. COHEN, A. S. GOLDMAN, J. J. COSTANZI & M. C. MCDANIEL. 1974. Transplant. Proc. In press.

THYMOSIN-INDUCED DIFFERENTIATION OF MURINE THYMOCYTES IN ALLOGENEIC MIXED LYMPHOCYTE CULTURES *

Geraldine H. Cohen, John A. Hooper, and Allan L. Goldstein

Division of Biochemistry
Department of Human Biological Chemistry and Genetics
University of Texas Medical Branch
Galveston, Texas 77550

Introduction

It has been postulated that there are two distinct subpopulations of thymic-derived (T) lymphocytes, designated T_1 and T_2 by Raff and Cantor.[1] The two populations are thought to represent successive stages of thymocyte maturation with T_2 being more mature than T_1.[1] Recent studies suggest that the more immature T_1 population is steroid-sensitive, enriched in θ and TL, H-2-poor, responsive to Concanavalin-A (Con-A), and located in the cortical region of the thymus.[1, 2] The T_2 population is located primarily in the medullary region of the thymus and has been characterized as being steroid-resistant, θ-poor, TL-negative, H-2-enriched, reactive to phytohemagglutinin (PHA), pokeweed mitogen (PWM), Con-A, and to allogeneic cells in the mixed lymphocyte reaction (MLR), graft-versus-host (GvH) reaction and cytotoxic cell assay.[1, 2] A number of laboratories [3–6] have recently described partially or fully purified thymic humoral factors which can convert precursor "pre-T" cells into more mature (T_1 or T_2?) cells *in vitro,* as manifested by increased expression of θ and TL surface antigens on treated cells of various subpopulations of murine bone marrow and spleen. We now describe an activity of a calf thymosin fraction that appears to convert immature T_1 thymocytes into functionally immunocompetent T_2 thymocytes, as judged by the markedly enhanced one-way allogeneic MLR of murine thymocytes treated with this fraction *in vitro.* Based on this finding, we present a relatively simple, rapid and quantitative *in-vitro* microculture bioassay for inducers of T-cell differentiation, and propose that thymosin treatment in the presence of antigen induces the two step T-cell maturational sequence of pre-T $\rightarrow T_1 \rightarrow T_2$.

Materials and Methods

Preparation of Calf Thymosin for Biological Testing

See Hooper *et al.*[7] in this Annal for the preparation and chemical properties of thymosin fractions used in this study.

For use in cell cultures, concentrated protein solutions were made by dissolving the lyophilized fraction in sterile water, and the protein content was

* These studies were supported by grants from the National Cancer Institute (CA 14108 and CA 15419) and the John Hartford Foundation, Inc.

determined using bovine serum albumin as the standard in the assay by Lowry *et al.*[8] The protein solution was appropriately diluted at least 10-fold with the culture medium and sterilized by means of Millipore filtration (0.22 μ pore size).

Animals

Six- to 12-week-old male CBA/J and C57B1/6J mice were obtained from Jackson Laboratories, Bar Harbor, Maine.

Preparation of Cells

Aseptic technique was used throughout these procedures. Single cell suspensions were prepared in a disposable plastic petri dish by mashing thymus, spleen, or lymph nodes (axillary, inguinal, and mesenteric) against a 100 wires/inch stainless steel mesh screen using the flat end of a plastic disposable 1 cc syringe plunger (B-D no. 8048). The screen was bathed in 2 ml of cold Medium 199 (Grand Island Biological Corp.) supplemented with 2% heat-inactivated (56° C, 30 minutes) human AB serum (v/v).

The cell suspension, kept at 4–10° C during processing, was washed into a 15 ml conical tube via a funnel lined with nylon monofilament cloth (15 μ pore size, NITEX HC-15). The tube was filled with 2% heat-inactivated human AB serum-Medium 199 and centrifuged at $200 \times g$ for 10 minutes. The medium was then discarded, and the cell pellet was resuspended in fresh medium. After a second wash, the cell pellet was resuspended in 25 mM HEPES-buffered RPMI-1640 medium (HRPMI) (GIBCO, Grand Island, N.Y.) containing 5% heat-inactivated human AB serum, fresh 2 mM L-glutamine, 100 units/ml penicillin and 100 μg/ml streptomycin. The cell density was measured with a Coulter Counter and the suspension was adjusted to the appropriate cell concentration. The bone marrow cell suspension was similarly prepared, except that the marrow cells were removed from femurs by aspiration with a syringe equipped with a 26 gauge ½ in. needle before being filtered through the nylon monofilament cloth.

Target Spleen Cells

Cell suspensions were prepared from CBA/J or C57B1/6 mice in Medium 199 (no serum) as described above. After the first wash in Medium 199, cells were suspended in Medium 199 at $10\text{–}20 \times 10^6$ cells/ml and incubated for 25 minutes with 25 μg/ml mitomycin-C (Sigma Chemical Co., St. Louis, Mo.) at 37° C in a humidified 5% CO_2 atmosphere. The cells were then pelleted at $200 \times g$, washed once in Medium 199, once in HRPMI, and finally resuspended in HRPMI that contained 7.5% heat-inactivated human AB serum (v/v). Cell density was measured with a Coulter Counter and adjusted to appropriate levels.

Mixed Lymphocyte Reactions

Triplicate cultures were prepared in microtiter trays (Cooke Engineering, Alexandria, Va.) with each well containing a total volume of 0.2 ml HRPMI and a final concentration of 5% heat-inactivated human AB serum, 2 mM fresh L-glutamine, 100 units/ml penicillin and 100 μg/ml streptomycin. Each well received 4×10^5 mitomycin-C-blocked target spleen cells and 4×10^5 to 8×10^5 CBA responder cells as detailed in the figures. Cultures were maintained for 120 hours in a humidified 5% CO_2 atmosphere at 37° C, and at 113 hours, 1 μCi [^{3}H]thymidine (New England Nuclear Corp., Boston, Mass., 1.9 Ci/mM specific radioactivity) was added to each well. Cultures were harvested with normal saline solution onto glass fiber filter paper with a multiple automated sample harvester (MASH) according to the methods of Thurman *et al.*[9] and the radioactivity retained by the dried filter paper was measured in Liquifluor scintillation fluid (New England Nuclear Corp., Boston, Mass.) in a Nuclear Chicago scintillation counter. The mean CPM of triplicate cultures plus or minus the standard error of the mean (SEM) is presented in the text and figures. The SEM is shown on the figures only when it exceeded the size of the circles.

Materials

Lipopolysaccharide (LPS) from *E. coli* (Difco 0111:B4) was obtained from Difco Laboratories, Detroit, Michigan. Freeze-dried erythropoietin, step 1 (CMRL) was from Connaught Medical Research Laboratories, Willowdale, Ontario, Canada. N^6-2′-O-dibutyryl-adenosine-3′,5′-monophosphate, cyclic, monosodium salt was obtained from Boehringer Mannheim Corp., New York, N.Y. Bovine serum albumin, fraction V, A4503, was obtained from Sigma Chemical Co., St. Louis, Mo.

Results and Discussion

The one-way mixed lymphocyte reaction by CBA thymocytes cultured with mitomycin-C-blocked spleen cells is markedly enhanced by thymosin fraction 5 (Figure 1a). This enhancement cannot be explained simply as increased survival and proliferation of the treated thymocytes, since the MLR of the syngeneic cell cultures does not increase with added thymosin.

When the experimental conditions were most optimal for the MLR of the untreated CBA spleen, lymph node, or bone marrow responder cells, thymosin treatment depressed the MLR, but only in the cultures that contained allogeneic cell combinations. At first glance, it appears that the allogeneic MLR in cultures containing 4×10^5 CBA lymph node responder cells (Figure 1c) may have been enhanced by thymosin addition. But these data are difficult to interpret because the stimulation index (allogeneic cpm/syngeneic cpm) obtained in the absence of thymosin is 30.52 (37,302 ± 202 cpm/1,222 ± 99 cpm) compared to 2.58 (129,188 ± 4,831 cpm/50,025 ± 6,602 cpm) obtained in the presence of thymosin. We do not know the significance of the pronounced increase in [^{3}H]thymidine incorporation by the CBA lymph node cells responding to the mitomycin-C-blocked CBA spleen cells (Figure 1c). The uptake may represent a change in cell permeability or may have resulted from proliferation of (T or B?) cells.

The feasibility of using the MLR of thymocytes as a bioassay for the thymic hormone and other inducers of T-cell differentiation is shown in Figure 2, which is a dose-response curve for thymosin fraction 7A.[7] This thymosin

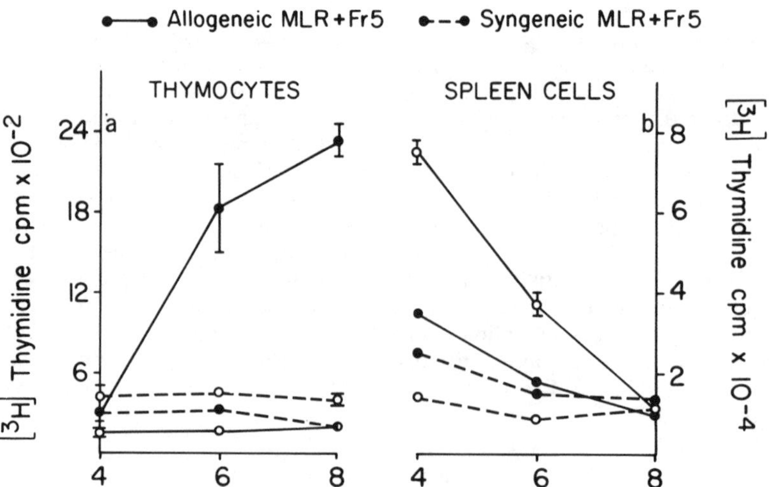

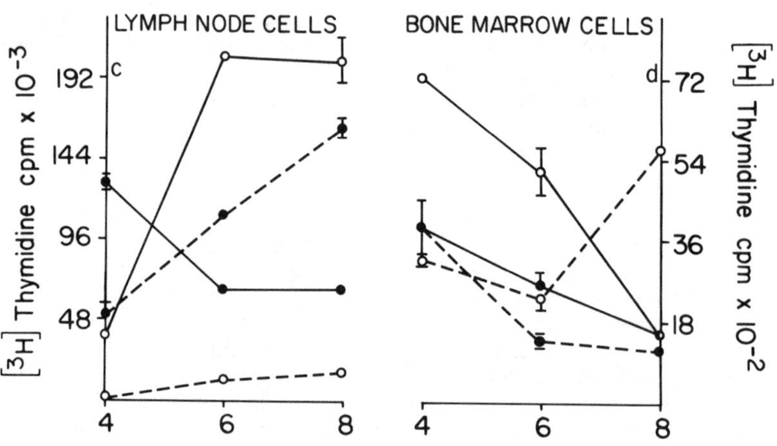

FIGURE 1. Effect of thymosin fraction 5 on the one-way MLR of CBA lymphoid cells. See MATERIALS AND METHODS for details of cell preparation and culture conditions. For the allogeneic one-way MLR, 4×10^5 mitomycin-C-treated C57Bl/6J spleen cells were present in each well. For the syngeneic one-way MLR, 4×10^5 mitomycin-C treated CBA spleen cells were present in each well. The one-way MLR of various numbers of CBA thymocytes in the presence or absence of thymosin fraction 5 is shown in panel a. The one-way MLR of various numbers of CBA spleen cells in the presence or absence of thymosin fraction 5 is shown in panel b. The one-way MLR of various numbers of CBA lymph node cells in the presence or absence of thymosin is shown in panel c. The one-way MLR of various numbers of CBA bone marrow cells in the presence or absence of thymosin is shown in panel d. Solid circles indicate presence of thymosin throughout the culture time. Circles indicate absence of thymosin. Solid lines denote allogeneic cell combinations. Broken lines denote syngeneic cell combinations.

fraction is a highly purified, but not homogeneous, fraction from calf thymus. Bovine serum albumin and partially purified sheep plasma erythropoietin at concentrations ranging from 100 μg/ml to 1 μg/ml were found to be inactive in this kind of bioassay, as was dibutyryl-cAMP at concentrations ranging from 10^{-9} M through 10^{-3} M at 10-fold increments. Material from liver and spleen of normal calf prepared in a manner identical to that for thymosin fraction 5 contained MLR-enhancing activity, but we have not yet quantitated yields or investigated whether the activity can be recovered from these same tissues from thymectomized animals, nor have we determined whether any nonhematopoietic tissue such as muscle or brain contains the activity. Some thymosin-like activity in crude preparations from spleen and other tissues has been previously noted by our laboratory and others.[5, 10–12] Lipopolysaccharide (LPS) in nanogram amounts enhanced the allogeneic MLR markedly with little, if any, increase in the syngeneic MLR by thymocytes (manuscript in preparation). The effects of endotoxin (e.g. LPS) in the MLR, however, should be readily distinguishable from those of a thymic protein, since only the latter would be highly susceptible to degradation by proteolytic enzyme treatment.

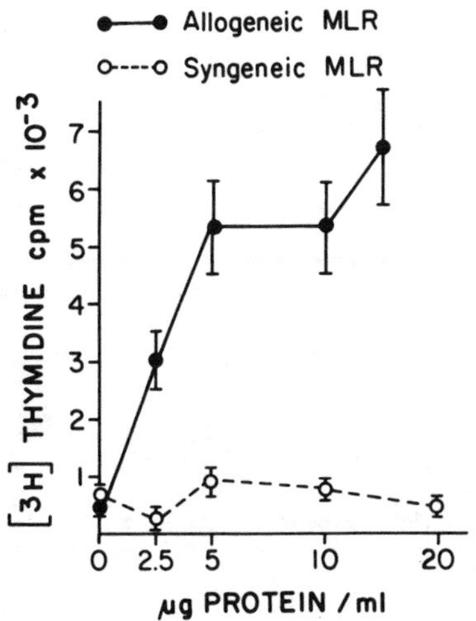

FIGURE 2. Bioassay of thymosin fraction 7A. Dose-response curve obtained with thymosin fraction 7A in a one-way MLR by CBA thymocytes. Varying concentrations of thymosin fraction 7A (see Hooper *et al.* in this volume for preparation) were present in each well throughout the culture period. Cultures, in triplicate, contained 8×10^5 CBA thymocytes and 4×10^5 mitomycin-C-treated C57Bl/6J spleen cells (in allogeneic cultures) or 4×10^5 mitomycin-C-treated CBA spleen cells (syngeneic cultures). See MATERIALS AND METHODS section for details of the cell preparation and culture conditions.

Results obtained with the MLR can often be correlated with those obtained with the GvH reaction.[13, 14] Trainin and colleagues[15–17] have recently described a stimulatory effect by a high-speed supernatant fraction of thymus (THF) on thymic-derived cells in the GvH reaction *in vitro* and *in vivo*. They can achieve this effect either with responder thymocytes or with responder spleen cells from neonatally thymectomized, but not normal, mice. Our inability to obtain a thymosin-enhanced MLR with spleen cells or with bone marrow cells may be related to an inappropriate ratio of T_1- to T_2-cells, the cell types believed to be synergistically involved in the MLR.[13] For example, there may be too many T_2-cells generated by thymosin in the mixed lymphocyte cultures containing responder spleen cells, and hence, neonatal thymectomy might produce a population of thymic-derived spleen cells in which the ratio of T_1- to T_2-cells in thymosin-supplemented cultures would be more favorable to the MLR. By using albumin density gradients similar to those employed by Komuro and Boyse,[3, 4] we may be able to isolate a subpopulation of spleen or bone marrow cells which would respond to thymosin and undergo increased reactivity in an MLR.

It should also be noted that an alternative explanation for the enhancement of the thymocyte MLR in the presence of thymosin may be a direct proliferation of T_2-cells already existing in the thymus. Since it is estimated that about 5% of the thymus cells are T_2,[1] a doubling of their number might be sufficient to enhance the allogeneic MLR by synergy with T_1-cells, but not sufficient in magnitude to be detected by increased [^{3}H]thymidine incorporation in the syngeneic MLR.

The apparent suppression of the spleen cell MLR (FIGURE 1b) by thymosin correlates with the findings of Kiger *et al.*[18] with respect to the *in vivo* GvH reaction. When they treated murine spleen cells with a 42% ethanol-soluble

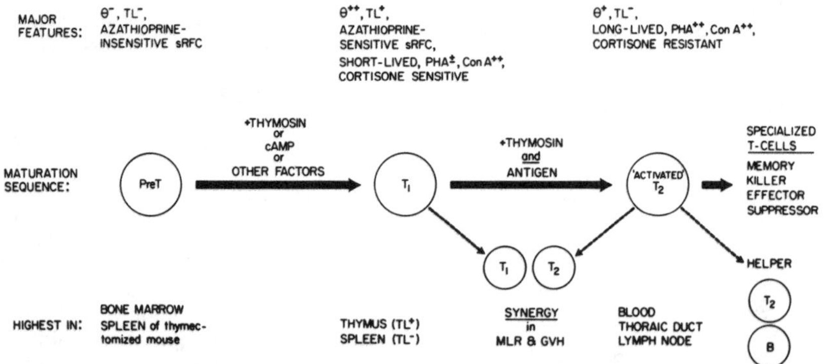

FIGURE 3. Hypothetical sites of thymosin action in murine thymic (T) cell maturation. See text for explanation.

fraction from lamb thymus, they observed a depression in their ability to produce a GvH-response *in vivo*.

The results of the present studies indicate that a major role of thymosin in thymic (T) cell differentiation is to convert immunologically immature lymphoid cell populations (T_1-cells) into immunocompetent lymphocytes (T_2-cells). A similar conclusion has been reached recently by Trainin and colleagues,[15–17] who, working with a high-speed supernatant fraction of thymus (THF), were able to enhance significantly the ability of thymocytes to implement the GvH reaction *in vivo* and *in vitro* and to confer higher cortisone resistance upon thymocytes.[19]

In FIGURE 3, we present our current hypothesis of thymosin action: The precursor T-cell (Pre-T) corresponds to a stem cell in the bone marrow that may or may not be pluripotential. Recent experiments by Boyse *et al.*[3, 4] indicate that this cell seems to be genetically poised to become a T-cell, that is, to express T-cell surface markers such as θ and TL. A variety of agents including thymosin,[5] thymin,[6] cyclic AMP (cAMP), poly I:C and endotoxin[5] can induce expression of these antigens on cells of various isolated subpopulations of bone marrow, spleen, and fetal liver,[4] and even on cells obtained from congenitally athymic "nude" mice.[4]

The conversion of a θ^- lymphoid cell to one with θ^{++} appears to be a feature also of the thymosin-induced conversion of azathioprine-insensitive spontaneous rosette-forming cells (sRFC) into azathioprine-sensitive sRFC in murine bone marrow and in spleen from thymectomized mice.[12, 20] This latter spleen sRFC population is rather labile (i.e. short-lived or reverts to pre-T state?), disappearing within a few days following neonatal or adult thymectomy[20–22] and reappearing shortly after supplementation of the athymic animal with thymosin or other thymus extracts.[23] In agreement with findings related to θ-induction reported jointly by the laboratories of Boyse and A. Goldstein,[5] Bach *et al.* have reported that cAMP is able to mimic thymosin in this capacity,[24] as does the "thymosin-like activity" (T.A.) detected in the serum of normal young adults (murine and human) possessing a thymus gland.[25, 26]

The simplest explanation for the thymosin-enhanced one-way mixed lymphocyte reaction (MLR) observed in allogeneic, but not in syngeneic, thymocyte cultures is that T_1-cells, in the presence of thymosin and antigen, are driven to immunocompetent "educated" T_2-cells. The possible existence of such a substance has been proposed by Raff and Cantor.[1] We hypothesize that thymosin must be present at or very near the time of antigen presentation for the realization of the T_1 to T_2 conversion. It may be required to prolong survival of T_1, to prevent T_1 from reverting to pre-T, or to participate more directly in antigen processing. Evidence for or against this hypothesis may be provided by experiments designed to determine whether thymocytes, exposed *in vitro* to thymosin for a short period of time and then thoroughly washed, can produce an MLR comparable to that attained when thymosin is added and present in the cell culture during the entire course of the MLR. Most of the positive studies with thymosin reported to date have been experiments where the hormone was present at the time of antigen challenge, i.e., the responding animals are injected with thymosin, or the responding cells are incubated *in vitro* with thymosin for brief periods, and then these unwashed cells are concentrated and injected into host animals for assessment of immunocompetence. Yet, there are major exceptions in which positive effects on immune function by thymic extracts are demonstrated although the nonimmunocompetent cells are treated with the preparation for only a brief period *in vitro* and then washed before testing for immunocompetence (challenged with antigen) in the absence of thymosin. An interesting case in point is the attempt by two different groups to convert bone marrow cells into immunocompetent lymphocytes through short-term exposure of the cells to thymic factors *in vitro*. Conflicting results are reported: Miller *et al.*[27] were able to obtain increased helper T-cell activity *in vivo* (i.e. plaque-forming cell, PFC, increase following sRBC challenge) after pretreating bone marrow cells with thymosin *in vitro* and injecting the washed cells into lethally irradiated (not thymectomized) syngeneic mice, whereas Trainin's group[17] was not able to detect such increased immunocompetence when the THF treated, washed bone marrow cells were injected into thymectomized, irradiated host mice. Since recent reports by Balch and Feldman[28] indicate that the nonthymectomized, lethally irradiated rat has residual thymic function as compared to the thymectomized, lethally irradiated rat, it is not inconceivable that such conflicting results could be obtained. The reticuloepithelial cells of the thymus are thought to secrete most of the reported thymus humoral factors[29, 30] and these cells would be expected to be less radiosensitive than the majority of thymic lymphocytes.

In contrast to the lack of an effect of THF on production of PFC to SRBC, Small and Trainin[31] also reported that parental bone marrow cells, incubated in 200 μg/ml THF and concentrated by centrifugation before injection into thymectomized, irradiated F_1 mice, could give rise to a positive GvH response. It should be noted, however, that the THF-treated cells were not washed, but merely concentrated, before injection into the host mice.

It is more difficult, however, to explain how the short term exposure of thymocytes to 2 mg/ml THF *in vitro,* followed by washing of the treated cells, converted thymocytes into immunocompetent cells capable of inducing an enhanced GvH *in vitro* in the absence of thymic extracts.[16] The thoroughness of the cell wash would be critical here, since very low concentrations of THF might suffice to facilitate the antigen-driven differentiation from T_1 to T_2.

We suggest that in the absence of antigen there are a number of ways to convert bone marrow pre-T to T_1 cells, some of which are far more efficient than others, an encounter with thymosin, for example. Indeed Balch and Feldman[28] have shown that F_1 bone marrow cells initially having no T-cell markers can subsequently acquire T-cell surface markers after infusion into a thymectomized, irradiated parental rat. The infused bone marrow cells used here were not pretreated with any thymic agents. In mitogen stimulation assays, however, Balch and Feldman observed that acquisition of T-cell surface markers need not be associated with proportional increases in immunocompetence.[28]

Following T-cell marker expression (pre-T $\rightarrow T_1$), the amount of thymosin required to facilitate T_1 to T_2 conversion in the presence of antigen may be lower than that required to convert Pre-T to T_2 cells. If it is possible to enrich for a subpopulation of bone marrow or spleen cells that are pre-T (θ and TL negative), as Boyse's group[3, 4] has done, then one may be able to test the hypothesis that less thymosin is required to convert these cells into T_2 states, the pre-T cells having been converted to T_1 first *in vitro* (in the absence of antigen) by thymosin or other agents. Thymosin application in the presence of antigen would result in the conversion of these not fully competent T_1 cells into competent T_2 cells. Since we have observed both T-cell marker induction[3–5] and MLR enhancement with partially purified thymosin fractions, it is not known if the same molecule is responsible for both activities.

Summary

Calf thymosin is shown to enhance the one-way MLR of CBA thymocytes cultured with allogeneic mitomycin-C-treated C57Bl/6J spleen cells. Thymosin does not enhance the one-way MLR of CBA thymocytes cultured with syngeneic mitomycin-C-treated spleen cells. Based on this finding we present a relatively simple, rapid, and quantitative *in vitro* microculture bioassay for inducers of T-cell differentiation and propose that thymosin treatment, when accompanied by antigen presentation, induces the two-step maturational sequence of pre-T $\rightarrow T_1 \rightarrow T_2$.

ACKNOWLEDGMENTS

We are indebted to Dr. Gary Thurman for introducing cell microculture techniques into this laboratory, and to Ms. Janet Anderson, for her skilled technical assistance.

REFERENCES

1. RAFF, M. C. & H. CANTOR. 1971. *In* Progress in Immunology. B. Amos, Ed. 83–93. Academic Press. New York.
2. MOSIER, D. E. & C. W. PIERCE. 1972. J. Exp. Med. **136:** 1484–1500.
3. KOMURO, K. & E. A. BOYSE. 1973. Lancet **i:** 740–743.
4. KOMURO, K. & E. A. BOYSE. 1973. J. Exp. Med. **138:** 479–482.
5. SCHEID, M. P., M. K. HOFFMAN, K. KOMURO, U. HAMMERLING, J. ABBOTT, E. A. BOYSE, G. H. COHEN, J. A. HOOPER, R. S. SCHULOF & A. L. GOLDSTEIN. 1973. J. Exp. Med. **138:** 1027–1032.
6. GOLDSTEIN, G. 1974. Nature **247:** 11–14.
7. HOOPER, J. A., M. MCDANIEL, G. B. THURMAN, G. H. COHEN, R. S. SCHULOF & A. L. GOLDSTEIN. 1974. This volume.
8. LOWRY, O. H., N. J. ROSENBROUGH, A. L. FARR & R. J. RANDALL. 1951. J. Biol. **193:** 265–275.
9. THURMAN, G. B., D. M. STRONG, A. AHMED, S. S. GREEN, K. W. SELL, R. J. HARTZMAN & F. H. BACK. 1973. Clin. Exp. Immunol. **15:** 289–303.
10. GOLDSTEIN, A. L., Y. ASANUMA, J. R. BATTISTO, J. QUINT, M. A. HARDY & A. WHITE. 1970. J. Immunol. **104:** 359.
11. GOLDSTEIN, A. L., S. BANERJEE, C. L. SCHNEEBELI, T. F. DOUGHERTY & A. WHITE. 1970. Rad. Res. **41:** 579–593.
12. BACH, J. F., M. DARDENNE, A. L. GOLDSTEIN, A. GUHA & A. WHITE. 1971. Proc. Nat. Acad. Sci. U.S. **68:** 2734–2738.
13. COHEN, L. & M. L. HOWE. 1973. Proc. Nat. Sci. U.S. **70:** 2707–2710.
14. LAFFERTY, K. J. & M. A. S. JONES. 1969. Aust. J. Exp. Biol. Med. Sci. **47:** 17–54.
15. LONAI, P., B. MOGILNER, V. ROTTER & N. TRAININ. 1973. Eur. J. Immunol. **3:** 21–26.
16. GLOBERSON, A., V. ROTTER, I. NAKAMURA & N. TRAININ. 1973. *In* Microenvironmental Aspects of Immunity. : 183–189. B. D. Jankovic & K. Isakovic, Eds. Academic Press. New York, N.Y.
17. ROTTER, V., A. GLOBERSON, I. NAKAMURA & N. TRAININ. 1973. J. Exp. Med. **138:** 130–142.
18. KIGER, N., I. FLORENTIN & G. MATHE. 1973. Transplantation **16:** 393–397.
19. TRAININ, N., Y. LEVO & V. ROTTER. 1974. J. Exp. Med. In press.
20. BACH, J. F. & M. DARDENNE. 1972. Cell. Immunol. **3:** 11–21.
21. BACH, J. F. & M. DARDENNE. 1973. Cell. Immunol. **6:** 394–406.
22. BACH, J. F., M. DARDENNE & A. J. S. DAVIES. 1971. Nature New Biol. **231:** 110–111.
23. DARDENNE, M. & J. F. BACH. 1973. Immunology **25:** 343–352.
24. BACH, M. A. & J. F. BACH. 1974. Immunology. In press.
25. BACH, J. F. & M. DARDENNE. 1973. Immunology **25:** 353–366.
26. BACH, J. F., M. DARDENNE, M. PAPIERNIK, A. BARIOS, P. LEVASSEUR & H. LE BRIGAND. 1972. Lancet **ii:** 1056–1058.
27. MILLER, H. C., S. K. SCHMIEGE & A. RULE. 1973. J. Immunol. **111:** 1005–1009.
28. BALCH, C. M. & J. D. FELDMAN. 1974. J. Immunol. **112:** 87–95.
29. STUTMAN, O., J. YUNIS & R. A. GOOD. 1969. J. Nat. Cancer Inst. **43:** 499–508.
30. HAYS, E. F. 1969. J. Exp. Med. **129:** 1235–1246.
31. SMALL, M. & N. TRAININ. 1971. J. Exp. Med. **134:** 786–800.

EXAMINATION OF LYMPHOCYTE MEMBRANES OF ATHYMIC "NUDE" MICE BY SCANNING ELECTRON MICROSCOPY *

Gary B. Thurman, Paul S. Baur, and Allan L. Goldstein †

Divisions of Biochemistry and Cell Biology
Department of Human Biological Chemistry and Genetics
University of Texas Medical Branch
Galveston, Texas 77550

INTRODUCTION

The immunological system has two functionally distinguishable types of lymphocytes [4] known as T-cells and B-cells. These cell types in addition to acting separately can also function in a cooperative manner.[5] They have specific surface receptors [6–9] and distinct surface antigens,[10, 11] which enable them to be differentiated from each other.[12] Recently, Polliack et al.[1] and Lin et al.,[2] studying human cells, have presented new evidence of surface differences between B- and T-lymphocytes as seen by scanning electron microscopy (SEM). They report that T-cells are smaller and smoother with fewer and shorter microvilli and B-cells are larger and have a "hairy" appearance caused by a multiplicity of long microvilli extending from the surface. These studies are based primarily on the capacity of smooth cells to form rosettes (T-cells), "hairy" cells having receptors for the third component of complement (B-cells), and T and B classifications of cultured cell lines.

A general correlation was reported as existing [1] between human lymphocytes classified into the T or B category by generally accepted immunological techniques, and human lymphocytes classified into the T or B category by examining their surface morphology by SEM.

These findings led us to examine the surface morphology of mouse lymphocytes, including those of the congenitally athymic [13] hairless mouse mutant [14] called "nude" (nu/nu), and to study the influence of thymosin on surface morphology. Nude mice, as a result of being thymusless, are lacking in cellular immunity. They show an absence of lymphocytes from those areas in lymphoid organs that are known to be T-cell dependent.[15] The white blood cell count of adult mice is about 30% that of phenotypically normal littermates.[16] They lack mature T-lymphocytes, as shown by the low numbers of lymphocytes having θ or TL antigen on their surfaces,[17] and are immunologically deficient as shown by their inability to reject human or animal tumor implants,[18, 19] their acceptance of skin allografts and xenografts,[16, 20–22] their lack of contact sensitization to oxazolone,[23] and their failure to exhibit virus plaque producing cells.[24] Without mature T-lymphocytes, nude mouse spleen cells do not respond to those plant lectins known to stimulate only T-cells,

* These studies were supported by grants from the National Cancer Institute (CA 14108 and CA 15419) and the John A. Hartford Foundation, Inc.

† Author to whom all correspondence should be addressed.

such as phytohemagglutinin-P (PHA-P) and Concanavalin A (Con-A).[25] Nude mice do have a functional humoral immune system (B-cells) as indicated by near-normal levels of serum IgM antibodies[26] and by responses to certain antigens.[27] Their spleen cells do show a response to mitogens that stimulate B-cells such as pokeweed mitogen (PWM) and bacterial lipopolysaccharide (LPS).[25] Because of the lack of T-cells, the humoral immunity cannot function entirely normally as indicated by the lack of antibody response to T-cell-dependent antigens[28] and the absence of a secondary (IgG) antibody response.[26]

The rationale of the present study was predicated on the preceding information which has established that the B-cell system of the nude mouse is intact and the T-cell system is essentially absent. If T- and B-cells have different surface morphology as has been proposed, nude lymphocytes should be grossly different when compared by SEM to lymphocytes obtained from normal thymus-bearing mice. This assumption was found not to be the case and is the basis for this report.

Materials and Methods

Nude mice of the outbred Swiss variety were obtained from the colonies of Dr. Beppino Giovanella, St. Joseph Hospital, Houston, Texas. They were kept in sterile cages covered with nonwoven polyester filters, and their drinking water was supplemented with vitamins and antibiotics as previously described.[29] The cages were changed and all treatments were performed with sterile equipment in a laminar flow hood. Normal littermates were also treated in an identical manner. CBA/J mice were obtained from Jackson Laboratories and were housed in conventional animal-care facilities.

Bovine thymosin was isolated by modification[30] of a procedure previously outlined.[31]

Lyophilized fractions were dissolved in sterile pyrogen-free saline and sterilized by filtration through a 0.22 μ Millipore filter. Thymosin concentrations were based on protein/ml. Bovine thymosin, fraction 6 was prepared at 0.1 mg protein per ml, and bovine, fraction 8 at 0.05 mg/ml and 0.005 mg/ml. The nude mice used to measure mitogenic responses were injected intraperitoneally three times at 24-hour intervals with 0.5 ml aliquots of the appropriate suspension.

The lymphocyte cultures were prepared and harvested as previously described.[32] In brief, lymphoid organs were removed using sterile precautions, placed in plastic petri dishes containing RPMI 1640 (with 25 mM HEPES buffer, 100 μg/ml penicillin, 100 μg/ml streptomycin and 2 mM L-glutamine) and gently minced using fine curved tweezers or stainless steel mesh screens. Single cell suspensions were obtained by sequential passage through 20 GA, 25 GA and 27 GA needles. The cells were washed once, counted using a Coulter Counter Model Z and suspended to give a concentration of 6×10^6 lymphocytes/ml with 10% fetal calf serum (GIBCO; Grand Island, New York). Cultures were prepared in flat bottom microtiter plates by placing 0.10 ml of the cell suspension into each well. Control cultures received 0.10 ml of RPMI 1640 and the stimulated cultures received 0.10 ml of PHA-P (Difco; Detroit, Michigan) Con-A (Calbiochem; Oxnard, California), PWM (GIBCO; Grand Island, New York) or *E. coli* LPS (Difco; Detroit, Michigan) all made up in RPMI 1640. Cultures were pulsed by adding 1 μCi tritiated thymidine, 1.9 Ci/mM (Schwarz/Mann; Orangeburg, New Jersey), in 0.02 ml of RPMI 1640 24 hours before culture termination. Cultures were harvested utilizing the Multiple Automated Sample Harvester (Microbiological Associates; Bethesda, Maryland) as previously described.[32] The resulting filter spots were dried and placed in 1 dram opticlear vials (Kimble Glass Co.; Toledo, Ohio) to which was added 3 ml of a scintillation cocktail. The vials were stoppered, inserted in lidless polyethylene scintillation vials, and the tritiated thymidine incorporation analyzed by scintillaton spectrophotometry. Processing of the data and necessary statistical tests are performed on a Wang 700C Advanced Programming Calculator (Wang Labs; Tewksbury, Massachusetts).

The technique used for examining lymphocyte surface ultrastructure was almost identical with the technique reported by Polliack et al.[1] Single cell suspensions were fixed for at least 30 minutes with 1% gluteraldehyde (pH 7.3, 320 mOsmol), rinsed twice with buffer (pH 7.3, 320 mOsmol), postfixed in 1% osmium tetroxide (pH 7.3, 320 mOsmol) for an hour, subsequently rinsed twice in distilled water and dehydrated in a graded series of alcohol for 5 minutes each. The cells were then removed from suspension by filtration through Whatman 115 cellulose filters. The filters, bearing the cells on their upper surfaces were then prepared for critical point drying by dehydrating the sample through a graded series of amyl acetate/absolute alcohol and then absolute amyl acetate for 5 minutes each. The soaking specimen was quickly transferred to a critical point drying apparatus. After the amyl acetate had been dissipated by carbon dioxide, the chamber temperature was raised to 50° C with the resultant pressure reaching approximately 1,500 lb/in^2. The chamber was vented slowly and the dried specimen removed.

Portions of the filters were attached to stubs using double-sided sticky tape and coated with a thin layer of carbon (100–200 Å) and gold (250–300Å) on a rotary stage. The specimens were then stored under vacuum until examination.

A Cambridge S4 scanning electron microscope was used to examine the specimens. An accelerating voltage of 20 kV was used. Micrographs were recorded on Polaroid type 55 P/N films at direct magnifications from × 1,000 to 14,000. Resolution of the SEM was in the order of 100 angstroms. Thousands of cells were scanned on the SEM in order to obtain an evaluation of cell size and surface morphology of the entire population before recording micrographs.

Results

Mitogenic Responses on Thymosin-treated Nude Mice

Untreated nude mouse lymphocytes do not respond by [^{3}H]TdR uptake when cultured with PHA-P and Con-A as shown in Table 1. However, when treated *in vivo* with thymosin, nude lymphocytes begin showing evidence of T-cell development by a small but significant response of their splenic lymphocytes to PHA-P and Con-A as shown in Table 1. Lower than normal optimal concentrations of mitogens had to be used to observe mitogenic stimulation, indicating that the lymphocytes from thymosin-treated mice are more sensitive to mitogens. Normal nude lymphocytes mounted a small response to PWM and a larger response to LPS. Responses to PWM and LPS were changed little by *in vivo* thymosin treatment.

TABLE 1

STIMULATION OF NUDE MOUSE LYMPHOCYTES BY MITOGENS * FOLLOWING THYMOSIN TREATMENT *In Vivo*

Treatment	Amount †	Uptake of [^{3}H] TdR (cpm+S.E.) §				
		Control	PHA-P	Con-A	PWM	LPS
none (saline)	—	8121 ± 238	7513 ± 168	6977 ± 303	16267 ± 224	89297 ± 650
thymosin, fraction 7	.05 mg	12346 ± 923	15954 ± 882	16749 ± 153	22262 ± 864	85875 ± 6514
thymosin, fraction 8	.025 mg	22626 ± 756	29445 ± 504	31551 ± 731	35578 ± 416	124130 ± 623
thymosin, fraction 8	.0025 mg	**14938 ± 313**	18921 ± 459	22302 ± 360	27983 ± 512	100123 ± 2508

* Final concentrations were: PHA-P, 0.025%; Con-A, 1.25 μg/ml; PWM, 0.25%; and LPS, 10 μg/ml.
† The amount of protein injected daily for 3 days.
§ Lymphocytes harvested at 24 hours of culture.

Scanning Electron Microscopy of Lymphocytes of Athymic "Nude" and Normal Mice

Lymphocyte types present in the spleen and lymph nodes of CBA/J and NLM were also found in the respective organs of nude mice. Nudes have fewer lymphocytes than do normal mice, but the distribution of surface morphology appears similar to that of normal thymus-bearing mice. FIGURES 1

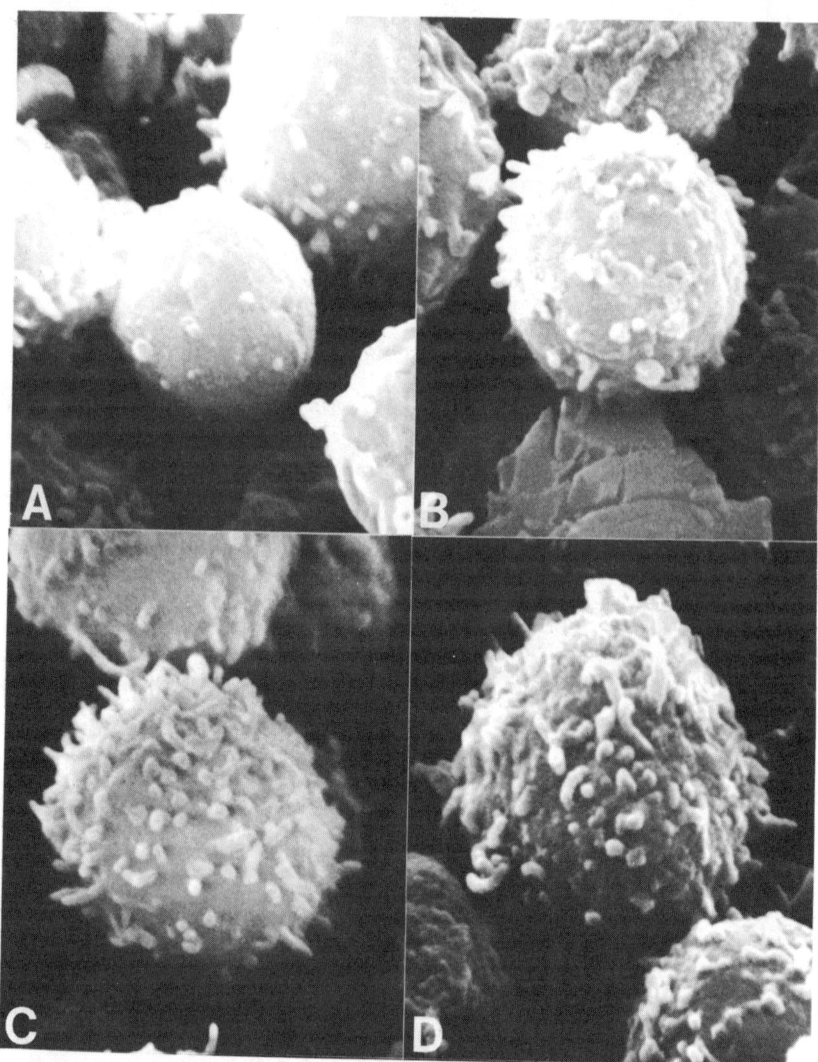

FIGURE 1. Illustration of the variety of cell surface morphology evident in the lymph node cells of normal littermate (*nu*/+) mice. The cell-surface range was: A–fairly smooth, B and C–intermediate, and D–mostly covered with microvillous projections (× 14,000)

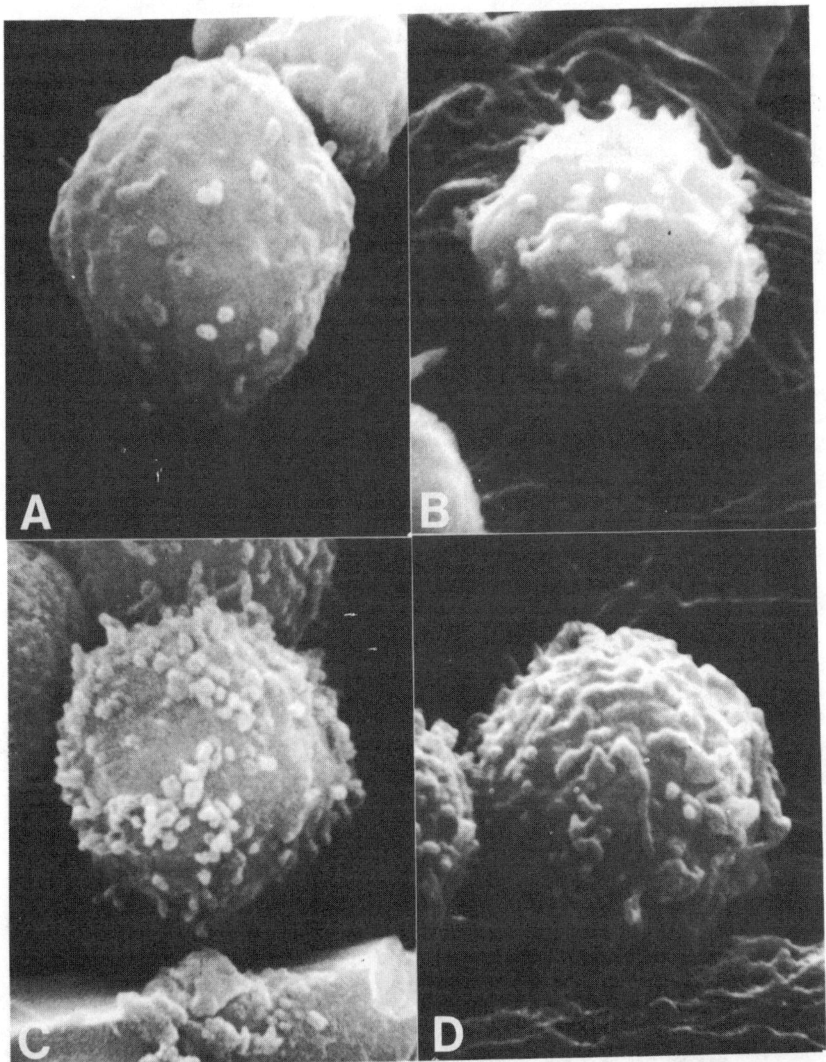

FIGURE 2. Spleen cells from normal littermates ($nu/+$). Cells A–D represent typical observed cells ranging from smooth to covered with microvilli (× 14,000)

and 2 show the typical range of cell morphologies found in lymph node and spleen of $nu/+$ mice. We found that lymphocytes from CBA/J mice were almost identical to those seen in $nu/+$ mice. FIGURES 3 and 4 show the ranges of cell morphology seen in nude lymph node and spleen. No gross differences or absence of certain cell-surface morphologies were observed. It was observed that cells with long microvilli on their surface tended to clump together. Whether this is an artifact of processing or a natural phenomenon is not yet known. An example of such clumping is shown in FIGURE 5.

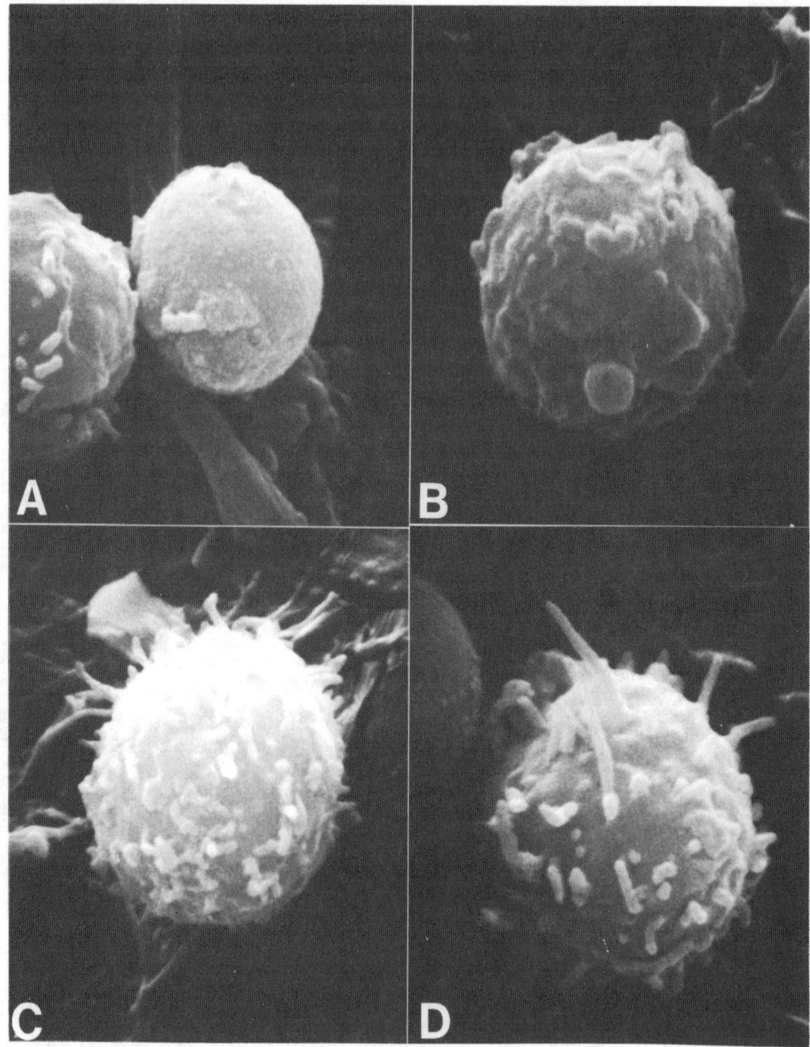

FIGURE 3. Lymph node cells from athymic nude (*nu/nu*) mice. The gamut of cell types ranging from smooth (A) to "hairy" (D) is again obvious. No gross variation between the incidence of the different types was obvious when these cells were compared to the cells shown in FIGURE 1 (× 14,000)

DISCUSSION

The results of the present investigation indicate that the T and B classification as proposed by Polliack et al.[1] and Lin et al.[2] based upon human lymphocyte surface morphology under the scanning electron microscope is questionable in a mouse model. Genetically athymic "nude" mice have many "smooth" cells in their lymph nodes and spleen although they have very few, if any, mature functional T-cells.[16–24]

Our finding that short-term (3 days) administration of thymosin to nude mice increases the responsivity of their lymphocytes to T-cell mitogens supports the contention of Bach et al.[38] and Scheid et al.[39] that thymosin-sensitive stem cells (predetermined T-cells) are present in nude mice and can be rapidly

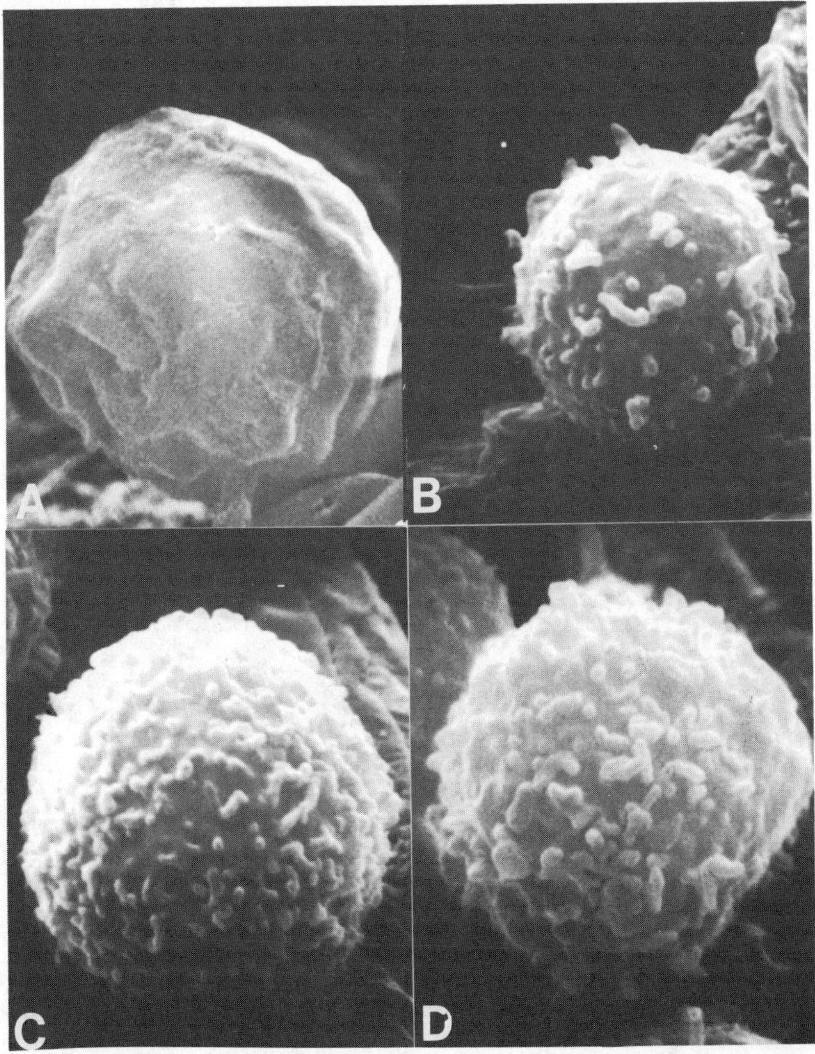

FIGURE 4. Spleen cells from athymic nude (*nu/nu*) mice. Cell types shown are typical of those observed. Smooth cells (A) were again obvious, and the cell surface morphology showed all the intermediate stages (B and C) as well as cells mostly covered with microvilli (D). (× 14,000)

activated by thymosin. These studies also support the findings of Lowenberg et al.[37] who found that thymosin could reconstitute the capacity of spleen cells derived from nude mice to elicit an *in vitro* graft-versus-host response. From the initial studies with nude mice it would appear that nude mice could become an ideal model for testing the potency of extracted thymus hormones.

Recently Pritchard and Micklem [33] have found that nude bone marrow has a similar capacity to that of normal littermate and CBA bone marrow to reprieve lethally irradiated mice and restore colony-forming units (CFU). They also found that thymus glands from CBA-T6T6 mice (with the marker

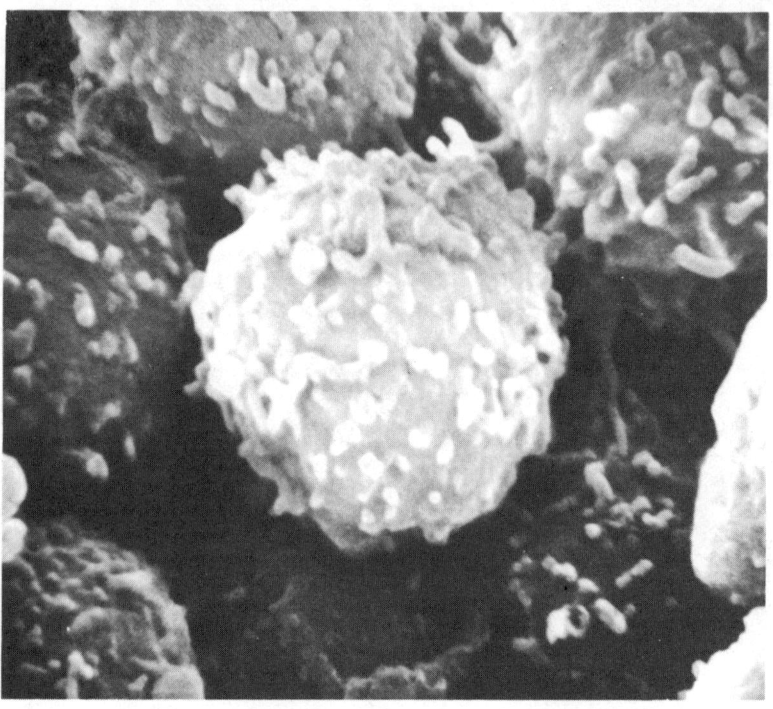

FIGURE 5. Evidence of clumping by cells of the type with the longest microvilli on their cell surface (× 17,500)

chromosome T6T6) transplanted into nude mice are entirely repopulated (after about 30 days) with lymphocytes not bearing the T6T6 marker. Conversely, CBA-T6T6 mice, lethally irradiated but reprieved with nude bone marrow, exhibit lymphocytes in the repopulated thymus that do not have the T6T6 marker. The lymph node cells responding to oxazolone also do not have the T6T6 marker. These findings would support the conclusion that the failure of thymic development in nude mice is not due to an absence of thymocyte precursors in the bone marrow, or to any physiological effect that prevents their differentiation but is due to the thymus epithelium developing inadequately or defectively. In contrast, Zspori and Trainin [34] have reported that nude bone marrow cells have less of a radioprotective effect than control cells. They found lower responses to SRBC in chimeras reprieved with nude bone marrow. They suggest that nude mice suffer from an intrinsic defect in the proliferative capacity of their bone marrow colony-forming cells. These conflicting studies are more understandable when it is realized that only outbred nudes were used. Much of this work needs to be done in inbred strains as they become available. Loor and Kindred [35] have found that when a thymus from an AKR mouse (TL−, θAKR) is grafted into a Balb/c-*nu/nu* mouse (TL2, θC3H), repopulation of the grafted thymus (as identified by immunofluorescence) begins at 2 weeks and is virtually complete within 4 weeks. After 4 weeks a Balb/c-*nu/nu* mouse implanted with an AKR thymus could not be distinguished from a normal Balb/c mouse on the basis of the number of TL2 positive thymocytes or θC3H positive lymphocytes in thymus, spleen, or lymph nodes. These experiments are strong evidence for existence of precursor cells for the T-cell compartment in nude mice and suggest involvement of host-derived T-cells in the recovery of some T-cell functions by nude mice grafted with allogeneic thymus glands.

The latest work by Stutman,[36] reports an inability to reconstitute nudes using other thymic extracts. This is in contrast to the work reported here using thymosin to increase mitogenic responsivity of the lymphocytes from nude mice. Dr. Marc Weksler (personal communication) has also been successful in inducing a small PHA-P and a Con-A response as well as to increase the number of θ-bearing cells in nude mouse lymphocytes by pretreating the animals with thymosin *in vivo*. Our findings indicate the presence of a stem cell population in nude mice, capable of differentiating into T-cells.

Our observations of nude mice lymphocytes using SEM have indicated that both "smooth" and "hairy" lymphocyte cell populations are clearly present. Nude lymphocytes have all of the types of cell-surface morphologies seen in mice bearing thymus glands. These findings indicate that the criteria of distinguishing human T- and B-cells may not be valid for distinguishing mouse T- and B-lymphocytes. It is a temptation to speculate that perhaps the smooth cells observed in the nude mice are T-cell precursors. It is just as feasible at present, however, that immature B-cells also have few, if any, microvilli on their surfaces. The development of microvilli on the surface may be a sequence of maturation of B lymphocytes. The presence of cells with smaller numbers of microvilli on supposedly enriched T-cell populations may be B-cells not yet sufficiently mature to be removed by the physical manipulations used to remove B-cells. In summary, discernment between B- and T-cells in mice by surface morphology is not as simple as it has been reported to be for human B- and T-cells.

Summary

Recent reports [1–3] have proposed that T-lymphocytes (thymus derived) could be distinguished from B-lymphocytes (thymus independent) by examining their features under the scanning electron microscope. T-cells were designated as having relatively smooth surfaced cells, whereas B-cells had "hairy" surfaces with many microvilli. We have examined this hypothesis in congenitally athymic "nude" mice, animals lacking T-cells,[4] and have not been able to confirm these reports. We have found that lymphocytes from nude (*nu/nu*) mice are indistinguishable from lymphocytes obtained from normal littermates (NLM) and CBA/J mice. We have found that in all the murine lymphoid tissue examined, including nude, the complete gamut of cell surface types, ranging from smooth to "hairy" are present. Our studies indicate that the proposed T- and B-cell classification based upon human surface morphology under the scanning electron microscope is questionable in a mouse model. It is presently unclear whether the smooth lymphocytes seen in nude mice are immature B-cells, pre-T-cells, or another unidentified population of cells.

References

1. Polliack, A., N. Lampen, B. D. Clarkson, E. De Harven, Z. Bentwich, F. P. Siegal & H. G. Kunke. 1973. Identification of human B and T lymphocytes by scanning electron microscopy. J. Exp. Med. **138:** 607–624.
2. Lin, P. S., A. G. Cooper & H. H. Wortis. 1973. Scanning electron microscopy of human T-cell and B-cell rosettes. N. Engl. J. Med. **289:** 548–551.
3. Sulliven, A. K., L. S. Adams, I. Silke & L. M. Jerry. 1974. "Hairy" B-cells and "smooth" T-cells. N. Engl. J. Med. **290:** 689–690.
4. Greaves, M. F., J. J. T. Owen & M. C. Raff. 1973. T and B lymphocytes, origins, properties and roles in immune responses. Excerpta Med.
5. Playfair, J. H. L. 1971. Cell cooperation in the immune response. Clin. Exp. Immunol. **8:** 839–856.
6. Lay, W. H., N. F. Mendes, C. Bianco & V. Nussenweig. 1971. Binding of sheep red blood cells to a large population of human lymphocytes. Nature **230:** 531–532.
7. Nussenzweig, V., C. Bianco, P. Dukor & A. Eden. 1971. Receptors for C_3 on B lymphocytes: possible role in the immune response. *In* Progress in Immunology, (First International Congress on Immunology, Washington, D.C.) : 73–82. B. Amos, Ed. Academic Press. New York, N.Y.
8. Makela, O., S. Sell, M. F. Greaves, H. Wigzell, G. L. Ada & W. E. Paul. 1970. Antigen binding lymphocyte receptors. Transplant. Rev. **5:** 3–166.
9. Basten, A. J. Sprent & J. F. A. P. Miller. 1972. Receptor for antibody antigen complexes used to separate T cells from B cells. Nature New Biol. **235:** 178–180.
10. Raff, M. C. 1969. Theta isoantigen as a marker of thymus-derived lymphocytes in mice. Nature **224:** 378–379.
11. Raff, M. C., S. Nase & N. A. Mitchison. 1971. Mouse specific bone marrow-derived lymphocyte antigen as a marker for thymus–independent lymphocytes. Nature: 230–250.
12. Wioland, M., D. Sabolovic, & C. Burg. 1972. Electrophoretic mobilities of T and B cells. Nature New Biol. **237:** 274–276.
13. Pantelouris, E. M., 1968. Absence of thymus in a mouse mutant. Nature **217:** 370–371.
14. Flanagan, S. P. 1966. 'Nude,' a new hairless gene with pleiotropic effects in the mouse. Genet. Res. (Camb.) **8:** 295–309.
15. De Sousa, M. A. B., D. M. V. Parrott & E. M. Pantelouris. 1969. The lymphoid tissues in mice with congenital aplasia of the thymus. Clin. Exp. Immunol. **4:** 637–644.
16. Wortis, H. H. 1971. Immunological responses of "nude" mice. Clin. Exp. Immunol. **8:** 305–317.
17. Raff, M. C. & H. H. Wortis. 1970. Thymus dependence of θ-bearing cells in the peripheral lymphoid tissues of mice. Immunology **18:** 931–942.
18. Rygaard, J. & C. O. Povlsen. 1969. Heterotransplantation of a human malignant tumor to "nude" mice. Acta Pathol. Microbiol. Scand. **77:** 758–760.

19. Giovanella, B. C., S. O. Yim, J. S. Stehlin & L. J. Williams 1972. Development of invasive tumors in the "nude" mouse after injection of cultured human melanoma cells. J. Nat. Cancer Inst. **48:** 1531–1533.
20. Rygaard, J. 1969. Immunobiology of the mouse mutant "nude." Acta Pathol. Microbiol. Scand. **77:** 761–762.
21. Pantelouris, E. M. 1971. Observations of the immunobiology of "nude" mice. Immunology **20:** 247–252.
22. Pennycuik, P. R. 1971. Unresponsiveness of nude mice to skin allografts. Transplantation. **11:** 417–418.
23. Pritchard, H. & H. S. Micklem. 1972. Immune responses in congenitally thymusless mice. I. Absence of response oxazolone. J. Exp. Immunol. **10:** 151–161.
24. Kano, S., B. R. Bloom, & M. L. Howe. 1973. Enumeration of activated thymus-derived lymphocytes by the virus plaque assay. Proc. Nat. Acad. Sci. U.S. **70:** 2299–2303.
25. Thurman, G. B., B. B. Silver, J. A. Hooper, B. C. Giovanella & A. L. Goldstein. 1974. *In vitro* mitogenic responses of spleen cells from "nude" mice following thymosin administration *in vivo. In* 1st International Workshop on Nude Mice. J. Rygaard & C. O. Povlsen, Eds. : 105–117. Gustav Fischer Verlag. Stuttgart, West Germany.
26. Bloemmen, J. & H. Eyssen. 1973. Immunoglobulin levels of sera of genetically thymusless (nude) mice. Eur. J. Immunol. **3:** 117–118.
27. Manning, J. K., D. Reed & J. W. Jutila. 1972. Antibody response to *Escherichia coli* lipopolysaccharide and Type III pneumococcal polysaccharide by congenitally thymusless (nude) mice. J. Immunol. **108:** 1470–1472.
28. Sjoberg, O., J. Anderson & G. Moller. 1972. Lipopolysaccharide can substitute for helper cells in the antibody response *in vitro.* Eur. J. Immunol. **2:** 326–331.
29. Giovanella, B. C. & J. S. Stehlin. 1973. Heterotransplanatation of human malignant tumors in "nude" thymusless mice. I. Breeding and maintenance of nude mice. J. Nat. Cancer Inst. **51:** 615–619.
30. Hooper, J. A., G. H. Cohen, R. S. Shulof, A. White & A. L. Goldstein. 1973. Thymic hormones: chemical and biological properties of human and bovine thymosin. Fed. Proc. **32:** 489(Abs.).
31. Goldstein, A. L., A. Guha, M. M. Zatz, M. A. Hardy & A. White. 1972. Purification and biological activity of thymosin, a hormone of the thymus gland. Proc. Nat. Acad. Sci. U.S. **69:** 1800–1803.
32. Thurman, G. B., D. M. Strong, A. Ahmed, S. S. Green, K. W. Sell, R. J. Hartzman & F. H. Bach. 1973. Human mixed lymphocyte cultures: evaluation of a microculture technique utilizing the multiple automated sample harvester (MASH). Clin. Exp. Immunol. **15:** 289–301.
33. Pritchard, H. & H. S. Micklem. 1973. Haemopoietic stem cells and progenitors of functional T lymphocytes in the bone marrow of "nude" mice. Clin. Exp. Immunol. **14:** 597–607.
34. Zipori, D. & N. Trainin. 1973. Defective capacity of bone marrow from nude mice to restore lethally irradiated recipients. Blood **42:** 671–678.
35. Loor, F. & B. Kindred. 1974. *In* 1st International Workshop of Nude Mice. Immunofluorescence study of T cell differentiation in allogeneic thymus-grafted nudes. J. Rygaard & C. O. Povlsen, Eds. : 141–145. Gustav Fischer Verlag. Stuttgart, West Germany.
36. Stutman, O. 1974. Inability to restore immune functions with humoral thymic function. Fed. Proc. **33:** 736.
37. Lowenberg, B., H. T. M. Nieuweskerk & D. W. Van Bekkum. 1972. Effect of thymus extracts on *in vitro* graft virus host activity in nude mouse spleen cells. Annual Report of the Radiobiological Institute THO: 105–111. Rijswijk, Netherlands.

ISOLATION AND QUANTIFICATION OF LSH * AND THE EVALUATION OF RELATED SERUM BASIC PROTEINS IN NORMAL ADULTS AND CANCER PATIENTS

T. D. Luckey and B. Venugopal

Department of Biochemistry
University of Missouri School of Medicine
Columbia, Missouri 65201

The recent isolation of several thymic hormones will undoubtedly stimulate further work and understanding of the enigmatic thymus. Although many thymic hormones have been proposed, those isolated in pure form are: LSH_h (lymphocyte stimulating hormone) isolated by Hand et al. in 1967;[8] thymosterin by Potop and Milcu in 1970;[21] LSH_r was first announced by Robey et al.[23] to the 1st International Congress for Immunology in 1971; thymosin purification reported by A. Goldstein et al. in 1972;[5] and thymin I and II were purified by G. Goldstein in 1974.[6] The ambiguous role and/or purity of other compounds such as HTH (homeostatic thymic hormone) of Comsa,[2] the thymic hypocalcemia factor of Mizutani,[20] and the human thymus specific protein of Tallberg et al.[24] allow their omission from the above listing; hopefully these, or others, may be added to the list of pure thymic hormones during the course of this conference.

The availability of pure thymic hormones will expedite the full development of thymology (FIGURE 1). The importance of the thymus as a central immune organ has overshadowed the importance of the thymus in theoretical biology and classical endocrinology.[12] The latter was substantially rectified by the review of hormonal interactions of the thymus by Comsa.[3] The role of the thymus in immunology suggested a model for differentiation and molecular communication as components of a general communication theory.[13] The timing of cell potentials for such activity was suggested as a general phenomenon in which the initiation of recognition was an important step in molecular imprinting under a variety of conditions in nature. The cytocrine activity of thymic factors has importance in the differentiation of stem cells and presumably the differentiation of T-cells. Injection of one microgram of LSH_r increases circulating lymphocyte counts in mice. The role of the thymus in differentiation is demonstrated by the increased lymphocyte to polymorph (L/P) ratio caused by the addition of either LSH_h or LSH_r to neonate mice. Potop and Milcu[21] have pioneered in relating the thymus to both metabolism and cancer. All of these aspects of thymology are reviewed in detail.[12]

In 1910, Klose and Vogt[10] suggested that the thymus was a central organ in immunity. The continuation of this work by Hellman and White[9] in 1930 is of particular interest because Glimsted's main germfree research with guinea pigs[4] was performed to confirm the function of "Hellman reaction centers." His work culminated in a monograph on the lymphatic system of the germfree

* LSH=lymphocyte stimulating hormone.

guinea pig. In retrospect, our work paralleled that of Glimsted.[1, 10] Addition of either live bacteria, dead bacteria, or soluble antigens to germfree mice led to a dramatic change in the size and cell structure of lymph nodes in germfree mice (FIGURE 2). The weight of a single, cervical lymph node doubled within 13 hours, and the number of cells must have increased much faster than this. Histologic examination showed tremendous numbers of cells in mytoses; a great number of small cells began to define small reaction centers that were previously nebulous. This rapid, generalized proliferation of lymphocytes constitutes an early reaction to injected antigen; the specific reaction to antigen, which culminates in specific cells producing specific antibodies, follows this generalized stimulation of lymphopoiesis.

The lymphopoietic reaction of germfree mice to antigen focused our atten-

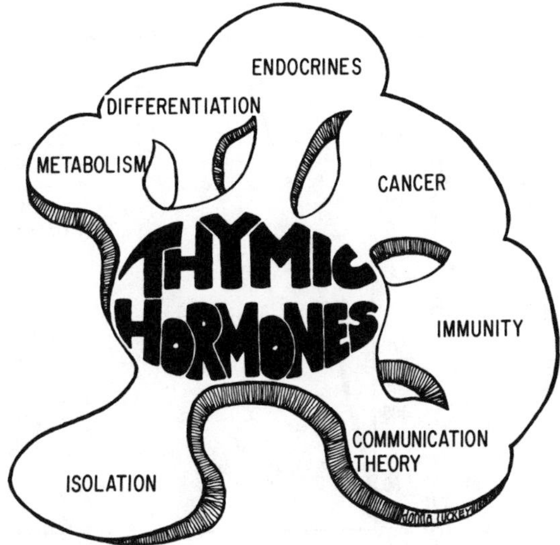

FIGURE 1. The isolation of pure thymic hormones provides opportunity to investigate many interlocking areas of thymology.

tion upon the importance of the thymus in antibody production. The involvement of thymus extracts in lymphopoiesis, suggested by Gregoire[7] in 1934 followed by Roberts and White[22] and Metcalf,[16, 17] indicated that thymus extracts would also cause lymphopoiesis. Metcalf[18] suggested that the lymphopoietic-stimulating factor (LSF) could be the same as the competence-inducing factor (CIF) of Miller.[19] A modified Metcalf assay was used to isolate our first thymic hormone named lymphocyte stimulating hormone (LSH), after LSF of Metcalf.[16] Following chemical fractionation, microgram quantities of a pure active protein were eluted from analytic gel electrophoretic columns by Hand et al.[8] Although it is often criticized because nonspecific substances affect it, the simplicity and reproducibility of this assay using the L/P ratio allowed isolation of compounds from thymus that are active in submicrogram quantities whereas the less specific compounds (i.e., phytohemogglutinin) must be utilized in quantities a thousand times greater. Note that a single injection of only 0.1 μg per mouse was active in this assay (FIGURE 3).

Subsequently, Robey et al.[23] isolated a second LSH from bovine thymus; therefore, the two compounds were designated as LSH_h and LSH_r after the responsible persons. The chemical fractionation scheme of Robey allowed milligram quantities of pure active protein to be isolated. Some of the physical-chemical characteristics of these two compounds are indicated in TABLE 1. The biological activity of LSH_r (FIGURE 4) illustrates both stimulatory and inhibitory characteristics. Humoral activity for initiating immune competence

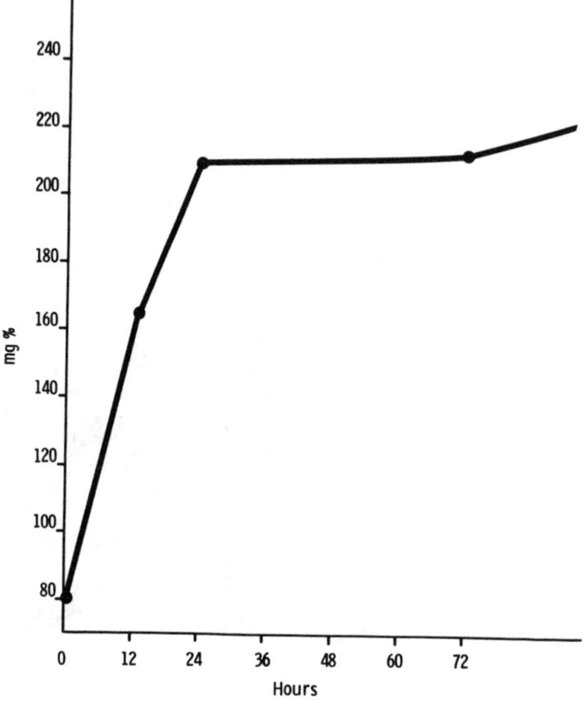

FIGURE 2. Weight of cervical lymph nodes per 100g body weight of mice. Germ-free mice were orally inoculated at zero hours with *Streptococcus sp.*

in mice was shown by the increased number of plaque-forming cells in spleen and serum antibody titer against sheep RBC. Further activity of both compounds to increase the L/P ratio suggests that they may be cytocrines and affect the differentiation of stem cells early in lymphocytopoiesis. It is unfortunate that quantities lower than 5 ng per mouse have not been tested.

The involvement of thymic hormones in cancer suggested that this component of the immune system could be a factor in cancer susceptibility. It seemed to be feasible that persons with a relative deficiency of LSH_r might be more susceptible to cancer than healthy persons.

Availability of pure LSH_r allowed the development of a quantitative elec-

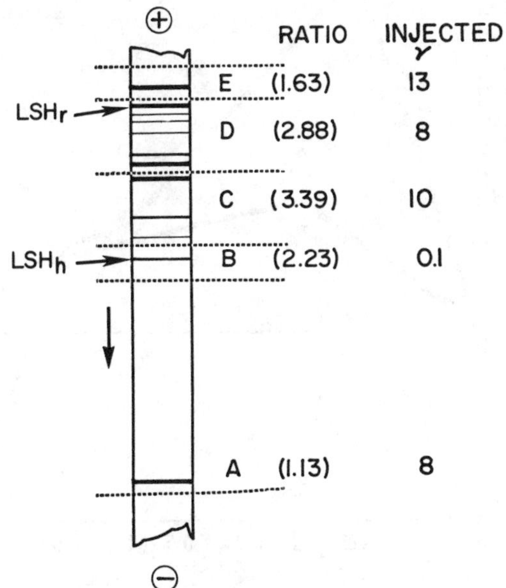

FIGURE 3. Diagram of gel electrophoresis bands of bovine thymus showing the relative position of LSH_r, LSH_h and the L/P ratios developed in mice from a single injection of fractions eluted from gels. Band E may be related to GEM 126 from serum.

trophoretic assay for LSH_r and related compounds.[15] Graded microgram amounts of LSH_r were electrophoresed on gels and stained with amido black 10B. The resulting pattern provided a standard curve for quantitative determination of this, or comparable proteins. Since pure LSH_r is not readily available, alpha chymotrypsinogen A, which gives equal color density of the band under identical conditions, was used as a secondary standard. This standard has a somewhat faster mobility, so it is developed only one hour whereas other gels are developed 2 hours. Either of these standards can be used for LSH_r assay in a variety of biologic material. FIGURE 5 shows the density evaluation

TABLE 1

CHARACTERISTICS OF PURE THYMIC HORMONES

	LSH_h	LSH_r	Thymosin	Thymin I	Thymin II	Thymosterin
molecular wt. (daltons)	15,000	80,000	12,000			Steroid
isolated	1967	1971	1972	1974	1974	1970
protein	+	+	+	+	+	Steroid
activity,* μg/gm	<1	<1	1+	<1	?	?
heat stable	—	+	+	+	+	+
wasting prev.	?	?	+	?	?	?
lymphopoetic	±	+	+	?	?	+
WBC differentiation	+	+	?	+	+	?
AB production	+	+	—	?	?	+
cell-mediated immunity	?	?	+	?	?	?

* Per mouse.

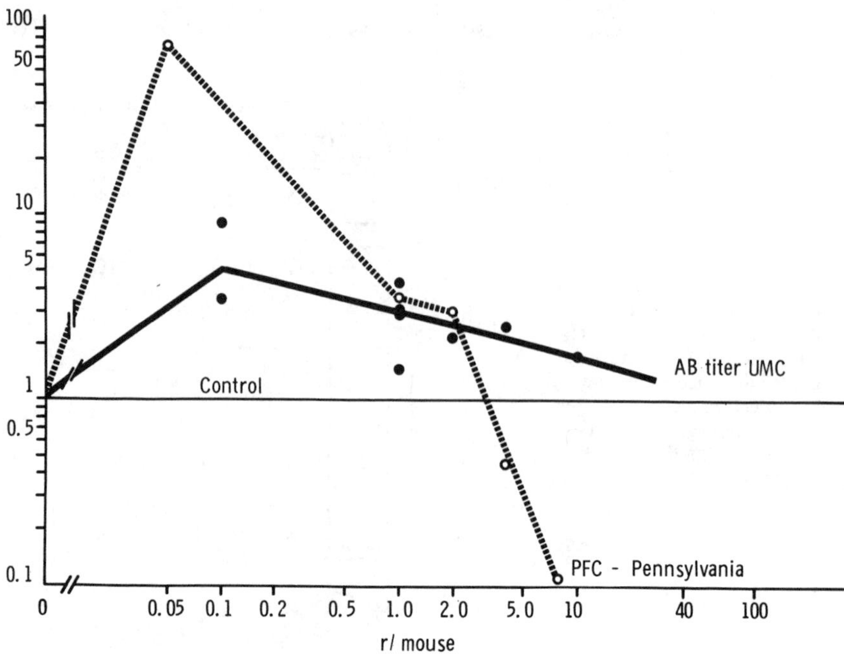

FIGURE 4. Biologic activity of LSH_r when a single injection (μg/mouse is given on the abscissa) was administered during the first 24 hours of life. Note that large quantities are expected to be inhibitory.

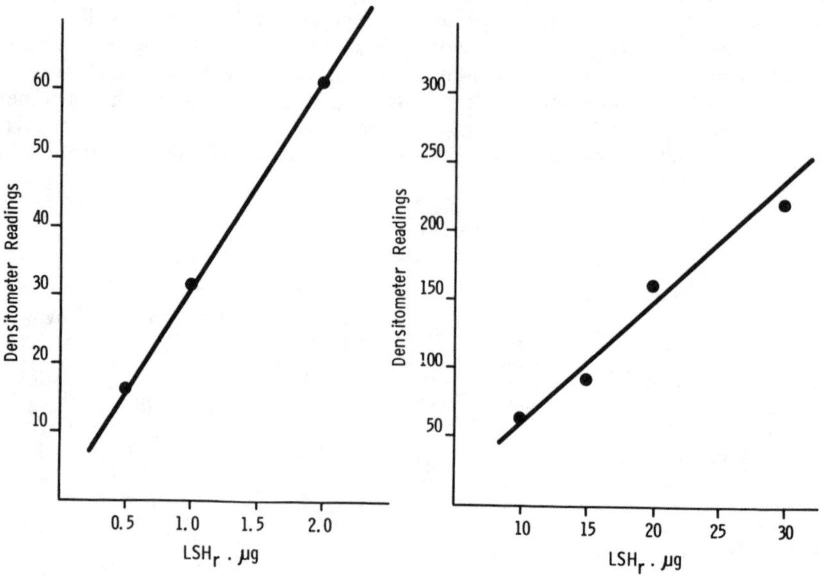

FIGURE 5. Density gradient curves obtained with different slit widths read directly from gels containing graded quantities of LSH_r.

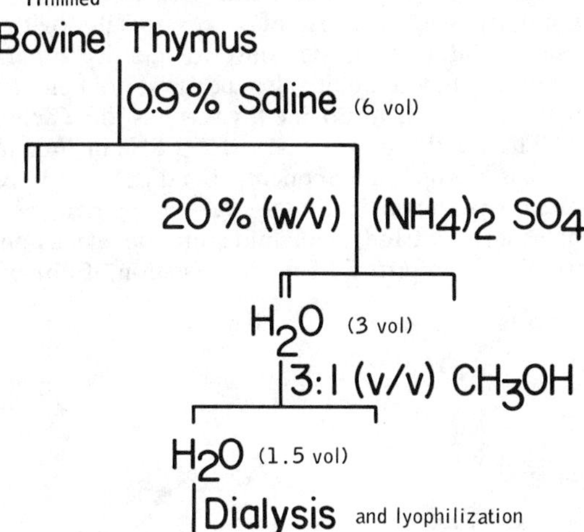

FIGURE 6. Fractionation scheme for treatment of tissues prior to electrophoresis. Serum is treated directly with $(NH_4)_2SO_4$.

using a strip densitometer with two different slit widths. Either this objective system or visual comparison can be used to determine the relative quantity of this or comparable proteins in serum.[26]

Tissues or biologic fluids were fractionated using a modification of the fractionation scheme of Hand (FIGURE 6), electrophoresed on the analytical gel system, stained and compared to the standard for quantitative evaluation. When this assay was utilized for natural tissues,[15] thymus was found to have approximately 15 bands. Other tissues (TABLE 2) had 5 to 10 bands whereas serum and saliva had 2 and 3 bands, respectively. No bands were found in urine. Although LSH_h was not found in human or bovine serum it was present in high quantity in beef thymus and in higher quantities in chick bursa. High concentrations of LSH_r were found in bovine and chick thymus and chick bursa. Possibly the two components of immune competence may be identified

TABLE 2

NONHISTONE, BASIC PROTEINS IN MATERIALS

	Human			Beef		Chick	
	Serum	Saliva *	Urine	Thymus	Serum	Thymus	Bursa
number	29	3	3	1	1	2	2
GEM-126	0.67	0.87	0	3.9	0.73	1.4	0
	(0.00–1.33)	(0.73–0.06)				(1.1–1.6)	
LSH_r	2.04	0.21	0	6.1	1.2	1.5	3.9
	(0.20–4.00)	(0.16–0.27)				(1.3–1.6)	
LSH_h	0	0.30	0	1.6	0	0	1.9
		(0.16–0.53)					(1.6–2.1)

* Presumptive identity of these salivary proteins has not been made. Data are given as mg LSH_r equivalents per g fresh material. (Data taken from Luckey et al.[15])

by differences in LSH content. LSH_r may be associated with the cell-mediated immunity whereas LSH_h may be associated with humoral immunity. Thus, this assay could be used not only to identify other basic proteins in tissues, i.e., thymosin, but it could also be used to help identify the bursa-equivalent in mammalian tissue. Bovine thymus has some activity.

The electrophoretic assay for LSH_r in human sera revealed the presence of two basic protein components; the difference in response obtained from different humans is shown in FIGURE 7.[14] Treatment of serum in this manner suggests that the two bands remaining on the electrophoretic column represent basic proteins from serum. The identification of one of these is indicated in FIGURE 8.

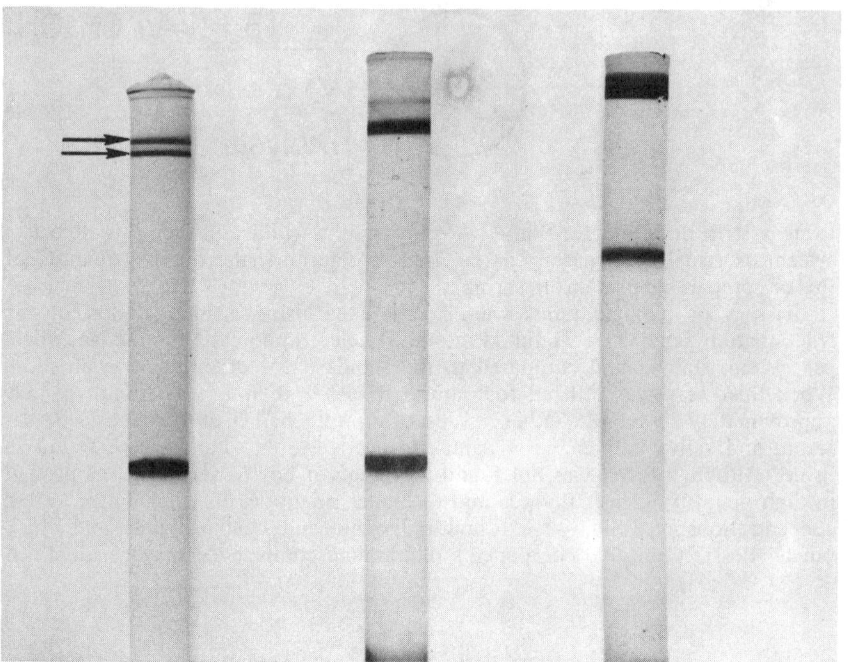

FIGURE 7. Variation noted in patterns of serum basic protein for different individuals.[15]

The fast-moving component in serum moves at the same rate as does LSH_r. When serum and LSH_r are mixed together, the top band appears to be diluted whereas the fast-moving band appears to be augmented; therefore LSH_r is judged to have reinforced the fast-moving (lower) band. When this protein was eluted from a non-dyed gel, it was found to show a precipitin line when diffused in agarose against anti-LSH_r serum. It was tentatively identified as LSH_r. The slow-moving band has tentatively been called GEM 126 because of its gel electrophoretic mobility.[15]

More extensive study was made of the basic serum proteins in adults[14] (TABLE 3). Occasionally no GEM 126 is found in human serum. In about

TABLE 3

HUMAN SERUM BASIC PROTEINS *

Category		mg Protein/ml serum					
		GEM-126		LSHr		Both	
	n-1/5	M	s.e.	M	s.e.	M	s.e.
healthy	23	0.67	0.09	2.04	0.13	2.70	0.12
untreated ca.	37	0.64	0.07	2.03	0.08	2.70	0.11
treated ca.	26	0.43	0.08	2.17	0.10	2.60	0.14
surgery ca.	37	0.65	0.08	2.05	0.09	2.72	0.14

* Data reported in detail by Luckey, et al.[14] These data were obtained in collaboration with Dr. C. Say, Ellis Fischel Cancer Research Center, Columbia, Mo.

10% of subjects, the mobility represented by this band shows two serum proteins and occasionally LSH_r is represented by two distinct bands. These limited data provide a standard which needs further extensive investigation, particularly confirmation and extension to the very young and to the aged. It will be especially important to observe the variations in these two components under different clinical circumstances. The average of 2.0 milligrams of LSH_r in human serum is unusually high for a highly active hormone that shows bio-

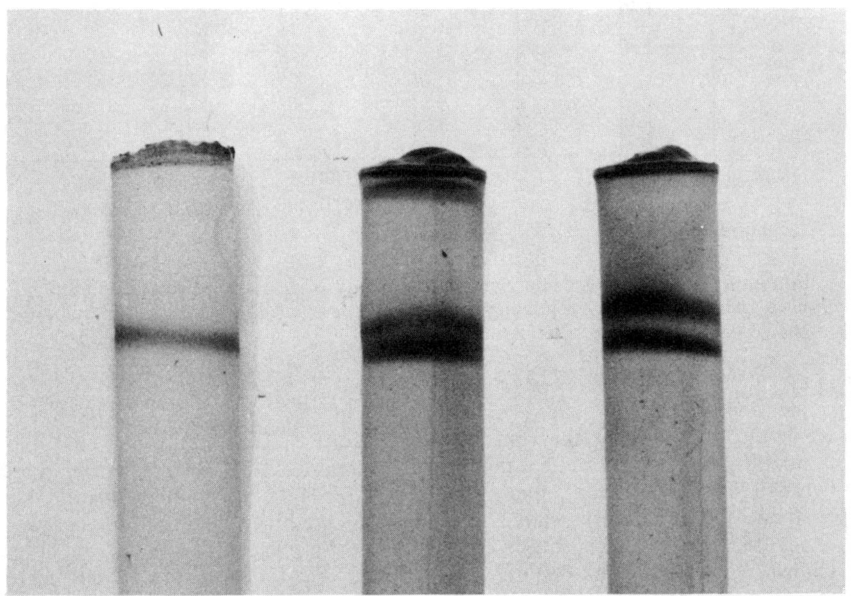

FIGURE 8. Presumptive identity of the fast-moving ocmponent (lower band) with LSH_r.[14] Only pure LSH_r was added to the left gel. Only processed human serum was added to the right gel. The two were mixed and added to the middle gel.

logical activity when injected into mice in nanogram quantities. The logical conclusion from such data is that serum LSH_r is acting as an inhibitor at these concentrations. It is appropriate to recall the limited data of Rushing (FIGURE 9), which suggest that LSH stimulates protein synthesis and effectively counteracts hydrocortisone for this activity.

A summary of the data of Luckey et al.[14] in human cancer also is presented in TABLE 3. No consistent differences were noted when males and females were compared nor when proven healthy adults were compared with untreated cancer patients or with surgery cancer patients for LSH_r, GEM 126, or the totals. As noted in the table, however, cancer patients who have been

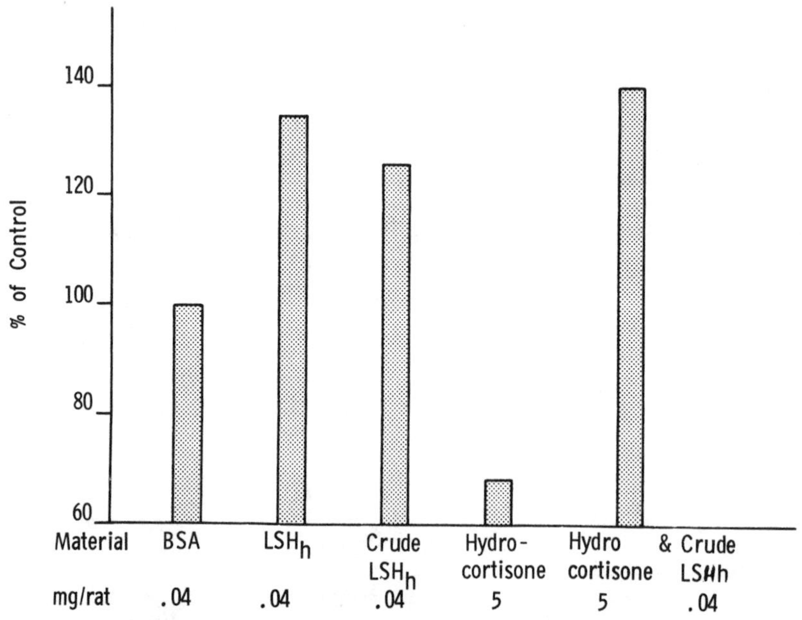

FIGURE 9. Rat spleen protein synthesis. Activity of LSH preparations to stimulate *in-vitro* protein synthesis following *in-vivo* injections of the materials in quantities indicated below the figure. Data from Rushing.[24]

treated with radiation and chemotherapy had low quantities of GEM 126 compared with any of the other three categories. Thus it appears that this dramatic treatment does affect this protein component. The lack of correlations between cancer and the quantity of serum LSH_r suggests that this thymic hormone is not directly related to cancer susceptibility. Correlation between either of these thymic proteins, particularly LSH_r should be found in other clinical conditions. The quantity of LSH and GEM 126 should be related to the ontogeny and function of the thymus. And it should be expected that a variety of thymic disorders would be reflected in the LSH component of serum. This and other disease entities remain to be examined. We apparently have a diagnostic test for an undesignated disease.

The similarity between LSH_h and thymosin, isolated by A. White et al.,[5] poses an important issue. The characteristics of these and other active fractions from the thymus should be compared in a single thymology laboratory using standardized conditions. Until this is done, even conferences such as this cannot truly resolve all the problems; there are too many differences in technique, state of purity, animal strains, and conditions.

References

1. CASTER, P., R. GARNER & T. D. LUCKEY. 1966. Antigen-induced morphological changes in germfree mice. Nature **209:** 1202–1204.
2. COMSA, J. 1973. Thymus replacement and HTH the homeostatic thymic hormone. *In* Thymic Hormones. T. D. Luckey, Ed. : 39–58. University Park Press. Baltimore, Md.
3. COMSA, J. 1973. Hormonal interactions of the thymus. *In* Thymic Hormones. T. D. Luckey, Ed. : 59–96 University Park Press. Baltimore, Md.
4. GLIMSTED, G. 1936. Bakterienfreie Meerschweinchen, Aufzucht, Lebensfahigkeit und Wachstum, nebst Untersuchungen uber das lymphatische Gewebe. Acta Pathol. Microbiol. Scand. [Suppl.] **30:** 1–295.
5. GOLDSTEIN, K. L., A. GUHA, M. M. ZATZ, M. A. HARDY & A. WHITE. 1972. Purification and biological activity of thymosin, a hormone of the thymus gland. Proc. Nat. Acad. Sci. U.S. **68:** 1800–1803.
6. GOLDSTEIN, G. 1974. Isolation of bovine thymin: a polypeptide hormone of the thymus. Nature **247:** 11–14.
7. GREGOIRE, C. 1935. Recherches sur la symbiose lymphoepitheliale au niveau du thymus de mammifere. Arch. Biol. **46:** 717–720.
8. HAND, T., P. CASTER & T. D. LUCKEY. 1967. Isolation of a thymus hormone, LSH. Biochem. Biophys. Res. Commun. **26:** 18–23.
9. HELLMAN, T. & G. WHITE. 1930. Des verhatten des lymphatischen Gewebes wahrend eines Immunisierungsprozesses. Virchows Arch. **287:** 221–257.
10. HUDSON, A. & T. D. LUCKEY. 1964. Bacteria-induced morphologic changes. Proc. Soc. Exp. Biol. Med. **116:** 628–631.
11. KLOSE, H. & H. VOGT. 1910. Klinik und Biologic der Thymus druse. Bietr. Klin. Chem. **69:** 1–200.
12. LUCKEY, T. D. 1973. Thymic Hormones. University Park Press. Baltimore, Md.
13. LUCKEY, T. D. 1973. Perspective of thymic hormones. *In* Thymic Hormones. T. D. Luckey, Ed. : 275–314. University Park Press. Baltimore, Md.
14. LUCKEY, T. D., C. C. SAY, J. S. SPRATT, JR. & B. VENUGOPAL. 1975. Occurrence LSH_r and GEM 126 in serum of normal and cancerous adults. J. Surg. Oncol. Submitted.
15. LUCKEY, T. D., B. VENUGOPAL, R. LEGRAND & E. MILITZER. 1975. Quantification of two basic proteins related to a thymic hormone (LSH). J. Surg. Oncol. Submitted.
16. METCALF, D. 1956. The thymic origin of the plasma lymphocytosis-stimulating factor. Brit. J. Cancer **10:** 442–457.
17. METCALF, D. 1958. The thymic lymphocytosis-stimulating factor. Ann. N. Y. Acad. Sci. **73:** 113–119.
18. Metcalf, D. 1965. Functional interactions between the thymus and other organs. *In* The Thymus. V. Defendi & D. Metcalf, Eds. : 53–73. Wistar Institute Press. Philadelphia, Pa.
19. MILLER, J. F. A. 1964. The lymphoid tissues and immune responses of neonatally thymectomized mice bearing thymus tissue in millipore diffusion chambers. J. Exp. Med. **119:** 177–194.
20. MIZUTANI, A. 1973. A thymic hypocalcemic component. *In* Thymic Hormones. T. D. Luckey, Ed. : 193–204. University Park Press. Baltimore, Md.

21. Potop, I. & S. M. Milcu. 1970. Isolation of a antiblastic factor from the bovine thymus. Rev. Roum. Endocrinol. **7:** 253.
22. Roberts, S. & A. White. 1949. Biochemical characterization of lymphoid tissue protein. J. Biol. Chem. **178:** 151–156.
23. Robey, W. G., B. J. Campbell & T. D. Luckey. 1972. Isolation and characterization of a thymic factor. Infect. Immunol. **6:** 682–688.
24. Rushing, D. R. 1968. Ph.D. Thesis. University of Missouri. Columbia, Mo.
25. Tallberg, T., S. Nordling & K. Cautell. 1968. On the biological activity of human thymus protein. Scand. J. Clin. Lab. Invest. **21:** 36.
26. Venugopal, B. & T. D. Luckey. 1973. Isolation and characterization of serum proteins similar to lymphocyte stimulating hormone (LSH_r). Abstract. Ninth Intern. Cong. Biochem. Stockholm, Sweden. 1973 : 310.

THE ISOLATION OF THYMOPOIETIN (THYMIN) *

Gideon Goldstein †

Irvington House Institute and the Department of Pathology
New York University School of Medicine
New York, New York 10016

Previous papers have described the isolation of[1] and biological studies on[1–3] thymin I and II, two closely related polypeptide hormones of the thymus, each of molecular weight 7,000. Objections have been raised to the name thymin, since it is readily confused with the pyrimidine base thymine;[4] we have therefore elected to change our terminology and in the light of our further knowledge of the actions of these polypeptide hormones of the thymus, thymin has been renamed thymopoietin.[5] Thymopoietin, in subnanogram concentrations, induces the differentiation of prothymocytes to thymocytes[3, 6, 7] and our present evidence suggests that it is produced by thymic epithelial cells and effects this differentiation within the thymus.

Thymopoietin was not isolated using this physiological effect as a bioassay, but rather by a presumably secondary effect on neuromuscular transmission, which was brought to light in the course of studying the human disease myasthenia gravis.[1, 2, 8–20]

Myasthenia Gravis, the Thymus and Neuromuscular Block

Myasthenia gravis is a disease in which patients have symptoms of motor weakness due to a partial failure of neuromuscular transmission. It has long been known to be associated with pathology of the thymus and thymectomy has been found on an empirical basis to cure or provide substantial remission to a large proportion of patients.

The analogy between curare-poisoning and the neuromuscular block of myasthenia gravis led to the use of anticholinesterase therapy for the disease. This was followed up by a large body of *unsuccessful* experimental work looking for a curare-like agent in the serum and urine and especially in thymus of myasthenic patients and normals (reviewed in reference 21). My work, which eventually converged on this same premise of a thymic substance causing the curare-like neuromuscular block, developed from different origins.

The concept that autoimmune thymitis was central in myasthenia gravis was developed from a study of the clinical, histopathological and immunological features of the human disease.[8, 9] This led to a body of experimental work which culminated in the isolation of thymopoietin.[1]

The hypothesis concerning autoimmune thymitis in myasthenia gravis was tested by developing an animal model of autoimmune thymitis by immunization

* Supported by grants from the United States Public Health Service (NS 09173), the Muscular Dystrophy Association, The New York Cancer Research Institute, and the Sackler Research Fund.

† Present address: Memorial Sloan-Kettering Cancer Center, New York, N.Y. 10021.

with thymic antigens in Freund's complete adjuvant.[10, 11, 13, 15–20] Experimental autoimmune thymitis was shown by a number of diverse criteria to be associated with a neuromuscular lesion similar to that of myasthenia gravis. It was further shown that the neuromuscular block was caused by a humoral substance released from the thymus. This was established by studying neuromuscular transmission in animals thymectomized prior to immunization,[10] or at the height of the neuromuscular block,[19] and also by cell and serum transfer experiments.[20] Final proof was obtained by the isolation of thymopoietin which, purified, produced neuromuscular block at extremely low concentrations.[1]

Knowing that a neuromuscular blocking substance was released from the thymus in thymitis, it was further established that this substance was being released by the normal thymus, since studies of neuromuscular transmission in thymectomized and in syngeneic thymus-grafted animals showed clear differences from controls.[14]

Thus these studies, based on a hypothesis concerning autoimmune thymitis in myasthenia gravis, had revealed a thymic hormone causing neuromuscular block and thymopoietin (previously thymin) appeared to be the curare-like agent sought by earlier investigators.

Despite application of these newer concepts, thymus extracts still failed to produce a curare-like neuromuscular block when applied to neuromuscular preparation *in vitro*.[12] It was only when extracts were injected *in vivo* that neuromuscular impairment could be detected after a delay of at least one day.[12] This delayed appearance of neuromuscular impairment has served as the bioassay to monitor the fractionation of thymus extracts and isolate thymopoietin.[1]

Isolation of Thymopoietin

The isolation of thymopoietin I and II has been described previously.[1] These two closely related polypeptides were isolated to homogeneity from calf thymus by saline extraction and heating, by molecular sizing on membranes, and by molecular sieve chromatography, adsorption chromatography on hydroxyl-apatite and ion-exchange chromatography on QAE-Sephadex.® Thymopoietin I and II show a consistent difference on ion-exchange chromatography and also on disc electrophoresis on polyacrylamide gels. Yet they are similar, for they show a line of identity in Ouchterlony plate immunodiffusion with antisera to either and behave similarly in functional tests of their neuromuscular and thymopoietic effects.[1, 3]

We have not yet resolved whether thymopoietin I and II are variant forms of the same hormone or whether they are two separate hormones closely related by common gene ancestry.

The chemical criteria of homogeneity for thymopoietin include a single band when 200 μg loads are run by disc electrophoresis on polyacrylamide gels at pH 8.9 and pH 4.3 (FIGURE 1) and single residues at the N-terminus (glycine) and the C-terminus (lysine).[22] The extreme potency of thymopoietin in biological assays (active at 3×10^{-12} M *in vitro*) suggests that the major homogenous polypeptide we have isolated is indeed the active molecule and that activity is not due to some contaminant present in amounts not detectable by chemical criteria ($<2\%$).

Thymopoietin I and II caused a detectable neuromuscular effect in mice in doses down to 4ng and 32ng per mouse, respectively.[1] An important feature of their neuromuscular action is that the effect is delayed, appearing after 18 hours and persisting through five days. Since thymopoietin has no direct or early effect on neuromuscular transmission, these findings suggest that modulates a chronic regulatory mechanism at the neuromuscular synapse and does not combine directly with the acetylcholine receptor as does curare.

The isolation of a thymic hormone affecting neuromuscular transmission raised two possible alternatives. Firstly, there could be a thymic hormone system affecting neuromuscular transmission and independent of the major function of the thymus—the induction of prothymocyte to thymocyte differentiation. Secondly, thymopoietin could be a hormone exerting this inductive function, with the effects on neuromuscular transmission being secondary. Experiments on the localization of thymopoietin in thymus supported this latter hypothesis, which was directly confirmed experimentally.[3, 6, 7]

Thymopoietin Localization in the Thymus

The site of secretion of thymopoietin in the normal thymus was determined by the following experiments:

Fractions from the hydroxyl-apatite stage of the thymopoietin isolation were separated by polyacrylamide disc electrophoresis on polyacrylamide gels at pH 8.9 as described previously. Unfixed gels were sliced, and the gel fragments representing Rf 0.26–0.35 with respect to the bromphenol blue dye marker were homogenized in phosphate buffered saline and emulsified with Freund's complete adjuvant.

These fragments contained thymopoietin I and II but no major contaminants since no other bands could be visualized in this region in parallel gels fixed and stained with Coomassie blue. Three rabbits were immunized intradermally in the footpads and multiple sites on the back and reimmunized four weeks later. After one week, they were bled and the serums tested for antibodies by the indirect immunofluorescence technique, using crystat sections of normal tissues as substrate.

One rabbit failed to develop antibodies and each of the other two showed a distinctive pattern of reactivity. Immunofluorescence was detected only in the thymus and not in control sections of liver, kidney, spleen, lymph node, muscle or thyroid. The reactivity was not species specific in that a similar pattern of reactivity could be found with cryostat sections of normal thymus from guinea pig, man, mouse, rat, and calf.

One rabbit reacted exclusively with the cytoplasm of most epithelial cells in the cortex (FIGURE 2). Lymphocytes and nuclei were not stained. The serum was active to 1/80. Serum obtained before immunization, and other control serums were negative. The other rabbit reacted exclusively with the cytoplasm of epithelial cells in the medulla (FIGURE 3). Hassall's corpusules were not stained. This serum was active to 1/160.

Unfortunately, these antisera were consumed in experiments and further antisera of sufficient avidity for immunofluorescence have not yet been obtained. These studies therefore require confirmation. If true, they suggest the possibility that thymopoietin I and II may arise from different epithelial cells in the thymus; furthermore, these studies suggested that the thymopoietins may be involved in thymopoiesis since they are being secreted by the majority of thymic epithelial cells and these cells have processes closely related to the developing thymocytes.

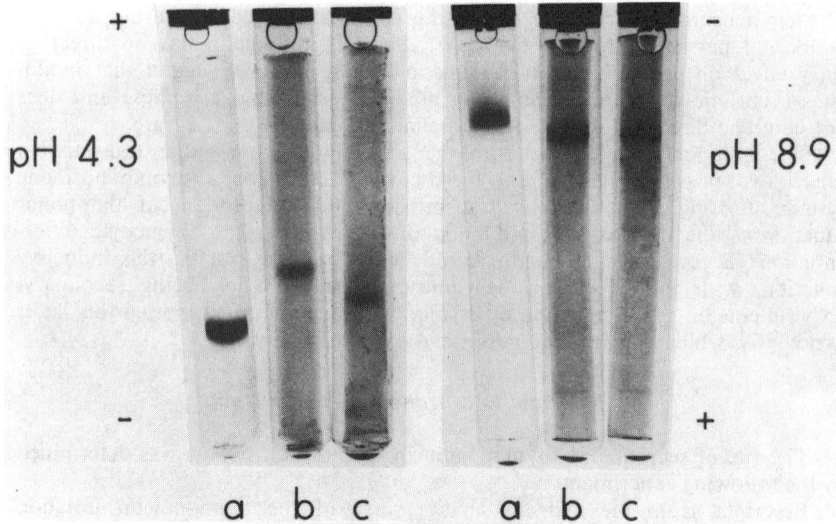

FIGURE 1. Polyacrylamide gels from disc electrophoresis at pH 4.3 and pH 8.9 of 200 μg loads of (a) UBIP, (b) thymopoietin II and (c) thymopoietin I. Each polypeptide shows a single band with a characteristic and distinctive mobility at each pH.

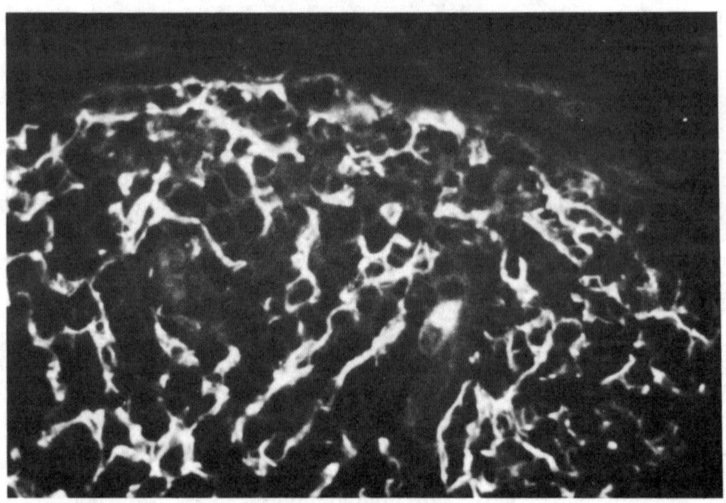

FIGURE 2. Indirect immunofluorescent section of normal guinea pig thymus incubated with rabbit antihymopoietin serum and visualized with fluorescein-labeled goat antirabbit immunoglobulin. There is immunofluorescence of the cytoplasm of cortical epithelial cells. This antiserum showed no staining of thymocytes or medullary epithelial cells and nonthymic tissues were also negative. Magnification: $\times$ 246.

Thymopoiesis

The prime role of the thymus is to induce the differentiation of prothymocytes derived from hemopoietic tissues to thymocytes, and eventually permit the development of a line of thymus-derived T-cells.

Experiments with purified thymopoietin I and II have shown them to be capable of inducing *in vitro,* in subnanogram concentrations, the differentiation of bone marrow or spleen prothymocytes, as judged by the development of characteristic differentiation antigens [3, 6, 7] or acquisition of the functional capacity to response by increased DNA synthesis to the plant lectins concanavalin-A and phytohemagglutin.[6]

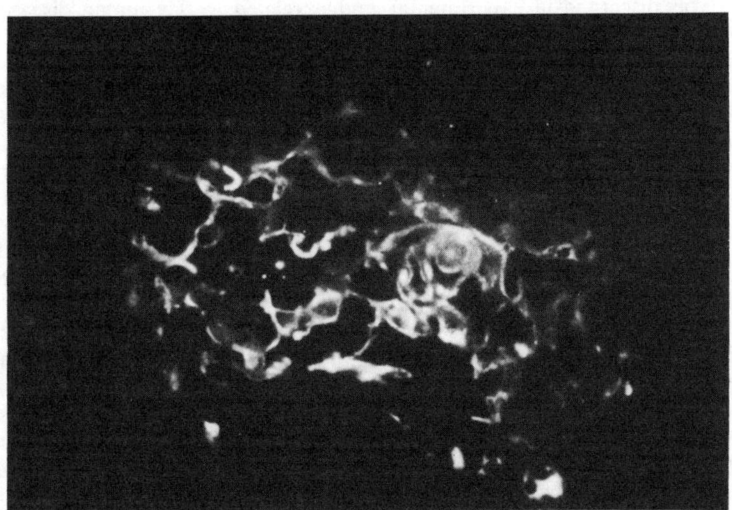

FIGURE 3. Indirect immunofluorescent section of normal guinea pig thymus incubated as in FIGURE 2. This antiserum shows immunofluorescence of the cytoplasm of epithelial cells in an island of medulla. There is no staining of thymocytes or cortical epithelial cells and nonthymic tissues were also negative. Magnification: × 246.

In the course of isolating thymopoietin I and II, a third polypeptide (FIGURE 1) was isolated.[23] This was the major component of the 4,000–12,000 molecular weight fraction of thymus prepared during the thymopoietin isolation. This polypeptide, which does not affect neuromuscular transmission, is widely distributed in all tissues of the body and indeed in many species. It also is capable of inducing, in subnanogram concentrations, the differentiation of T-cells and, unlike thymopoietin, the differentiation of B-cells.

This polypeptide is widespread in living cells and almost ubiquitous; since it is capable of inducing the differentiation of, or "producing," immunocytes of both T-cell and B-cell lineage we have termed it ubiquitous immunopoietic polypeptide (UBIP).

These findings highlight our good fortune in using the presumably secondary neuromuscular effect of thymopoetin to monitor its isolation since the nonthymus-specific agent UBIP, which is capable of activity in the assays of T-cell induction, is present in extracts of thymus in far greater amounts than thymopoietin.

Summary

The isolation from bovine thymus of two closely related polypeptides, thymopoietin I and II, is described. These are considered to be thymic hormones, which physiologically induce the differentation of prothymocytes to thymocytes within the thymus.

The isolation of the thymopoietins was monitored not by their differentiative effects, but by a presumably secondary effect on neuromuscular transmission. This was discerned in experimental studies related to the human disease myasthenia gravis in which it was suggested that autoimmune thymitis was regularly present. In an animal model, experimental autoimmune thymitis, the thymic disease was shown to result in the release of a substance that depressed neuromuscular transmission and this substance was shown to be also secreted in small amounts by the normal thymus. A bioassay was developed, this being the delayed appearance of neuromuscular impairment after *in vivo* injection of the active material, and this bioassay was used to monitor the fractionation of thymus extracts and isolate thymopoietin.

Pure thymopoietin was active at subnanogram concentrations, both in producing its effect on neuromuscular transmission and in inducing the differentiation of prothymocytes to thymocytes.

This potency of activity of the purified polypeptide, as well as its specificity in inducing the differentiation of T-cells and not B-cells, support the consideration that thymopoietin is a physiological inducing hormone produced by the thymus. This is further supported by the evidence that thymopoietin is only produced in the thymus: neuromuscular blocking effects are not present in extracts of other tissues and immunofluorescent localization of thymopoietin shows it to be present only in thymic epithelial cells.

Acknowledgments

Excellent technical assistance was provided by Mr. Ronald King and Ms. Miriam Siegelman. I appreciate the kind collaboration of Drs. R. S. Basch, M. P. Scheid, U. Hammerling, E. A. Boyse, D. H. Schlesinger, and H. D. Niall.

References

1. GOLDSTEIN, G. 1974. Isolation of bovine thymin: A polypeptide hormone of the thymus. Nature **247:** 11–14.
2. GOLDSTEIN, G. & A. MANGANARO. 1971. Thymin: A thymic polypeptide causing the neuromuscular block of myasthenia gravis. Ann. N.Y. Acad. Sci. **183:** 230–240.
3. BASCH, R. S. & G. GOLDSTEIN. 1974. Induction of T cell differentiation *in vitro* by thymin, a purified polypeptide hormone of the thymus. Proc. Nat. Acad. Sci. U.S. **71:** 1474–1478.

4. ROTH, M. 1974. Matters arising. Nature **249:** 863.
5. GOLDSTEIN, G. 1974. Matters arising. Nature **249:** 863–4.
6. BASCH, R. S. & G. GOLDSTEIN. 1974. Antigenic and functional evidence for the *in vitro* inductive activity of thymopoietin (thymin) on thymocyte precursors. Ann. N.Y. Acad. Sci. This volume.
7. SCHEID, M. P., G. GOLDSTEIN, U. HAMMERLING, & E. A. BOYSE. 1974. Lymphocyte differentiation from precursor cells *in vitro.* Ann. N.Y. Acad. Sci. This volume.
8. GOLDSTEIN, G. 1967. Thymic germinal centres in myasthenia gravis. A correlative study. Clin. Exp. Immunol. **2:** 103–107.
9. GOLDSTEIN, G. 1966. Thymitis and myasthenia gravis. Lancet **2:** 1164–1167.
10. GOLDSTEIN, G. & S. WHITTINGHAM. 1966. Experimental autoimmune thymitis. An animal model of human myasthenia gravis. Lancet **2:** 315–318.
11. GOLDSTEIN, G. & S. WHITTINGHAM. 1967. Histological and serological features of experimental autoimmune thymitis in guinea pigs. Clin. Exp. Immunol. **2:** 257–268.
12. GOLDSTEIN, G. 1968. The thymus and neuromuscular function. A substance in thymus which causes myositis and myasthenic neuromuscular block in guinea pigs. Lancet **2:** 119–122.
13. GOLDSTEIN, G. & W. W. HOFMANN. 1968. Electrophysiological changes similar to those of myasthenia gravis in rats with experimental autoimmune thymitis. J. Neurol. Neurosurg. Psychiat. **31:** 453–459.
14. GOLDSTEIN, G. & W. W. HOFMANN. 1969. Endocrine function of the thymus affecting neuromuscular transmission. Clin. Exp. Immunol. **4:** 181–189.
15. GOLDSTEIN, G., A. J. L. STRAUSS & S. PICKERAL. 1969. Antigens in thymus and muscle effective in inducing experimental autoimmune thymitis and the release of thymin. Clin. Exp. Immunol. **4:** 3–16.
16. OPPENHEIM, J. J. & G. GOLDSTEIN. 1969. Enhanced thymic lymphocyte response to phytohaemagglutinin in experimental autoimmune thymitis. Nature **222:** 192–193.
17. KALDEN, J. R., W. G. WILLIAMSON, R. J. JOHNSTON & W. J. IRVINE. 1969. Studies on experimental autoimmune thymitis in guinea pigs. Clin. Exp. Immunol. **5:** 319–340.
18. KALDEN, J. R. & W. J. IRVINE. 1969. Experimental myasthenia gravis. Lancet **2:** 638–639.
19. KALDEN, J. R., W. G. WILLIAMSON & W. J. IRVINE. 1970. The effect of thymectomy, hemi-thymectomy and sham thymectomy on experimental myasthenia gravis in guinea pigs. Clin. Exp. Immunol. **6:** 519–530.
20. KAWANAMI, S. & R. MORI. 1972. Experimental myasthenia in mice. The role of the thymus and lymphoid cells. Clin. Exp. Immunol. **12:** 447–454.
21. GOLDSTEIN, G. & I. R. MACKAY. 1969. The human thymus. William Heinemann. London, England.
22. SCHLESINGER, D. H., G. GOLDSTEIN & H. D. NIALL. Submitted for publication.
23. GOLDSTEIN, G., M. P. SCHEID, U. HAMMERLING, E. A. BOYSE, D. H. SCHLESINGER, & H. D. NIALL. Isolation of a polypeptide which has lymphocyte-differentiating properties and is probably represented universally in living cells. Proc. Nat. Acad. Sci. U.S. In press.

DISCUSSION OF THE PAPER

DR. A. RULE (*Tufts University School of Medicine, Boston, Mass.*): I direct my comments and questions to Dr. G. Goldstein. Thymectomies performed in myasthenia gravis often show no germinal centers after surgery.

In certain patients thymectomy does not yield the expected result; i.e. there is no remission of the disease. However, in many patients remission after thymectomy occurs within 5 to 7 years. In view of the fact that your factor worked on the electrical stimulus between the 18th hour and two days, and in view of the fact that our group has found delayed hypersensitivity both to muscle and central nervous tissue, how can you be sure that the effect of your thymic hormone is not on some mechanism directed towards relieving symptoms of delayed hypersensitivity and antibody production in these patients?

DR. G. GOLDSTEIN: That question really dates back to very early changes in the sequence of events and I have direct answers for them. First of all, the polypeptide nature has been established by biochemical criteria. Secondly, these polypeptides, which are in the process of being sequenced, are active in several assay systems at extremely low concentrations. We have calculated the dose as less than 300 molecules per cell for potency. The development of neuromuscular impairment occurs at 18 hours, the time we first detect it. Thus we are getting an effect which clearly precedes the immunological effects in healthy animals. This happens at a concentration which in endocrinological terms means an extremely high avidity. Thus the receptors must have an extremely good fit and hold this polypeptide hormone. Now the questions that you raise about myasthenia gravis are appropriate. I did not go into it, but that was the basis of my original histological study. I developed a quantitative analysis of the density of thymic germinal centers and found that in fact they were not related to the disease's severity, the presence of antibody or other parameters but decreased with age so that my hypothesis was that this was an autoimmune reaction in older patients. These are some clues as to why patients don't all improve after thymectomy. First of all, about 20% of normal people have ectopic thymus tissue which is not surgically removed. The second point is that progressive disease is partly reversible, but partly irreversible changes occur with long-standing disease. It was long recognized that the prognosis after thymectomy decreased if the disease went on too long. Thus I think these factors account for the clinical findings. Let us emphasize that 70 or 80 percent of the patients have remarkable improvements.

DR. H. MILLER: Have you or either Dr. Bach or Dr. Goldstein attempted to use the radioimmunoassay to detect the factor that Dr. Bach is working with?

DR. A. GOLDSTEIN: We have not as yet looked at Dr. Bach's fraction with our radioimmunoassay. We have looked at Dr. G. Goldstein's fraction and it does not cross-react with our fraction.

DR. W. CEGLOWSKI: May I add one point to Dr. Bach's comments. He had 5 possibilities concerning the relationship between thymosin and TF. I would like to add a sixth. There may be different factors, i.e. multiple factors, which have similar biological activities produced by the thymus. Also I believe it is much too early to ask all thymus "purifiers" to explain everything, but if Dr. Gideon Goldstein's immunogenically active peptide is present and ubiquitous in many substances, including celery and carrots, what is the basis for most of the thymic deficiencies that we see?

DR. G. GOLDSTEIN: Thymopoiten, as I emphasized, is unique to the thymus and has been isolated on the basis of another property which does not overlap with another tissue extracts; they have been shown (a) to be secreted physiologically in rats, and (b) to have two effects, one being the neuromuscular effect in excess. My colleagues have shown the extraordinary potency of these extracts in systems with differentiating prothymocytes, in which they seem to have a unique thymopoiten receptor that can interact with many antagonists.

Now this other ubiquitous material, the polypeptide, was isolated in the course of these experiments but then found to be also present in other tissues. It actually acts via the β-adrenergic receptor. This seems to be an extraordinary peptide which has been conserved in living cells right through higher plants, bacteria, yeasts, and man. It does not seem to be secreted because nude mice have it in their tissues but don't transform their prothymocytes to thymocytes even though they have β-adrenergic receptors. Thus I believe that this peptide and the β-adrenergic system evolved very early in life within cells and had functions long before cell to cell communications.

ISOLATION, BIOCHEMICAL CHARACTERISTICS, AND BIOLOGICAL ACTIVITY OF A CIRCULATING THYMIC HORMONE IN THE MOUSE AND IN THE HUMAN

Jean-François Bach, Mireille Dardenne, Jean-Marie Pleau, and Marie-Anne Bach

Hôpital Necker
75730 Paris Cedex 15 France

Introduction

The secretion of a hormone by the thymus was envisaged when the role of the thymus gland in cell-mediated immunity was discovered.[1,2] Experiments were then performed showing that it was possible to restore the immunocompetence of neonatally thymectomized mice by grafting a thymus within a cell-impermeable millipore chamber that allowed the passage of macromolecules.[3,4] However, these millipore chambers (0.45 μ pore) proved to be incompletely impermeable. A few years later, more direct experiments were performed by Trainin in Israel [5,6] and Goldstein and White in New York: [7,8] cell-free thymus extracts prepared in the calf were injected into neonatally thymectomized mice. These mice recovered the capacity to reject skin grafts or to induce a graft-versus-host (GvH) reaction. On the basis of these assays, or of other assays, the thymic extracts were fractionated and a protein with a molecular weight (MW) of 12,500 that contained the biological activity was isolated by Goldstein and White and called *thymosin.*[8] In fact, these experiments were open to some criticism, three main points being raised: (1) the extracts were all of heterologous origin (for obvious practical reasons, due to the small size of mouse thymus). It is known that injection of large amounts of heterologous proteins may induce a nonspecific immunostimulation; (2) the extracts were sometimes contaminated by endotoxin,[9] secondary to bacterial proliferation, which is difficult to avoid during long and complicated fractionation procedures. It is known that endotoxins are powerful immunological adjuvants; and (3) the spleen extracts that were used as controls were not satisfactory controls of thymic extracts because, even if there was indeed a thymic hormone present in the thymic extract and absent from the spleen extract, there were many other differences of composition between the two types of extracts; this criticism is emphasized by the significant activity demonstrated by spleen extracts in certain experiments. Moreover, the presence of an active principle in the thymus, did not imply that the product in question was exclusively or even predominently secreted by the thymus.

In summary, experiments with millipore chambers and thymic extracts strongly suggested the existence of a thymic hormone, but did not provide a definitive demonstration.

Our approach to the problem was perceptibly different from that mentioned above. We had demonstrated that a large percentage of rosette-forming cells (RFC) are thymus-dependent and bear the θ antigen, specific to T-cells.[10–12] Conversely, other RFC, thymus-independent, do not bear the θ antigen and include both B-cells and T-cell precursors. We first showed that thymic extracts (given by Goldstein and White, and Trainin) induced the appearance of the θ antigen on certain RFC from the bone marrow.[11, 13, 14] Similarly, spleen cells from adult thymectomized mice, which had lost the θ antigen,[13, 16] recovered their sensitivity to anti-θ serum after *in vivo* or *in vitro* treatment by thymic extracts. These experiments, perhaps more analytical than the previous ones by Goldstein and White, and Trainin, were however submitted to the same specificity criticism, even if spleen extracts were essentially inactive. The demonstration that there was a substance in normal mouse serum with the same activities as thymic extracts that was absent in the serum of thymectomized mice brought the definitive proof of the specificity of the phenomenon.[17, 18] Besides, the action of the hormone on RFC provided a simple and reproducible bioassay that allowed us to isolate and characterize the serum thymic hormone. As will be detailed in this article, this hormone appears to be a peptide with a MW of about 1,000; i.e. 10 times lower than that of the thymosin of Goldstein and White, but also 10 to 1,000 times more active for the same molarity. We have temporarily called this peptide "thymic factor" and not "thymosin" because the thymic factor and thymosin are obviously two distinct entities, even if they may be biochemically related.

This article presents a synthetic review of the data collected in our laboratory on the serum thymic hormone. Detailed experimental data are partly published elsewhere. We shall first present experimental data obtained from animals, mainly mice and pigs, and then some clinical data collected from normal subjects in relation to age and in various immunopathological conditions.

The Rosette Assay for the Detection of Thymic Hormone

The principle of the assay, which has already been mentioned, consists in the induction of the θ-antigen on θ-negative T-cell precursors after incubation with the thymic hormone, or more precisely, with the serum sample of the thymic extracts supposed to contain it. For practical reasons we usually prefer to use spleen cells from mice thymectomized 10–20 days before the test, rather than normal bone marrow cells. We also prefer to use azathioprine (AZ) instead of anti-θ serum. We had previously shown that AZ inhibited a large percentage of spontaneous RFC as found in the normal spleen,[19, 20] and that the AZ-sensitive RFC population disappeared after adult thymectomy, as did the population of θ-positive spleen RFC. We had demonstrated that in all conditions tested, AZ and anti-θ serum appeared to inhibit the same RFC, which proved to be T-RFC.[11, 16] We prefer AZ to anti-θ serum because AZ is a chemically pure product with a MW of 266, whereas anti-θ serum is a biological product of variable potency. Its preparation is time consuming and its activity difficult to evaluate when large quantities are needed. In our thymic hormone experiments we have never seen any differences between AZ and anti-θ serum. For each experiment, however, we have verified that anti-θ serum gave identical results to AZ.

C57Bl/6 mice are thymectomized at the age of 8–10 weeks. Ten to 20 days later spleen cells are collected, dissociated, washed twice, and incubated in Hanks medium to which is added the sample supposed to contain the factor, at variable log 2 dilutions. When serum is tested, more than 98% of the molecules with MW over 100,000 are excluded by diafiltration on CF 50 Amicon membrane, which is done in order to remove a high MW inhibitor and is discussed below. AZ is then added at a concentration of 10 μg/ml; i.e., a concentration intermediate between that inhibiting spleen or normal thymus rosettes (1 μg/ml) and that inhibiting spleen RFC in adult thymectomized mice (5 μg/ml).[16] After a 90-minute incubation at 37° C, sheep red blood cells (SRBC) are added and the cell suspension is centrifuged at 4° C and resuspended gently. Rosettes are read in a hemocytometer. In the absence of thymic factor, rosette formation is not inhibited by the AZ concentration selected. However, in the presence of thymic factor, AZ inhibits rosette formation as it would do at a concentration of 10 μg/ml for spleen or thymus RFC from normal mice. The lowest concentration of the tested sample which induces sensitivity to AZ is then taken as the active concentration of thymic hormone. It is expressed in dilution or in protein concentration evaluated by Lowry's method or eventually by ninhydrin after hydrolysis (18 h, 110° C in 6 N HCl). As mentioned above, anti-θ serum can be used in the test instead of AZ with absolutely identical results.

The sensitivity of the assay is assessed by the activity of the purest fraction, which shows activity at a concentration of 1 pg/ml. This sensitivity allows easy testing of fractions resulting from biochemical fractionation, since the tested sample can always be diluted at least 100 times and yet retain biological activity as measured by the assay. The reproducibility of the assay is reliable, since on two consecutive testings in a blind study we did not find a difference of more than one log 2 dilution in 130 out of 134 tested samples. Moreover, in studies made in collaboration with Stutman [21] and Davies, we had the opportunity of testing coded serum samples of normal, thymectomized, and thymectomized thymus-grafted mice, and found no error in the evaluation of serum thymic hormone; normal mice, sham thymectomized mice and thymus-grafted mice showed high levels, and thymectomized mice no significant serum activity.

Demonstration of a Circulating Thymic Hormone

Cell-free extracts given by Goldstein and White, and Trainin give back to spleen RFC from adult thymectomized mice the sensitivity to AZ and anti-θ serum that they had lost 5–7 days after thymectomy.[13, 14] Conversely, cell free extracts prepared from spleen, muscle, or brain do not have this property.[13]

Normal mouse serum previously filtered on Amicon membrane CF 50 to remove macromolecules has the same action on spleen RFC from adult thymectomized mice as that described above for thymic extracts. This effect is significant in C57Bl/6 mice for serum dilutions lower than 1/256, but a complete normalization in RFC sensitivity to AZ up to 1 μg/ml needs 1/16 dilution and at 10 μg/ml AZ concentration as routinely used, maximum serum active dilution is 1/64.

Thymic factor serum level varies with mouse strain. At the age of 3 months, the blood level of the thymic factor is 1/128 in the Swiss strain, 1/64 in C57Bl/6, CBA, A, and AKR mice, and 1/32 in Balb/c and C3H mice.

Concentration of TF in normal mice serum by ultrafiltration on UM2 membrane can raise TF level to 1/10,000. Nude mice serum shows no TF activity at any age tested (1 to 3½ months) even after concentration. As will be detailed later, autoimmune strains of mice, such as NZB, B/W, and Swan mice, show premature cessation of the thymic hormone production and a low level at the age of 3 months.

Decrease of Thymic Hormone Production with Aging: Relationship to Autoimmunity

The level of serum thymic hormone depends on age, as does thymus weight. The thymic hormone level is stable in most strains of mice until the age of 6 months, after which it progressively declines. After the age of 12 to 15 months serum activity is no longer detectable. This decrease of thymic hormone level that parallels the decrease in thymus weight, precedes by several months the diminution of cell-mediated immunity and eventually humoral immunity observed with aging. (Figure 1).

Thymic hormone is already at the adult level at birth. The fact that thymic hormone is secreted by the fetus, already suggested by its high level at birth, is

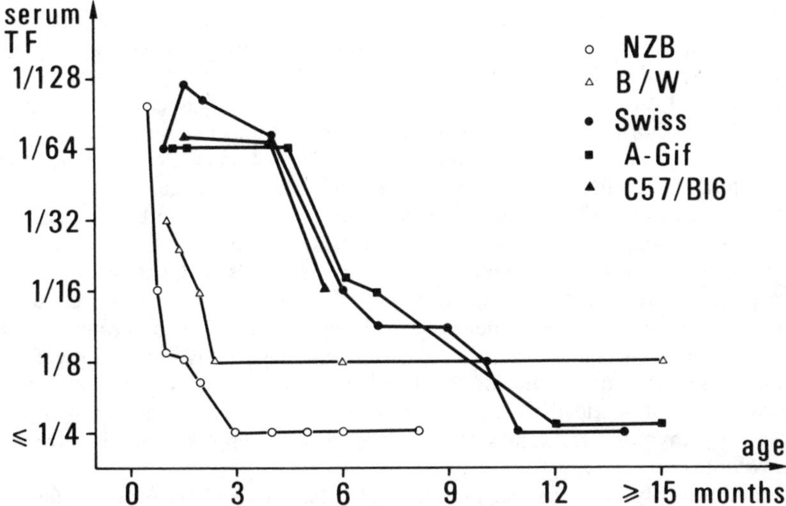

Figure 1. Age-dependence of serum TF level in NZB. B/W and nonautoimmune strains of mice (see Bach *et al.* 1973. Clin. Exp. Immunol. **14:** 247). Note the premature decline of TF secretion in NZB and B/W mice.

further confirmed by the reappearance of the serum thymic hormone in the blood of pregnant thymectomized mice (personal unpublished data). In these mice no activity is detected until the 14th or 15th day of gestation, after which there is a progressive increase in TF level, with a peak immediately before parturition. In the hours following parturition, the TF level becomes nil again. These data, which are very much in favor of TF secretion by the fetal thymus after the 15th day of gestation (that is the time when the thymic epithelium is already well formed and eventually colonized by a few lymphoid stem cells) would need more direct demonstration, however, since one cannot exclude TF activity in the mothers' serum due to various secretions related to the pregnancy, including placental secretion.

NZB and B/W (F1) hybrids have a normal level of serum TF at birth, but this level decreases prematurely between the 3rd and 6th week of life[22] (FIGURE 1). At two months NZB and B/W (F1) mice have no significant circulating TF. Six weeks after the decline of serum TF, NZB mice show disappearance of θ-positive lymph node RFC and two weeks later, progressive decrease in spleen RFC sensitivity to anti-θ serum and AZ, as present in neonatally thymectomized mice.[11] Interestingly, the normal AZ and anti-θ serum sensitivity of spleen and lymph node RFC is reconstituted by *in vitro* and *in vivo* treatment by thymic extracts.[22] This early fall in TF level is in keeping with the early abnormality reported by De Vries and Hijmans in NZB thymic medullar epithelial cells[23] which, as we shall see later, are the TF-secreting cells.

The etiology of the thymic lesions causing premature disappearance of serum hormonal activity is not known. That thymocytotoxic auto-antibodies, present early in life in NZB mice,[24] play a role is one among several possible hypotheses. Such antibodies, however, do not act (if they do play a role) by the elimination of hormone produced in normal amounts, since injection of thymic extracts corrects both serum TF and sensitivity of spleen and lymph node RFC to AZ and anti-θ serum in NZB mice.[22] Moreover, when grafting a neonatal NZB thymus into young or old NZB mice, one can very rapidly reconstitute a normal level of serum TF (our unpublished results). Interestingly, the duration of the reconstitution is between 2–4 weeks, which is identical to the spontaneous life span of thymus secretion of NZB mice. This short life span is at contrast with the long life span of thymus grafts in other strains.

T-cell deficiency is well documented in NZB and B/W mice. Decrease in the level of recirculating lymphocytes, in responsiveness in GvH reactions and in responsiveness to phytohemagglutinin and alloantigens are also well documented.[25] These T-cell deficiencies occur later than the fall in serum TF, but might be due to the same basic cause. A current hypothesis involves the T-cell deficiency in the hyperactivity of B-cells through the loss of suppressor T-cells. These considerations lead to the possibility of treating NZB mice with thymic extracts or thymus grafts in order to prevent autoimmune diseases (Talal, this volume).

Spontaneously autoimmune mice can also be obtained by genetic selection for spontaneous antibody production against nuclear antigens. Such mice have been obtained by Monier *et al.* by genetic selection bearing on an initial stock of outbred Swiss mice.[26] Autoimmune mice thus obtained exhibit high titers of antinuclear antibodies at the age of 3 months and ultimately glomerulonephritis with immune complex deposits. Interestingly, the genetic selection also induces an early cessation of TF production, similar to that noted in NZB mice.[27] As a control for these experiments, it has been shown that Swiss mice, genetically selected as "high" and "low" responders for anti-sheep RBC hemagglutinin production, showed no difference from ordinary Swiss mice with regard to serum TF level.[27] This observation is compatible with previous results showing that the selection thus obtained mainly induces changes in B-cell or macrophage reactivity without T-cell modification.[28] It is interesting to note that recent data in Swan mice have focused the attention on the thymus and on T-cells. Thus, it has been reported that Swan spleen cells showed a premature decrease in responsiveness to phytohemagglutinin[29] and that the thymus of Swan mice showed epithelium atrophy as that described in NZB mice and the presence of unexpected crystals.[30]

Epithelial Origin of the Serum Thymic Factor

The thymic origin of the circulating factor assessed by the rosette assay, is demonstrated by the rapid disappearance of TF from the serum after thymectomy and its rapid reappearance after thymus grafting (whether subcutaneous or intraperitoneal). A lag-time of 2 to 3 days is however observed before the reappearance of a normal serum factor level, probably due to the initial necrosis of the thymus graft. As mentioned above, grafting a neonatal thymus in a thymectomized mouse leads to a very long-lasting recovery of a normal serum TF level [21] (Figure 2).

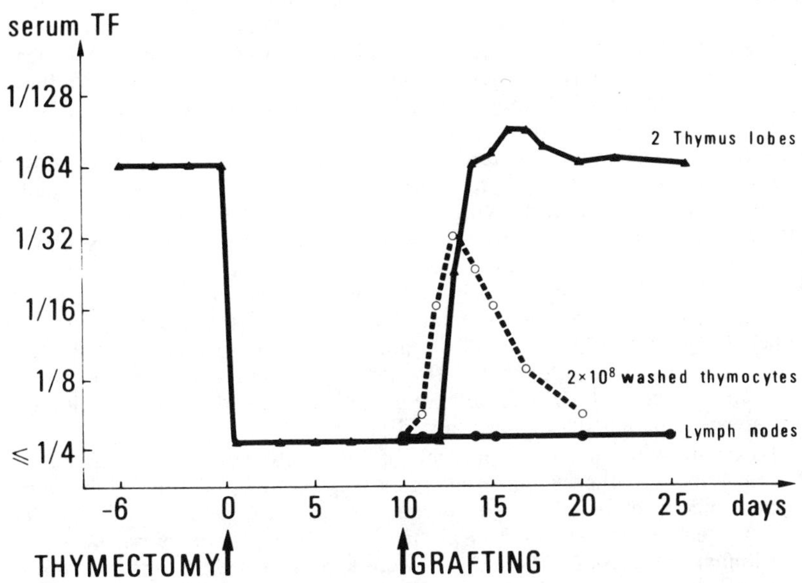

Figure 2. Effect of thymectomy and thymus (or lymph node) grafting in adult C57Bl/6 mice. Grafting integral thymus provides a more long-lasting recovery of TF level than dissociated thymocytes. Mice were splenectomized before thymectomy which eliminates the plateau noted in normal mice after thymectomy (see text).

It is also possible to induce the reappearance of a normal TF level in the serum of thymectomized mice by injecting dissociated thymocytes, but large numbers of thymocytes must then be injected,[18] since thymus-cell dissociation leads to the loss of a majority of the epithelial cells, which are not easily separated from the reticular epithelium. Lastly, injection of thymic extracts can also induce a restoration of the TF level. The injection of thymic cell-free extracts, however, only restores the TF level temporarily.[14]

Confirming the thymic origin of serum TF, nude mice with congenital lack of the thymus, do not have detectable TF in their serum, even at the age of 1 or 2 months, as mentioned above. Normally, when the serum of normal mice is concentrated on UM 0.5 Amicon filters, which do not allow passage of molecules with MW higher than 500, one can increase TF concentration up to 10,000. Conversely, no activity appears after the "concentration" of nude or thymectomized mice serum, which suggests the total absence of TF in these sera and the exclusive secretion of TF by the thymic gland.

The thymus contains two cell types: lymphocytes and epithelial cells. The epithelial origin of TF could be suspected in view of the secretory activity of normal thymic epithelial cells demonstrated in electron microscopy[31] and in view of the absence of serum TF in young adult NZB mice, which exhibit as mentioned above, an early atrophy of the thymus epithelium. This epithelial origin has been demonstrated by the significant reconstitution of serum TF level in adult thymectomized mice obtained by grafting a relatively small number of epithelial cells. These pure epithelial cells were obtained after *in vivo* incubation of two neonatal thymus lobes within a millipore chamber in an intermediate host for 7 days. The absence of lymphocytes was verified histologically. Whether grafted directly into adult thymectomized mice or within the millipore chamber, the epithelial thymus restored significant levels of serum TF within 2 days, and the restoration was even more clearcut 5 days after grafting.[21] Similarly, grafting thymectomized mice with 10^6 epithelial thymoma cells resulted in a highly significant recovery of serum TF. Grafting an identical number of normal thymocytes (mainly including lymphocytes) did not produce detectable level of TF. In addition only transient restoration was obtained with 2×10^6 thymocytes. More generally, these data outline the important function of epithelial thymic cells: it may be recalled in this respect that epithelial cells appear first in the fetal thymus before lymphoid cells,[32] and that epithelial thymus grafts are rapidly repopulated by lymphocytes.[33] Moreover, it has been shown that epithelial thymoma cells and thymuses placed in a millipore chamber, which become mainly epithelial, could reconstitute immunocompetence in neonatally thymectomized mice.[34]

To obtain a more direct approach of this problem, we have studied with Martine Papiernik the changes undergone by spleen cells from adult thymectomized mice after incubation on thymic reticular epithelium cultures.[35] Thymus fragments were explanted in plastic flasks in Eagle's medium, mixed with 10% human AB serum. The cultures were kept at 37° C and the medium was renewed twice a week. Rings of epithelial cells were visible at the explant periphery within 2–3 days, reaching 0.5–1 cm diameter after 7 to 10 days. No more lymphocytes were then found in the culture at 7 days. Electron microscopy studies, performed after 8 days of culture, confirmed the absence of lymphoid cells and the epithelial nature of the remaining cells in which tono filaments were seen. Fibroblasts cultures were used as controls. Sixty cultures of between 6 and 30 days duration were tested for the ability to induce the appearance of sensitivity to anti-θ serum in RFC from the spleen of adult thymectomized mice. In 23 cases the anti-θ serum rosette inhibition titer increased up to the titer observed with spleen or thymus RFC from normal mice. Control fibroblast cultures did not induce any significant changes in anti-θ serum sensitivity of spleen RFC. Interestingly, significant differences were noted in the ability of epithelial cells to modify spleen RFC according to the duration of culture. Forty-eight percent of the tests were positive between 7 and 15 days after the beginning of the culture, but, conversely, no positive results were obtained with 17 cultures of more than 15 days, in spite of the absence of any abnormality of the epithelial cells in light microscopy. Similar results were obtained when the spleen cells were placed within a millipore chamber on the culture, avoiding direct contact between epithelial cells and spleen cells.

Biochemical Characteristics of the Serum Thymic Factor

TF activity found in normal mouse serum persists after diafiltration of the serum through CF 50, PM 30, and PM 10 Amicon membranes. Conversely, no significant activity is found after filtration through UM 2 and UM 0.5 membranes. These data, although only indicative, suggest that the molecular weight (MW) of TF might range between 500 and 5,000 daltons.

When normal mouse serum is submitted to dialysis, using cellophane or cuprophane membranes, TF disappears from the serum sample within 8 hours at 4° C against distilled water or phosphate buffer (0.2 M) with a half life of less than 4 hours, the equilibrium being reached at 24 hours. In order to obtain accurate results, a dialysis system using a Cordis dialysis unit was used in the pig. It was verified, using markers of various MW, that MW of TF ranged between 500 and 3,000.

Serum TF stability at various temperatures is very weak when using total serum.[18] Thus, if TF is stable at −20° C and +4° C for several days, conversely the product is not stable at higher temperatures since most of the activity has disappeared after 5 hours at room temperature, 2 hours at 37° C, and a few minutes at 80° C (as opposed to thymic extracts such as thymosin which are heat stable). However, when TF is purified, as will be described later, it is much more stable since it is possible to maintain TF activity for more than 8 hours at 37° C. Interestingly, TF resists lyophilization, which provides an easy method for storage of TF and chemical procedures. TF is relatively resistant to extreme pH since we have shown that it was possible to keep most of the activity at pH ranging from 2 to 10. Lastly, TF adheres strongly to glass but not to plastic.

Proteolytic enzymes inhibit rosette formation at relatively low concentrations (our unpublished results). As some of these enzymes have a MW less than 20,000 daltons, they are difficult to remove from the sample before application of spleen cells. To avoid this difficulty, we have used enzymes coupled to insoluble particles such as carboxymethyl-cellulose and polyacrylamide. Using this method we have observed that TF was destroyed by trypsin, chymotrypsin, and pronase after a 60-minute incubation at 37° C at pH of 7.3. Control experiments included non-TF-containing Hanks samples treated in the same way, and TF incubated in identical conditions without enzyme. Ribonuclease used in similar conditions did not alter TF activity. Destruction of TF by proteolytic enzymes has been obtained both for mouse and pig TF and was obtained on crude serum preparations as well as on purified factor.

Mouse and pig TF-containing serum has been fractionated on various Sephadex® columns. In all cases the serum samples were first purified on Amicon membranes, (consecutively PM 30 and PM 10) and then concentrated 10 to 40 times on UM 2 membranes. It was shown, both in the mouse and in the pig that TF is eluted with the void volume in G 10 and is separated from the bulk of proteins in other Sephadex beads (G 15, G 25, G 50). The best separation is obtained with Sephadex G 25 (Figure 3) where TF is eluted after cytochrome and peroxydase and with angiotensin in phosphate buffer (0.02 M pH 6.3). A small amount of TF may be eluted with proteins in Sephadex

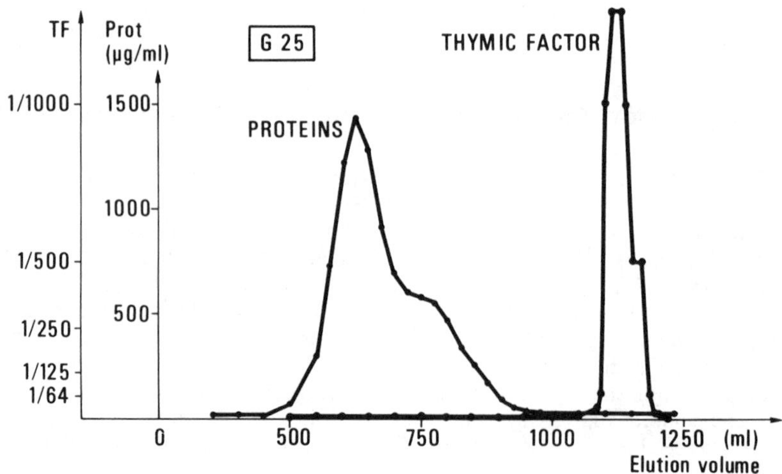

FIGURE 3. G 25 Sephadex chromatography of a pig serum ultrafiltrate (previously concentrated on UM2 Amicon membrane). Phosphate buffer pH 7.3/0.2 M.

G 25 and especially in Sephadex G 50. This protein-associated TF is variable in intensity from one experiment to another and is particularly important with buffers of low molarity, suggesting that TF binds to proteins. These Sephadex data, which have been confirmed using Sephadex G 25 with acetic acid 50%, suggest that the MW of TF is between 700 and 2,000.

TF binding to CM and DEAE cellulose was first examined by incubating 1 ml of mouse serum CF 50 ultrafiltrate with 1 ml of DEAE or CM cellulose previously equilibrated with phosphate buffer (0.01 M of various pH). After 60 minutes of incubation at 4° C in a hemolysis tube, the preparation was centrifuged and TF activity was evaluated in the supernatant. TF proved to bind to CM cellulose at pH lower than 7.0 and to DEAE cellulose at pH higher than 9.0. When applied to a CM cellulose column, mouse or pig TF was bound to the cellulose and was eluted with sodium chloride at a molarity of 0.12 M in phosphate buffer pH 6.3. TF was not retained on DEAE cellulose, at pH 8.3.

When electrophoresis was performed using the CM cellulose eluate, it was shown that TF had a pHi of 7.5 in pyridine acetate buffer (FIGURE 4).

In summary, serum TF appears to be a polypeptide, relatively neutral (pH of 7.5) with a MW of about 1,000.

ISOLATION AND PURIFICATION

Isolation of the polypeptide has been achieved by these successive operations: (1) defibrination, (2) dialysis, (3) concentration on UM 2 Amicon membrane, (4) G 25 Sephadex filtration, (5) CM cellulose chromatography, (6) thin layer chromatographies, and (7) electrophoresis. Each of these steps will be described briefly.

The routine fractionation procedure utilizes a starting batch of 8 liters of pig blood, but it must be realized that to obtain 20 μg of pure TF 180 liters of blood must be used. Normal 3–4 month old pigs are bled lethally at a local abattoir where blood is immediately defibrinated by mechanical agitation. The blood is then cooled at 4° C and transported to the laboratory where it is centrifuged to obtain the serum. Biological activity of the serum as determined by the rosette assay after defibrination is 1/128.

Dialysis is the following step: 3.6 liters of serum are dialyzed in the cold room in ultrafiltration conditions (positive pressure in the membrane, no liquid on the outside of the membrane. The membrane used is a polyacrylonitrile membrane (a product of Rhône Poulenc), with a total surface of 1.02 m2. The serum is circulated with a pump, and the ultrafiltrate is collected in the outside compartment of the dialyzer by a second pump equipped with an automatic outflow and pressure device (N. K. Man, to be published). The biological activity of the ultrafiltrate is 1/128.

Four-hundred ml of the serum ultrafiltrate are placed in each of seven Amicon diafiltration chambers at the continuous pressure of 50 psi. After 8 hours, when the membrane is dry, the chamber is filled with phosphate buffer and agitated to take up the product into the buffer. The activity is enriched to 1/25 000.

The pooled samples are then applied on a G 25 Sephadex and eluted with phosphate buffer 0.2 M, pH 7.3. Fractions active in the rosette assay are found with an elution volume between 2 and 2.5. Active fractions show activity up to the dilution of 1/256 000.

The active fractions obtained in the Sephadex chromatography are desalted using Amicon UM 2 membranes, and the retentate is then applied on a CM cellulose column equilibrated by phosphate buffer (0.01 M, pH 6.3). TF is eluted with a step-wise NaCl gradient from 0.05 M to 0.4 M. Active fractions are eluted for NaCl molarity of 0.1 to 0.15 M and show activity diluted 1/500,000.

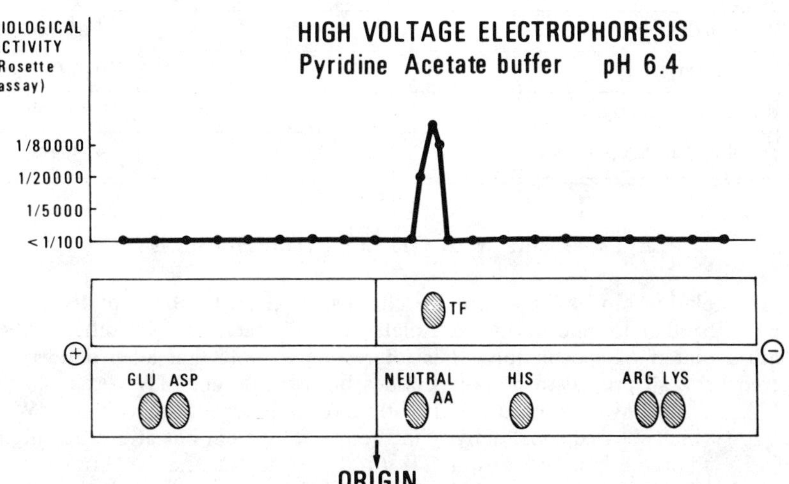

FIGURE 4. Paper electrophoresis at pH 6.4. TF was eluted (with water) from the area showing a spot after fluorescein staining. An amino acid mixture has been tested in identical conditions for comparison.

CM cellulose eluates are then separated on 3 successive thin-layer chromatographies (TLC) including chromatography in butanol pyridine, methanol chloroform ammonia and rechromatography in the latter solvent. (J.-M. Pleau *et al.*, in preparation)

The last stage of purification involves high voltage electrophoresis in diluted formic acid at pH of 1.9.

The product thus obtained appears to be pure in TLC performed in 5 different solvents using fluorescein staining. Studies are in progress to ascertain whether the product is indeed a pure entity (determination of amino acid terminals and amino acid composition). It should be emphasized that all these fractionation procedures are made easy by the very high sensitivity of the rosette assay and that, at the end, the amount of the material recovered from serum is low which complicates direct TF characterization. TABLE 1 summarizes the different phases of the fractionation and shows the progressive enrichment obtained. The products used in biological studies treated further have been fractionated to the 5th step, that is to say the CM cellulose chromatography.

TABLE 1

ISOLATION OF SERUM TF IN THE PIG

	Minimum Active Concentration
Defibrination	800 μg/ml
Dialysis	4 μg/ml
Amicon UM2 concentration	2 μg/ml
G 25 Sephadex	4 ng/ml
CM Cellulose	50 pg/ml
Thin layer chromatography	20 pg/ml
High voltage electrophoresis	4 pg/ml

RELATIONSHIP WITH OTHER THYMIC HORMONES

The relationship of the serum TF characterized on the basis of the rosette assay with other thymic hormones isolated and characterized by other authors is still a matter of speculation. It is interesting to note that all products considered have all proved to be polypeptides but of different MW. A. Goldstein and A. White have reported the isolation of a polypeptide with a MW of 12,500 [8] which showed some activity in the rosette system but at a much higher molarity than the purified serum TF (100 ng/ml for the best fraction [13]). Similarly G. Goldstein reported the isolation of three proteins with respective MW of 11,000 (prothymin) and 7,000 (thymin I and thymin II).[36] These products, isolated on the basis of their activity on neuromuscular transmission, did show some activity on lymphocytes (θ conversion of θ-negative spleen cells). However, they proved inactive in our hands in the rosette assay. These results must however be considered with caution since the products were used in the presence of BSA, which might have inhibited the activity in our system, although it did not in other θ assays.[37] Lastly, one may mention the thymic humoral factor (THF) isolated by Trainin and Kook[38] on the basis of an *in vitro* GvH assay[5,6] which appears to be a polypeptide with a MW between 1 and 3,000. This latter product is certainly the closest to ours.

Several hypotheses can be put forward to explain the possible relationship between thymosin or thymins with serum TF. It may be that thymosin or thymin are polymers or aggregates of TF. It is also possible that thymin or thymosin are precursors of TF since they are obtained from the thymus gland itself, whereas we work with serum (however, one must note that Trainin's THF is also obtained from the thymus gland). Lastly, it is possible that thymosin or thymin and TF are different entities, either both active in the rosette assay (at least for thymosin) or TF contaminating thymosin, as suggested by the fact that thymosin is an acidic protein whereas TF is a basic peptide. It is difficult to choose at the present time between these various possibilities. One may note, however, that few biological activities have been reported for these products, or at least few biological activities not submitted to the criticism of specificity. It is noteworthy that in our hands thymosin has proved to be much less active than serum TF. When thymosin was injected into thymectomized mice, "TF-like" activity recovered in the serum was higher than predicted from the *in vitro* activities, which goes with the idea that active molecules are splitting from precursors. However, this assumption will have to be confirmed after investigation of a possible enzymatic production of split products from thymosin. As will be detailed later, TF is indeed rapidly degradated and eliminated and only gets a half-life over a few minutes when bound to a vehicle like BSA or CM cellulose. It would be interesting to know for example whether thymosin releases active metabolites when bound to CM cellulose.

We have ourselves been engaged in the preparation of thymic extracts in the pig using N. Trainin's technique which includes dialysis as a first step.[5] Results showed that some "TF-like" activity was recovered in the dialysate but that amount of active products recovered for one whole thymus gland was not much more than that recovered from half a liter of serum. This might be due again to the predominant presence in the thymus of precursors which rapidly release the active product once split. It might also be due to the binding of active factors to other molecules from which they are not separated by fractionation procedures.

Serum TF Inhibitor

Total mouse serum examined in the test described above does not possess the activity reported for serum ultrafiltrate. This activity only appears after elimination of molecules with MW between 100,000 and 300,000 as assessed by diafiltration on Amicon membrane.[18] Therefore, there seems to exist a TF inhibitor with high MW present in normal serum and separable from TF by simple dialysis or diafiltration. The molecule responsible for this inhibitory activity of normal serum is not known, but it has been shown that it was active at very low concentrations since total serum diluted 1/5000 keeps its inhibitory activity.[18]

The thymic origin of the serum inhibitor has been investigated in the mouse

(TABLE 2). It was first thought that the inhibitor might be of thymic origin, since when mixing directly retentate of thymectomized mouse serum on XM 100 Amicon membrane with normal serum ultrafiltrate one did not see any inhibitory activity in the retentate. The disappearance of inhibitory activity after thymectomy paralleled that of TF.[18] However, when incubating "thymectomized" retentate and "normal" ultrafiltrate for 30 minutes at 37° C before adding it to spleen cells from adult thymectomized mice for the rosette assay, the inhibitory activity was recovered.[18] The extrathymic origin of the TF inhibitor has been confirmed by the demonstration that nude mice injected with serum TF recovered serum activity within a few hours after the injection when tested after diafiltration, but that nondialyzed serum did not show any activity (our unpublished results).

TABLE 2

TA INHIBITORY ACTIVITY IN SERA FROM TX MICE AND NUDE MICE *

Filtered Fraction (MW <50,000)	Retained Fraction (MW. >100,000)	TA	
		Immediate Testing	Delayed Testing
normal	normal	$\leqslant 1/4$	$\leqslant 1/4$
normal	O	1/64	1/64
O	normal	$\leqslant 1/4$	$\leqslant 1/4$
Tx	Tx	$\leqslant 1/4$	$\leqslant 1/4$
Tx	O	$\leqslant 1/4$	$\leqslant 1/4$
O	Tx	$\leqslant 1/4$	$\leqslant 1/4$
normal	Tx	1/64	$\leqslant 1/4$

* Sera have been filtered on a XM 100 Amicon membrane. Mixtures of filtered and retained fractions have been added to spleen cells from adult thymectomized mice for TA evaluation, either immediately or after a 60-minute preincubation at 37° C.[18]

These data suggest that TF binds to the inhibitory molecule, as is the case for thyroxin, the *in vitro* function of which is inhibited by its specific binding protein,[39] an hypothesis supported by the data presented in the next paragraph of TF metabolism.

METABOLISM OF SERUM TF

Serum TF level decreases rapidly after thymectomy, and no more TF activity is found in serum after 6 days. However, this decrease is biphasic. During the first 6 hours, serum TF varies from 1/64 to 1/8 with a half-life of 2½ hours. It remains at this level for 5 days. One the 6th day a new fall is observed down to the dilution of ½–¼. The second fall on the 6th day is a significant one and occurs simultaneously with a drop in spleen RFC sensitivity to AZ and AθS. Similar results have been obtained in Swiss, CBA, C3H, and AKR strains. In all cases sera collected 8–10 days after thymectomy showed TF levels lower or equal to ¼.

Although splenectomy alone has no effect on serum TF when it is performed 2 days before thymectomy, it modifies serum TF kinetics following thymectomy. Splenectomy suppresses the plateau observed between day 1 and day 6 after thymectomy alone. The significance of this effect of splenectomy is not known but may be eventually explained by the binding and protection of TF in the spleen with slow and progressive release after thymectomy. It is interesting to note that the relatively slow decrease of TF level after thymectomy has also been observed in other species, such as the pig or the human.

When normal mouse serum is injected i.p. into adult thymectomized mice, one can observe the reappearance of serum TF for a few hours. Similar data are obtained with serum filtrated through XM 300 or XM 100 membrane, with MW cutoffs of 300,000 and 100,000, respectively. However, when serum is ultrafiltrated through CF 50 (MW cutoff:50,000), PM 30 or PM 10 membranes (MW 30,000, and 10,000) no more activity is found in the serum, except if one uses the i.v. route and looks at the serum within the first 5 minutes after the injection.

This rapid elimination of TF represents a difficult problem when using purified TF completely separated from other serum proteins, since no *in vivo* effects of ultrafiltrated TF are noted in keeping with the absence of serum activity. To avoid these difficulties in using *in vivo* purified TF, various vehicles have been tried in order to bind and protect the TF from degradation. Among these vehicles, CM cellulose, Dextran, BSA, and serum from thymectomized mice, CM cellulose proved to be the most efficient (our unpublished observation). The best prolongation of TF half-life was obtained with CM cellulose equilibrated at pH 6.3 in phosphate buffer 0.01 M, that is the exact conditions of the CM cellulose chromatography used in the isolation procedure. CM cellulose-bound TF half-life is of 4–6 hours. Interestingly, when a sufficient half-life is obtained, the *in vivo* effects previously noted with thymic extracts or total serum, are obtained again (correction of the normally low sensitivity to AθS of the spleen RFC). This method of injection of serum TF has been adopted in all *in vivo* biological studies reported further using purified TF.

Species Specificity

The activity of thymic extracts and sera from various species have been tested on mouse RFC. A TF-like activity has been found in thymic extracts of mice, calves, pigs, and humans as well as in the sera of calves, sheep, pigs, rats, and men. For pig and human sera, the disappearance of TF-like activity after thymectomy allowed the ascertainment that the biological activity detected was due to thymic secretion. Biochemical studies have so far shown no difference between TF characteristics in the mouse, the pig, and the human.

Serum TF has also recently been shown to be present in the serum of Urodeles. This data was obtained in 60 normal and thymectomized *Triturus alpestris, Pleurodeles Waltlii* and *Ambystoma Mexicanum.*[40] Sera of these Urodeles contains a factor with TF-like activity, which disappears after thymectomy. This activity of amphibian TF in the mouse is reminiscent of the activity of certain mammalian hormones in amphibians.

Biological Activities

The serum TF isolated on the basis of the rosette assay has been tested by several *in vitro* and *in vivo* biological tests (Table 3).

Theta conversion has been obtained not only at the level of RFC but also at the level of the overall lymphocyte population using a cytotoxic assay as is reported elsewhere in this volume.[41] In short, when spleen cells from normal (or adult thymectomized) mice were fractionated on a BSA discontinuous gradient the less dense cell layer was found to contain only few θ-positive cells (less than 5% in most experiments). When these cells were incubated with purified serum TF for 2 hours at 37° C (in the absence of fetal calf serum, which probably inhibits TF by binding) and then AθS was added to the cells, a significant increase in the number of θ-positive cells was noted. Conversely, no increase was noted in cell layers where θ-positive cells were already present before incubation in percentages higher than 25%. These data on our factor confirm the data published by Komuro and Boyse[42, 43] with thymic extracts. However, one should emphasize that this experimental system is a difficult one, with some variability in the efficiency of cell separation and in the percentage of nonspecific cell deaths. It is only when these two factors were well controlled that θ conversion was regularly observed for TF concentrations as low as 10 ng/ml.

In vitro response to mitogens of nude spleen cells under TF influence was also investigated in collaboration with P. Haÿry. Nude spleen cells were incubated with TF (100 ng/ml) for 2 hours at 37° C then washed and Concavalin A and PHA were added. Three days later mitotic and blast cells were evaluated by a method previously described.[44] Significant Con-A responsiveness was obtained in 4 consecutive experiments. Conversely, responses to PHA were much weaker and not statistically significant (our unpublished observations).

Thymocytes include two cell subpopulations, one mainly present in the cortex which is sensitive to the *in vivo*[45] and *in vitro*[46] lytic action of steroids, the other predominant in the thymus medulla which is corticoresistant. It has been reported by Trainin[47] that *in vitro* incubation of thymus cells with the dialysable thymus humoral factor decreased the sensitivity of thymocytes to *in vitro* cortisol-induced lysis. We have investigated this experimental system by studying the *receptors for steroids* present on the surface of thymocytes in collaboration with D. Duval. These receptors, which are detected by their property of binding triated dexamethasone, are specific for cortisol.[48] They are located in the cell cytosol from which they are extracted.[48] We have examined the effect of *in vitro* TF treatment of thymocytes on the expression of steroid

Table 3

Induction of θ-Positive Cells by *In Vivo* Treatment of Nude Mice (Means ± S.D.)

	% θ + Cells (Cytotoxic Assay)	Rosette Inhibition Titer AθS
no treatment	2% ± 2%	1/5
T F (+ CMC) 200 ng	18% ± 3%	1/40
CMC	3% ± 1%	1/5

TABLE 4

SUMMARY OF BIOLOGICAL ACTIVITIES OF PURIFIED THYMIC FACTOR

In Vitro
- —Theta conversion
  - Rosette-inhibition assay
  - Cytotoxic assay
- —Induction of concanavalin-A responsiveness
- —Decrease in density of steroid receptors on thymocytes
- —Induction of capping in spleen cells from adult thymectomized mice

In Vivo
- —Theta conversion
- —Promotion of rejection of MSV-Moloney virus-induced sarcoma in thymectomized mice.

receptors. Purified TF was shown to induce a 70% inhibition of steroid-specific uptake by thymus cells, suggesting that decrease in the number or in the availability of receptors for steroids is one of the mechanisms by which T-cells lose their high steroid sensitivity as they mature. Our experiments also indicate that such changes might be due to TF action.

The last *in vitro* system that we have currently investigated (with J. Charreire) deals with antigen-induced redistribution of antigen-binding receptors at the surface of T-cells. It has been reported [49] that rosette-forming cells (like radiolabeled antigen-binding cells) redistribute their antigen-binding receptors after 15 minutes incubation at 37° C with the antigen in question. We have shown that such "capping" could be observed at the T-RFC level in the spleen and that adult thymectomy depleted the capacity of these T-spleen RFC to cap. Interestingly, *in vitro* treatment with purified TF rapidly restored normal capping characteristics when added to the spleen cells simultaneously with the SRBC. Whereas normal mouse serum also showed that effect, serum from adult thymectomized mice and nude mice did not exhibit it.

In vivo studies of TF activity have been performed first in systems where TF had been shown to possess *in vitro* activity. Purified serum TF was injected into adult thymectomized, thymectomized irradiated bone marrow reconstituted, and nude mice, after binding to CM cellulose as previously described. Twenty-four hours later several changes were observed including: (1) normalization of RFC sensitivity to azathioprine and antitheta serum; (2) increase in the number of θ-positive cells assessed by a classic cytotoxic assay; (3) correction of capping by T-RFC as described above for *in vitro* experiments; all changes observed both in adult thymectomized mice with 20 ng of TF and in nude mice with 200 ng per mouse.

A last and important *in vivo* TF activity concerns the rejection of virus-induced sarcomas (studied in collaboration with J. C. Leclerc and E. Gomard). Thymectomized irradiated bone marrow reconstituted C57/B16 mice were injected in the thigh with MSV Moloney virus and treated by the purified serum TF (40 ng of TF 4 times a week, bound to CM cellulose, s.c.). The treatment was begun the day of MSV-virus injection and was continued for 25 days. Controls included normal mice and thymectomized irradiated bone marrow reconstituted mice injected with CMC alone. There was a high percentage of sarcoma incidence in normal mice as is well documented[50] and all the tumors were rejected within 20 days after virus injection. In thymectomized mice treated with CMC alone, there was no rejection and the mice with tumors ultimately died. Conversely, in the TF treated group of thymectomized mice, 85% of mice had rejected their tumors at day 25 when TF treatment was stopped. However, a large percentage of tumors reappeared 20–40 days after treatment stopped, whereas there was no tumor recurrence in normal mice. These data indicate that serum TF has enabled the mice to reject the tumors, probably through recruitment of cytotoxic cells, but that this recruitment has been reversible. It is interesting to note in this context that thymus grafts also rapidly restore the capacity of thymectomized mice to reject MSV-induced sarcomas, more rapidly than they restore the capacity to respond to phytohaemagglutinin or to reject skin grafts (Davies, personal communication).

TF Mode of Action

Mode of Action at the Cellular Level

Serum TF effects on rosette-forming cells are obtained in a matter of minutes, at 37° C. Similarly Basch and Goldstein[37] have reported, using a cytotoxicity inhibition test, that thymin induced changes in θ antigen in less than 30 minutes. This effect is reversible. Thus, after *in vivo* injection of purified TF or of thymic extracts (thymosin), the θ-RFC changes do not last more than 48 hours. One may also note that the promotion effect noted on tumor immunity was reversible within a few days after treatment stopped.

Interesting information on the mode of action of TF has been gained from studies concerning the cyclic AMP system[51–53] as is detailed elsewhere in this symposium.[41] In short, we have shown that cyclic AMP, or products increasing cAMP level in lymphocytes, such as prostaglandin PGE_1, or PGE_2, had a TF-like effect on RFC (inducing sensitivity to AθS in θ-negative RFC). Synergism was demonstrated between cAMP and TF for that effect. It is interesting that decrease of θ expression was obtained by altering cyclic AMP level in theta positive cells either increasing it by dibutyryl cAMP treatment or decreasing it by indomethacin treatment. Prostaglandins might act as intermediates between TF-induced stimulation and cAMP synthesis, since indomethacin, a potent prostaglandin synthetase inhibitor, inhibits TF effects. These data suggest the involvement of cAMP and eventually of prostaglandins in the regulation of θ expression, under TF control. This tentative interpretation, which is discussed more in detail elsewhere,[41] obviously needs a direct demonstration with an intralymphocyte measurement of cAMP level after cell incubation in the presence of TF. This is not an easy matter, since the TF target cell would have first to be physically separated from other cells. One may note in these lines, the recent finding of Kook and Trainin showing adenylcyclase stimulation in thymocytes incubated with dialysed extracts of thymic tissue.[54] In summary, little is known about the mode of action of TF, but the involvement of prostaglandins and of the cyclic AMP system is suspected in the development of its relatively rapid and reversible effects.

Determination of the TF Target Cell

Theta-conversion experiments concern spleen cells from normal, adult thymectomized, or nude mice. However, as mentioned above, nude mouse spleen cells are less sensitive to TF than cells from normal or adult thymectomized mice (TABLE 5). This fact is in keeping with Stutman's work, which suggests that thymic epithelial function is mainly active in the periphery on "postthymic cells."[4, 55] It may be that TF is only active physiologically on stem cells present in nude mice at high concentrations, only present in the thymus gland itself.

The mechanisms of T-cell maturation are still largely unknown. We have just mentioned that TF might be involved in the first stages of this maturation, especially on the postthymic cells. Conversely, TF is probably not involved in the last stages of maturation of long lived PHA-responsive cells. This is suggested by the fact that it takes several weeks to obtain restoration of lymphocytes' ability to respond to PHA, to reject skin allografts, or to produce antibodies after grafting a syngeneic thymus in thymectomized irradiated bone marrow reconstituted mice[56, 57] even if the graft has been removed after 7–10 days.[58, 59] Conversely, we have reported early reconstitution of the ability of such mice to reject MSV-Moloney virus-induced sarcomas. Finally, one may postulate the existence of two different T-cell populations with different times of maturation and life-spans.[12, 16] The short life-span of the T-cell subpopulation is suspected by the early effect of adult thymectomy on spleen θ-positive RFC. TF action on the maturation of suppressor T-cells is not known, although premature cessation of TF secretion in NZB mice which rapidly lose suppressor T-cell function[60] would also suggest TF action on these suppressor cells. Let us lastly mention the problem of the relationship of TF with various factors secreted by activated T-cells, some of them may be active in the rosette assay.[61, 62, 63] We have verified that such allogeneic factors were completely distinguishable by molecular weight and electric charge from serum TF.[63]

TABLE 5

DIFFERENCE IN SENSITIVITY TO PURIFIED THYMIC FACTOR OF SPLEEN RFC FROM NUDE AND ADULT THYMECTOMIZED MICE (MEANS±2 S.D.)

	In Vitro Minimum Active TF Concentration	*In Vivo* Minimum Active Dose
Adult Tx mice	10 pg/ml ± 3	50 ng ± 15
Tx, Rx BM-reconstituted mice	40 pg/ml ± 5	60 ng ± 20
Nude mice	200 pg/ml ± 25	250 ng ± 40

Clinical Applications

Demonstration of the Existence of TF in Human Serum; Relationship with Aging

Human serum shows TF activity when applied in the mouse rosette inhibition assay described above. We have not yet performed detailed studies on the biochemical characteristics of human TF, but it is already established that human TF behaves like mouse or pig TF for diafiltration through Amicon membranes of various molecular weight cutoffs, and also binds to CM cellulose at pH 6.3 and not to DEAE cellulose at pH 7.3.

Human TF disappears from the serum after thymectomy in myasthenic patients,[64] with a half-life of less than 6 hours. As in the mouse, TF level depends on age. Serum TF is stable until the age of 15–20 years and declines progressively afterwards (Figure 5), to become insignificant in most subjects over 30 years of age.

One should emphasize at this stage that TF is heat labile and unstable in

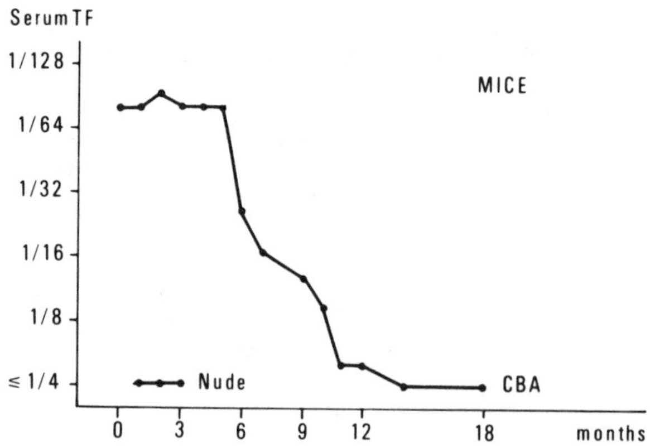

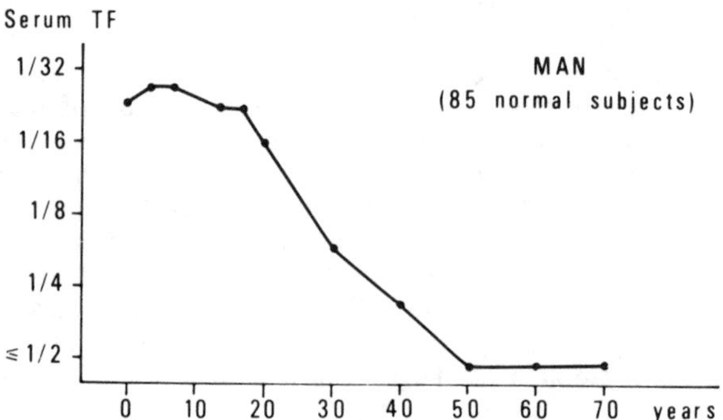

Figure 5. Comparison of age dependency of serum TF in mice and in man.

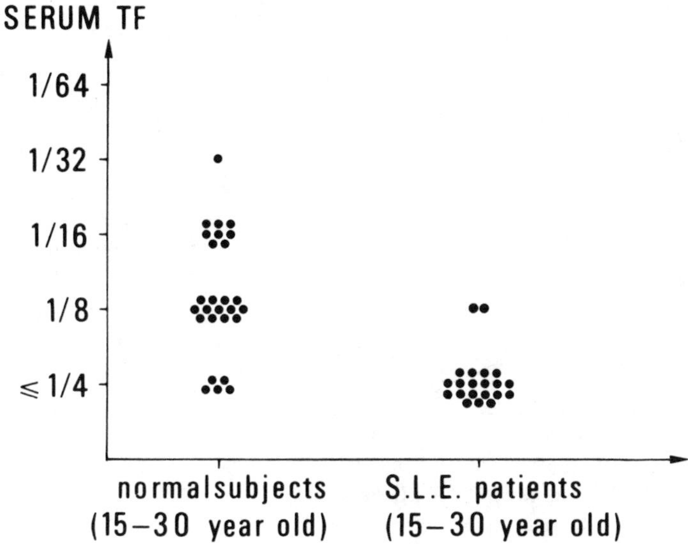

FIGURE 6. Serum TF level in systemic lupus erythematosus.

crude serum, probably because of serum proteolytic enzymes, hence the need for strict precautions for the storage of samples especially those from young children in whom, for still unknown reasons, TF is particularly unstable. In practice, one should collect blood on heparin (Liquemin) at 0° C, centrifuge at 4° C and immediately put the plasma sample at –20° C. The sample can then be lyophilised, which does not alter TF activity (as opposed to thawing, which may do so).

One should also be aware of the possible existence of false positives due to serum allogeneic factors secreted by activated T-cells (such as in organ allotransplantation or infections) which may provoke some difficulties in interpretation.[63]

Results in Some Immunological Diseases

In systemic lupus erythematosus serum TF has consistently been found at a low level (FIGURE 6), before any treatment and in young patients under 25, an age where control subjects still show high hormone levels. These data are in keeping with the low TF level found in NZB mice[22] and would suggest that TF secretion deficiency might play a role in S.L.E. pathogenesis.[65]

Conversely, normal or high TF levels have been found in rheumatoid arthritis, particularly in patients over 40 who showed in 65% of cases a hormone level significantly higher than normal controls of the same age (FIGURE 7). In keeping with these data, T-cells evaluated by sheep cell spontaneous rosette formation showed normal or high values in most cases with correlation with TF level.[66]

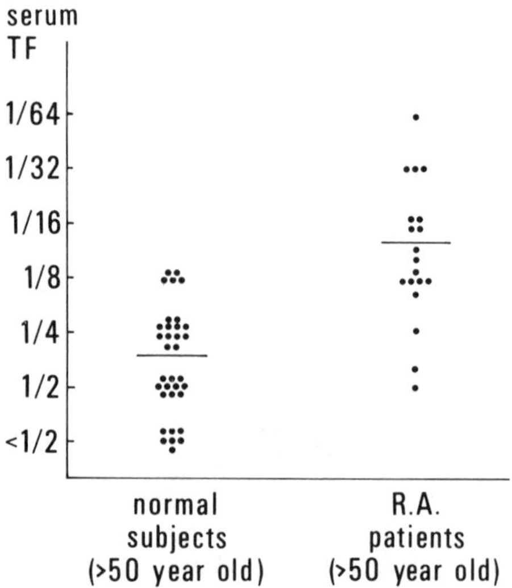

FIGURE 7. Serum TF level in rheumatoid arthritis (patients over 50 years old).

In immunodeficiency states, TF level was strictly normal in pure agammaglobulinemia (6 cases studied) but TF was undetectable (as in nude mice) in two cases of Di George's syndrome. Normal or decreased (but not zero) TF levels have been found in ataxia telangectasia and variable immunodeficiencies with variable onset (TABLE 6).

In myasthenia gravis, TF levels were normal in patients less than 20 years old but tended to be high (although inconsistently so) in older patients.[64]

SUMMARY

The circulating thymic factor (TF) is exclusively secreted by the thymic epithelium. TF is a basic polypeptide with a molecular weight close to 1,000. Purified TF, isolated on the basis of a θ-conversion assay, has been shown to possess several other biological activities, including induction of responsiveness

TABLE 6

THYMIC HORMONE EVALUATION IN IMMUNODEFICIENCY *

	Number	Serum TF
Normal children (aged 1–10)	22	1/16–1/64
Sex-linked agammaglobulinemia	5	1/16–1/32
Di George's syndrome	2	⩽1/4
Ataxia-telangectasia	6	1/4–1/32
Variable immunodeficiency with variable onset	2	1/16–1/32

* In collaboration with C. Griscelli.

to mitogens and promotion of antitumor immunity. TF is active on nude mouse precursor cells, but is active at lower concentrations on more differentiated "postthymic" T-cell precursors. TF production decreases with aging. Premature cessation of TF secretion is observed in spontaneously autoimmune mice. TF is found in human serum; serum TF levels are low in T-cell immunodeficiencies and in S.L.E. and high in rheumatoid arthritis.

References

1. Miller, J. F. A. P. 1961. Immunological function of the thymus. Lancet **2:** 748.
2. Dalmasso, A. P., C. Martinez & R. A. Good. 1962. Failure of spleen cells from thymectomized mice to induce graft versus host reaction. Proc. Soc. Exp. Biol. Med. **110:** 205.
3. Osoba, D. & J. F. A. P. Miller. 1963. Evidence for humoral thymus factor responsible for the maturation of immunological faculty. Nature **199:** 653.
4. Stutman, O., E. Yunis & R. A. Good. 1970. Studies on thymus function. I. Cooperative effects of thymic function and lymphohemopoietic cells in restoration of neonatally thymectomized mice. J. Exp. Med. **132:** 583.
5. Trainin, N. & M. Small. 1970. Studies on some physicochemical properties of a thymus humoral factor conferring immunocompetence on lymphoid cells. J. Exp. Med. **132:** 885.
6. Trainin, N. & M. Small. 1973. Thymic humoral factors. *In* Contemporary Topics in Immunobiology. **:** 321. A. J. S. Davies & R. L. Carter, Eds. Plenum Press. New York, N.Y.
7. Goldstein, A. L. & A. White. 1973. Thymosin and other thymic hormones: their nature and roles in the thymic dependency of immunological phenomena. *In* Contemporary Topics in Immunobiology. **:** 339. A. J. S. Davies and R. L. Carter, Eds. Plenum Press. New York, N.Y.
8. Goldstein, A. L., A. Guha, M. M. Zatz, M. A. Hardy & A. White. 1972. Purification and biological activity of thymosin a hormone of the thymus gland. Proc. Nat. Acad. Sci. U.S. **69:** 1800.
9. Kruger, J., A. L. Goldstein & B. Waksman. 1970. Immunologic and anatomic consequences of calf thymosin injection in rats. Cell. Immunol. **1:** 51.
10. Bach, J. F. & M. Dardenne. 1972. Antigen recognition by T-lymphocytes. I. Thymus and bone marrow dependence of spontaneous rosette forming cells in normal and neonatally thymectomized mice. Cell. Immunol. **3:** 1.
11. Bach, J. F. & M. Dardenne. 1972. Antigen recognition by T-lymphocytes. II. Similar effects of azathioprine, ALS and antitheta serum on rosette forming lymphocytes in normal and neonatally thymectomized mice. Cell. Immunol. **3:** 11.
12. Bach, J. F. 1973. Thymus dependency of rosette forming cells. *In* Contemporary Topics in Immunobiology. **2:** 189. A. J. S. Davies & R. L. Carter, Eds. Plenum Press. New York, N.Y.
13. Bach, J. F., M. Dardenne, A. Goldstein, A. Guha & A. White. 1971. Appearance of T-cell markers in bone marrow rosette forming cells after incubation with purified thymosin, a thymic hormone Proc. Nat. Acad. Sci. U.S. **68:** 2734.
14. Dardenne, M. & J. F. Bach. 1973. Studies on thymus products. I. Modification of rosette forming cells by thymic extracts. Determination of the target RFC subpopulation. Immunology **25:** 343.
15. Bach, J. F., J. Y. Muller & M. Dardenne. 1970. *In vivo* specific antigen recognition by rosette forming cells. Nature **227:** 1251.
16. Bach, J. F. & M. Dardenne. 1973. Antigen recognition by T-lymphocytes.

III. Evidence for two populations of thymus-dependent rosette forming cells in spleen and lymph nodes. Cell. Immunol. **6:** 394.

17. BACH, J. F. & M. DARDENNE. 1972. Thymus dependency of rosette forming cells. Evidence for a circulating thymic hormone. Transplant. Proc. **4:** 345.
18. BACH, J. F. & M. DARDENNE. 1973. Studies on thymus products. II. Demonstration and characterization of a circulating thymic hormone. Immunology **25:** 353.
19. BACH, J. F. & M. DARDENNE. 1971. Activities of immunosuppressive agents *in vitro* I. Rosette inhibition by azathioprine. Eur. J. Clin. Biol. Res. **8:** 770.
20. BACH, J. F., M. DARDENNE & C. FOURNIER. 1969. *In vitro* evaluation of immunosuppressive drugs. Nature **222:** 998.
21. DARDENNE, M., M. PAPIERNIK, J. F. BACH & O. STUTMAN. 1974. Studies on thymus products. III. Epithelial origin of the thymic hormone. Immunology **27:** 209.
22. BACH, J. F., M. DARDENNE & J. C. SALOMON. 1973. Studies on thymus products. IV. Absence of serum "thymic activity" in adult NZB and (NZB × NZW)F1 mice. Clin. Exp. Immunol. **14:** 247.
23. DEVRIES, M. J. & W. HIJMANS. 1967. Pathological changes of thymic epithelial cells and autoimmune disease in NZB, NZW (NZB/NZW)F1 mice. Immunology **12:** 179.
24. SHIRAI, T. & R. C. MELLORS. 1971. Natural thymocytotoxic autoantibody and reactive antigen in NZB and other mice. Proc. Nat. Acad. Sci. U.S. **68:** 1412.
25. TALAL, N. & A. D. STEINBERG. 1974. The pathogenesis of autoimmunity in New Zealand Black mice. In press.
26. MONIER, J. C., J. THIVOLET, A. J. BEYVIN, J. C. CZYBA, D. SCHMITT & D. SALUSSOLA. 1971. Les souris Swan (Swiss antinucléaires). Modèle animal pour l'étude du lupus érythémateux disséminé et de l'amylose. Etude immunopathologique. Pathol. Eur. **6:** 357.
27. DARDENNE, M., J. C. MONIER, G. BIOZZI & J. F. BACH. 1974. Studies on thymus Products. V. Influence of genetic selection based on antibody production on thymus hormone production. Clin. Exp. Immunol. **17:** 339.
28. BIOZZI, G., C. STIFFEL, D. MOUTON, Y. BOUTHILLIER & C. DECREUSEFOND. 1972. Genetic regulation of the function of antibody producing cells *In* Progress in Immunology. : 509. B. Amos, Ed. Academic Press. New York, N.Y.
29. MONIER, J. C., J. CZYBA M. ROBERT & D. SCHMITT. 1974. Defective T-cell functions in autoimmune Swan mice. Ann. Immunol. **125**(C)**:** 527.
30. SCHMITT, D. 1974. Inclusions cristallines dans les cellules réticuloépithéliales du thymus des souris Swan avec anticorps antinucléaires. C. R. Acad. Sci. (Paris). **278:** 1649.
31. CLARK, S. L. 1968. Incorporation of sulfate by mouse thymus, its relation to secretion by medullar epithelial cells and to thymic lymphopoiesis. J. Exp. Med. **128:** 927.
32. OWEN, J. J. T. 1972. The origin and development of lymphocyte populations. *In* Ontogeny of acquired immunity. Excerpta Med. : 35.
33. HAYS, E. F. 1969. The effect of epithelial remnants and whole organ grafts of thymus on the recovery of thymectomized irradiated mice. J. Exp. Med. **129:** 1235.
34. STUTMAN, O., E. J. YUNIS & R. A. GOOD. 1969. Carcinogen-induced tumors of the thymus. IV. Humoral influences of normal thymus and functional thymomas and influence of post-thymectomy period on restoration. J. Exp. Med. **130:** 809.
35. PAPIERNIK, M., B. NABARRA & J. F. BACH. 1975. *In vitro* secretion of a humoral factor by human thymic epithelial cells. Clin. Exp. Immunol. In press.
36. GOLDSTEIN, G. 1974. Isolation of bovine thymin; a polypeptide hormone of the thymus. Nature **247:** 11.
37. BASCH, R. S. & G. GOLDSTEIN. 1974. Induction of T-cell differentiation *in vitro*

by thymin, a purified polypeptide hormone of the thymus. Proc. Nat. Acad. Sci. U.S. **71:** 1474.
38. Kook, A. I., C. Carnaud & N. Trainin. 1973. Hormone-like activity of thymus humoral factor (THF) on lymphoid cells. *In* Joint Meeting of European Societies for Immunology. Strasbourg, 1973. Abstract : 43.
39. Robbins, J. & J. E. Rall. 1960. Proteins associated with the thyroid hormones. Physiol. Rev. **40:** 415.
40. Dardenne, M., A. Tournefier, J. Charlemagne & J. F. Bach. 1973. Studies on thymus products. VII. Presence of thymic hormone in urodele serum. Ann. Immunol. **124c:** 465.
41. Bach, M. A., C. Fournier & J. F. Bach. 1974. Regulation of theta antigen expression by agents altering cyclic AMP level and by thymic factor. Ann. N.Y. Acad. Sci. This volume.
42. Komuro, K. & E. A. Boyse. 1973. *In vitro* demonstration of thymic hormone in the mouse by conversion of precursor cells into T lymphocytes. Lancet **i:** 740.
43. Komuro, K. & E. A. Boyse. 1973. Induction of T-lymphocytes from precursor cells *in vitro.* J. Exp. Med. **138:** 479.
44. Häyry, P., M. C. Andersson, S. Nordling & M. Virolainen. 1972. Allograft response *in vitro.* Transplant. Rev. **12:** 91.
45. Blomgren, H. & B. Andersson. 1969. Evidence for a small pool of immunocompetent cells in the mouse. Exp. Cell. Res. **57:** 185.
46. Claman, H. N., J. W. Moorhead & W. H. Benner. 1971. Corticosteroids and lymphoid cells *in vitro.* I. Hydrocortisone lysis of human, guinea pig and mouse thymus cells. J. Lab. Clin. Med. **78:** 499.
47. Trainin, N., Y. Levo & V. Rotter. 1974. A thymic humoral factor increases the hydrocortisone resistant cell population of the thymus. Eur. J. Immunol. **4:** 634.
48. Baxter, J. D., A. W. Harris & G. M. Tomkins. 1971. Glucocorticoid receptors in lymphoma cells in culture: relationship to glucocorticoid killing activity. Science **171:** 189.
49. Ashman, R. F. & M. C. Raff. 1973. A direct demonstration of theta-positive antigen binding cells with antigen-induced movement of T-cell receptors. J. Exp. Med. **137:** 69.
50. Fefer, A., J. L. McCoy & J. P. Glynn. 1967. Induction and regression of primary Moloney sarcoma virus-induced tumors in mice. Cancer Res. **27:** 1626.
51. Bach, M. A. & J. F. Bach. 1973. Studies on thymus products. VI. The effects of cyclic nucleotides and prostaglandins on rosette forming cells. Interactions with thymic factor. Eur. J. Immunol. **3:** 778.
52. Bach, M. A. & J. F. Bach. 1972. Effects de l'AMP cyclique sur les cellules formant les rosettes spontanées. C.R. Acad. Sci. (Paris). **275:** 2783.
53. Bach, M. A. 1974. Disparition de l'antigène theta sous l'action de produits modifiant le métabolisme de l'AMP cyclique intralymphocytaire. C.R. Acad. Sci. (Paris). **278:** 3023.
54. Kook, A. & N. Trainin. 1974. Hormone-like activity of a thymus humoral factor on the induction of immune competence in lymphoid cells. J. Exp. Med. **139:** 193.
55. Stutman, O. & R. A. Good. 1973. Thymic hormones. *In* Contemporary Topics in Immunobiology. : 299. A. J. S. Davies & R. L. Carter, Eds. Plenum Press. New York, N.Y.
56. Doenhoff, M. J. & A. J. S. Davies. 1971. Reconstitution of the T-cell pool after irradiation of mice. Cell. Immunol. **1:** 82.
57. Cross, A. M., E. Leuchars & J. F. A. P. Miller. 1965. Studies on the recovery of the immune response in irradiated mice thymectomized in adult life. J. Exp. Med. **119:** 837.
58. Cross, A. M., A. J. S. Davies, B. Doe & E. Leuchars. 1964. Time of action of the thymus in the irradiated adult mouse. Nature **201:** 1045.

59. Stutman, O., E. J. Yunis & R. A. Good. 1972. Studies on thymus function. III. Duration of thymic function. J. Exp. Med. **135:** 339.
60. Barthold, D. R., S. Kysela & A. D. Steinberg. 1973. Decline in suppressor T-cell function with age in female NZB mice. J. Immunol. In press.
61. Bach, J. F. & M. Dardenne. 1974. Direct demonstration of a serum factor produced by activated T-cells. Exp. Haematol. In press.
62. Bach, J. F., M. Dardenne & J. M. Pleau. 1974. Mise en évidence de deux facteurs de faible poids moléculaire sécrétés l'un par le thymus, l'autre par les cellules T activées, confèrant l'antigène theta à des lymphocytes theta-négatifs. C.R. Acad. Sci. (Paris). **278:** 335.
63. Bach, J. F. & M. Dardenne. Direct demonstration of a serum factor produced by activated T-cells. Submitted for publication.
64. Bach, J. F., M. Dardenne, M. Papiernik, A. Barois, P. Levasseur & H. Le Brigand. 1972. Evidence of a serum factor produced by the human thymus. Lancet **2:** 1056.
65. Bach, J. F. & M. Dardenne. 1972. Absence d'hormone thymique dans le sérum de souris NZB et NZB-NZW et de malades atteints de lupus érythémateux disséminé. J. Urol. Néphrol. **78:** 994.
66. Bach, J. F., M. Dardenne & J. Clot. 1974. Evaluation of serum thymic hormone and T-cells in rheumatoid arthritis and systemic lupus erythematosus. *In* Proc. Intern. Symp. Immunological Aspects Rheumatological Diseases. J. Clot & J. Sany, Eds. Karger. Basel, Switzerland. In press.

FURTHER CHARACTERIZATION OF AN ANTIBODY-STIMULATING FACTOR ISOLATED FROM BOVINE THYMUS *

W. Gerry Robey

National Cancer Institute
Bethesda, Maryland 20014

Introduction

The early studies of Metcalf [1] showed that cell-free extracts of mouse and human thymus contained material(s) capable of inducing lymphocytosis in neonatal mice. Hand *et al.*[2] described a fractionation method of bovine thymus whereby a single polypeptide was isolated; microgram quantities increased the lymphocyte-polymorphonuclear leukocyte ratio in intact neonatal mice. The protein was named Lymphocyte Stimulating Hormone (LSH). Additional reports [3, 4] have appeared further characterizing the immunological properties of LSH preparations in various degrees of homogeneity. The methanol precipitate fraction of Hand *et al.*[2] was found to contain a second, unrelated, protein capable of accelerating the appearance of specific hemolysin in neonatal mice. The isolation, purification, and initial characterization of this single, active protein was described by Robey *et al.*[5] The nomenclature of LSH_r was adopted to distinguish this protein from the protein formerly isolated. The former preparation was designated LSH_h. Luckey *et al.*[6] have compared the properties of both polypeptides. The characteristics of rabbit antiserum prepared against purified LSH_r and the tissue distribution of this material are described here.

Methods and Results

Fresh bovine thymus was prepared by the method described by Hand *et al.*[2] and as further purified by Robey *et al.*[5] Briefly, trimmed thymus was homogenized in 6 volumes of saline at −20 C. Subsequent steps were performed at 4 C. The homogenate was clarified by centrifugation and precipitated by the addition of crystalline ammonium sulfate to 20% (w/v). This precipitate was dissolved in a volume of distilled water equal to one-half the volume of saline used for homogenization. This suspension was clarified by centrifugation. The supernatant was then precipitated by the addition of 3 volumes of absolute methanol. The methanol precipitate was collected by centrifugation and resuspended in one-fourth the volume of saline used for homogenization, clarified

* This work was partially supported at the University of Missouri with funds from the Research Council of the University of Missouri Graduate School, Eli Lilly and Co., and by Public Health Service Training Grant GM-01239 from the National Institute of General Medical Sciences. This work was partially supported at The Pennsylvania State University by funds from the Damon Runyon Memorial Fund for Cancer Research (DRG-1037AT), the National Science Foundation (GB-25996), and the American Cancer Society, Inc. (IC-19G).

by centrifugation, and dialyzed against distilled water. Any insoluble material was removed by centrifugation, and the supernatant was lyophilized to dryness. This and subsequent preparations were stored at —20 C over anhydrous calcium chloride. Methanol precipitates of bovine thymus, spleen, kidney and serum were prepared in this manner. The methanol precipitate of thymus was subjected to further purification by column chromatography. LSH_r was eluted from diethylaminoethyl-cellulose (DEAE) by 0.05 M tris(hydroxymethyl) aminomethane-hydrochloric acid (Tris-HCl) buffer, pH 6.9, that contained 0.40 M NaCl. This preparation contained 5 of the original 15 proteins contained in the methanol precipitate as determined by polyacrylamide gel electrophoresis.[2, 5, 7] This DEAE fraction was then chromatographed on Sephadex® G-150 equilibrated with 0.002 M Tris-HCl buffer, pH 8.0. The fraction containing LSH_r contained two minor components that were removed by rechromatography on the same Sephadex G-150 column. The final preparation contained one component as determined by polyacrylamide gel electrophoresis. The yields of the major purification steps are summarized in TABLE 1, and the electrophoretic patterns of the methanol precipitate and the LSH_r preparation purified by column chromatography are shown in FIGURE 1.

This LSH_r preparation was then analyzed for homogeneity.[5] Polyacrylamide gel electrophoresis using 100 μg of protein per gel showed a single band with a mobility of 0.108 relative to the ion front[7] as shown in FIGURE 1. A sedimentation velocity analysis by the method of Schachman[8] showed a single symmetrical peak with a S_{20} value of 3.92. A sedimentation equilibrium analysis using the method of Yphantis[9] was used to assess both the degree of homogeneity and the whole-cell average molecular weight of the purified protein. These methods indicated that LSH_r consisted of a single macromolecular species having a molecular weight of 79,950 ± 940.

Further analysis of LSH_r by the method of Lowry *et al.*[10] indicated that the molecule was 97.7% protein, did not contain detectable carbohydrate, and exhibited an absorption spectrum typical of a protein. Furthermore, the biological activity of LSH_r was shown to be heat-stable at 60 C and sensitive to pronase digestion.[5]

Antiserum to purified LSH_r was prepared in the following manner. Ten mg of the purified material was emulsified with 2.0 ml of Complete Freunds Adjuvant (Gibco). One ml of the emulsion was injected intradermally into each of 2 New Zealand white rabbits (2.5 kg) in several depots along the flank. Thirty days later the rabbits were challenged with 1.0 mg of LSH_r injected intravenously. This was repeated three additional times on a weekly basis.

TABLE 1

YIELDS IN THE THYMUS FRACTIONATION PROCEDURE USED TO ISOLATE AND PURIFY LSH_r

Purification Step	Yield
thymus	1000 g
methanol precipitate	100 mg
DEAE-cellulose	7.0 mg
first Sephadex G-150	1.8 mg
second Sephadex G-150	1.1 mg

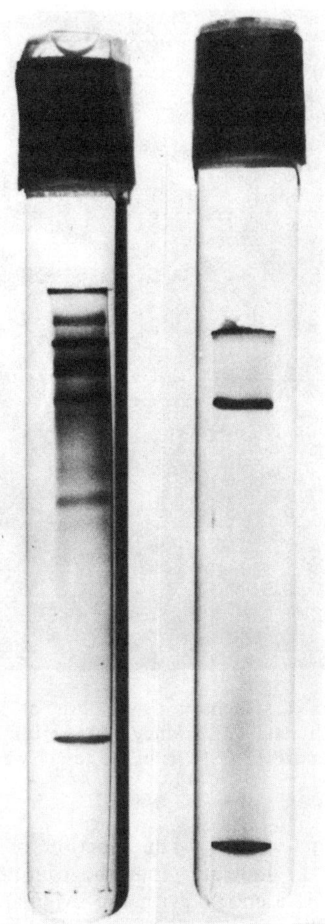

FIGURE 1. Polyacrylamide gel electrophoresis patterns of the methanol precipitate fraction of bovine thymus (left) and purified LSH_r (right).

Sixty days after the initial challenge, the animals were bled by cardiac puncture. Serum was collected, aliquoted, and stored at −20 C in sealed ampules. Both rabbits responded weakly when 10 μl of undiluted immune serum was diffused against 100 μg of LSH_r in 10 μl of buffer. Commercially prepared immunodiffusion plates (Immuno-Plate. Pattern C. Hyland Laboratories) were used for the Ouchterlony analyses.

In order to determine the distribution of this material in other bovine tissues, the methanol precipitate fractions from bovine thymus, spleen, kidney, and serum were prepared according to the procedure described earlier. Each methanol precipitate was prepared to a concentration of 5.0 mg/ml and clarified by centrifugation. The supernatants were used as the antigens. Ten μl of each were diffused against 10 μl of immune serum and incubated 3 days at 25 C. The results of this experiment are shown in FIGURE 2. LSH_r was shown to be present in the methanol precipitates of thymus (FIGURE 2, number 2) and spleen (FIGURE 2, number 5). LSH_r appears to be present in lower concentration in the spleen than in the thymus and not detectable in either the kidney

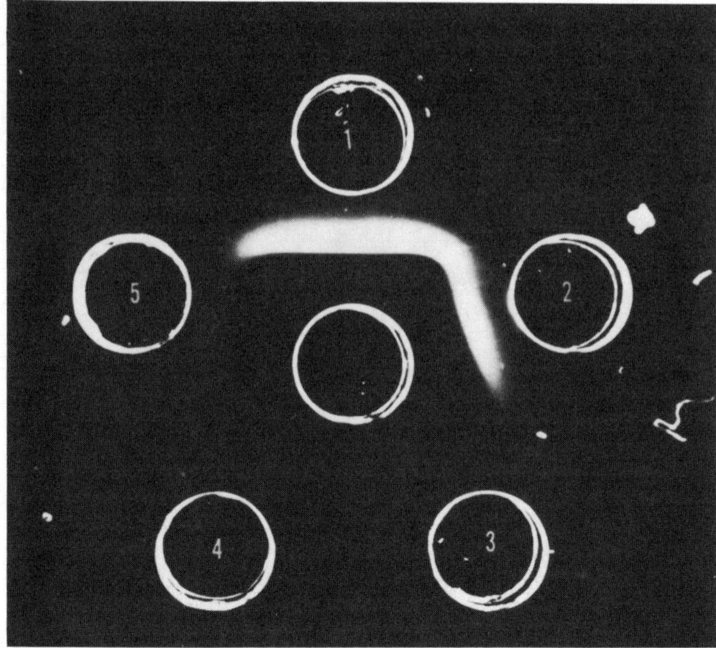

FIGURE 2. Ouchterlony analysis of LSH_r (1) and the methanol precipitates of bovine thymus (2), kidney (3), serum (4) and spleen (5). Rabbit antiserum prepared to purified LSH_r is in the center well.

or serum extracts. The reaction of the positive control, LSH_r, (FIGURE 2, number 1) indicates that the immunoprecipitable component in these tissue extracts is identical with the original immunizing agent. LSH_r did not cross-react with rabbit antiserum (Schwarz Mann) prepared against bovine serum albumin.

To further characterize the location of LSH_r in the lymphatic system, and to further understand its role in accelerating the development of the humoral immune response in neonatal mice, mouse thymus, spleen, and bone marrow cells were incubated in the presence of rabbit antiserum to LSH_r and guinea-pig complement. Experiments were conducted with unabsorbed heated antiserum and heated antiserum that had previously been absorbed by mouse liver powder. Adult ICR mice were used as the source of cells. The tissues were removed and mechanically teased into a monocellular suspension. The cells were then washed with Hank's salts and adjusted to a final concentration of 2×10^6 cells/ml. Initial viabilities and then after 2 hours of incubation at 37 C were determined by the trypan blue exclusion method. Each experimental reaction mixture consisted of 0.5 ml of cells, 25 μl of either unabsorbed or absorbed antiserum to LSH_r and 25 μl of reconstituted guinea-pig complement. Three sets of control reaction mixtures were used. They were (1) cells plus Hank's salts, (2) cells plus antiserum, and (3) cells plus complement. The control values shown the table are those from cells plus Hank's salts as no differences were observed in any of the other control reaction mixtures. The results of these experiments are shown in TABLE 2. The initial study with unabsorbed antiserum indicated that one-half of the thymus cells were lysed and no bone marrow cells were lysed. It also appeared that a few spleen cells were subject to complement mediated lysis. However, using the absorbed antiserum, the number of susceptable thymus cells decreased and no spleen cells were affected. This observation indicated that LSH_r, as isolated from bovine thymus, appears to be an antigenic component present on the surface of approximately one-fourth of the thymus cells in the adult ICR mouse. Furthermore, this component does not appear on the surface of spleen or bone marrow cells as measured by this method. The cytotoxic effects of this antiserum on neonatal thymus cells is unknown.

Two biological assays were used to assess the effect of LSH_r on hemolysin development in the intact neonatal mouse. The first was the hemolytic immunoplaque assay [11] used to measure the number of cells in the spleen of immunized mice that were producing hemolysin to sheep erythrocytes (SRBC), and the second method measured the hemolysin present in the serums of immunized mice. The immunoplaque assay was used to assess the tissue distribution of LSH_r, and the serum hemolysin assay was used to study hemolysin production as a function of dosage.

Newborn mice received the appropriate thymus extracts within 12 hours of birth in 0.02 ml injected subcutaneously. At various times later, 0, 7, 14 or 21 days after birth, the mice were challenged with 0.1 ml of a 50% suspension of washed SRBC. Four days after immunization the animals were killed and their spleens removed. Excised spleens were mechanically teased into monocellular suspensions. A volume of 0.1 ml of freshly prepared spleen suspension suspended in Hank's salts was mixed with 2.0 ml of melted 0.9% Noble agar which contained dextran and SRBC. This mixture was poured over the surface of a previously prepared Petri plate containing 10 ml of solidified 1% Noble agar. The plates were incubated at 37 C for 1 hour and then flooded with a 1:20 dilution of reconstituted guinea-pig complement. The plates were then incubated for an additional 30 minutes at 37 C. The resulting zones of hemolysis were regarded as being due to hemolysin secreted by individual antibody-forming cells. Usually two or three dilutions of spleen cells were plated in duplicate to facilitate accurate counts of the number of plaque forming cells (PFC). The numbers of PFC in the experimental groups are expressed as a ratio to the number of PFC in the control group. The optimum time for

TABLE 2

CYTOTOXIC EFFECT OF RABBIT ANTISERUM PREPARED AGAINST PURIFIED LSH_r ON THYMUS, SPLEEN AND BONE MARROW CELLS FROM ADULT ICR MICE

	Percentage of Lysis			
Cell Source	Control	Unabsorbed Antiserum	Control	Absorbed Antiserum
thymus	3	51	3	28
spleen	3	7	3	4
bone marrow	0	4	—	—

antigenic challenge for the ICR mouse was found to be 14 days of age.[12, 13] To determine the tissue specificity of LSH_r, the methanol precipitates of bovine thymus and spleen were compared using this assay system. The mice were injected with approximately 100 μg of each preparation within 12 hours of birth, immunized on day 14, and assayed on day 18. The results shown in TABLE 3 show that the greatest activity was observed in the group that received the extract of thymus. It appeared that the spleen showed marginal activity with extracts of kidney and serum producing no enhancement of hemolysin production. This observation was consistent with the gel diffusion pattern in FIGURE 2, in that the immunoprecipitable material detected in the thymus and spleen extracts was responsible for the increase in ability to produce hemolysin the SRBC.

A second series of experiments was used to determine the effect of increasing amounts of LSH_r on the development of the immune response in intact neonatal mice. The assay method used was the determination of serum hemolysin titers in immunized mice.[5, 6] Intact neonatal ICR mice were used to construct a standard curve for the development of the ability to produce hemolysin to SRBC. Test or control solutions were injected subcutaneously into the mice within 12 hours of birth. Protein concentrations were such that 0.02 ml contained the appropriate amount of protein in sterile buffer. At various times later, 4, 7, 10 or 14 days after birth, the mice were immunized intraperitoneally with 0.02 ml of a 10% suspension of washed SRBC. Seven days after immunization, serums were collected and stored at 4 C. Endogenous complement was heat-inactivated and serum hemolysin titers were determined using the Microtiter Dilution System (Cooke Engineering Company) and the ratio of reactants described by Mayer.[14] The optimum time for antigenic challenge in the ICR mice was found to be 10 days of age for this assay method. Increasing amounts of LSH_r were tested in both ICR and Swiss Webster mice. The hemolysin titers shown in TABLE 4 show that LSH_r in the ICR mice produced an appreciable increase at 0.1 μg per mouse, but much less at 1.0 and 10.0 μg. This same trend is observed more dramatically in the Swiss Webster mice. Thus LSH_r accelerated the appearance of hemolysin at all levels tested, but the optimum concentration may be less than 0.1 μg per mouse. The difference in the data obtained from the two strains of mice studied must be a function of variability inherent to each strain. The Swiss Webster control mice responded to SRBC on day 10, whereas the ICR mice did not unless they were injected with LSH_r. In a previous report[5] the increase in hemolysin titers was

TABLE 3

THE EFFECTS OF EXTRACTS OF BOVINE THYMUS, SPLEEN, KIDNEY AND SERUM ON THE IMMUNE RESPONSE TO SHEEP ERYTHROCYTES IN THE NEONATAL ICR MOUSE

Methanol Precipitate Source	PFC *
bovine thymus	7.2
boine serum	2.3
bovine kidney	1.6
bovine serum	0.5

$$* \text{ Ratio} = \frac{\text{Number of PFC in immunized treated group}}{\text{Number of PFC in immunized untreated group}}$$

TABLE 4

SERUM HEMOLYSIN RESPONSE TO INCREASING DOSAGES OF LSH_r INJECTED INTO NEONATAL ICR AND SWISS WEBSTER MICE

Experimental Group	Geometrical Mean Titers	
	ICR Mice	Swiss Webster Mice
control	1.0	3.3
0.1 μg LSH_r	5.8	22.2
1.0 μg LSH_r	2.2	7.1
10.0 μg LSH_r	2.8	—

shown to be specific to the purified thymus extract and not due to nonspecific antigenic stimulation.

Summary and Discussion

The results of this study indicate that bovine thymus contains a protein capable of accelerating the production of specific hemolysin when injected into intact neonatal ICR and Swiss Webster mice. Results obtained indicate that the optimal activity may be less than 0.1 μg per mouse when serum hemolysin is measured.

The physical analyses indicated the protein to be homogeneous. Sedimentation velocity, sedimentation equilibrium and polyacrylamide gel electrophoresis determinations suggested the presence of only one macromolecular species. Rabbit antiserum to the purified LSH_r produced only one precipitin band when diffused against the immunogen.

The specificity of this protein in relationship to extracts of other bovine tissues was determined. Of the tissue extracts tested, thymus, spleen, kidney and serum, only thymus and spleen contained detectable immunoprecipitable material. Of these, the thymus contains considerably more than spleen. This relationship is further verified by the biological activities of the crude methanol precipitates (TABLE 3) in which thymus showed the highest activity while spleen exhibited marginal activity and kidney and serum did not enhance PFC development.

The complement-mediated cytotoxicity data obtained showed that a substantial number of adult ICR thymus cells have a component on their surface that is either LSH_r or similar enough to its antigenic properties that it cross-reacts with antiserum specific to LSH_r. Spleen cells and bone marrow cells do not have this component on their cell membranes at levels which are sufficient for antibody dependent complement-mediated cytolysis. At present this relationship is unclear. Studies should be done in which thymus cells from neonatal mice, weanlings and adult mice are compared as to their susceptability to lysis in the presence of this antiserum. Also the relationship of LSH_r to the θ antigen should be investigated by comparing the singular and additive effects of anti-θ and anti-LSH_r serums on thymus cells.

Other reports concerning the various effects of this group of proteins on the humoral immune response [3, 4, 12] have not been able to demonstrate any effect in adult mice. That the thymus is required for the development of the normal response to heterologous erythrocytes is well established.[15–17] It may be that events early in the ontogeny of murine immunocompetence include the establishment of this particular component on the membrane of some thymus cells, which in some as yet unrecognized manner enables the mouse to respond to this class of particulate antigen.

Of the many reported thymus extracts reviewed by Luckey,[18] only antiserum prepared against thymosin[19] has shown similar cytotoxic effects toward thymus cells. Thymosin however, has not been shown to have any effect on the humoral immune response.[20] This may be due to a dose dependency as the concentrations they tested were relatively high when compared to dosages we have tested. Initially, it was reported that our methanol precipitate contained a high molecular weight inhibitor[3] which subsequently was shown to stimulate at low levels but inhibit hemolysin production at the levels originally tested. The other alternative may be that this is an example of the thymus containing different factors required for different functions.

The biochemical stability or uniformity of LSH_r is fairly good from batch to batch, although occasionally, after storage for several months at —20 C, a second minor band appears upon electrophoresis that has a slightly slower mobility than the major component. Variations in Ouchterlony patterns have also been observed when the antigen preparations have been stored for several years.

The biological uniformity of LSH_r has been extremely variable. Although every effort was made to collect thymus glands from animals of the same sex and age or weight, some preparations have exhibited high activity in our assays but others contained marginal or no activity. Uniformly poor results have been obtained from thymus glands purchased frozen from a commercial supplier. Another difficult variable is the inherent ability of newborn mice to respond to the sheep erythrocyte antigen used in these studies. This variable is discussed by Dr. W. S. Ceglowski in this volume.

It is this author's opinion that large quantities of any thymus extract should be prepared before it is standardized by a given biological assay. Assuming that all other variables can be controlled, this would be a step in the direction of comparing the numerous thymic factors reported and perhaps establishing interrelationships between these activities and the function of the thymus in the total physiology of the experimental animal.

Acknowledgments

The author thanks Drs. W. S. Ceglowski, T. D. Luckey and B. J. Campbell for their input into this research. Gratitude is also extended to R. LeGrande, G. LaBadie and N. Musulin for their respective contributions to this work.

References

1. Metcalf, D. 1958. Ann. N.Y. Acad. Sci. **73:** 113–119.
2. Hand, T., P. Caster & T. D. Luckey. 1967. Biochem. Biophys. Res. Commun. **26:** 18–23.
3. Hand, T., W. S. Ceglowski & H. Friedman. 1970. Experientia **26:** 653–655.

4. Hand, T., W. S. Ceglowski, D. Damrongsak & H. Friedman. 1970. J. Immunol. **105:** 442–450.
5. Robey, G., B. J. Campbell & T. D. Luckey. 1972. Infection and Immunity. **6:** 682–688.
6. Luckey, T. D., W. G. Robey & B. J. Campbell. 1973. *In* Thymic Hormones. : 167–183. T. D. Luckey, Ed. University Park Press. Baltimore, Md.
7. Reisfeld, R. A., R. J. Lewis & D. E. Williams. 1962. Nature **195:** 281–283.
8. Schachman, H. K. 1957. *In* Methods in Enzymology. S. P. Colowick & N. O. Kaplan, Eds. **4:** 32–103. Academic Press. New York, N.Y.
9. Yphantis, D. A. 1964. Biochemistry **3:** 297–317.
10. Lowry, O. H., N. J. Rosebrough, A. L. Farr & R. J. Randall. 1951. J. Biol. Chem. **193:** 265–275.
11. Jerne, N. K. & A. A. Nordin. 1963. Science **140:** 405–407.
12. Ceglowski, W. S., T. L. Hand & H. Friedman. 1973. *In* Thymic Hormones. : 185–192. T. D. Luckey, Ed. University Park Press. Baltimore, Md.
13. Robey, G., W. S. Ceglowski, T. D. Luckey & H. Friedman. 1973. *In* Microenvironmental Aspects of Immunity. : 295–300. B. D. Jankovic & K. Isakovic, Eds. Plenum Press. New York, N.Y.
14. Mayer, M. M. 1961. *In* Experimental Immunochemistry. : 133–240. E. A. Kabat & M. M. Mayer, Eds. Charles Thomas Co. Springfield, Ill.
15. Lischner, H. W. & A. M. DiGeorge. 1969. Lancet **2:** 1044–1049.
16. Takeya, K. & K. Nomoto. 1969. J. Immunol. **99:** 831–836.
17. Weissman, I. L. 1970. *In* Developmental Aspects of Antibody Formation and Structure. J. Sterzl & I. Riha, Eds. **1:** 55–67. Academic Press. New York, N.Y.
18. Luckey, T. D., Ed. 1973. Thymic Hormones. University Park Press. Baltimore, Md.
19. Hardy, M. A., J. Quint, A. L. Goldstein, A. White, D. State & J. R. Battisto. 1969. Proc. Soc. Exp. Biol. Med. **130:** 214–219.
20. Goldstein, A. L. & A. White. 1970. *In* Biochemical Actions of Hormones. G. Litwack, Ed. **1:** 465–502. Academic Press. New York, N.Y.

A HYPOCALCEMIC AND LYMPHOCYTE-STIMULATING SUBSTANCE ISOLATED FROM THYMUS EXTRACTS, AND ITS PHYSICOCHEMICAL PROPERTIES

Akira Mizutani, Michihiko Shimizu, Ikukatsu Suzuki, Takayuki Mizutani, and Shigeru Hayase

Faculty of Pharmaceutical Sciences
Nagoya City University
Nagoya, Japan

The presence of a hypocalcemic substance in the thymus gland has been reported by Nitschke,[1] Scholtz,[2] and many other workers. In 1944, Ogata, Ito, and Mizutani[3,4] reported that a fraction obtained from calf thymus lowered serum calcium in rabbits. Later, Ito and Mizutani[5] showed that the preparation obtained earlier had a high phosphorus content. A few years later, we began studies on the hypocalcemic substance (calcium-active substance) obtained from the thymus to see whether it was a nucleoprotein or one of the ordinary proteins; it was thereby found that this calcium-active substance was an ordinary protein.[6] During the course of this study, the important role of the thymus in immune reaction became known, and the reports of Comsa,[7,8] Goldstein,[9] Metcalf,[10] and Luckey[11] on lymphocyte stimulation especially prompted us to examine the presence of lymphocytotic activity in our fraction. Some of our results were reported at the First International Congress of Immunology held in Washington, D.C., in 1971,[12] and details have been reviewed in *Thymic Hormones* edited by Dr. Luckey.[13] However, the preparation described in that paper failed to show good purity by polyacrylamide gel disc electrophoresis. Therefore, we attempted to purify the extract completely. The present paper describes the method for this purification, and some of the biochemical and biological properties of the preparation.

Materials and Methods

All the fractionation procedures were carried out in a cold room at about 5° C or under ice cooling, and toluene was added to the buffer solution as a preservative.

Materials

Acetone-dried powder was prepared from fresh thymus gland of a mature steer by the method of Mizutani *et al.*[14] The yield of the powder was about 3.8% of the gland. The extract from the powder with 0.9% NaCl solution was fractionated with $(NH_4)_2SO_4$ by using a slightly modified method of Mizutani *et al.*,[15] and the fraction precipitating at 15% or 20% of $(NH_4)_2SO_4$ concentration was used as the starting material for further purification. The yields of the 15% $(NH_4)_2SO_4$ and 20% $(NH_4)_2SO_4$ fractions were about 1.7 and 2.8% of the powder, respectively.

Bioassay

Hypocalcemic activity was assayed by the method described previously.[15] Mature male rabbits were divided into 2 groups of 6 animals each, deprived of food for about 24 hours, and a physiological saline solution of a sample was injected into the aural vein, in a dose of 0.5 ml/kg. Blood was drawn before the injection, and 4, 5, and 6 hours after injection. The amount of serum calcium was titrated with EDTA solution, using Dotite NN as an indicator. Out of three serum samples taken after the injection, the value of maximum lowering in calcium was taken, and its percent decrease was calculated against the calcium value before injection, then averaged for the six animals. The difference between this mean value and the mean of control values obtained from animals injected with physiological saline was examined by the t-test, and the value giving a significant difference at below 5% probability was taken as being effective.

Lymphocyte-stimulating activity was assayed mostly by the Metcalf method,[16] as modified by Luckey.[11] Litter mates of neonatal mice were divided into two groups, one group being used as a control by interperitoneal injection of physiological saline and the other injected intraperitoneally with a physiological saline solution of a sample. Blood was obtained from the tail before the injection, and 6, 10, and 14 days after the injection. Differential white cell counts were made using Wright's stain. The mean value of the increment against the initial ratio was counted for each of blood samples obtained from the control and test groups, and the difference in the increment between the two groups for the same day was examined by the t-test. If one of these blood samples showed a significant difference at less than 5% probability, the sample tested was considered to be effective.

TABLE 1

BUFFER SYSTEM USED FOR CHROMATOGRAPHY ON DEAE CELLULOSE

Buffer Number	Component	pH	μ
I	0.007 M Phosphate buffer	7.7	0.02
II	0.033 M Phosphate buffer	7.0	0.07
III	0.067 M Phosphate buffer	6.8	0.13
IV	0.067 M Phosphate buffer—0.1 M NaCl	6.5	0.23
V	0.067 M Phosphate buffer—0.2 M NaCl	6.3	0.33
VI	0.067 M Phosphate buffer—0.4 M NaCl	6.1	0.43

Chromatography on DEAE Cellulose

DEAE cellulose (exchange capacity, 0.97 meq/g) activated by the conventional method[17] was fully equilibrated with buffer 1 in TABLE 1 and packed into a chromatographic column. The sample of 15% $(NH_4)_2SO_4$ or 20% $(NH_4)_2SO_4$ fraction was dissolved in the buffer 1 (centrifuged, if necessary), the clear solution was loaded on the column, and eluted stepwise successively with the buffer system shown in TABLE 1. The eluted fractions were dialyzed against deionized water and lyophilized.

Gel Chromatography on Sepharose® 4B or 6B

Sepharose was equilibrated with 0.05M phosphate buffer (pH 7.0, 0.1 μ) and packed in columns. A fraction purified by DEAE cellulose chromatography was dissolved in the buffer solution and centrifuged to remove insoluble materials, and the supernatant was loaded on the column. Elution was performed with the same buffer solution by the ascending method, at a water pressure of about 50 cm.

Preparative Polyacrylamide Gel Disc Electrophoresis

A commercial apparatus, Toyo Model CD-50, was modified for this purification procedure. Polyacrylamide gel and buffer solution used for the procedure were the same as used for analytical polyacrylamide gel disc electrophoresis.

Polyacrylamide Gel Disc Electrophoresis for Analysis and Isoelectric Focusing

In order to examine the homogeneity of the protein fraction, analytical polyacrylamide gel disc electrophoresis was carried out by the Davis method.[18] The resulting gels were submitted to recording by an autodensitometer, Fuji-Riken Model FD-A-IV. Isoelectric focusing was carried out by an apparatus of Model KLB-8101 with 0.5% Ampholine in the range of pH 5–7 according to the Vesterberg and Svensson method.[19]

Molecular Weight Determination by SDS Polyacrylamide Gel Electrophoresis

Electrophoresis by the split gel method of Dunker and Reuckert [20] was carried out in 10% polyacrylamide gel in 0.1% SDS. The molecular weight of the purified material was calculated by comparing its mobility with those of a set of proteins (Schwarz-Mann Product) of known molecular weight. Gel staining followed the method of Weber and Osbon.[21] A part of the protein sample was submitted to electrophoresis without mercaptoethanol.

Amino Acid Analysis

The purified material was hydrolyzed at 110 ± 2° C with 6N HCl, and the dried hydrolyzate was submitted to analysis by the Hitachi Model KLA-3B amino acid analyzer.[22] Values obtained from the hydrolyzates for 24, 36, and 72 hours were corrected by extrapolation to 0 hour and the amounts of amino acids were determined. The amounts of tryptophan were determined by the Spies and Chambers method.[23]

Determination of Sugar and Protein

Sugar in the purified material was determined as glucose by the phenol-H_2SO_4 method.[24] Protein concentration in the sample solutions was estimated by measuring optical density of the solutions at 280 nm, or by the method of Lowry *et al.*,[25] using bovine albumin as a standard.

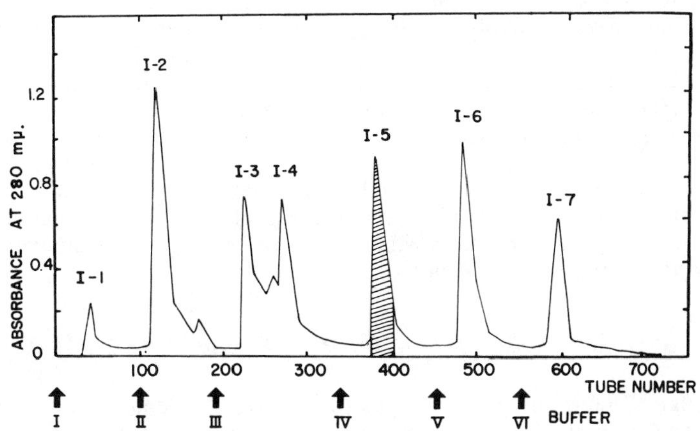

FIGURE 1. Chromatography of the 15% $(NH_4)_2SO_4$ fraction on DEAE cellulose. Sample: T–28∼32A. 4.1 g/300 ml. Column size 2.5×145 cm. Flow rate 6 ml/cm²hr. One tube=15 ml.

RESULTS

Chromatography on DEAE Cellulose

FIGURE 1 shows the chromatographic pattern of the 15% $(NH_4)_2SO_4$ fraction on DEAE cellulose. Fractions obtained from this chromatography were designated as I-1 through I-7 from left to right. The calcium activity of these fractions is shown in TABLE 2. The activity and yield of fractions I-5 and I-6 were relatively great. Disc electrophoresis of these fractions on 7.5% polyacrylamide gel is shown in FIGURE 2. The left-hand side is the pattern of 15% $(NH_4)_2SO_4$ fraction and numerous bands (about 7) are seen. Fraction I-5 and I-6 also gave several bands and further purification was carried out on these fractions.

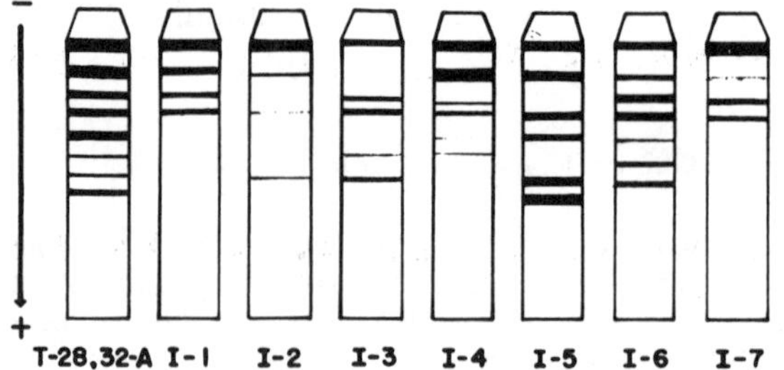

FIGURE 2. Disc electrophoresis of the fractions obtained from chromatography of the 15% $(NH_4)_2SO_4$ fraction on DEAE cellulose.

Gel Chromatography of Fraction I-5 on Sepharose 4B

The solution of the fraction I-5 was loaded on a column of Sepharose 4B and was eluted with 0.05M phosphate buffer. The pattern thereby obtained is shown in FIGURE 3. This effluent was divided into three fractions designated as G4B-1, G4B-2, and G4B-3, as shown in the graph. Fraction G4B-2, shown by the hatched area, had an especially strong activity in a dose of 0.1 mg/kg, but the disc electrophoresis of this fraction still showed three bands in its pattern (TABLE 3, FIGURE 4). This fraction was rechromatographed over Sepharose 6B, and the fraction, G4B-2.G6B-2, was obtained. Fraction G4B-2.-G6B-2 gave an almost single band in disc electrophoresis, but the densitometric tracing of this gel showed poor symmetry. This fraction was further fractionated by preparative disc electrophoresis.

Preparative Disc Electrophoresis of Fraction G4B-2.G6B-2

FIGURE 5 shows the pattern of the preparative electrophoresis of this fraction. The disc electrophoresis of fraction E-1 (designated as TP1) in this graph

TABLE 2

YIELD AND HYPOCALCEMIC ACTIVITY OF THE FRACTIONS OBTAINED FROM CHROMATOGRAPHY OF THE 15% $(NH_4)_2SO_4$ FRACTION ON DEAE CELLULOSE

Fraction Number	Yield mg	Yield %	Dose mg/kg	Percent Decrease in Serum Calcium Mean ± S.E.
I–1	23.1	0.6	0.5	7.2 ± 1.8
I–2	182.6	4.5	0.5	3.7 ± 1.8
I–3	50.9	1.2	0.5	8.7 ± 1.5 *
I–4	69.8	1.7	0.5	4.8 ± 1.8
I–5	130.0	3.2	0.5	13.8 ± 2.1 *
I–6	259.6	6.3	0.5	12.3 ± 0.9 *
I–7	107.7	2.6	0.5	9.7 ± 1.0 *
T–28.32–A †	—	—	1.0	14.8 ± 2.2 ‡

* Significantly different from control: $p < 0.01$.
† $(NH_4)_2SO_4$ 15% fraction.
‡ Significantly different from control: $p < 0.05$.

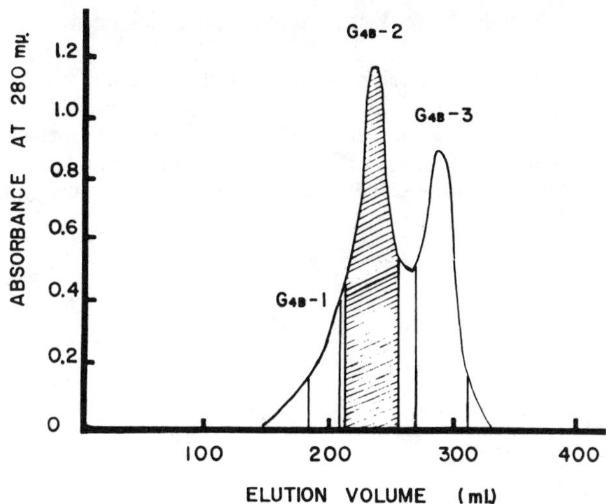

FIGURE 3. Gel chromatography of the fraction (T–28∼32A·I–5) on Sepharose 4B. The fraction (T–28∼32A·I–5) was obtained from chromatography of the 15% $(NH_4)_2SO_4$ fraction on DEAE cellulose. Sample: 117 mg in 5 ml of 0.05 M phosphate buffer (pH 7.0). Column size: 1.7×120 cm. One tube=5.0 ml.

TABLE 3

YIELD AND HYPOCALCEMIC ACTIVITY OF THE FRACTIONS OBTAINED FROM GEL CHROMATOGRAPHY ON SEPHAROSE 4B

Fraction Number	Yield mg	Yield %	Dose mg/kg	Percent Decrease in Serum Calcium Mean ± S.E.
G_{4B}–1	20.4	17.4	0.1	9.9 ± 1.0 *
G_{4B}–2	33.3	28.5	0.1	17.1 ± 1.9 *
G_{4B}–3	25.5	21.8	0.1	4.1 ± 0.7

* Significantly different from control: $p < 0.01$.

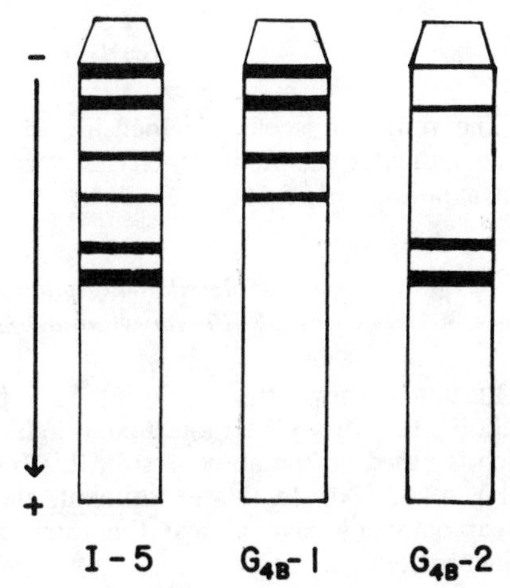

FIGURE 4. Disc electrophoresis of the fractions obtained from gel chromatography of the sample (T–28∼32A·I–5) on Sepharose 4B. Sample (T–28∼32·A·I–5) was obtained from chromatography of the 15% $(NH_4)_2SO_4$ fraction on DEAE cellulose.

gave a single band and the calcium activity of this fraction was significant in a dose of 0.005 mg/kg. Later, gel chromatography was carried out on Sepharose 6B alone instead of 4B, and the resulting fraction was further purified by preparative electrophoresis. A fraction giving a single band in disc electrophoresis was obtained (FIGURE 6b) and its densitometric tracing showed good symmetry (FIGURE 6a).

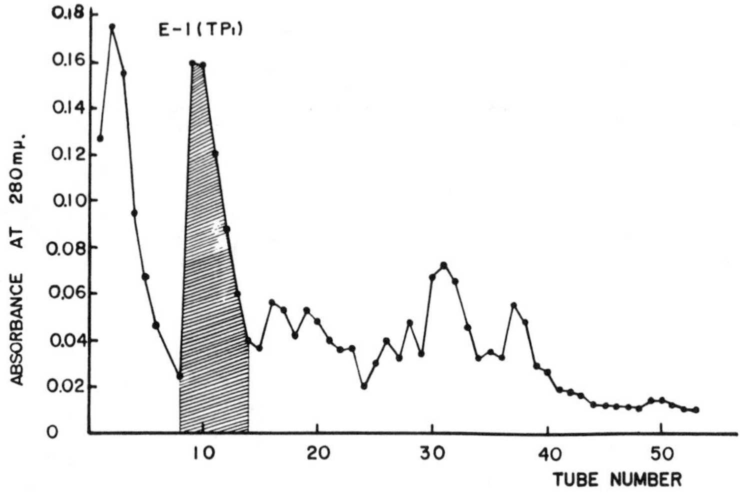

FIGURE 5. Preparative disc electrophoresis of the sample purified by gel chromatography. For separation 7.5% polyacrylamide gel was used. Sample: T–41∼47A·I–5·G4B·G6B. Solution of 73.5 mg of the sample in 10 ml of buffer was loaded. Buffer: Tris-glycine, pH 8.6 μ: 0.05. Condition: 2.93∼3.67 mA/cm,[2] 800∼720 V.

Isoelectric Focusing

The result of isoelectric focusing of fraction TP1 is shown in FIGURE 7, which indicates the homogeneity of this sample and the presence of an isoelectric point at pH 5.65.

Molecular Weight Determination by SDS Polyacrylamide Gel Electrophoresis

FIGURE 8 shows the results of SDS polyacrylamide gel electrophoresis of fraction TP1. From the molecular weight calibration curve shown in FIGURE 9, which is based on the above result, this fraction was found to be a protein with a MW of 68,000. In this experiment. electrophoresis after preincubation with mercaptoethanol gave almost the same result as electrophoresis without the preincubation.

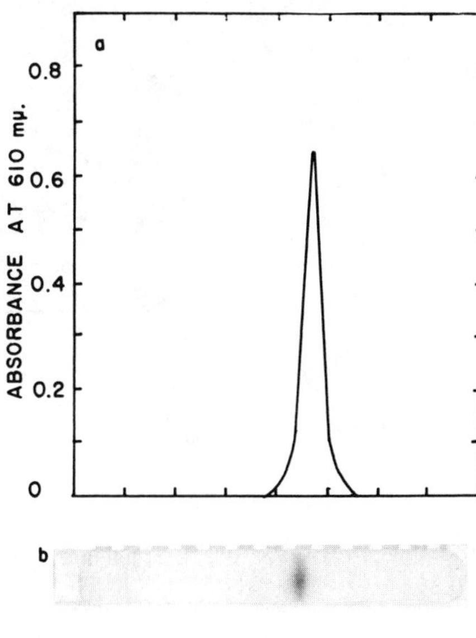

FIGURE 6. (a) Densitometric tracing of disc electrophorogram of the fraction (T–51∼53A·I–5·G6B·E). (b) Disc electrophoresis of the fraction (T–51∼53A·I–5·G6B·E).

Amino Acid Analysis

TABLE 4 gives the result of amino acid analysis and each amino acid is expressed by molar ratio, taking the MW of this protein as 68,000. The amino acid composition of the protein showed no remarkable feature.

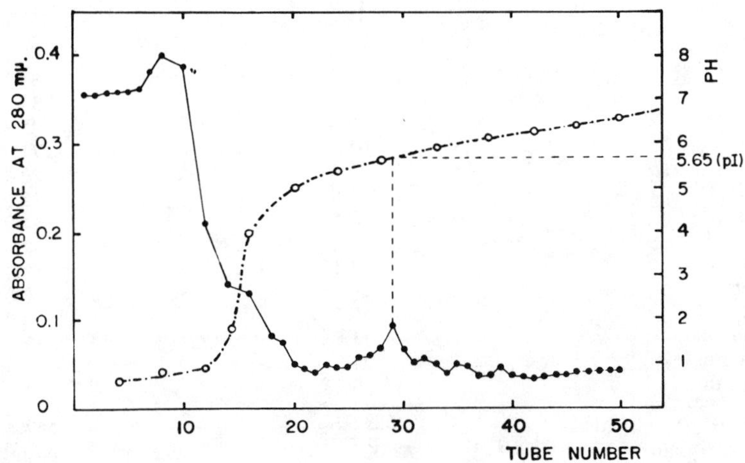

FIGURE 7. Isoelectric focusing of the purified sample. Sample: T–41∼47·A·I–5·G4B·G6B·E–1 (TP_1). The solution of 1 mg of the sample was loaded. Ampholyte: pH 5∼7. —·—○—·— pH; —●— 280 mμ.

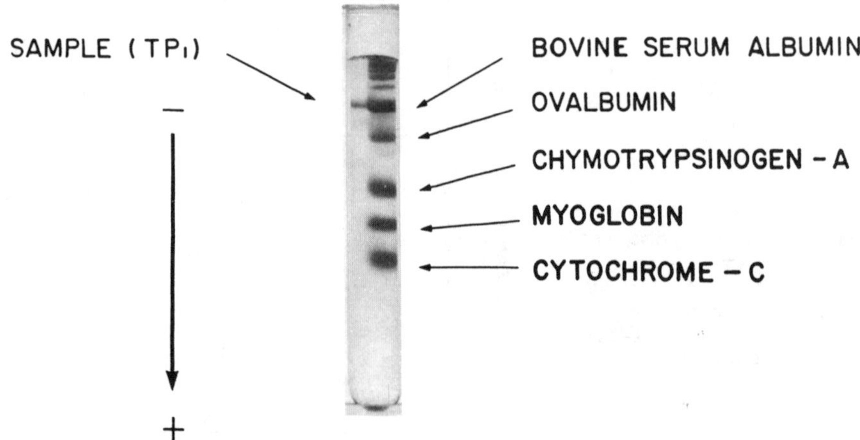

FIGURE 8. Electrophoresis on 10% polyacrylamide gel in 0.1% SDS by the split gel technique.

TABLE 4
AMINO ACID COMPOSITION OF THE PURIFIED SAMPLE (TP_1)

Amino Acid	Moles/Mole of protein TP_1	B.S.A.*
Lysine	45.1	55.3
Histidine	13.0	16.5
Arginine	23.7	21.7
Aspartic acid	65.4	52.5
Cystine/2	13.5	31.5
Threonine	37.2	31.4
Serine	50.2	25.8
Glutamic acid	65.1	71.8
Proline	35.1	26.4
Glycine	68.8	15.6
Alanine	50.5	44.9
Valine	42.8	32.4
Methionine	2.1	3.4
Isoleucine	24.5	12.8
Leucine	50.2	60.0
Tyrosine	11.8	17.9
Phenylalanine	21.7	25.6
Tryptophan †	3.23	1.8
Totals	623.93	547.3
Molecular weight	68,000	64,000

* Bovine serum albumin: Data are taken from Advan. Protein Chem. **18:** 227 (1963).

† Tryptophan was determined by the method of J. R. Spies and D. C. Chambers.

Determination of Sugar

The sugar in fraction TP1 was determined by the phenol-H_2SO_4 method, and the content was 2.43%.

Purification of Fraction I-6

This fraction was purified by gel chromatography on Sepharose 6B and then by preparative electrophoresis, and a fraction (designated as TP2) giving a single band in analytical disc electrophoresis was obtained. The densitometric tracing of this gel and the second gel chromatography of this fraction on Sepharose 6B gave peaks with good symmetry in both the patterns.

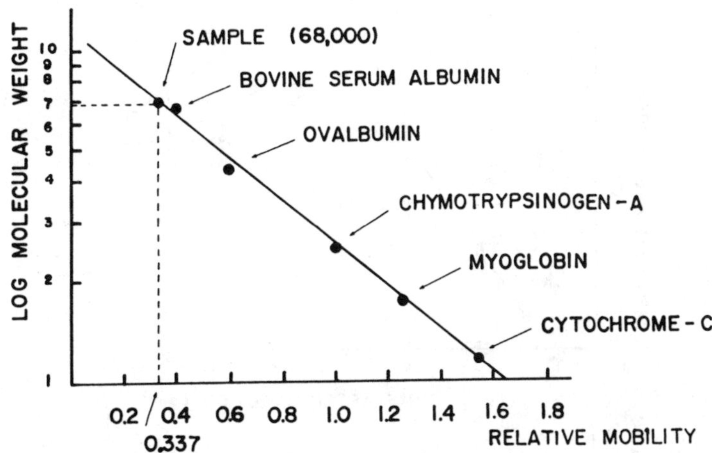

FIGURE 9. Molecular weight calibration curve for SDS polyacrylamide gel electrophoresis. Sample: T–51∼53·A·I–5·G6B·E (TP_1).

Isoelectric Focusing of Fraction TP2

In isoelectric focusing using 4.3 mg. of the sample, the single peak was given and the isoelectric point of this protein was at pH 5.4. The fraction obtained from this procedure showed a calcium activity when administered in a dose of 0.025 mg/kg but it was lower than that of the fraction TP1.

Molecular Weight of Fraction TP2

This protein was found to have a molecular weight of 57,000 from the molecular weight calibration curve.

Lymphocyte-stimulating Activity of the Fraction Obtained from Thymus Extracts

FIGURE 10a shows the daily variation in L/P ratio when a dose of 0.2 μg/mouse was injected, using the fraction T-28.32A.I-5.G4B.G4B from fraction I-5 of DEAE cellulose chromatography, purified further by gel chromatography on Sepharose 4B. The difference between the test and control groups became significant 6 and 10 days after the injection, while the values in two groups became close after 30 days. FIGURE 10b shows the daily variation in L/P ratio when a dose of 0.1 μg/mouse was injected, using fraction T-70.74A.1-6.-G6B.E.G6B from fraction I-6 of the DEAE cellulose chromatography purified consecutively by gel chromatography, preparative electrophoresis, and second gel chromatography. Significant difference between the two groups was found 6, 10, and 14 days after the injection.

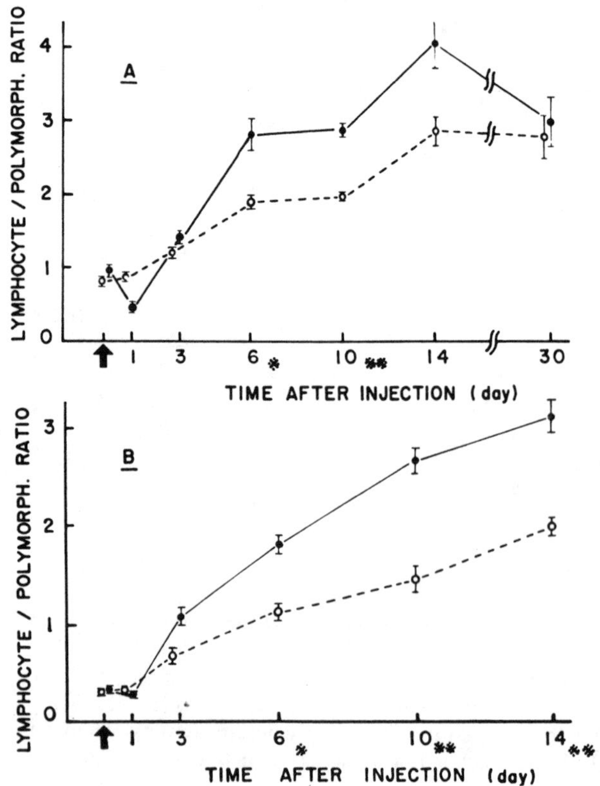

FIGURE 10. Time course of increase of lymphocyte/polymorph ratio in mice. (A) Sample: T–28∼32 A·I–5·G4B·G4B; Dose 0.2 μg/mouse. (B) Sample: T–70∼74 A·I–6·G6B·E·G6B; Dose 0.1 μg/mouse. —●—: sample; ---○---: control; ※ significantly different from control: $p < 0.05$; ※ ※ significantly different from control: $p < 0.01$. ₸: Mean ± S.E.

TABLE 5

HYPOCALCEMIC ACTIVITY AND LYMPHOCYTE/POLYMORPH RATIO ACTIVITY OF THE FRACTIONS OBTAINED FROM THYMUS EXTRACTS

Sample	Hypocalcemic Activity		L/P ratio activity	
	Dose mg/kg	Percent Decrease in Serum Calcium Mean ± S.E.	Dose μg/ mouse	Ratio Mean ± S.E
1 T–72.73	10	8.9 ± 0.9 *	20	2.4 ± 0.2 †
2 T–28∼32A·15	1	14.8 ± 2.2 *	10	3.1 ± 0.3 *
3 T–60∼68A·20∼25	1	9.9 ± 1.9 *	10	2.2 ± 0.1
4 T–60∼68A·25∼satu.	0.5	2.0 ± 0.9	10	2.6± 0.1 *
5 T–28∼32A·I–2	0.5	3.7 ± 1.8	5	1.1 ± 0.1
6 T–28∼32A·I–5	0.5	13.8 ± 2.1 *	5	2.9 ± 0.1 *
7 T–28∼32A·I–5G_{4B}·G_{4B}	0.01	19.1 ± 1.8 *	0.2	2.7 ± 0.1 *
8 T–41∼47A·I–5·G_{4B}·G_{6B}E(TP_1)	0.005	8.3 ± 1.4 †	0.2	2.4 ± 0.2 *
9 T–28∼32A·I–6	0.5	12.3 ± 0.9 †	5	2.4 ± 0.2 †
10 T–60∼68A·I–6·G_{6B}	0.1	17.2 ± 3.2 *	1	3.2 ± 0.2 *
11 T–70∼74A·I–6·G_{6B}·E·G_{6B} (TP_2)	0.05	8.0 ± 0.6 *	0.1	3.1 ± 0.1 *
12 Bovine serum albumin	1	6.3 ± 0.9	20	1.6 ± 0.1

* Significantly different from control: $p < 0.01$.
† Significantly different from control: $p < 0.05$.

Calcium activity and L/P ratio activity of various fractions are summarized in TABLE 5. Number 1 shows the result of acetone-dried powder. Numbers 2–4 show the results of fractions precipitated with $(NH_4)_2SO_4$ at concentrations of 15%, 20%, and 25% saturation, respectively. Numbers 5 and 6 are the results of fractions obtained from DEAE cellulose chromatography. Fraction T-28.32A.I-5 showed calcium activity in a dose of 0.5 mg/kg in the rabbit and L/P ratio activity in a dose of 5 μg/mouse. Number 8 is the result of fraction TP1, 9 that of fraction I-6 from DEAE-cellulose chromatography, and 10 that of the fraction purified by gel chromatography of fraction I-6 on Sepharose 6B, 11 that of fraction TP2, and 12 is a test as control with bovine serum albumin, which showed activity at neither 1 mg/kg or 20 μg/mouse. From this table, it can be seen that both the calcium activity and L/P ratio activity tended to increase with progress in purification. With respect to the calcium activity, however, that of fraction TP2 (11) was lower than that of fraction TP1 (8), though there was no great difference between them in L/P ratio activity. Since these two fractions were homogeneous in disc electrophoresis, they may retain two kinds of activity, though there is a difference in their potency. It cannot be said that all of the fractions have both activities, as seen in this table, and the fractions may have one of two activities, or neither of the activities.

DISCUSSION

Two kinds of active protein fraction were separated from bovine thymus extracts. Since the first protein (TP1) showed that its mobility in disc electrophoresis was close to that of bovine serum albumin (BSA) and its MW obtained from SDS electrophoresis was 68,000, it is very similar to BSA; but its strong calcium activity and L/P ratio activity, difference in amino acid composition, especially the higher content of glycine, serine, and tryptophan in fraction TP1 than in that of BSA, and the difference in K_{av} value obtained from gel chromatography on Sepharose 6B (TP1, K_{av} 0.53; BSA, K_{av} 0.65) all suggest that it is a protein different from BSA. From the value of K_{av} 0.53, the MW of fraction TP1 was estimated as 100,000, whereas the MW was 68,000 by SDS electrophoresis. This may be due to the fact that protein of 68,000 is a subunit of the protein of 100,000, or to the large dissymmetry of the protein molecule. The pattern of disc electrophoresis was almost the same whether a preincubation with 8M urea was carried out before electrophoresis or not. This also was the case in preincubation with mercaptoethanol before SDS electrophoresis. From these observations, it would be hard to consider that the protein with MW of 68,000 is a subunit or that it can easily be dissociated into smaller units. Consequently, we think that this protein has a fairly large dissymmetry of the molecule.

The second protein TP2 considerably differed from the first TP1 in calcium activity but its L/P ratio activity showed no great difference (TABLE 5). The observed disc electrophoresis mobility was smaller for fraction TP2 than for TP1, and the K_{av} value of TP2 (about 0.45) in gel chromatography on Sepharose 6B was also smaller. The molecular weight of TP2 (57,000) differed from that of TP1. However, the molecular weight of TP2 estimated from K_{av} 0.45 gave a fairly large value of 170,000. The reason for this difference, including that of the first protein TP1, must await further study.

Calcitonin, known as the hormone lowering serum calcium, is said to be a peptide with molecular weight of 4,000.[26] The two principles with hypocalcemic activity separated from the thymus are now known to be far larger proteins. When fraction TP1 was injected into the aural vein of rabbits, their serum

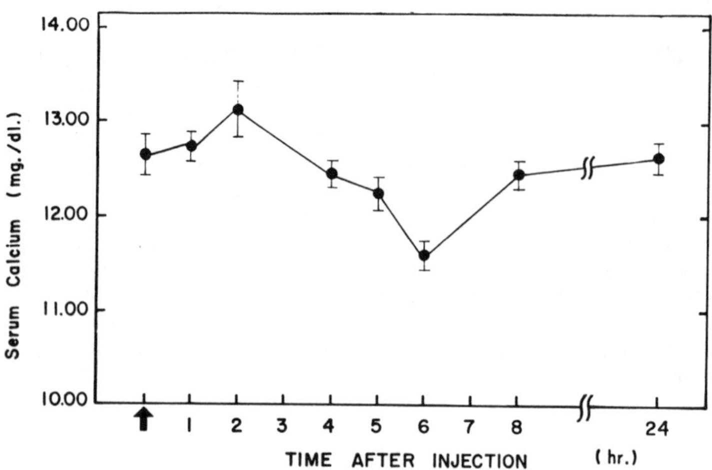

FIGURE 11. Time course of purified fraction (TP_1). Each point represents the mean of 6 rabbits ± S.E. Dosage of TP_1: 5 μg/kg intravenous injection.

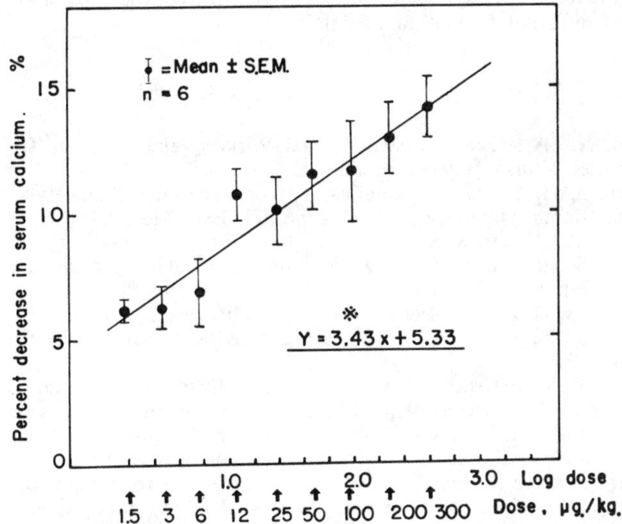

FIGURE 12. Dose-response curve of the fraction purified by gel chromatography on Sepharose 6B.

※ Linearity of regression was found from the analysis of variance. Regression coefficient (b=3.43) differed from 0 at a significance level of 0.05 in t-table.

calcium level reached a minimum about 6 hours after the injection, but the periodical effect of calcitonin [27] differed somewhat from that of fraction TP1, though it depends on the kind and dose of calcitonin (FIGURE 11).

The dose-response curve of a fraction purified from the thymus extracts showed that the regression of hypocalcemic response on log dose may be effectively linear over a moderate range of doses (FIGURE 12).

We have isolated a protein fraction with hypocalcemic activity from the bovine parotid gland, and this fraction also showed a strong L/P ratio activity.

SUMMARY

Two kinds of active protein fraction, TP1 and TP2, were isolated from bovine thymus extracts. Both these fractions showed a single band in polyacrylamide gel disc electrophoresis. Though these two fractions showed a difference in potency, they both lowered serum calcium in rabbits and increased lymphocytes in mice. Molecular weight determination by SDS polyacrylamide gel electrophoresis gave the values of 68,000 for TP1 and 57,000 for TP2. Amino acid composition of TP1 did not show marked characteristics but was clearly different from that of bovine serum albumin. Isoelectric focusing showed the isoelectric point at pH 5.65 for TP1 and pH 5.4 for TP2. Dose-response relation in serum calcium-lowering activity was examined with a sample purified from the extracts, and a linear dependence of the response to log dose was recognized over a moderate range of doses. The time-course measurement of the hypocalcemic activity showed that the action of TP1 is somewhat different from that of calcitonin.

References

1. Nitschke, A. 1928. Darstellung und Wirkung eines aktiven Thymusdrusenextraktes. Klin. Wochenschr. **7:** 2080.
2. Scholtz, H. G. 1932. Beeinflussung von experimentellem Hyperparathyroidismus durch Thymuspraparate. Zentralbl. Exp. Med. **85:** 547.
3. Ogata, A., Y. Ito & A. Mizutani. 1944. Studies on salivary gland hormones. IV. Separation of an active fraction from bovine parotid gland. J. Pharm. Soc. Jap. **64:** 325.
4. Ogata, A. & Y. Ito. 1944. Studies on salivary gland hormones. V. Bioassay method based on the thypocalcemic activity in rabbits. J. Pharm. Soc. Jap. **64:** 332.
5. Ito, Y. & A. Mizutani. 1952. Studies on salivary gland hormones. XVII. Comparison of properties of parotin and various organ extracts acting like parotin on serum calcium level. J. Pharm. Soc. Jap. **72:** 1468.
6. Mizutani, A., Y. Saito, H. Sato & M. Saito. 1970. The search for a hypocalcemic factor in thymus gland. I. Separation of fractions producing hypocalcemia in rabbits from bovine thymus gland by precipitation with calcium chloride. J. Pharm. Soc. Jap. **90:** 445.
7. Comsa, J. 1957. Consequences of thymetomy upon the leucopoiesis in guinea pigs. Acta Endocrinol. **26:** 361.
8. Comsa, J. 1966. Zur Reindarstellung des Thymushormones. Arzneimittelforschung. **16:** 18.
9. Goldstein, A. L., F. D. Slater & A. White. 1966. Preparation, assay, and partial purification of thymic lymphocytopoietic factor (thymosin). Proc. Nat. Acad. Sci. U.S. **56:** 1010.
10. Metcalf, D. 1956. A lymphocytosis stimulating factor in the plasma of chronic lymphatic leukemic patients. Brit. J. Cancer **10:** 169.
11. Hand, T., P. Caster & T. D. Luckey. 1967. Isolation of a thymus hormone, LSH. Biochem. Biophys. Res. Commun. **26:** 18.
12. Mizutani, A. 1971. Hypocalcemic components of thymus gland. Presented at the First International Congress of Immunology, in Washington, D.C., August 4, 1971.
13. Mizutani, A. 1973. A thymic hypocalcemic component. *In* Thymic Hormones. T. D. Luckey, Ed. **:** 193. University Park Press. Baltimore, Maryland.
14. Mizutani, A., M. Terada, Y. Toda & K. Yamamoto. 1969. The search for hypocalcemic factor in thymus gland. III. Fundamental experiment for an improved method of the extraction of substance producing hypocalcemia in rabbits. Ann. Rep. Pharm. Nagoya City Univ. **17:** 16.
15. Mizutani, A., K. Yamamoto, H. Sato, Y. Saito, H. Kitsugawa & H. Yamamoto. 1971. The search for a hypocalcemic factor in thymus gland. II. Improved method for the purification of the substance producing hypocalcemia in rabbits. J. Pharm. Soc. Jap. **91:** 297.
16. Metcalf, D. 1959. The thymic lymphocytosis stimulating factor and its relation to lymphatic leukemia. *In* Proceedings Third Canadian Cancer Conference. **:** 351. Academic Press. New York, N.Y.
17. Peterson, E. A. & H. A. Sober. 1956. Chromatography of proteins. I. Cellulose ion-exchange adsorbents. J. Am. Chem. Soc. **78:** 751.
18. Davis, B. J. 1964. Disc electrophoresis-II. Method and application to human serum proteins. Ann. N.Y. Acad. Sci. **121:** 404.
19. Vesterberg, O. & H. Svensson. 1966. Isoelectric fractionation, analysis, and characterization of ampholytes in natural pH gradients. IV. Further studies on the resolving power in connection with separation of myoglobins. **20:** 820.

20. Dunker, A. K. & R. R. Rueckert. 1969. Observations on molecular weight determinations on polyacrylamide gel. J. Biol. Chem. **244:** 5074.
21. Weber, K. & M. Osborn. 1969. The reliability of molecular weight determinations by dodecyl sulfate-polyacrylamide gel electrophoresis. J. Biol. Chem. **244:** 4406.
22. Spackman, D. H., W. H. Stein & S. Moore. 1958. Automatic recording apparatus for use in the chromatography of amino acids. Anal. Chem. **30:** 1190.
23. Spies, J. R. & D. C. Chambers. 1949. Chemical determination of tryptophan in proteins. Anal. Chem. **21:** 1249.
24. Dubois, M., K. A. Gilles, J. K. Hamilton, P. A. Reber & F. Smith. 1956. Colorimetric method for determination of sugars and related substances. Anal. Chem. **28:** 350.
25. Lowry, O. H., N. J. Rosebrough, A. L. Farr & R. J. Randall. 1951. Protein measurement with the Lowry phenol reagent. J. Biol. Chem. **193:** 265.
26. Potts, J. T., R. A. Reisfeld, P. F. Hirsch, A. B. Wasthed, E. F. Voelkel & P. L. Munson. 1967. Purification of porcine thyrocalcitonin. Proc. Nat. Acad. Sci. U.S. **58:** 328.
27. Maier, P., R. Neher, W. Rittel & M. Staehelin. 1969. Comparison of the hypocalcemic response between human and porcine calcitonins. *In* Calcitonin 1969. Proceedings of the Second International Symposium. July, 1969. London, England : 381. William Heinemann Medical Books, Ltd. London, England.

IMMUNOSUPPRESSIVE α GLOBULIN FROM BOVINE THYMUS AND SERUM: MODE OF ACTION UPON AFFERENT AND EFFERENT ARCS OF THE MOUSE IMMUNE RESPONSE *

S. Michael Phillips,† Charles B. Carpenter,†§
and Patricia Lane ‡

† *Immunology Laboratory, Renal Division*
Department of Medicine
Peter Bent Brigham Hospital, Harvard Medical School
Boston, Massachusetts 02115

‡ *Division of Communicable Disease and Immunology*
Walter Reed Army Institute of Research
Washington, D.C. 20012

Introduction

The original observations of Kamrin that a serum α-2 globulin fraction could promote the survival of allogeneic parabiotic rats [1] and skin grafts [2] has led to a growing interest in the immunosuppressive potential of these naturally occurring substances. The subsequent observation of a generalized elevation of α globulins in the serum of transplant recipients prompted Mowbray to attempt further purification in order to determine the nature and function of such suppressive globulins. Subsequently, a subfraction "Fraction C," obtained by adsorption and elution from DEAE cellulose of bovine serum α globulins, was found to have potent immunosuppressive potential *in vivo* and *in vitro*.[3, 4] Using similar fractionation techniques other laboratories have confirmed the existence of these α glycoproteins in both human serum [5, 6] and bovine thymus.[7] Recently, interest has been focused on growth control factors isolated from various tissues, including thymus [8, 11] lymph node [12] and spleen.[10] Such "chalones" are generally defined by their tissue-specific, but not species-specific, suppression of cell proliferation.[10] Previous work from this laboratory has shown that bovine thymus suppressive globulin is functionally similar to that obtained from bovine serum. Both products have predominant effects upon DNA synthesis and proliferation of lymphocytes, while not blocking antigen recognition and macrophage migration inhibition factor (MIF) release from sensitized cells.[13]

The present study delineates more sharply the kinetics of cellular responses *in vitro* in the presence of both serum and thymus derived α globulins and investigates the effects of these fractions on the specific immune events involved in allogeneic recognition and cell mediated alloimmune cytotoxicity *in vitro*. Comparative studies on thymus and serum fractions were made with *in vitro* systems selected to define the recognition (afferent), proliferative, and effector (efferent) phases of the immune response.

* Supported in part by National Institutes of Health Grant AI-09059.
§ Investigator, Howard Hughes Medical Institute.

Materials and Methods

Preparation of Immunosuppressive α Globulin

Lyophilized defatted bovine thymus powder (Nutritional Biochemicals Corp. lot 3786) was extracted in buffered saline, acidified and the soluble proteins adsorbed to DEAE cellulose in sodium acetate, 0.03M. pH 5.0 as previously described.[7] Fractions were serially eluted at salt concentrations of 0.1, 0.2, and 0.5M, and are referred to as Fractions A, B, and C, respectively. Identically prepared fractions from bovine serum were provided by Dr. James Mowbray (B6C, MRC69). Protein concentrations were determined by the Lowry method and by the OD 280 mμ, corrected for presence of nucleic acid by the OD 260 mμ reading.[7]

Lymphocyte Cultures

Mouse cultures were performed as previously described.[14, 15] Briefly, mitogenic stimuli included phytohemagglutinin (PHA, P Difco), PPD (Weybridge), and allogeneic cells (MLC). Cultures were performed in both sealed Virtis vials under 10% 0_2–85% air–5% CO_2 or in microtiter plates (Falcon 3040). Animals sensitized to PPD were tested for their *in vitro* response 4 weeks later. The synthesis of DNA, RNA, protein and membrane phospholipid was assessed by the addition of 1 μCi [^{3}H]thymidine, [5-^{3}H]uridine, DL[^{14}C]leucine, and [^{3}H]myoinositol, respectively, to cultures during the last 4 hours of incubation. Samples were terminated and washed on glass fiber filters and assessed for isotope incorporation by liquid scintillation. Results represent the mean and 95% confidence interval of 4 replicates.

Lymphocyte-mediated Alloimmune Cytotoxicity

Mixed lymphocyte cultures (MLC) were performed as previously described with modification.[14] Medium consisted of RPMI-1640 with Hepes buffer (0.005M), 10% fresh heat-inactivated normal human serum (40 minutes at 56° C), 5×10^{-5}M 2-mercaptoethanol, penicillin, streptomycin, and amphotericin B (Gibco). 50×10^6 splenic mononuclear cells were incubated with 50×10^6 irradiated (1250 R 60_{Co} Gammacell) target cells in 20 ml volumes in tightly capped upright flasks (Falcon 3012). After 4½ days of incubation, the cells were layered on a Ficoll-Hypaque gradient and assayed for cytotoxic potential using freshly prepared ^{51}Cr-labeled normal thymocytes as targets as previously described in detail.[16] Results are expressed as the percent specific chromium release:

$$\frac{\text{cpm experimental supernatant} - \text{cpm spontaneous release}}{\text{cpm freeze-thaw supernatant} - \text{cpm spontaneous release}} \times 100$$

Macrophage Inhibition Factor Release

MIF activity was assessed upon peritoneal macrophages obtained from guinea pigs as described previously.[13] Lymph node lymphocytes were incubated with Weybridge PPD (15–20 μg/ml). Percent migration was determined by the formula:

$$\frac{\text{area without antigen} - \text{area with antigen}}{\text{area without antigen}} \times 100 = \%\ \text{inhibition}$$

T-cell Rosettes

Normal human peripheral blood lymphocytes (10^6 cells in 25 μl) were mixed with 25 μl fetal calf serum (absorbed with sheep red blood cells (SRBC)), and 50 μl of 2% washed SRBC. After centrifugation at $150 \times g$ for 5 minutes, the cells were left undisturbed for 1 hour at room temperature, gently resuspended, and examined under the microscope. This modification of Wybran's method[17] results in the formation of rosettes with 55–65% of human peripheral blood lymphocytes.

Results

Studies on Afferent Arc of the Immune Response

Effect of α Globulins upon the Proliferative Response

As shown in Figure 1, α globulins were able to affect a variety of *in vitro* responses. These included the response to PHA (a nonspecific mitogen), to PPD (an *in vitro* "secondary" response to antigen, following *in vivo* sensitization), and to allogeneic cells in MLC (an *in vitro* "primary" response). In addition, the effects of both thymic derived (T31C) and serum derived (B6C) α globulins were dose-dependent. In low concentrations, stimulation of all responses occurred and in higher concentrations suppression was observed. Additional studies indicated that the response to Concanavalin-A, Pokeweed mitogen, and sheep red blood cells (following *in vivo* sensitization) were similarly affected by these fractions. In addition, the blastogenic response to lipopolysaccharide was inhibited by the serum α globulin. Hence, it is clear that a variety of antigenic and mitogenic stimuli can be augmented or suppressed by these species nonspecific globulins.

Additional data on the effects of the globulins were obtained by the addition of these fractions to mixed lymphocyte cultures (MLC) at various intervals following their inception. Table 1 illustrates that the low dose (30 μg/ml) stimulatory effect of both fractions apparently requires intervention early, as addition after 24 hours of culture fails to demonstrate augmentation. In contrast, the suppressive effect of the α globulins at high doses (1000 μg/ml) appears to be active when added at 24 hours or later. Addition of the fractions as late as 48 hours still results in significant suppression of the response. These results with an MLC confirm our previous report on PHA stimulation of human lymphocytes, showing that cells can be suppressed 24 hours after PHA stimulation, at a time when protein and RNA synthesis are active and the cell is enlarging, but before the onset of the S phase.[13] These metabolic observations are confirmed and extended by studies with the mouse MLC as shown in Figure 2. Results are expressed as percentage change from the baseline MLC,

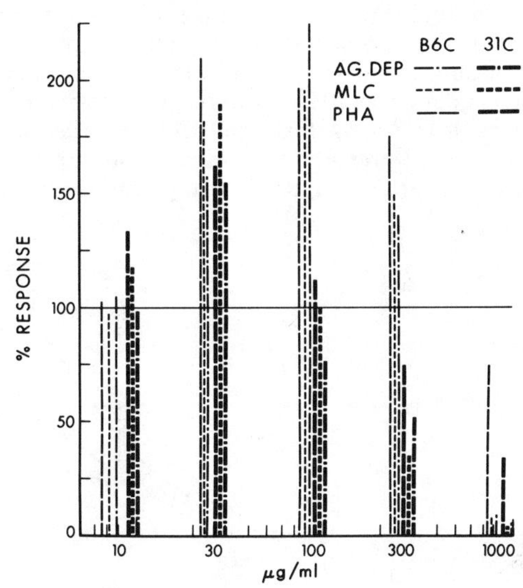

FIGURE 1. Effect of immunosuppressive α globulins upon *in vitro* blastogenic responses. Various concentrations of thymic (T31C) and bovine (B6C) derived α globulins were added to cultures of C57B1/6 spleen cells containing either medium, 15 μg/ml PPD (Ag. Dep.), 1.2 μg/ml PHA, or BALB/c spleen cells (MLC). The concentration of each fraction is plotted against the resulting degree of isotope incorporation (determined by [^{3}H]thymidine) as a percentage of the untreated control. Note a dose-dependent stimulatory and suppressive effect by both α globulins on all responses. Mean cpm of unstimulated cultures: 1480 ± 315 at 48 hours (PHA), 1690 ± 427 at 72 hours (MLC and Ag. Dep.). No significant direct effect was observed upon spontaneous isotope incorporation of unstimulated cultures by the addition of the fractions.

with the fractions present during the entire culture period. Both the stimulatory and suppressive aspects of the fraction illustrated (T31C) are reflected most significantly by alterations of DNA synthesis. Lesser percentage alterations occur in overall protein and phospholipid synthesis, and minimal effects on RNA synthesis are observed. The isotopic methods employed indicate only precursor incorporation into macromolecular moieties, and do not, of course, reflect the possibility of qualitative changes in synthetic events. The data shown

TABLE 1

In Vitro EFFECTIVENESS OF IMMUNOSUPPRESSIVE α GLOBULIN VARIES WITH TIME OF ADDITION TO CULTURES

Fraction		Time of Addition to Mixed Lymphocyte Cultures * 0 †	12	24	48	72
B6C	30 μg	214 ± 24 ‡	149 ± 11	109 ± 12	102 ± 6	98 ± 7
B6C	1000 μg	4 ± 2	4 ± 1	16 ± 4	69 ± 8	90 ± 6
T31C	30 μg	163 ± 25	128 ± 14	93 ± 12	106 ± 12	112 ± 14
T31C	1000 μg	3 ± 1	7 ± 3	28 ± 11	79 ± 10	81 ± 9

* C57B1/6 + BALB/c.
† Hours after culture initiation.
‡ Percentage of control MLC ± S.D. Control MLC=32,400 ± 4800, unmixed cells=2010 ± 730. cpm [^{3}H]thymidine incorporation at 72–76 hours.

in FIGURE 2 are representative of results obtained with both thymus and serum fractions, and with either allogeneic or mitogenic stimulation.

A number of α globulin preparations were tested for their ability to augment or suppress an *in vitro* proliferative response. TABLE 2 illustrates the effect of 2 serum and 6 thymus-derived extracts upon the *in vitro* response of mouse lymphocytes to PHA. Although all fractions were not tested at all concentrations, it is evident that considerable variation exists with regard to the potency of different preparations. In addition, there is no obvious relationship between the dose producing optimal augmentation and that causing suppression of the

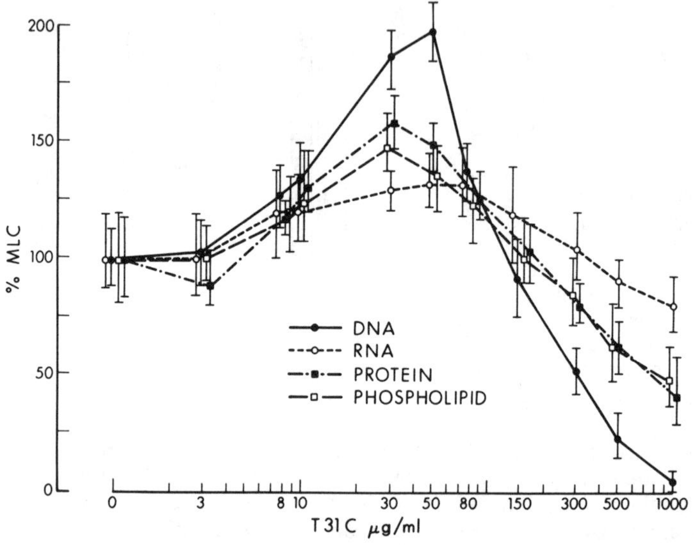

FIGURE 2. Effect of immunosuppressive α globulin on MLC. 75×10^6 C57B1/6 $+75 \times 10^6$ BALB/c spleen cells were incubated *in vitro* in the presence of various concentrations of immunosuppressive α globulin. After 68 hours of incubation [^{3}H] thymidine, [5-^{3}H]uridine DL [^{14}C]Leucine, or [^{3}H]myoinositol were added to replicate cultures which were terminated at 72 hours. The concentration of fraction is plotted against the resulting degree of isotope incorporation shown as a percentage of the untreated control. Each point represents the mean and 95% confidence interval of replicates. Note the dose-dependent stimulation and suppression of all four synthetic rates; however, the most profound effects are upon DNA synthesis.

PHA response for a given fraction. Taken together with the results in TABLE 1 showing a different time dependency for the stimulating activity compared to the suppressive effect, these data suggest the presence of two factors in these preparations.

Effect of α Globulins upon the Development of Lymphocyte-mediated Alloimmune Cytotoxicity

FIGURE 3 illustrates the effect of a serum α globulin upon proliferation, assessed by DNA synthesis, and upon the subsequent development of cytotoxic

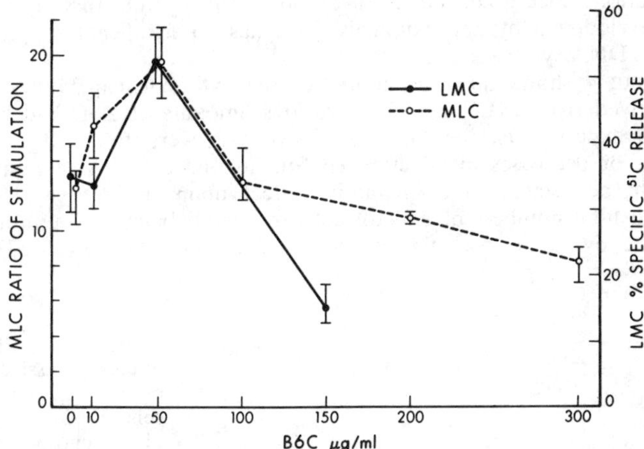

FIGURE 3. Effect of immunosuppressive α globulin upon MLC and subsequent effector cell development. Various concentrations of immunosuppressive α globulin were added to MLC upon initiation (BALB/c+C57B1/6 irradiated spleen cells) and the resultant cell population tested for MLC activity by [^{3}H]thymidine incorporation and LMC by ^{51}Cr release. The ratio of stimulation and percent specific chromium release is plotted against concentrations of immunosuppressive (B6C) α globulins added to culture. Note the dose-dependent correlation of stimulation and suppressive effects upon both phenomena. MLC cpm mixture, 34,300 ± 4500; C57B1/6 irrad, 220 ± 150; BALB/c, 2650 ± 310. LMC cpm freeze-thaw, 3920 ± 36 cpm, spontaneous release, 1283 ± 71 cpm.

effector cells directed against ^{51}Cr-labeled target cells that are syngeneic to the irradiated targets of the MLC. As can be seen, low concentrations of the fraction stimulate both cell division and the subsequent development of effector cells, whereas higher concentrations of the fraction are suppressive to both. In this experiment, the ability of the fraction to suppress the specific development of effector cells appears to be greater than its ability to suppress total

TABLE 2

VARIATION OF EFFECTIVENESS OF IMMUNOSUPPRESSIVE α GLOBULINS

Fraction		μg/ml Added to Mouse PHA Cultures 10	30	100	300	1000	2000
Serum	B6C	104 *	210	204	132	73	0.8
	MRC69	98	111	124	103	74	11.2
Thymus	T38B	98	102	113	146	17	2.1
	T38C	106	98	108	159	102	5.6
	T36B	—	—	174	152	62	1.9
	T37B	—	—	102	124	61	5.7
	T23C	—	—	186	197	125	4.2
	T31C	137	184	112	71	35	2.6

* Percentage of PHA control, [^{3}H]thymidine incorporation mean cpm, cells alone 1480 ± 315, PHA 47,810 ± 4190.

proliferation, since a concentration of B6C (150 μg/ml) that suppresses cytotoxic development by approximately 50% has no significant suppressive effect upon net DNA synthesis.

FIGURE 4 shows the time course of the cytotoxic capabilities of effector cells derived from MLCs to which various amounts of B6C had been added. In these experiments, the kinetics of cytolysis were followed to see if the increases or decreases in effector cell function measured at 4 hours (FIGURE 3) might be related to a qualitative effect upon the rate of ^{51}Cr release. Although total numbers of effector cells recovered from each culture were the same, the cytotoxic potential varied considerably when assessed kinetically

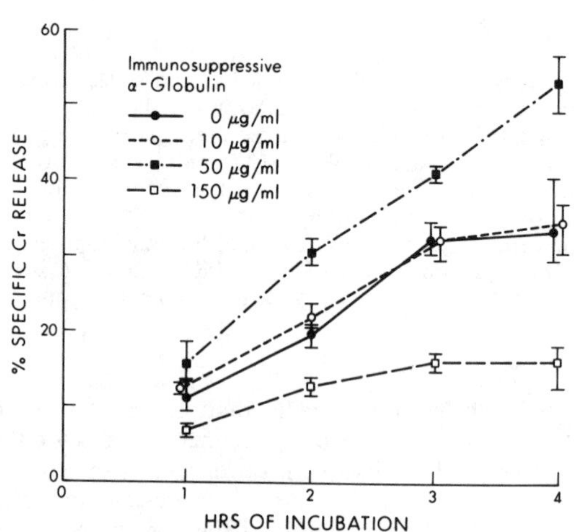

FIGURE 4. Effect of immunosuppressive α globulins on development of effector cells. Various concentrations of immunosuppressive α globulins were added to MLC upon initiation (BALB/c +C57Bl/6 irradiated spleen cells) and the resultant cell population tested for cytotoxicity against chromium labeled C57Bl/6 and BALB/c cells. The percent specific chromium release by cells from each incubation mixture is plotted against time of incubation. Note the dose-dependent stimulation and suppression of cytotoxic potential. Mean cpm of C57Bl/6 freeze-thaw, 3920 ± 36. Spontaneous release 290 ± 14, 570 ±16, 820 ± 23, 1283 ± 71 cpm at 1, 2, 3, and 4 hours, respectively. No significant cytotoxicity was observed against BALB/c cells.

over time, and increases or decreases were present at all time intervals. Whether these differences are due to qualitative or quantitative differences in the effector cell populations is under active study.

Effect of α Globulins on Formation of T-cell Rosettes

When concentrations of B6C, MRC69, and T31C up to 2000 μg/ml were preincubated for 15 minutes with normal human peripheral blood lymphocytes, no inhibition of rosette formation occurred when SRBC were subsequently added to the lymphocyte-globulin mixture.

Studies on the Efferent Arc of the Immune Response

We have previously reported that concentrations of immunosuppressive α globulin that were highly effective in suppressing blastogenesis have no apparent effect upon the release of MIF by tuberculin presensitized guinea pig cells nor upon the effectiveness of that MIF upon normal guinea pig peritoneal macrophages.[13] TABLE 3 confirms this lack of effect upon preestablished MIF effector capability. In addition, lymphocyte-mediated cytotoxicity, developed *in vitro* (MLC) is not altered by the addition to the assay of a wide range of concentrations of immunosuppressive serum and thymus α globulins, and the fractions were not directly toxic to the target cells. When the cytotoxic potential was studied kinetically as shown in TABLE 4, no significant effect was observed upon the addition of either serum or thymus-derived immunosuppressive α globulins. The concentration of glycoprotein employed (1000 μg/ml) had been previously shown to suppress virtually all blastogenic reactivity in MLC.

DISCUSSION

These studies confirm and extend previous observations on the mechanism of action *in vitro* of serum and thymus-derived immunosuppressive α globulins.[7, 13, 18, 19] We have previously reported the ability of immunosuppressive α globulins to both stimulate and suppress the response of human cells to PHA *in vitro*. It would appear that mouse cells show similar sensitivity, emphasizing the species nonspecificity of these agents. In addition, the present studies extend the spectrum of *in vitro* reactivity to include a number of nonspecific mitogens and specific antigens, PPD, SRBC, and allogeneic cells. This broad range of *in vitro* activity would be predicted from the previously observed *in vivo* suppressive effect upon the response to a variety of diverse antigens.[4, 7, 20]

The significance of the biphasic dose-dependent effect of the immunosuppressive α globulins is not known, and *in vivo* studies have demonstrated primarily suppressive effects. The various preparations demonstrate no necessary relationship between suppressive and augmentative potential. Furthermore, kinetic experiments would indicate that the stimulatory effect is confined to an earlier period in the *in vitro* proliferative response than is the suppressive effect. These observations would argue for the presence of at least two moieties in these preparations, and further purification will be necessary to determine this possibility. It may also be that the same globulin stimulates proliferation in low doses and suppresses in high doses, and that the variations from product to product are related to the modifying influences of contaminants. In any event, the essential functional identity of the bovine serum and bovine thymus preparation is established. Both must be administered 10–20 hours prior to antigen administration in the mouse for immune suppression,[7, 20, 21] and both have similar characteristics in mitogen-stimulated lymphocyte cultures.[13, 22] Furthermore, in this and in previous studies, effects on afferent and efferent aspects of the immune response have been identical.[13, 19] The rather specific locus of inhibitory action upon DNA synthesis is also of importance. Although qualitative alterations in RNA, protein and membrane phospholipid synthesis may be present, the overall net synthetic effect on stimulated cells is upon [^{3}H]thymidine incorporation. When alloimmune lymphocyte-mediated cytotoxicity, an effector function that depends upon a degree of T-cell proliferation,

TABLE 3

EFFECT OF IMMUNOSUPPRESSIVE α GLOBULIN ON PREEXISTING EFFECTOR CAPABILITY

Assay	Fraction	μg/ml Fraction Added to Assay 0	30	100	300	1000	3000
LMC *	B6C	2709 ± 115 †	2592 ± 201	2609 ± 106	2463 ± 8	2590 ± 175	2391 ± 69
	T31C		2801 ± 6	2558 ± 63	2668 ± 156	2815 ± 46	2493 ± 106
MIF ‡	B6C	60,66 §	60,68	59,63	65,69	64,68	56,62
	T31C		57,61	58,66	62,68	58,64	56,60

* Lymphocyte mediated cytotoxicity.

† Cpm ^{51}Cr release at 4 hours (freeze-thaw cpm=4651 ± 35; spontaneous cpm=1265 ± 25).

‡ Macrophage migration inhibition factor.

§ Percentage inhibition of migration (2 experiments): cells from guinea pigs sensitized to complete Freund's adjuvant. 15 μg/ml Weybridge PPD in assay, read at 30 hours. Control migration inhibition: 2.6 ± 0.7%, without PPD; 1.9 ± 1.2%, unsensitized cells + PPD.

is assessed, a parallel dose-response relationship can be demonstrated between DNA synthesis and the degree of cytolysis subsequently produced. On the other hand, large concentrations of α globulin cannot block the cytolytic action of aggressor cells in the LMC assay. In the light of previously described ribonuclease (RNAse) activity possessed by these fractions [20] and the increasing recognition of the importance of RNA in various immune reactions such as macrophage-antigen interaction [23] and transfer factor activity,[24] it remains to be determined what the relationship is, if any, of RNAse to the mechanism and locus of action of these naturally occurring immunoregulatory α globulins. The present studies serve to emphasize relative selectivity of the immunosuppressive bovine α globulins upon the immune response. Antigenic recognition by sensitized cells and by thymus-dependent rosette-forming cells is not impaired; furthermore, the cytolytic action of preformed effector lymphocytes is not blocked. It is the proliferative response to antigen and mitogens that is profoundly modulated by the α globulins. When similar preparative tech-

TABLE 4

EFFECT OF ADDITION OF IMMUNOSUPPRESSIVE α GLOBULIN UPON KINETICS OF LYMPHOCYTE-MEDIATED CYTOTOXICITY BY ALLOSENSITIZED CELLS

	Hours of Incubation			
	1	2	4	8
Fraction *				
none	3.2 ± 0.1 †	23.0 ± 0.5	41.0 ± 0.8	60.0 ± 2.4
T31C	1.6 ± 0.2	25.0 ± 0.2	44.0 ± 0.5	57.0 ± 4.1
B6C	4.1 ± 0.1	22.0 ± 0.7	37.0 ± 1.8	54.0 ± 2.3

* Fraction added, 1000 μg/ml, at time of attacking and target cell mixture.

† Percentage specific ^{51}Cr release. cpm freeze-thaw=4651 ± 35. Spontaneous release=470 ± 21 (1 hour), 666 ± 13 (2 hours), 1265 ± 18 (4 hours), 2901 ± 18 (8 hours).

niques have been applied to human plasma, Cooperband *et al.*[25–28] have prepared an immunoregulatory α globulin (IRA) with many *in vivo* and *in vitro* similarities to the bovine products. However, their IRA does interfere with antigen recognition, as it prevents MIF release from sensitized cells [26] and blocks formation of T-cell rosettes.[29] Hence, it appears that human α globulin is a different molecule, or more likely, that there is an additional factor in the IRA preparation that is lacking in the bovine products. The recent finding that the IRA active molecule is in fact a peptide [28] represents a significant step in purification of that material. A number of laboratories have been reporting recently on immunosuppressive and inhibitory factors obtained from thymus, serum, and other tissues. These include thymus extracts [11, 30] and serum globulins from mice,[31] cows,[32] and humans.[33] The molecular and functional relationships among these various products are presently unknown. There may be a number of regulatory factors, some of them tissue-specific chalones. On the other hand, our finding that bovine thymus and serum α globulins in a partially purified form are functionally identical suggests that a number of these extracts may, in fact, contain the same moieties.

Summary

Immunosuppressive bovine α globulins of both serum and thymus origin were analyzed for *in vitro* effects upon the afferent and efferent arcs of the immune system. Although considerable variation in potency occurs between preparations, the functional identity of thymus and serum fractions is apparent. Antigenic recognition and effector capability are not altered whereas the proliferative lymphocyte response is either augmented or suppressed, depending upon the concentration of alpha globulin. A rather selective effect is noted on DNA synthesis and is followed by parallel changes in the development of effector capability, as measured by the development of alloimmune cytotoxic lymphocytes.

Acknowledgments

We thank Nikki Korkatti, Rasma Niedra, David Pollard, Chris Dammers, Ruth Kostick, and Kathy George for excellent technical assistance. The guidance and support of Dr. John P. Merrill and Dr. James F. Mowbray are much appreciated.

References

1. Kamrin, B. B. 1958. Ann. N.Y. Acad. Sci. **73:** 848.
2. Kamrin, B. B. 1959. Proc. Soc. Exp. Biol. Med. **100:** 58.
3. Mowbray, J. F. 1963. Transplantation **1:** 15.
4. Mowbray, J. F. 1963. Immunology **6:** 217.
5. Cooperband, S. R., H. Bondevik, K. Schmid & J. A. Mannick. 1968. Science **159:** 1243.
6. Riggio, R. R., G. H. Schwartz, F. G. Bull, K. H. Stenzel & A. L. Rubin. 1969. Transplantation **8:** 689.
7. Carpenter, C. B., A. W. Boylston, II & J. P. Merrill. 1971. Cell. Immunol. **2:** 425.
8. Kiger, N., I. Florentin & G. Mathe. 1973. Nat. Cancer Inst. Monograph **38:** 91.
9. Kiger, N., I. Florentin & G. Mathe. 1973. Transplantation **16:** 393.
10. Houck, J., H. Irausquin & S. Leikin. 1971. Science **173:** 1139.
11. Trainin, N., C. Carnaud & D. Ilfeld. 1973. Nature New Biol. **245:** 253.
12. Moorhead, J. F., E. Paraskova-Tchernozenska, A. J. Pirrie & C. Hayes. 1969. Nature **224:** 1207.
13. Carpenter, C. B., S. M. Phillips & J. P. Merrill. 1971. Cell. Immunol. **2:** 435.
14. Phillips, S. M., C. B. Carpenter & J. P. Merrill. 1972. Cell. Immunol. **5:** 235.
15. Phillips, S. M., C. B. Carpenter & J. P. Merrill. 1972. Cell. Immunol. **5:** 249.
16. Phillips, S. M., C. B. Carpenter & T. B. Strom. 1973. Transplant. Proceed. **5:** 1669.
17. Wybran, J., S. Chantler & H. H. Fudenberg. 1973. Lancet **1:** 126.
18. Carpenter, C. B. 1971. *In* Proc. 4th Leukocyte Culture Conf. O. R. McIntrye, Ed. : 317. Appleton Century Crofts. New York, N.Y.
19. Carpenter, C. B., S. M. Phillips, A. W. Boylston II & J. P. Merrill. 1971. Transplant. Proc. **3:** 929.

20. Mowbray, J. F. & D. C. Hargrave. 1966. Immunology **11:** 413.
21. Boylston, A. W. II, J. F. Mowbray & J. R. W. Ackermann. 1968. *In* Advance in Transplantation. J. Dausset, J. Hamburger & G. Mathe, Eds. : 189. Munksgaard. Copenhagen, Denmark.
22. Milton, J. D. 1971. Immunology **20:** 205.
23. Fishman, M. & F. L. Adler. 1973. Cell Immunol. **8:** 221.
24. Gottlieb, A. A., L. G. Foster, S. R. Waldman & M. Lopez. *In* Lymphocyte Recognition and Effector Mechanisms. K. Lindahl-Kiessling & D. Osoba, Eds. : 191. Academic Press, New York, N.Y.
25. Cooperband, S. R., A. M. Badger, R. C. Davis, K. Schmid & J. A. Mannick. 1972. J. Immunol. **109:** 154.
26. Cooperband, S. R., R. C. Davis, K. Schmid & J. A. Mannick. 1969. Transplant. Proc. **1:** 516.
27. Glasgow, A. H., J. P. Menzoian, S. R. Cooperband, R. B. Nimberg, K. Schmid & J. A. Mannick. 1973. J. Immunol. **111:** 272.
28. Occhino, J. C., A. H. Glasgow, S. R. Cooperband, J. A. Mannick & K. Schmid. 1973. J. Immunol. **110:** 685.
29. Glasgow, A. J., S. R. Cooperband & J. A. Mannick. 1972. Fed. Proc. **31:** 3314.
30. Goldstein, G. 1974. Nature **247:** 11.
31. Veit, B. & J. G. Michael. 1973. J. Immunol. **111:** 341.
32. Karpas, A. B. & D. Segre. 1973. Proc. Soc. Exp. Biol. Med. **144:** 141.
33. Nelken, D. 1973. J. Immunol. **110:** 1161.

ACTIVATION OF IMMUNE COMPETENCE BY THYMUS FACTORS *

Amiela Globerson, Tehila Umiel, and David Friedman

Department of Cell Biology
The Weizmann Institute of Science
Rehovot, Israel

The significance of the thymus for proper development of the immune system has become quite unequivocal.[1] However, the increasing volume of information on the occurrence of various lymphoid cell populations with distinct immunological functions, i.e., the thymus-processed T-cells, cells not processed by the thymus, B-cells, and their subclasses—T1, T2 [2] and B1, B2 [3]—raises the question of what cells are the targets of thymus activity. It has been suggested that development of T1 cells is more dependent on thymus factors than that of T2 cells.[3] On the other hand, it has been reported that development of the capacity to produce a graft-versus-host (GvH) response, which is considered to involve both T1 and T2 cells,[4] is under certain conditions not thymus-dependent, but rather thymus-influenced.[5, 6] Thus, the question whether functional expression of cells inducing a GvH response generally requires activation by thymus factors remains unresolved. In addition, it has not yet been critically established what controls differentiation of B-cell populations that are not processed by the thymus, and whether any of the early phases of their development during ontogeny is triggered by thymus factors. Furthermore, the various lymphoid populations are characterized by their distinct patterns of circulation.[7] Hence, it seems important to find out whether this cell traffic plays any determining role in dictating differentiation or whether development of the cells is predetermined before circulation.

Ideally, a critical analysis of these questions should be performed *in vitro,* to enable examination of the various cell populations under controlled conditions. We have therefore attempted to find out whether establishment of immunocompetence of both T- and B-cells depends on thymus factors. We employed organ culture techniques permitting differentiation of lymphoid cells [8, 9] for eliciting a GvH response,[10] and for the production of antibodies.[11, 12] Analysis of ontogenic development of B-cells was performed in mouse embryonic liver, using antigens capable of induction of T-independent responses.[13] We found that the capacity to elicit the splenomegaly component of a GvH response is in general conferred by thymus factors (THF) prepared according to Trainin and Small.[14] In contrast, development of B-cell activity as expressed in antibody production seems to require factors other than, or additional to THF.

* This work was supported by a grant from the Talisman Foundation, Inc., New York, N.Y.

Materials and Methods

Mice

C57BL/6, (BALB/c × C57BL/6)F_1 and (C3H/eb × C57BL/6)F_1 mice were used throughout this study. Experiments on aging were performed on (C3H/eb × C57BL)F_1 male mice.

Thymectomy

Thymectomy was performed on 6–8 week old mice under nembutal anesthesia. Thymuses were removed by suction.

Irradiation

Mice were exposed to total body irradiation from a ^{60}Co source (gamma beam 150 A, Atomic Energy of Canada, Ottawa), R/min, focal skin distance 34 inches.

Preparation of Thymus Extracts (THF)

Partially purified calf thymus extract was used as previously described.[14] For *in vitro* treatment, 0.2 mg/ml culture medium was added for the entire period of culture.[15]

Preparation of Cell Suspensions

Cell suspensions of embryonic or newborn mouse livers, and bone marrow and spleen from 6–8 week-old mice were prepared as previously described.[16]

In Vitro *Assay of GvH Reaction*

The method of Auerbach and Globerson [10] was employed. An inoculum of 10^6 test or control cells was added to the explants of newborn mouse spleen, unless otherwise specified. Cultures were considered reactive when the index of splenomegaly obtained after 4 days was $\geqslant 1.2$.[15]

In Vitro *Induction of a Response to α-dinitrophenyl-poly-L-lysine (DNP-PLL)*

We used the technique of Segal *et al.*[12] with the modification of Bernstein and Globerson.[17] Medium samples were pooled from 5 cultures of the same experimental treatment at 2-day intervals and diluted 1:10 before assay of antibodies. Antibodies were assayed by the technique of inactivation of the chemically modified bacteriophage DNP-T4, as previously described.[12, 18] In some cases medium samples were treated with 2-mercaptoethanol (2-ME) at a final concentration of 0.2 M for 30 min at room temperature, and subsequently assayed for inactivation of DNP-T4 bacteriophage.[12]

In Vivo *Immunization and Antibody Assay*

Polyvinyl pyrrolidone (PvP), K_{90} (molecular weight 360,000, Fluka, Switzerland) was dissolved in phosphate buffered saline (PBS), pH 7.4, and injected intravenously at a concentration of 0.25 γ/mouse. The number of direct plaque forming cells (PFC) in response to PvP was determined 7 days later, using sheep red blood cells (SRBC) coated with PvP.[13] The technique for assay of PFC was according to Jerne.[19]

Experimental

In the first series of experiments we tested whether thymus extracts in general affect the development of the ability to induce a GvH response. We

Table 1

GvH Response by Irradiated Spleens Treated *in Vitro* with Thymus Extract

Treatment to Spleen Donor	Extract	Incidence of Reactive Cultures *	% Reactive Cultures
550 R	thymus	3/6, 1/4, 0/4, 4/10, 2/7	32
550 R	spleen	0/4, 0/4, 0/4, 0/10, 0/9	0
550 R	—	0/6, 0/4, 0/4, 0/10, 0/9	0
Unirradiated control	—	3/6, 4/4, 2/4, 6/10, 3/6	60

* The figures represent results of 5 independent experiments.

studied a variety of conditions in which this response is either impaired or undeveloped. It has been previously demonstrated that spleens of x-irradiated mice could be activated upon culturing with thymus tissue across a Millipore filter barrier.[20] Furthermore, spleens of neonatally thymectomized mice acquired reactivity following incubation with THF.[15] We therefore wished to test whether spleens of x-irradiated mice can trigger a GvH response after *in vitro* treatment with THF. Spleens of C57BL mice were removed 24 hours after total body irradiation (550 R). Cell suspensions were made and added at a dose of 5×10^5 cells to explants of newborn (C3H $\times$ C57BL)F_1 spleens. One group of cultures was incubated with THF, whereas the other was left without any further treatment. Splenomegaly reaction was measured on days 3 and 4. As shown in Table 1, a positive GvH response was recorded in 32% of the THF-treated cultures, whereas cultures treated with spleen extracts as well as the untreated cultures did not react.

The second system involving impaired ability to produce a GvH response concerned aged mice. Since it has been demonstrated that the capacity to produce a GvH response declines with age,[21] and if reactivity of the cells

TABLE 2

In Vitro GvH RESPONSE INDUCED BY SPLEEN CELLS OF AGED MICE

Age (months)	Total Number of Cultures	Spleen Index (mean)	% Positive Cultures
2–3	32	1.36	79
12–15	12	1.28	58
23–26	8	1.06	25
32–33	16	1.05	18

depends on THF, then the decline in response may be related to insufficient thymus factor during aging. We therefore decided to investigate whether spleens of aged mice can be activated by THF. We first tested whether the failure to produce a GvH response by spleens of aged mice can be demonstrated *in vitro*. Spleens were removed from mice at ages 12–14, 23–26, and 32–34 months. Spleens of 2–3 month-old mice were assayed in parallel as controls. As indicated in TABLE 2, reactivity was remarkably lower in the 23–26 and 32–34 month group, as compared to the young mice. The next step was to determine whether THF exerts any effect on this system. Indeed, following treatment with THF, the percent of positive cultures, as well as spleen indices were significantly higher than those obtained in the untreated controls (TABLE 3). It could be argued that the THF causes replication of mature cells, thus increasing the number of reactive cells. If this explanation is correct, it is expected that activity of spleens of the young mice is also enhanced by THF. However, no overt effect of THF on young mice was observed (TABLE 3). It therefore appears that THF causes differentiation of cells that failed to mature, probably because of impaired thymus function. The failure to restore *in vivo* immune reactivity of aged mice by thymus grafts[22, 23] may be attributed to retarded hormonal activity of the grafts subjected to control mechanisms within the aged recipient.

Our next objective was to find out whether differentiation of immunocompetent cells during ontogeny follows the same pattern as described in this study for reactivation following x-irradiation and aging. We focused our attention on the development of immune reactive cells in the embryonic liver. It has been demonstrated that precursors of cells with properties of B populations

TABLE 3

In Vitro EFFECT OF THF ON INDUCTION OF A GvH RESPONSE BY SPLEEN CELLS OF AGED MICE

Age (months)	Treatment	Number of Cultures Assayed	Spleen Index (mean)	% Positive Cultures
23–26	THF	25	1.32 *	62
	none	25	1.03 *	17
2–3	THF	25	1.48	75
	none	25	1.49	79

* Highly significant difference ($p < 0.001$).

can be detected in the 18-day embryonic liver,[24] or in the newborn.[25] To ensure that the livers contain cells with the potential to produce antibodies, we first transferred embryonic (18-day or newborn) liver cells into thymectomized, total body irradiated (750 R) recipients. Two days after irradiation the mice were injected with PvP and their response was assayed 6 days later. As shown in FIGURE 1, there was no demonstrable response to PvP in the experimental group of the liver chimeras. To ascertain that cells capable of antibody production can manifest a response under such conditions, we treated thymectomized, irradiated mice with adult spleen cells. These mice did express a response to PvP, as reflected in the number of PFC obtained (FIGURE 1). We then repeated this experiment but waited 2 weeks after irradiation before immunization with PvP. Spleens of the liver chimeras (FIGURE 2, group A) did manifest a significant response to PvP, as did the bone marrow treated group (B) and the controls receiving spleen cells. These results suggest that the embryonic livers contain progenitors of B-cell populations. Yet, they do not rule out the possibility that precursors of T-helper cells may also derive from this tissue. Hence, we repeated the experiment, employing a T-cell dependent antigen, SRBC, to find out whether the liver tissue contains all the cell types required for this response. Thymectomized, irradiated adult (BALB/c $\times$ C57BL)F_1 mice were treated with liver cells of newborn mice and divided into 3 groups; the first did not receive any additional treatment, the second group received thymus cells, and the third was given THF. All mice were injected with SRBC. As shown

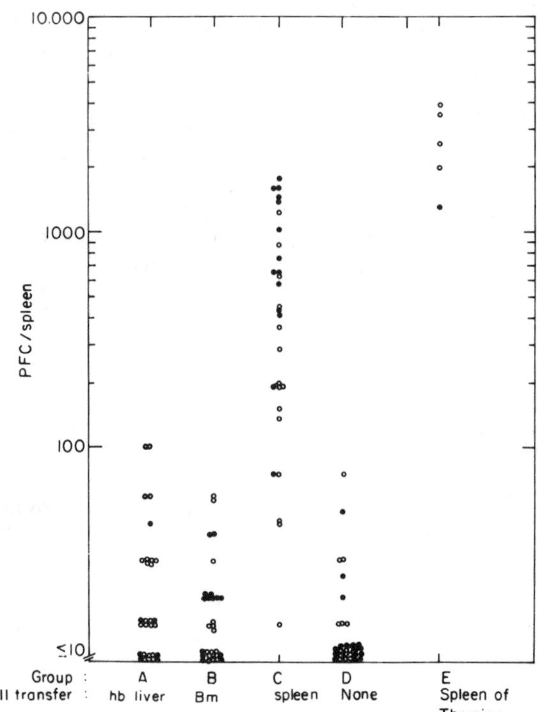

FIGURE 1. *In vivo* response to PvP by thymectomized, irradiated mice repopulated with newborn liver cells 2 days before immunization. Circles (● and ○) represent results of individual spleens in two unrelated experiments.

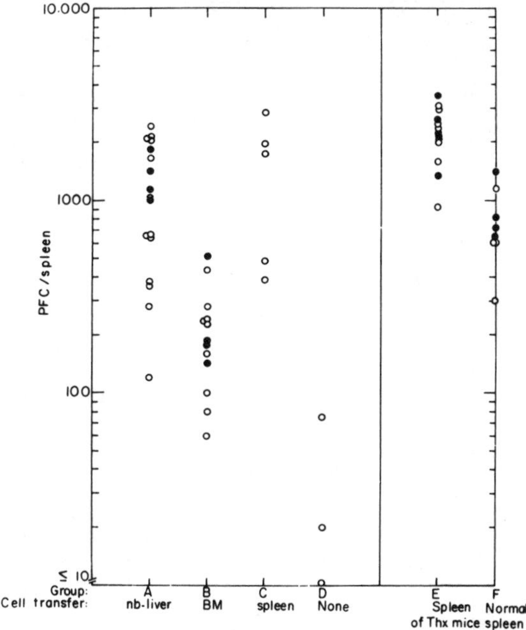

FIGURE 2. *In vivo* response to PvP by thymectomized, irradiated mice repopulated with newborn liver cells 2 weeks before immunization. Circles (○ and ●) represent results of individual spleens in 2 unrelated experiments.

in FIGURE 3, only the group receiving both liver and thymus cells produced a significant level of response to SRBC. The fact that neither the group treated with liver only, nor the group treated with liver and THF reacted to SRBC indicates that the liver does not contain any mature T-helper cells, nor precursors of T-cells which can be activated by THF.[26]

Since B antibody producing cells of liver origin can develop in the spleen of the irradiated recipients we wished to determine the minimal requirements for this differentiation. It has been demonstrated before that the capacity to induce a GvH response can be activated in embryonic livers by *in vitro* treatment with thymus tissue.[27] Furthermore, under certain conditions it appeared that this property could be expressed within the spleens of thymectomized, irradiated hosts, without any overt treatment with THF.[6] Hence, we decided to test whether spleens of x-irradiated mice might have any effect on the establishment of immune reactivity in these two systems.

Livers of 17- and 19-day old C57BL embryos were explanted and cultured either with fragments of irradiated spleens or singly isolated. Each of these groups was further divided into two, one receiving THF in the medium and the other without THF. One set of such cultures was treated with DNP-PLL, which can induce a T-independent response,[16, 28] to assay production of antibodies to the DNP haptenic determinant. Another set of cultures was sacrificed two days later, cell suspensions were made and their ability to initiate a GvH response *in vitro* was tested. TABLE 4 summarizes the results obtained in both types of immune responses. A GvH response was elicited by cultures treated with THF, in either the presence or the absence of irradiated spleen explants. Hence, THF seems to determine the establishment of this reactivity. On the

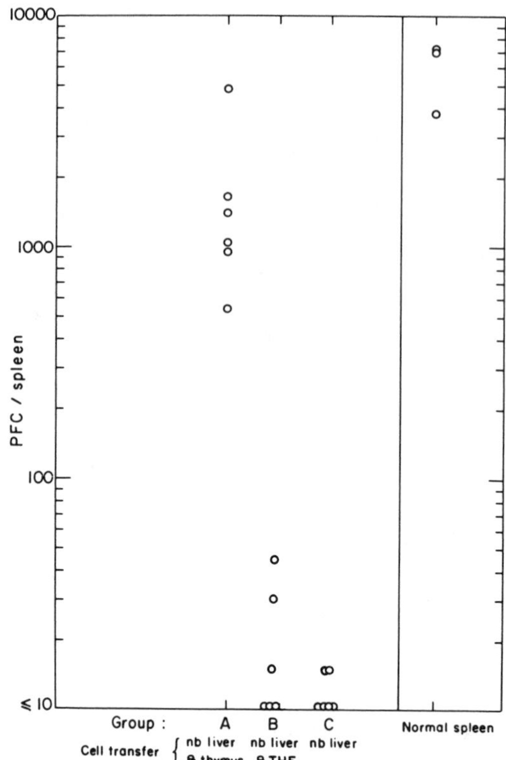

FIGURE 3. *In vivo* response to SRBC by thymectomized, irradiated mice repopulated with newborn liver and adult thymus cells.

TABLE 4

In Vitro EFFECTS OF THF AND IRRADIATED SPLEEN ON ESTABLISHMENT OF REACTIVITY OF EMBRYONIC LIVER CELLS IN A GvH RESPONSE AND PRODUCTION OF ANTIBODIES TO DNP-PLL

Culture Combination	Splenomegaly Index *		Incidence of Response to DNP	
	+ THF	− THF	+ THF	− THF
Liver + Irradiated spleen	1.35	1.18	3/12 †	0/5
Liver	1.25	1.05	0/25 ‡	0/25
Irradiated spleen	1.00	1.08	0/5	0/5
Normal adult spleen	N.T. §	1.78	4/5	4/5

* The figures represent mean values calculated from the results of 5 cultures in each group.

† Levels of response obtained: 61, 70 and 71% inactivation of DNP-T4 by medium samples pooled from 5 cultures and diluted 1:10.

‡ These are cumulative results from cultures of 17, 18 and 19 day embryos and newborn livers.

§ N.T. = not tested.

other hand, the spleen environment is not an essential requirement, although it may augment the response.

In contrast, reactivity to DNP-PLL did not manifest following treatment with THF (TABLE 4). Three out of 12 cultures exposed to both THF and irradiated spleen did produce antibodies. Although this appears to be a low level of response (60, 70 and 71% inactivation of DNP-T4 bacteriophage), it indicates that differentiation of antibody producing cells differs from that of cells involved in initiation of a GvH response. The antibody producing cells seem to require factors additional or alternative to THF. The spleen environment may be critical for this process.

DISCUSSION

The results obtained in this study suggest that activation of cells which elicit a GvH response can be triggered by THF, whereas a similar treatment has no effect on reactivity of cells producing antibodies. It has been previously demonstrated that the function of cells cooperating with B-cells in antibody production to SRBC is enhanced by THF.[26] Hence, B cells seem to have a different pattern of development, requiring alternative or additional factors, i.e., spleen microenvironment or factors emitted from T-cells.[29] These mechanisms, however, are related to later stages of B-cell maturation. The question of whether or not the early ontogenic establishment of B-cell populations depends on thymus factors remained unanswered. The fact that thymusless, nude mice can mount a B-cell response [30] could be considered as evidence that B-cells differentiate in the absence of the thymus. Yet, the possible effects of the mother's thymus factors cannot be ruled out. In fact, a reverse situation, namely, effects of the fetus' thymus on the thymectomized mother have been reported in the past.[31] Our findings indicate that even the early establishment of B populations is not obligatorily a THF-dependent process.

What is the mechanism by which THF confers activity on cells producing a GvH response? It has been previously reported that this effect manifests after incubation of the target cells with THF even for one hour only. In all probability, this would rule out dependency on immediate cell replication, since the replication cycle of lymphoid cells is 8–9 hours.[32] It thus offers a rapid inductive effect resulting in the expression of immune competence, possibly via changes in membrane properties. Which cells are the targets for this effect? It has been suggested that these are immature T1 cells.[33] Alternatively, this process may be based on blocking of cells which manifest suppressor functions. The possible existence in the embryonic liver cell population of cells interfering with establishment of a GvH response was indicated in recent experiments.[34] It was found that x-irradiated F_1 hybrid mice that were repopulated with parental strain embryonic liver did not manifest a GvH response when subsequently treated with normal adult spleen cells of the same strain as the liver donor. Hence, the adult spleen cells were inhibited within the liver radiation chimera from eliciting a GvH response. This possibility conforms with the finding that cells of 9-day old yolk sac can induce a GvH response,[35] whereas at subsequent stages of development the embryonic liver is unable to react unless activated by the thymus (see Umiel *et al.*[27] and the present study). The hypothesis that the embryonic liver contains cells which prevent the expression of the GvH producing cells could well explain this phenomenon.

If this possibility is correct, then both B- and T-cell populations may exhibit similar patterns of differentiation, yet final expression of T-cell functions may be determined by neutralizing the suppressing elements. Accordingly, THF may have a regulatory role in the functional expression of immune reactive cells.

Acknowledgments

We wish to thank Ms. Loya Abel, Ms. Ruth Goldman, Mr. N. Koller, and Mr. S. Leib for skillful technical assistance. The experiments on aging were performed by Miss Varda Kaiser as part of a research project for her Matriculation Certificate.

References

1. Miller, J. F. A. P. & D. Osoba. 1967. Current concepts of the immunological function of the thymus. Physiol. Rev. **47:** 437–520.
2. Raff, M. C. 1971. Surface antigenic markers for distinguishing T- and B-lymphocytes in mice. Transplant. Rev. **6:** 52–80.
3. Playfair, J. H. L. & E. C. Purves. 1971. Separate thymus-dependent and thymus-independent antibody forming cell precursors. Nature New Biol. **231:** 149–151.
4. Cantor, H. & R. Asofsky. 1972. Synergy among lymphoid cells mediating the graft-versus-host response. III. Evidence for interaction between two types of thymus-derived cells. J. Exp. Med. **135:** 764–779.
5. Cooper, M. D., R. D. A. Peterson, M. A. South & R. A. Good. 1966. The function of the thymus system and the bursa system in the chicken. J. Exp. Med. **123:** 75–102.
6. Umiel, T. 1971. Thymus influenced maturation of embryonic liver cells. Transplantation **11:** 531–535.
7. Harris, J. E., C. E. Ford, D. W. H. Barnes & E. P. Evans. 1964. Cellular traffic of the thymus: experiments with chromosome markers; evidence from parabiosis for an afferent stream of cells. Nature **201:** 886–887.
8. Auerbach, R. 1965. Experimental analysis of lymphoid differentiation in the mammalian thymus and spleen. *In* Organogenesis. R. DeHaan & H. Ursprung, Eds. : 539–557. Holt, Rinehart & Winston. New York, N.Y.
9. Globerson, A. 1965. *In vitro* studies on radiation lymphoid recovery of mouse spleen. J. Exp. Med. **123:** 25–32.
10. Auerbach, R. & A. Globerson. 1966. *In vitro* induction of the graft-versus-host reaction. Exp. Cell Res. **42:** 31–41.
11. Globerson, A. & R. Auerbach. 1966. Primary antibody resopnse in organ cultures. J. Exp. Med. **124:** 1001–1016.
12. Segal, S., A. Globerson, M. Feldman, J. Haimovich & M. Sela. 1970. *In vitro* induction of a primary response to the dinitrophenyl determinant. J. Exp. Med. **131:** 93–99.
13. Andersson, B. & H. Blomgren. 1971. Evidence for thymus-independent humoral antibody production in mice against polyvinyl pyrrolidone and *E. coli* lipopolysaccharide. Cell. Immunol. **2:** 411–424.
14. Trainin, N. & M. Small. 1970. Studies on some physicochemical properties of a thymus humoral factor conferring immunocompetence on lymphoid cells. J. Exp. Med. **132:** 885–897.
15. Trainin, N., M. Small & A. Globerson. 1969. Immunocompetence of spleen

cells from neonatally thymectomized mice conferred *in vitro* by a syngeneic thymus extract. J. Exp. Med. **130:** 765–775.
16. Umiel, T. & A. Globerson. 1974. Analysis of lymphoid cell types developing in mouse fetal liver. Differentiation **2:** 169–177.
17. Bernstein, A. & A. Globerson. 1974. Short pulses of antigen induce *in vitro* an antibody response to haptenic determinants. Cell. Immunol. **10:** 173–183.
18. Haimovich, J. & M. Sela. 1966. Inactivation of poly-DL-alanyl bacteriophage T4 with antisera specific toward poly-DL-alanin. J. Immunol. **97:** 338–343.
19. Jerne, N. K., A. A. Nordin & C. Hery. 1963. The agar plate technique for recognizing antibody producing cells. *In* Cell-Bound Antibodies. B. Amos & H. Koprowski, Eds. : 109–116. The Wistar Institute Press Inc. Philadelphia, Pa.
20. Globerson, A. & R. Auerbach. 1967. Reactivation *in vitro* of immunocompetence in irradiated mouse spleen. J. Exp. Med. **126:** 223–234.
21. Krohn, P. L. 1962. Heterochronic transplantation in the study of ageing. Proc. Royal Soc. B. (Biol. Sci.) **157:** 128–147.
22. Metcalf, D., R. Moulds & B. Pike. 1966. Influence of the spleen and thymus on immune responses in ageing mice. Clin. Exp. Immunol. **2:** 109–120.
23. Micklem, H. S., D. A. Ogden & A. C. Payne. 1973. Ageing, hemopoietic stem cells and immunity. *In* Ciba Found. Symp. on Hemopoietic Stem Cells. : 285–297. Elsevier, Excerpta Medica, North Holland Publishing Co. Amsterdam, Netherlands.
24. Nossal, G. J. V. & B. L. Pike. 1973. Studies on the differentiation of B-lymphocytes in the mice. Immunology **25:** 33–45.
25. Chiscon, M. O. & E. S. Golub. 1972. Functional development of the interacting cells in the immune response. I. Development of T-cell and B-cell function. J. Immunol. **108:** 1379–1386.
26. Rotter, V., A. Globerson, I. Nakamura & N. Trainin. 1973. Studies on characterization of the lymphoid target cell for reactivity of a thymus humoral factor. J. Exp. Med. **138:** 130–142.
27. Umiel, T., A. Globerson & R. Auerbach. 1968. Role of the thymus in the development of immunocompetence of embryonic liver cells *in vitro*. Proc. Soc. Exp. Biol. Med. **129:** 598–600.
28. Feldman, M. & A. Globerson. 1974. Reception of immunogenic signals by lymphocytes. Current Topics Devel. Biol. **8:** 1–40.
29. Schimple, A. & E. Wecker. Functional replacement of co-operating T-cell by a soluble factor in a humoral immune response *in vitro*. Advan. Exp. Med. Biol. **29:** 179–182.
30. Croy, B. A. & D. Osoba. 1973. Nude mice—a model system for studying the cellular basis of the humoral immune response. Cell. Immunol. **9:** 306–313.
31. Osoba, D. 1965. Immune reactivity in mice thymectomized soon after birth; normal response after pregnancy. Science **147:** 298–299.
32. Perkins, E. H., T. Sade & T. Makinodan. 1963. Recruitment and proliferation of immunocompetent cells during the log phase of the primary antibody. J. Immunol. **103:** 668–678.
33. Lonai, P., B. Mogilner, V. Rotter & N. Trainin. 1973. Studies on the effect of a thymic factor on differentiation of thymus-derived lymphocytes. Eur. J. Imunol. **3:** 22–25.
34. Umiel, T., F. Bach & R. Auerbach. 1973. Specific blocking factors prevent GvH response in fetal liver chimeras. Joint Meeting of European Immunol. Soc. Strasbourg, France. : 80.
35. Hofman, F. & A. Globerson. 1973. Graft-versus-host response induced *in vitro* by mouse yolk sac cells. Eur. J. Immunol. **3:** 179–181.

A T-CELL-PRODUCED MEDIATOR SUBSTANCE ACTIVE IN THE HUMORAL IMMUNE RESPONSE

E. Wecker, A. Schimpl, T. Hünig, and L. Kühn

Institut für Virologie der Universität Würzburg
8700 Würzburg, West Germany

This paper addresses itself to the question of T-B interaction in the *in vitro* system of humoral immune response as described by Mishell and Dutton.[1] The antigens used were heterologous blood cells, mostly SRBC. Let me briefly summarize some of the more pertinent results that have been already published.

Firstly, the *in vitro* immune response to SRBC is dependent on T-cells as shown by treatment with anti-θ serum and complement (TABLE 1).[2, 3]

Secondly, in addition to appropriate T-cells,[2, 4] 24-hour culture supernatants derived from mixtures of allogeneic mouse spleen cells also restore the *in vitro* IgM immune responses to various heterologous blood cells.[2, 5] This is possible not only in spleen cultures experimentally deprived of T-cells (TABLE 1), but also in those derived from the congenitally athymic nu/nu mouse (TABLE 2).[2, 5] Supernatants with an even higher biological activity can be obtained from normal spleen cells stimulated by Concanavalin A (TABLE 3).

Thirdly, no activity is found in supernatants of T-cell-deprived allogeneic spleen cells or T-cell-deprived cultures with Concanavalin A (TABLE 4).[5] Thus, the biologically active material is presumably a T-cell product and I shall henceforth refer to it as T-cell replacing factor or, for short, TRF.[5]

Finally, since IgG responses are particularly dependent on T-cell help, it was of crucial importance that TRF should also be able to restore an IgG response *in vitro*. This in fact was shown to be the case using a secondary *in vitro* system treated with anti-θ serum and complement (TABLE 5).[6, 7]

Some of the characteristics of TRF may be summarized as follows: (1) TRF is produced upon strong stimulation of T-cells either by histo-compatibility antigens or by T-cell mitogens, such as Concanavalin A. (2) TRF is not antigen-specific, i.e., it can restore immune responses equally well to all non-crossreacting heterologous red blood cells so far investigated as well as to TNP using a carrier system.[6, 8] (3) The biological activity of TRF does not seem to be strongly dependent on either the compatibility or incompatibility between producing T-cells and responsive B-cells, but this needs further clarification. (4) The biological activity is heat sensitive (1 hour, 60° C), destroyed by chymo-trypsin and trypsin, and partly destroyed by papain; protein is thus believed to be a decisive part of the molecule. Since the molecular weight is between 45,000 and 60,000 daltons TRF is not dializable.* We have concentrated TRF about 15-fold by ammonium sulfate precipitation and various column chromatographies.

I would now like to discuss briefly the question: at which point in the immune response does TRF exert its function? Theoretically, we may distinguish 3 steps: The first is the triggering of B-cells; the second, the prolifera-

* TRF produced in the absence of fetal calf serum shows a molecular weight of about 30,000 daltons.

TABLE 1

RECONSTITUTION OF T-CELL-DEPRIVED CULTURES BY SUPERNATANTS OF ALLOGENEIC LYMPHOCYTES

Spleen Cells	Treatment C	Anti-θ C_3H	TRF From	PFC/10^6 Day 4	PFC/10^6 Day 5
B6D 2	yes	no	—	680	2620
B6D 2	yes	yes	—	70	210
B6D 2	yes	yes	(DBA/2×C57BL/6) spleen	1580	9750
B6D 2	yes	yes	(DBA/2×C57BL/6) lymph-node	610	4850
B6D 2	yes	yes	(DBA/2×C57BL/6) thymo-cytes *	360	1110

* Concentrated 5-fold.

TABLE 2

RECONSTITUTION OF B-CELL CULTURES FROM NU/NU MOUSE SPLEENS BY ALLOGENEIC SUPERNATANTS

Spleen Cells	24-Hour Supernates From	PFC/10^6 Day 4
nude	—	175
nude	CBA	145
nude	C57BL/6J	157
nude	CBA×C57BL/6J	1680

TABLE 3

STIMULATION OF TRF PRODUCTION IN SYNGENEIC MOUSE SPLEEN CULTURES BY CONCANAVALIN A

Culture	Addition Day 2	PFC/10^6 Day 5	PFC/Culture Day 5
nu/nu spleen	—	66	275
nu/nu spleen	Con A	62	225
nu/nu spleen	Sup. allogenic	1070	4000
nu/nu spleen	Sup. Con A +α MM	2950	7900

TABLE 4

REQUIREMENT OF T-CELLS FOR PRODUCTION OF TRF

Spleen Cells	24-Hour Supernates From	PFC/10^6 Day 4	PFC/10^6 Day 5
F_1 control	—	480	2050
F_1 anti-θ	—	40	216
F_1 anti-θ	A * + B *	254	1830
F_1 anti-θ	A-anti-θ + B-anti-θ	36	174

* A: DBA/2J; B: C57BL/6J.

tion of B-cells; and the third is the commencement of antibody synthesis and antibody secretion.

From the very beginning of our experiments, we had noticed that TRF restored the immune response of T-cell-deprived cultures preferentially, indeed almost exclusively, if added at least one day after the onset of the culture and the addition of the antigen.[5, 8] Optimal results are routinely obtained when TRF is added on day 2 of a 5-day culture (FIGURE 1). This strongly suggests that TRF is not instrumental in the most early events, such as B-cell triggering.

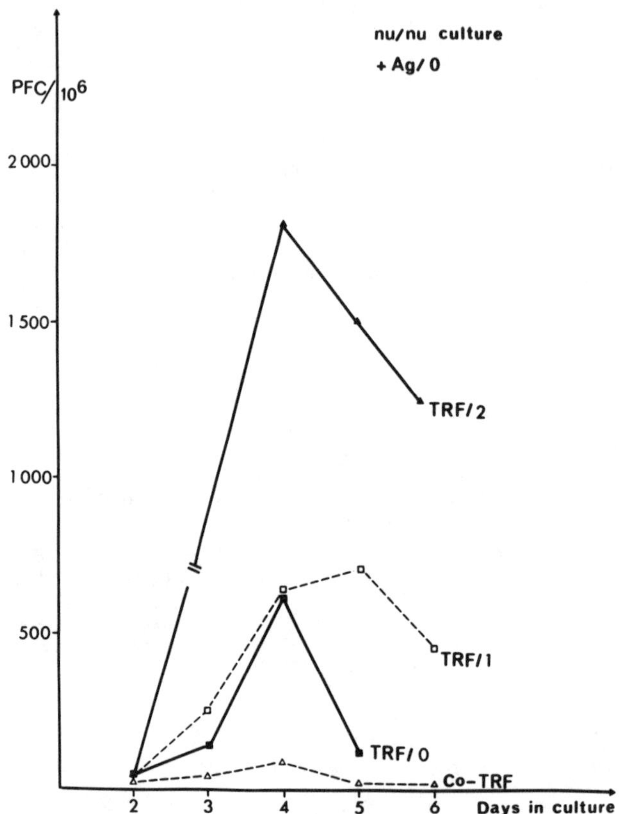

FIGURE 1. Reconstitution of B-cell cultures by TRF depending on time of addition.

In subsequent experiments, TRF was shown not to be a general B-cell mitogen on the following grounds:[8, 9] (1) TRF does not increase the thymidine incorporation of B-cell cultures; and (2) TRF does not increase the number of background plaques in the absence of the test antigens.

There remained, of course, the possibility that TRF acted as a specific mitogen which exclusively expands those B-cells that have reacted with their particular antigens.

In order to investigate this, we employed an autoradiographic technique.

TABLE 5

RECONSTITUTION BY TRF OF IGG PLAQUE RESPONSE IN T-CELL-DEPRIVED SECONDARY SPLEEN CULTURES

Spleen Cultures: 9 Days Primed *in Vivo*	Additions	PFC/10^6 Day 4 IgM	IgG
Control	—	10 500 (90)*	7 150 (350)*
Anti-θ GPS	—	140	120
Anti-θ GPS	Sup. A	150	170
Anti-θ GPS	Sup. A+B	3 220	3 050

* Figures in parenthesis: PFC/10^6 on day 0 of culture.

B-cell cultures were set up in the presence of antigen and received pulses of radioactive thymidine at various times during the ensuing days. All the pulses were terminated by a chase lasting to the end of the culture period. Hemolytic plaques were then developed, stained and autoradiographed. From the grains within each plaque center cell, it could be determined whether or not this particular cell had synthesized DNA and thus divided during the period when the label was available.[9]

It can be seen from FIGURE 2 that cells which later on become antibody

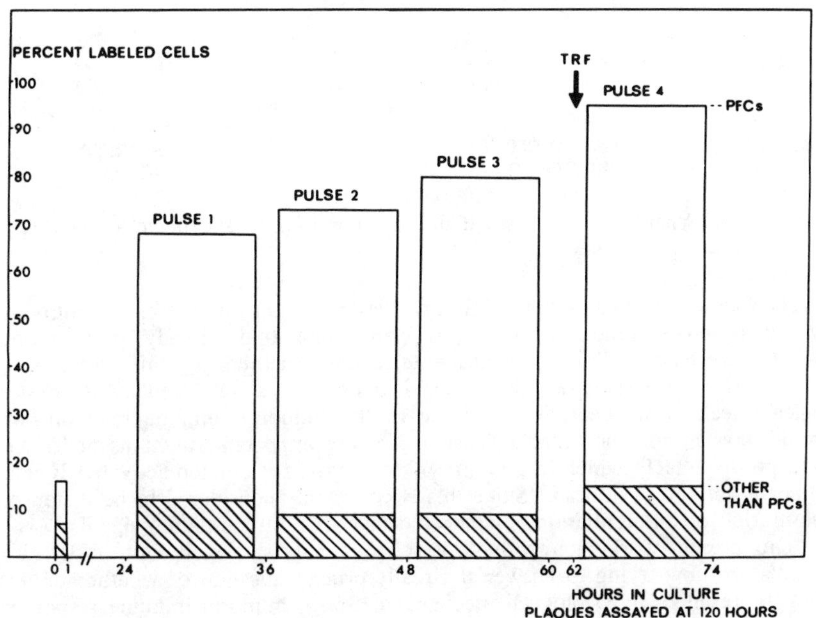

FIGURE 2. Autoradiographic evaluation of the proliferation of antigen-stimulated B-cells before and after TRF addition.

producing cells divide as early as 24 hours after the beginning of the culture, which is exactly what Dutton found using his elegant hot-pulse technique. The plaque precursor cells continue to divide throughout the culture period. The result most pertinent to our discussion is, however, that the cells divided in the absence of T-cells or TRF, respectively, triggered only by the blood cell antigens. Moreover, the rate of thymidine incorporation did not change significantly after the addition of TRF. Therefore, TRF did not noticeably influence the proliferation of the antigen-reactive cells, but, as pointed out before, it is essential for antibody production. Essentially the same results are obtained if FCS is omitted from the culture during the first 48 hours of incubation and only added together with TRF. Also, treatment of nude spleen cells with anti-θ serum and complement makes no difference.

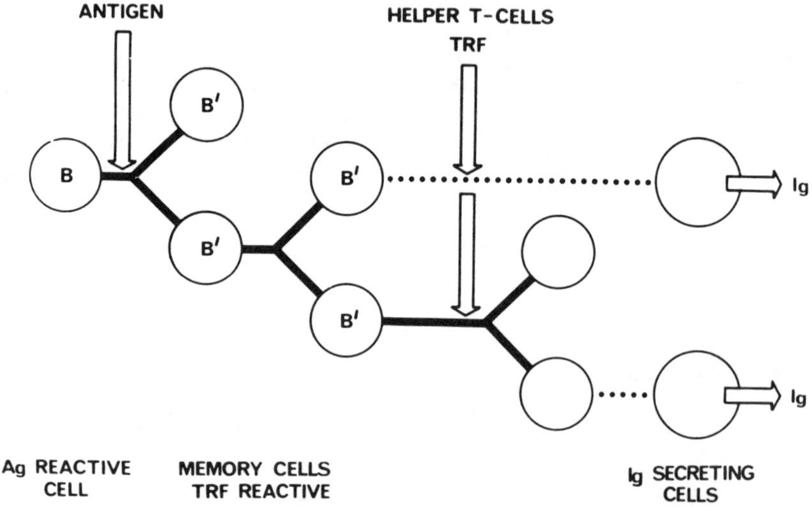

FIGURE 3. Scheme of the suggested site of action of TRF and/or helper T-cells.

This indeed indicates that TRF provides the signal that initiates antibody synthesis and secretion in antigen-triggered and thus already proliferating B-cells. We have additional experimental evidence supporting this notion.

If TRF, as investigated in this *in vitro* immune system, reflects a physiological mechanism generally occurring in the humoral immune reaction, we would have to conclude that at least one of the important functions of T-cells is to produce TRF, which in turn provides a signal for antigen-activated B-cells to begin antibody synthesis. Since this is commonly considered to be a step of maturation or differentiation, TRF would give this differentiation signal.

Our present working hypothesis is schematically shown in FIGURE 3.

We are now trying to answer the really crucial question of whether or not TRF represents a physiological mechanism. If so, humoral immune responses *in vivo* may be manipulated either positively or negatively by the administration of purified TRF or of an anti-TRF antibody.

References

1. MISHELL, R. J. & R. W. DUTTON. 1967. J. Exp. Med. **126:** 423.
2. SCHIMPL, A. & E. WECKER. 1971. 3. Tagung der Gesellschaft für Immunologie. Marburg, W. Germany.
3. SCHIMPL, A. & E. WECKER. 1970. Nature **226:** 1258.
4. SCHIMPL, A. & E. WECKER. 1971. Eur. J. Immunol. **1:** 304.
5. SCHIMPL, A. & E. WECKER. 1972. Nature New Biol. **237:** 15.
6. SCHIMPL, A. & E. WECKER. 1973. *In* Microenvironmental Aspects of Immunity. **:** 179. B. D. Jankovic, Ed. Plenum Press, Inc. New York, N.Y.
7. SCHIMPL, A. & E. WECKER. 1973. J. Exp. Med. **137:** 547.
8. ASKONAS, B. A., A. SCHIMPL & E. WECKER. 1974. Eur. J. Immunol. **4:** 164.
9. HÜNIG, TH., A. SCHIMPL & E. WECKER. 1974. J. Exp. Med. **139:** 754.

STIMULATION OF B-IMMUNOCYTES BY A T-CELL FACTOR PRODUCED IN MIXED LEUKOCYTE CULTURES *

Herman Friedman

Department of Microbiology
Albert Einstein Medical Center
Philadelphia, Pennsylvania 19141

Thymus derived "T" lymphocytes may serve as a "helper" for bone marrow derived "B" cells during the production of humoral antibody.[1–8] Synergism can be readily demonstrated between T- and B-lymphocytes during the antibody response to certain antigens, including sheep erythrocytes, hapten-carrier complexes and serum proteins. A number of different mechanisms have been proposed to explain how T-cells interact with B-lymphocytes during a specific antibody response. One explanation, based on both *in vivo* and *in vitro* studies, postulates that T-cells react, by means of a specific surface receptor, with an antigenic determinant and thus "focus" the antigen for subsequent interaction with another antigen receptor present on the surface of B-cells.[9, 10] Thus the T-cells are brought into close contact with the appropriate B-cell by means of a specific antigen "bridge." In this model, the interaction between T-cells and the immunogen increases the efficacy of antigen binding to the B-cell, producing an appropriate signal for the necessary differentiation and clonal proliferation of immunocytes.

The above hypothesis suggests that antigenic concentration by T-cells is important for triggering the activation of B-cells. However, it is also possible that factors elaborated by an antigen-reactive T-cell may indirectly affect potential antibody producing B-lymphocytes. In support of this, B-cells have on their surface distinct immunoglobulin (Ig) receptors that can interact directly with antigen, either in free-form or bound to other cells, including both T-cells and macrophages.[11–14] Nevertheless, the signal necessary for the activation and proliferation of specifically triggered B-cells after Ig receptors bind antigen is not understood. In this regard, recent studies from this and other laboratories concerning antibody formation to various antigens, including sheep erythrocytes, bacterial lipopolysaccharides (LPS) and proteins, have supported the view that T-cells may affect B-cells by means of a cell-free "factor(s)." For example, repopulation studies *in vivo* using a mixture of allogeneic lymphoid cells, as well as mixed lymphocytes cultures *in vitro* with allogeneic cells, have recently suggested that interaction of T-lymphocytes from histoincompatible individuals may enhance the immune response by B-lymphocytes.[13, 15–17]

Studies in this laboratory with mixed leukocyte cultures showed that *in vitro* antibody responses to sheep erythrocytes could be markedly affected by the interaction of T-lymphocytes *in vitro*. A supernatant factor produced in these mixed leukocyte cultures was responsible for the enhanced antibody responses to sheep erythrocytes by indicator spleen cells in culture.[18, 19] These experi-

* Supported in part by research grants from the United States National Science Foundation and the National Institute of Allergy and Infectious Diseases.

ments were based on earlier studies in which a mixed leukocyte reaction was utilized to detect cellular interactions by means of suppressed antibody responses.[20] For those studies, one strain of mice, considered the "target," was immunized with sheep erythrocytes; at the height of the expected antibody response, spleen cells from these "target" mice were cultured *in vitro* with splenocytes from another mouse strain, considered the "killer," which was sensitized by skin graft or injection of spleen homogenates from the target strain. The interaction between the target antibody-producing cells *in vitro* and the killer splenocytes resulted in a rapid reduction in the number of antibody forming cells in the culture chambers.[20] For example, when the target antibody forming cells are incubated *in vitro* either alone or with spleen cells from syngeneic mice, no significant reduction in the number of antibody-forming cells occurred as compared to the number of hemolysin-forming immunocytes in cultures without added spleen cells. However, when the target antibody-forming cells were incubated with splenocytes from allogeneic mice differing at the H2 locus there was a much more rapid decrease in the number of antibody forming cells. This reduction was most notable when the killer splenocytes were derived from mice specifically sensitized to the target mouse strain. The decrease in antibody-forming cells first became apparent within 4 to 6 hours after culture initiation, and by 24 to 48 hours after incubation the number of antibody-forming cells was markedly depressed as compared to control cultures.

These results indicated that incubation of antibody-forming cells with allogeneic spleen cells *in vitro,* even when the donor animals were not specifically sensitized, could result in a specific immunologic depression. Thus it seemed plausible that a similar immunocyte suppression might occur in an indirect manner when spleen cells from two histoincompatible mouse strains were incubated together with splenocytes from a third mouse strain immunized with sheep erythrocytes as an "indifferent" target. Thus, experiments were undertaken to determine whether a mixed leukocyte reaction between splenocytes from two strains of mice could affect the antibody response *in vitro* to sheep erythrocytes by a third mouse strain. Unexpectedly, a marked enhancement of the number of immunocytes was observed, rather than a depression. Such enhancement occurred when the mixed cultures contained splenocytes from mice differing at the H2 locus, regardless of the source of target spleen cells immunized with sheep erythrocytes. Further examination showed that supernatants from the mixed leukocyte reactions could markedly enhance the response by lymphocytes from RBC immunized donor mice and that the responding cells were B-lymphocytes. The supernatant factor was due to the interaction between allogeneic T-lymphocytes, since inactivation of the reacting cells by anti-θ serum abolished the reaction.

General Experimental Methods and Procedures

For these studies, a mixed leukocyte culture reaction was utilized. Spleen cells were obtained from several inbred mouse strains. The mice were purchased from Jackson Memorial Laboratories, Bar Harbor, Maine, or Huntingdon Farms, Conshohocken, Pa. The strains used included C57Bl, C3H, AKR, and Balb/c mice. All mice were 6 to 8 weeks of age at the start of an experiment and weighed approximately 18 to 20 grams each. For the mixed leukocyte reaction, mice were killed by cervical dislocation and their spleen obtained at autopsy; dispersed cell suspensions were prepared by the standard method of "teasing" with a sterile needle and forceps into cold sterile Hanks' solution. The cell suspensions were clarified and debris removed by passage through sterile gauze and several washes in the cold with sterile Hanks' solution. The resulting single cell suspensions were resuspended to a concentration of 10^7 viable nucleated splenocytes per ml using medium 199 containing 10% sterile fetal calf serum or isologous mouse serum. Individual cultures contained 5×10^6 spleen cells from each mouse source in 2.0 ml tissue culture medium. The culture tubes were incubated at 37° C in an atmosphere of 5% CO_2, 95% air in a roller apparatus.

The indicator antibody plaque-forming cells (PFC) consisted of spleen cells from donor mice immunized with 4×10^8 sheep erythrocytes 4 days before culture initiation. The splenocytes were prepared exactly as for the mixed leukocyte reaction, and 10^7 viable cells were incubated either alone or with equal numbers of spleen cells from one or both histoincompatible mouse strains in the culture tubes. To determine the effect of the mixed leukocyte reaction, samples of cells were harvested from each tube at daily intervals after culture initiation and tested for hemolytic PFCs by the agar gel procedure essentially as described initially by Jerne and Nordin.[21] In brief, 0.1 ml aliquots of the cell suspensions were added to 2.0 ml melted (42° C) Bacto agar, containing 1.0 mg DEAE-dextran and 0.1 ml of a washed suspension of 10% sheep erythrocytes. The agar-gel mixture was carefully poured onto the surface of a previously prepared base layer of 1.0% agar in 15×100 mm diameter Petri plates. When the upper layer had solidified, the plates were incubated at 37° C for one hour and then treated with approximately 5 ml guinea pig serum diluted 1:15 as a source of complement. The plates were incubated further for one hour at 37° C and the resulting zones of hemolysis were considered due to high efficiency 19S IgM PFC. The number of such PFC in 3 or more plates containing cells from a single culture were enumerated and used to calculate the number of PFC per million cells plated.

In order to test the effect of soluble products of mixed leukocyte cultures, spleen cells from two unrelated mouse strain were incubated together as for the mixed reaction, and 24 to 48 hours later the supernatants obtained by slow speed centrifugation. These supernatants were then added to the indicator PFC-forming spleen cell cultures. Control supernatants consisted of cultures of spleen cells from one mouse strain only or medium alone. In addition, the effects of various treatments on the spleen cell donors, as well as on target antibody-forming cells, were determined. For these purposes, donor mice were either thymectomized at birth, or thymectomized as adults followed by x-irradiation. In addition, other groups of donor mice were given 750 R whole-body x-irradiation 24 hours prior to sacrifice. In some experiments, the donor mice were injected i.v. either with 1.0 mg cortisone or 0.5 ml of a 1:10 dilution of polyvalent rabbit mouse antilymphocyte serum. The antisera used for this purpose were prepared by hyperimmunizing rabbits with pooled mouse thymocytes. Also, sera to murine Ig globulins were prepared after immunizing rabbits with ammonium-sulphate-precipitated and column-purified mouse Ig. Mouse anti-θ serum was obtained by immunizing AKR mice with C3H thymocytes. Anti-mouse marcophage serum was obtained by hyperimmunizing rabbits with pooled and washed mouse peritoneal exudate cells freed of nonadherent leukocytes by three cycles of absorption on glass plates. The antiserum was absorbed repeatedly with pooled mouse thymocytes and lymph node cells. *In vitro* treatment of test cell suspensions with these antisera was carried out by incubating 5×10^7 cells, either splenocytes to be used as killer cells or spleen cells from RBC-immunized mice used as target cells, for 30 to 60 minutes at 37° C with 0.1 ml of varying dilutions of the appropriate serum, plus 0.1 ml of a 1:10 dilution of sterile guinea pig serum as a source of complement.

The experimental design (FIGURE 1) consisted of using spleen cells from target mice immunized with sheep erythrocytes as the indicator of plaque formation *in vitro*. The target splenocytes were incubated in agar plates with sheep erythrocytes and the numbers of PFC appearing in these plates were

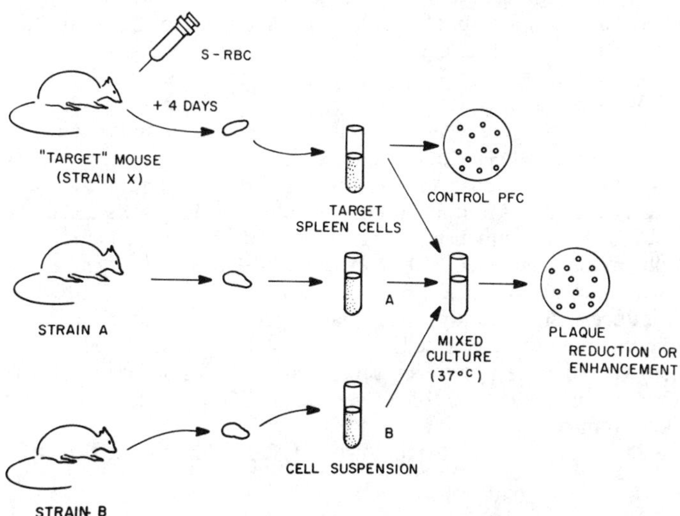

FIGURE 1. Schematic representation of the effect of mixed leukocyte cultures on hemolytic plaque formation *in vitro*. Spleen cells obtained from target mice immunized with sheep erythrocytes form PFC when incubated *in vitro*. Addition of splenocytes from normal allogeneic mice to the target spleen cells results either in antibody plaque reduction or, when mixed leukocyte cultures are prepared, in antibody plaque enhancement. Supernatants of the mixed cultures also are used for assessment of effects on antibody plaque formation by target spleen cells.

considered to be "100%." These target spleen cells were mixed with either the spleen cells from one mouse strain or with spleen cells from two strains of mice in mixed culture. After varying periods of time at 37° C, the number of PFC in the mixed cultures was determined by plating in agar gel and comparing the PFC response to that obtained in the control cultures containing target cells only. The effects of killer to target cell number, the length of incubation, and the effects of supernatants of mixed cultures on target PFC were determined in separate series of experiments. In addition, the effects of specific antisera on both target cells and mixed leukocyte cultures were assessed in terms of the PFC responses of the target cells.

Experimental Results

Incubation of spleen cells from SRBC-immunized donor mice with allogeneic splenocytes from one donor mouse strain resulted in a much more rapid plaque reduction than incubation of the cells with Medium alone or similar numbers of syngeneic splenocytes (TABLE 1). In initial experiments utilizing this model to detect an allograft reaction *in vitro* it was observed that the reduction in PFC *in vitro* was directly related to the histoincompatibility between the mouse strains used. For example, when splenocytes from A/J mice immunized with SRBC were incubated for up to 48 hours with spleen cells from normal C3H or C57Bl mice a much greater antibody plaque reduction occurred than when the same target cells were incubated with normal A/J splenocytes. The reduction in the number of PFC was directly related to the number of histoincompatible spleen cells added to the indicator culture. A ratio of 10:1 resulted in a much greater suppression of PFC than a lower ratio; however, even a 1:1 ratio resulted in a marked suppression (unpublished data). When allogeneic spleen cells were derived from mice sensitized to the target mouse strain there was an even greater plaque reduction (TABLE 1).

As shown in previous studies and confirmed in the present study, spleen cells from allogeneic mouse strains sensitized to the target mouse strain by either skin grafting or immunization with appropriate spleen cell homogenates generally resulted in a much more rapid antibody plaque reduction than spleen cells from unsensitized mice.[20] For example, the results in TABLE 1 show that splenocytes from C3H mice previously sensitized to A/J histocompatibility antigens induce a significantly faster plaque reduction, and ultimately very few PFC, as compared to spleen cells from normal C3H mice. Similarly, splenocytes from C57Bl mice previously sensitized to A/J skin grafts also induced a much more rapid reduction of target cell PFC than did splenocytes from normal C57Bl mice.

It was anticipated from the cultures of RBC-immunized target cells incu-

TABLE 1

ACCELERATED REDUCTION IN THE NUMBER OF HEMOLYTIC PFC BY SPLEEN CELLS FROM RBC-IMMUNIZED A/J MICE INCUBATED *in Vitro* WITH ALLOGENEIC SPLENOCYTES

Source of Spleen Cells Added to Cultures of A/J Splenocytes *	PFC/10^6 Spleen Cells (Time in Hours) †					
	0	3	6	12	24	48
None (controls)	515	503	431	265	123	65
A/J	538	521	503	336	186	73
C3H normal	593	465	338	150	62	15
C3H anti-A/J	520	416	260	105	21	10
C57Bl normal	518	426	319	130	35	18
C57Bl anti-A/J	546	412	295	78	30	10

* Spleen cells (5×10^6) from A/J mice immunized 4 days earlier with 4×10^8 sheep RBC cultured at 37° C *in vitro* with 5×10^6 splenocytes from indicated mouse strains; immunized mice given A/J skin grafts 2–3 weeks earlier.

† Average PFC response for 3–5 cultures at time interval indicated.

TABLE 2

ENHANCED HEMOLYTIC PFC FORMATION BY TARGET A/J SPLEEN CELLS FROM RBC-IMMUNIZED MICE CULTURED *in Vitro* WITH ALLOGENEIC SPLENOCYTES FROM TWO HISTOINCOMPATIBLE MOUSE STRAINS

Spleen Cells Added to Target A/J Cultures *	PFC/10^6 Spleen Cells (Time in Hours) † 4	12	24	48
None (controls)	596	312	140	96
A/J splenocytes (normal)	510	305	136	115
C3H splenocytes	550	215	95	31
C57Bl splenocytes	490	220	79	15
C3H plus C57Bl splenocytes	518	310	4870	7650

* Spleen cells (5×10^6) from A/J mice immunized 4 days earlier with 4×10^8 sheep RBC incubated *in vitro* with 5×10^6 spleen cells from indicated mouse strains.
† Average PFC response for 3–5 cultures at time indicated after culture initiation.

bated with splenocytes from only one mouse strain differing at the H2 locus that incubation of the same target splenocytes with spleen cells from two unrelated mouse strains would also result in a rapid PFC reduction. However, as shown in TABLE 2, a marked *enhancement* of antibody formation was observed in such cultures containing splenocytes from two different mouse strains. Incubation of spleen cells from the RBC-immunized A/J mice for a period of 24 to 48 hours *in vitro* with spleen cells from normal C3H in C57Bl mice resulted in a more marked decline in PFC numbers as compared to cultures incubated with normal A/J spleen cells. In contrast, when similar numbers of both C3H and C57Bl splenocytes were added to the cultures, there was a 10- to 15-fold enhancement in the number of PFC after the first day of culture (TABLE 2).

Supernatants of the mixed leukocyte cultures mediated the marked enhancement of PFC responsiveness in the target leukocyte cultures. Supernatants from cultures containing either syngeneic A/J splenocytes or allogeneic C3H or C57Bl splenocytes alone had no significant affect. As can be seen in TABLE 3, the target A/J spleen cells, when incubated alone, showed the usual moderate decline in PFC during the first few hours of culture, followed by the usual more rapid decrease. Incubation of these cultures with supernatants from either A/J, C3H or C57Bl spleens cultured for 24 or 48 hours alone did not result in a significant difference in the decline of antibody-forming cells. However, the supernatants of 24-hour cultures of mixed C3H and C57Bl splenocytes resulted in a marked enhancement in the number of PFC during the 24 to 48 hour culture period. As is evident in FIGURE 2, supernatants of the mixed allogeneic spleen cell cultures resulted in a relatively similar increase in the PFC response over the 24 to 48 hour period after culture initiation as compared to the direct effect of mixed leukocytes per se. The major difference was the magnitude of the enhancement, i.e., the mixed cultures resulted in significantly more PFC than the supernatants, even when used at a 1:1 concentration.

In order to investigate the cellular source of the supernatant factor which caused PFC enhancement, the mice used as donors of the mixed spleen cell cultures were treated in a variety of ways. When donor animals were thymectomized at birth or as adults followed by whole-body irradiation there was a marked diminution in spleen size and cell number. The cells that were obtained

TABLE 3

ENHANCED HEMOLYTIC PFC RESPONSE BY SPLEEN CELLS FROM A/J MICE IMMUNIZED WITH SHEEP ERYTHROCYTES AFTER INCUBATION *in Vitro* WITH SUPERNATANT FROM MIXED LEUKOCYTE CULTURES

Supernatants from Mixed Cultures Added to A/J Splenocytes *	PFC/10^6 Spleen Cells (Time in Hours) † 0	+3	+6	+12	+24	+48
None (controls)	496	410	320	184	69	21
A/J	464	441	385	221	73	40
C3H	444	391	315	178	65	25
C57Bl	481	325	290	150	59	31
C3H plus C57Bl	478	409	547	1173	1873	1040

* Supernatants from indicated cultures incubated with 5×10^6 spleen cells from A/J mice immunized 4 days earlier with 4×10^8 sheep RBC; indicated supernatants pooled from 3–5 cultures of spleen cells (5×10^7) incubated *in vitro* for 18–24 hours.

† Average PFC response of 3–5 cultures incubated at 37° C for indicated time period after addition of test supernatant.

from the spleens of these treated animals were markedly deficient in their ability to enhance either a primary or secondary PFC response *in vitro*. As can be seen in TABLE 4, spleen cells from thymectomized C3H and C57Bl mice, when mixed *in vitro* with target A/J splenocytes, did not result in the normal enhancement of the primary PFC response. Furthermore, spleen cells obtained from donor A/J mice primed with sheep erythrocytes 4–5 weeks before secondary challenge immunization with RBCs showed an even greater enhancement of IgG PFCs when incubated with mixed culture supernatants. Thymectomy of the C57 and C3H donor mice abolished the effect obtained with mixed

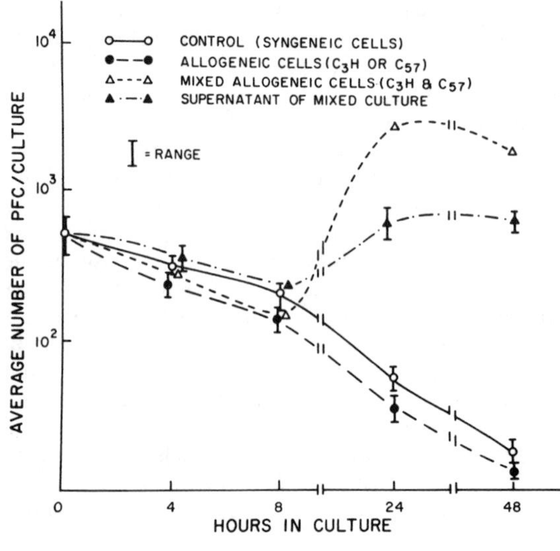

FIGURE 2. The effect of mixed allogeneic spleen cell cultures or supernatants of mixed cultures on antibody plaque formation by splenocytes from target A/J mice cultured *in vitro*. Each point represents the average PFC response of 3 to 5 cultures at the time indicated after incubation alone, with individual allogeneic cells, or with mixed allogenic cultures or their supernatants.

cultures. There was no significant effect on the IgM or IgG secondary PFC response by A/J spleen cells *in vitro*. Similarly, whole-body irradiation of the mice used as donors of the mixed leukocyte cultures also reduced this subsequent enhancement effect. Cortisone and antilymphocyte serum treatment of the donor mice also markedly suppressed the ability of the spleen cells from these animals to interact *in vitro* and enhance the antibody response of the target A/J spleen cells, either from primarily or secondarily immunized animals (TABLE 4).

In additional studies, spleen cells from the "killer" strains of mice used for mixed leukocyte cultures were incubated *in vitro* with a variety of antisera, plus complement, in order to determine which cell types were involved in the

TABLE 4

EFFECT OF TREATMENT OF SPLEEN CELL DONORS (C3H AND C57Bl MICE) ON SUBSEQUENT ENHANCEMENT OF TARGET HEMOLYTIC PFC RESPONSE *in Vitro* BY SPLEEN CELLS FROM A/J MICE AFTER PRIMARY OR SECONDARY IMMUNIZATION WITH SHEEP ERYTHROCYTES

Treatment of Spleen Cell Donors *	PFC Resopnse *in Vitro* (24 Hours) †		
	Primary	Secondary ‡	
	(19S IgM)	19S IgM	7S IgG
None (controls)	1165	975	5560
Thymectomy	285	335	1130
x-irradiation (750 R)	240	310	1300
Cortisone (1.0 mg)	220	405	1250
ALS (0.5 ml)	480	355	1150

* Spleen cell donors treated as indicated before obtaining splenocytes for mixed leukocyte cultures.

† Average PFC response of 3–6 cultures 24 hours after incubation of A/J spleen cells from either primary or secondary immunized mice with equal numbers of spleen cells from C3H and C57Bl mice treated as indicated; control cultures of A/J spleen cells only gave 72 ± 48 IgM PFC for primary response and 525 ± 32 IgM and 2160 ± 340 IgG PFC for secondary response.

‡ A/J mice primed with 4×10^8 sheep RBC 4 to 5 weeks before second immunization with same dose of RBC 4 days before culture initiation; IgG PFC determined by facilitation procedure with anti-Ig serum.

mixed leukocyte reactions resulting in enhancement of target PFC responses. Anti-θ serum treatment of the mixed leukocyte cultures *in vitro* for 30 minutes prior to incubation with the A/J spleen cells markedly diminished the expected enhanced PFC response (TABLE 5). Antilymphocyte serum also had a similar effect. On the other hand, anti-Ig serum was only slightly effective in suppressing the stimulatory effect on the target A/J cells. Similarly, antimacrophage serum also had only a slight effect. Normal rabbit serum and complement had no effect. When supernatants were obtained from mixed cultures 24 hours after initial incubation and treatment of the killer cells with the antisera, there was a similar effect on the subsequent PFC response by A/J splenocytes *in vitro* (TABLE 5). Only the treatment of the mixed leukocyte culture preparations with anti-θ sera or ALS plus complement affected the subsequent enhancement

TABLE 5

EFFECT OF TREATMENT OF MIXED LEUKOCYTE CULTURES *in Vitro* WITH ANTISERUM ON ENHANCEMENT OF HEMOLYTIC PFC RESPONSES OF TARGET SPLEEN CELLS FROM A/J MICE IMMUNIZED WITH SHEEP ERYTHROCYTES

In Vitro Treatment of Mixed Leukocyte Cultures *	PFC/10^6 Spleen Cells ($\times$ 24 Hours) † Direct Cultures	Supernatant Treated Cultures
None (control)	2650	1485
Normal rabbit serum + C^1	2730	1350
Anti-θ serum + C^1	385	310
Anti-Ig serum + C^1	2260	1165
ALS + C^1	315	320
Anti Mϕ serum + C^1	1800	3975

* Mixed spleen cell cultures from C57Bl and C3H mice (5×10^6 cells each) incubated *in vitro* for 30 minutes at 37° C with indicated antiserum, diluted 1:10, plus complement before incubation with target A/J spleen cells for direct assay or before preparation of 24-hour culture supernatants for indirect assay.

† Average hemolytic PFC response of spleen cells from A/J mice immunized 4 days earlier with 4×10^8 SRBC and cultured *in vitro* for 24 hours either with indicated mixed cultures or supernatants from mixed cultures; control cultures of A/J spleens cells only gave 285 ± 76 PFC when cultured for 24 hours at 37° C.

of the PFC response. The anti-Ig and the antimacrophage sera had only insignificant effects on enhancement.

In a further series of studies, similar antiserum preparations were tested as to their effects on the target or indicator splenocyte cultures (TABLE 6). For this purpose ALS, anti-Ig, anti-θ, or antimacrophage serum were incubated with the target A/J spleen cells from mice immunized with sheep erythrocytes

TABLE 6

EFFECT OF TREATMENT OF TARGET A/J SPLEEN CELLS *in Vitro* WITH ANTISERUM ON ENHANCEMENT OF HEMOLYTIC PFC RESPONSE *in Vitro* BY MIXED SPLEEN CELL CULTURES

In Vitro TREATMENT of Target A/J Spleen Cells (+ C^1) *	PFC per 10^6 Spleen Cells †
None (controls)	2250 ± 365
Normal serum	2340 ± 450
Anti-Ig	285 ± 76
Anti-θ sera	1970 ± 288
ALS	715 ± 93
Anti-Mϕ sera	1160 ± 195

* Target A/J spleen cells (5×10^6) incubated for 30 minutes at 37° C with 0.1 ml of 1:10 dilution of indicated serum plus G^1, before addition of equal numbers of C3H and C57B1 splenocytes.

† Average number of hemolytic PFC in cultures of A/J spleen cells after indicated treatment and incubation for 24 hours with mixed spleen cells; response of control A/J spleen cells alone was 181 ± 63 PFC at the same time.

4 days earlier. Thirty minutes later the splenocytes were washed and incubated with the mixed cultures of normal C3H and C57Bl splenocytes. Under these conditions, cultures containing the A/J spleen cells incubated with anti-Ig serum or ALS plus complement showed essentially no enhanced response to the mixed leukocyte cultures in terms of enhanced IgM PFCs (TABLE 6). The cultures treated with normal or anti-θ serum showed the expected enhanced PFC responses. Antimacrophage serum plus complement had a moderate suppressive effect on the responsiveness of the A/J splenocytes to the mixed leukocyte cultures, but the number of PFCs in these cultures was still much greater than those observed in the cultures of target spleen cells incubated with the anti-Ig serum or ALS.

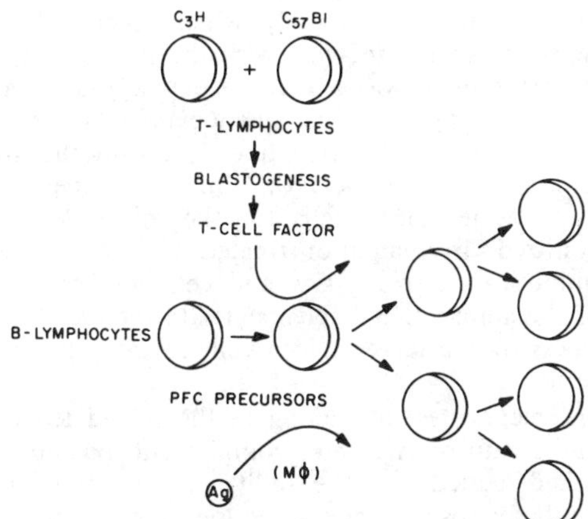

FIGURE 3. Schematic representation of the interaction of T-lymphocytes from allogeneic mouse spleen cells resulting in the release of a T-cell blastogenic factor (s) that can influence antigen-sensitized B-lymphocytes. The B-lymphocytes sensitized to antigen *in vivo* are reactive to the T-cell factor so as to form more antibody-producing cells than non-sensitized lymphocytes in culture.

Discussion and Conclusions

Thymus-derived cells play an important function in a variety of immune responses. Although much of the work to date has been concerned mainly with the role of T-cells in cell-mediated immunity in terms of responses of an individual to intracellular microorganisms, tumor antigens, and histocompatibility antigens, it is widely accepted that this class of lymphocytes may serve an important role as a helper for antibody formation by B-lymphocytes.[28] Whether or not the same T-cell population is involved in both cell-mediated immunity and as a helper for antibody formation is not known. Nevertheless, there has been much work in recent years concerning the mechanism whereby T-cells are involved in humoral immune responses. Recent studies have focused attention on subcellular factors released by T-cells that influence antibody formation.[13, 15, 20, 22–24] In the present study, a soluble factor derived from T-lymphocytes was found to markedly influence the antibody responsiveness by B-lymphocytes derived from antigen-stimulated donor mice. In this model antibody formation to sheep erythrocytes was assessed *in vitro* using the hemolytic plaque assay with spleen cells from RBC-immunized donor mice. When such splenocytes were incubated with either mixed cultures of spleen cells from mice allogeneic to the antibody-producing cells or, alternatively, with supernatants from such allogeneic mixed leukocyte cultures, markedly enhanced antibody responses occurred *in vitro*.

Evidence was obtained in the present study, as well as in previous studies in this laboratory,[18–21] that histoincompatibility between the different spleen cell populations in the cultures was necessary for the altered PFC responses. When antibody-forming splenocytes from one mouse strain were incubated *in vitro* with spleen cells from the same mouse strain that had not been immunized with sheep erythrocytes there was essentially no detectable effect on continued antibody formation *in vitro*. However, when the target antibody-producing cells were incubated with spleen cells from one allogeneic mouse strain there was an accelerated reduction in the number of PFC *in vitro* as a function of time, as well as cell number. Antibody plaque reduction occurred at even a greater speed when the killer splenocytes were obtained from donor mice specifically sensitized to the histocompatibility antigens of the target mouse spleen strain. In contrast, as found in the present study, when spleen cells from two unrelated mouse strains were incubated *in vitro* with the indicator spleen cells from the RBC-immunized mice there was a marked enhancement rather than depression in the number of PFC by the target splenocytes *in vitro*.

Enhancement was due to an interaction of T-lymphocytes during the mixed leukocyte reaction. This was shown by a variety of inhibition experiments. For example, when the donors of the spleen cells for the mixed leukocyte cultures were either thymectomized, irradiated or treated with cortisone or ALS, there was a marked diminution in spleen size and cell number as well as a concomitant depression of the ability of the splenocytes to interact *in vitro* and affect the PFC responsiveness by the target spleen cells forming hemolytic antibody.

It is noteworthy that when splenocytes interacting in the mixed leukocyte cultures were treated with anti-θ serum or ALS plus complement, but not with anti-Ig serum, there was a marked reduction in the ability of the surviving cell population to influence the antibody responsiveness by the target B-cells. In these experiments the spleen cells used for the mixed leukocyte cultures were first treated with the antiserum and complement at 37° C, then washed extensively with Medium and finally added to the target splenocytes *in vitro*. Addition of the same antisera directly to the mixed leukocyte cultures containing the target splenocytes also affected the PFC responsiveness *in vitro*. This appeared due to an effect of the antiserum on the target cells. To ascertain whether this was the case, separate experiments were performed whereby target spleen cells obtained from RBC-immunized mice were incubated *in vitro* with various antisera prior to addition to the mixed leukocyte cultures. Under these conditions it was readily apparent that the anti-Ig serum plus complement inactivated that cell population which could respond in the mixed leukocyte cultures or to the supernatants from such cultures. ALS also had this effect. Antimacrophage serum was only moderately effective. Anti-θ serum had essentially no effect on the responsiveness of the target PFC immunocytes in the mixed leukocyte cultures.

The results of these experiments suggest that the mixed leukocyte reaction involved interaction among histoincompatible T-cells, releasing a factor or factors which could stimulate an increased PFC response by committed B-lymphocytes present in the target spleen cell population. The anti-Ig serum apparently interacted with the immunoglobulin surface receptors of the B-cells. In the presence of complement such cells were inhibited or eliminated. Similarly, anti-θ serum apparently interacted with the specific θ antigen of the T-lymphocyte surface, similarly resulting in the depletion or inactivation of the functional activity of these cells in the cultures. The absence of functional T-cells resulted in the absence of the formation and/or release of the soluble supernatant factor(s) that enhanced PFC formation by the target B-cells.

It seems important to note that these studies differ in an important manner from other widely known studies using allogeneic cell *in vitro* or *in vivo*. For example, Schimpl and Wecker[22–24] have shown that supernatants of mixed leukocyte reactions, when added to T-cell depleted spleen cell cultures *in vitro*, can restore the ability of the cells to respond to *in vitro* challenge immunization with sheep erythrocytes. It seems likely that the supernatant factor from the mixed leukocyte cultures in that study influences the responsiveness of T-cell depleted splenocytes; no preexisting antigen-stimulated B-cells are involved. In the present study the B-lymphocytes were derived from mice actively sensitized with sheep erythrocytes. Culture of spleen cells at the time of the peak hemolysin response *in vitro* resulted in the continued appearance of PFC *in vitro* for a finite period of time. The largest numbers of PFC were present at the time of culture initiation, with a steady decline thereafter, apparently due either to the decrease in viability of the total spleen cell population *in vitro* or a diminution in the number or the functional capacity of the antibody-releasing cells. Addition of either two unrelated spleen cell populations or the supernatants thereof stimulated a rapid increase in the number of PFC, which were undoubtedly antibody releasing B-cells. This enhancement could be due either to the stimulation of the sensitized B-lymphocytes directly so that they replicated, or by affecting cells which had already been immunized to the RBCs but did not release enough antibody to be visible as a PFC.

It is noteworthy that the secondary IgG PFC response by spleen cells from RBC-stimulated spleen cells responded even better to the mixed leukocyte reaction or their supernatants than did the splenocytes obtained from mice forming only primary IgM antibody. It is widely accepted that thymus cells are considered essential for the formation of 7S IgG antibody as compared to the IgM antibody response to sheep erythrocytes. Thus it appears that the mixed leukocyte cultures or their T-cell supernatant product are more stimulatory for the secondarily stimulated B-cells than those involved in the primary response. Memory lymphocytes, rich in Ig receptors, are present in large numbers in the population of lymphocytes from RBC-primed mice challenged with sheep erythrocytes shortly before *in vitro* culture. In the presence of a mixed leukocyte reaction or supernatants these primed B-lymphocytes are stimulated to form large numbers of IgG PFCs.

The data presented in the present study is consistent with the hypothesis that the interaction of T-lymphocytes results in a blastogenic response and also releases certain cell kinins that influence B-lymphocytes sensitized to a T-dependent antigen such as sheep erythrocytes. The cells then appear to undergo much more rapid proliferation and/or differentiation into visible hemolysin-producing cells *in vitro*. Presumably these B-lymphocytes, both *in vivo* and *in vitro* after priming with sheep erythrocytes, become more responsive to the immunogen and develop more rapidly into IgG as well as IgM antibody-forming cells. In the presence of a mixed leukocyte reaction involving T-lymphocytes and the product of such reaction, i.e., a soluble factor, the B-lymphocytes stimulated to form much larger numbers of antibody-producing cells.

Since the factor derived from mixed leukocyte cultures is readily detectable in supernatants, it seems likely that various physicochemical means can be used to isolate and/or purify the active material for further study. This factor(s) may be either similar to the many well-defined kinins already described in terms of effector molecules in cellular immunity or a unique molecule. Regardless of the molecular nature of the factor or factors, it seems clear from the present studies that antigen-stimulated B-cells can be stimulated *in vitro,* and probably *in vivo,* to form more antibody. It would be of value to determine whether specific receptors are present on sensitized B-cells, as compared to normal cells, which can react or respond to this factor(s) preferentially. Numerous avenues of approach are available for additional studies concerning the nature and role of T-cell factors which modulate the immune response to antigens, both *in vivo* and *in vitro.*

Summary

Spleen cells derived from donor mice immunized to sheep erythrocytes continue to form hemolytic antibody plaques *in vitro;* these target spleen cells are reduced in number when incubated with splenocytes from normal or specifically sensitized allogeneic donor mice. Such depression is detectable within a few hours after incubation of the target spleen cells with the allogeneic splenocytes. In contrast, when spleen cell cultures from two unrelated mouse strains are incubated together with the target spleen cells there was a rapid enhancement rather than a depression of the antibody plaque response *in vitro.* Maximum enhancement of antibody formation occurred 24 to 48 hours after initiation of the mixed cultures *in vitro.* Enhancing activity was present in the supernatants of allogeneic spleen cell cultures and was maximal within 24 hours of culture initiation. The factor(s) derived from the supernatants of allogeneic spleen cells appeared to preferentially stimulate antigen-sensitized B-lymphocytes, especially those involved in secondary IgG antibody formation. Interacting T-lymphocytes as a source of the enhancing activity was readily demonstrated, since inactivation of the enhancing effect occurred when the cells involved in the mixed leukocyte reaction were treated with anti-θ serum or antilymphocyte serum and complement. The cells responding to the mixed cultures or the supernatants appeared to be B-lymphocytes, since they were readily suppressed by anti-Ig serum plus complement and not by the anti-θ serum. Additional investigations concerning the nature and mechanism of stimulation of B-lymphocyte responsiveness following treatment with supernatant factors from T-lymphocytes should be valuable in furthering knowledge concerning the nature of the collaboration of T- and B-lymphocytes during immunity and the role of T-lymphocytes in humoral antibody formation.

Acknowledgments

The excellent technical assistance of Mrs. Leony Mills and Miss Marsha Israel during various portions of these studies is acknowledged.

References

1. Claman, H. N., E. A. Chaperon & R. F. Triplett. 1966. J. Immunol. **97:** 28.
2. Miller, J. F. A. P. & D. Osoba. 1967. Physiol. Rev. **47:** 437.
3. Miller, J. F. A. P. & G. F. Mitchell. 1968. J. Exp. Med. **128:** 801.
4. Mitchison, N. A. 1967. Cold Spring Harbor Symp. Quant. Biol. **32:** 431.
5. Miller, J. F. A. P. & G. F. Mitchell. 1969. Transplant. Rev. **1:** 3.
6. Claman, H. N. & E. A. Chaperon. 1969. Transplant. Rev. **1:** 92.
7. Talmage, A. W., J. Radovich & H. Henningsen. 1972. Adv. Immunol. **12:** 271.
8. Abdow, H. N. & M. Richter. 1971. Adv. Immunol. **12:** 202.
9. Möller, G. 1970. Cell Immunol. **1:** 573.
10. Möller, G., O. Sjöberg & E. Möller. 1971. Ann. N.Y. Acad. Sci. **181:** 134.
11. Greaves, M. F. 1970. Transplant. Rev. **5:** 45.
12. Greaves, M. F. & Janossy. 1972. Transplant. Rev. **11:** 87.
13. Feldmann, M. & G. J. V. Nossal. 1972. Transplant. Rev. **12:** 3.
14. Raff, M. L., S. dePeters & M. Feldmann. 1973. J. Exp. Med. **137:** 1024.
15. Dutton, R. W., R. Falkoff, J. A. Herst, M. Hoffman, J. W. Kappler, J. R. Kettman, J. F. Lesley & D. Vann. 1971. *In* Progress in Immunology, I. Amos, Ed. : 355. Academic Press. New York, N.Y.
16. Schrader, J. W. 1973. J. Exp. Med. **138:** 1466.
17. Miller, J. F. A. P. 1975. Ann. N. Y. Acad. Sci. This volume.
18. Mills, L. & H. Friedman. 1972. Proc. IV. Intern. Congr. Transplant. Soc.
19. Mills, L. & H. Friedman. 1973. Fed. Proc. **32:** 1020.
20. Friedman, H. 1970. *In* Histocompatibility Testing. A. I. Terasaki, Ed. : 501. Munksgaard Co. Copenhagen, Denmark.
21. Jerne, N. K. & A. A. Nordin. 1963. Science. **140:** 405.
22. Schimpl, A. & E. Wecker. 1972. Nature New Biol. **237:** 15.
23. Schimpl, A. & E. Wecker. 1973. *In* Microenvironmental Aspects of Immunity. B. D. Jankovics, Ed. : 179. Plenum Pub. Co. New York, N.Y.
24. Schimpl, A. & E. Wecker. 1973. J. Exp. Med. **134:** 547.

Discussion of the Paper

Dr. A. B. Stavitsky (*Case Western Reserve University, Cleveland, Ohio*): Is fresh antigen added to the cultures?

Dr. H. Friedman: Not for the basic assay; only the mice are immunized and no antigen is added. For the secondary response we add antigen to the cultures and look for secondary plaque forming cells. Also, I believe antigen is still present when we take the spleen cells out of an antigen-primed mouse.

Dr. A. B. Stavitsky: We have performed similar experiments measuring antibody production with rabbit lymphoid cells. We added BSA and supernatants from KLH-stimulated lymphocytes to cultures of cells that have not been immunized to BSA; we have been able to increase anti-BSA production, although this would in a sense be a primary response.

INFLUENCE OF THYMOSIN ON THE INDUCTION AND REGULATION OF THE SECONDARY RESPONSE *IN VITRO* TO DIPHTHERIA TOXOID

Benjamin Wolf *

Department of Pathobiology
School of Veterinary Medicine
University of Pennsylvania
Philadelphia, Pennsylvania 19104

Introduction

It was previously demonstrated that normal rabbit thymus potentiated immunoglobulin synthesis by lymph nodes during the anamnestic response *in vitro.* Lymph node fragments from rabbits that had been secondarily injected with diphtheria toxoid were co-incubated with thymus fragments from normal 1 to 2 week old rabbits. Potentiation of both antibody and total immunoglobulin synthesis occurred, persisting up to three weeks in culture.[1] Thymus-stimulated lymph node fragments sensitized with toxoid *in vitro* also underwent an enhanced secondary response in culture. When heat-killed cells in thymus fragments or thymus fragments placed across cell-impermeable Millipore® filters were now assayed in this system, potentiation also was seen. This suggested the possibility that thymic humoral factors were involved.

A study was initiated to test the effects of thymosin, a highly purified calf thymus hormonal extract. Thymosin has been shown to have a number of interesting activities related to cell-mediated immunity (see A. Goldstein, this volume). It was important, however, to look for any activity in antibody-forming systems for which the secondary response *in vitro* could be a convenient model. Thymosin thus enhanced the secondary response *in vitro,* either when included in culture media or when added to antigen and then pulsed onto lymphoid cells for 2 hours. Potentiation by thymosin was dose-dependent, with enhancement inversely related to concentration, viz., 1.0 μg/ml > 10 μg/ml > 100 μg/ml. Further, although thymosin binding was seen on immunoglobulin-bearing rabbit ("B") lymphocytes, the actual binding was apart from immunoglobulin sites on the membrane. Although it is possible that thymosin can bind to rabbit thymus-derived ("T") cells as well, thymosin binding to B-lymphocytes would seem to be a minimal requisite for enhanced secondary antibody synthesis.

Methods

Primary Immunization

The hind foot-pads of adult (5–6 month old) New Zealand White rabbits were injected once with alum-precipitated diphtheria toxoid (60 Lf units/ml) for the primary injection.

* Supported by National Foundation Grant GB 28694.

Secondary Sensitization and Culture

Five to six months later, the animals were exsanguinated by heart puncture. Each popliteal lymph node was removed and cut into 60–80 fragments of equal size, each weighing 6–8 mg. These were combined and divided into several groups. Each group was sensitized with 5 Lf toxoid/ml for 2 hours in 10 ml Eagles minimal essential medium (MEM) containing supplements (see next paragraph) in 16 × 125 mm roller tubes on a rotary drum (12 rev/hr) at 37° C. Concurrently, a group of fragments were incubated without toxoid. Three fragments were cultured together in a 16 × 125 mm roller tube on the rotary drum after being covered by a thin pad of glass wool (0.5 cm) to attach them to the glass. A group of four replicate tubes was run. Into another set of tubes containing sensitized lymph node fragments, thymus fragments of the same size were planted. These had been pooled from four 1–2 week old normal rabbits. Normal lymph node and spleen from 3–4 week old rabbits were used in other sets of tubes to test for potentiation of the secondary response since these organs were too small in the younger rabbits. To minimize the variability in replicate tubes during antibody synthesis, the precautionary steps outlined in another report were taken.[1]

Thymosin (Fraction 3 or Fraction 5), a highly purified calf thymus hormone, was generously supplied to us by Dr. Allan Goldstein. Thymosin was freshly dissolved each time before use. When employed solely during culture conditions, thymosin Fraction 3, as well as the spleen and brain Fraction 3, were incorporated into the medium initially and whenever the medium was changed, i.e., every 2 or 3 days. When employed only for cell sensitization, thymosin was added together with toxoid for a two-hour pulse, and both were then washed free. The tissue culture fluid employed throughout these studies consisted of Eagle's minimal essential medium (MEM), MEM nonessential amino acids, hydrocortisone sodium hemisuccinate (Steraloid, New York) (1 μg/ml), insulin (Iletin, U-80, 0.01 unit/ml) and penicillin (100 units/ml). The hydrocortisone hemisuccinate concentration was determined by Ambrose[2] to be the most satisfactory in his study; the insulin concentration was 10-fold less than used by Ambrose, and experimentally concluded by us to be optimal. In the experiments in our laboratory to establish a cellular dependence upon these hormones during the secondary response, an absolute requirement for hydrocortisone was discovered, but only in certain rabbits was one established for insulin. The fluids were poured off every 2 or 3 days, so that antibody synthesized during each of these time intervals was an indication of *de novo* synthesis. *De novo* synthesis of both antibody and total immunoglobulin in cultures of this type was demonstrated in previous work by several criteria, including radioactive amino acid incorporation and quantitative measurement of antibody and immunoglobulin.[1,3]

Although a hemagglutination of toxoid-coated cells was employed here for serological assays, Jacobsen and Thorbecke[4] showed a good correlation between gel diffusion, binding of I^{125}-labeled diphtheria toxoid, and hemagglutination. Only the collected media were assayed because it had been previously determined that more than 95% of the total antibody is released from the tissues into the medium.[3]

Rosette Formation

Sheep erythrocytes were coupled with thymosin by use of a modification of the chromic chloride technique of Gold and Fudenberg, in which 0.15 M NaCl was buffered with 0.01 M tricine, pH 6.5.[5] The reagents were added in order: 0.03 ml 0.07% $CrCl_3.6H_2O$, 0.05 ml thymosin Fraction 5 (1 mg/ml), and 0.01 ml packed sheep erythrocytes. The mixture was incubated 5 minutes at room temperature, and the coupled erythrocytes were washed four times in phosphate-buffered saline 0.15 M, containing 0.5% bovine serum albumin. The erythrocyte concentration was adjusted to 0.4%. Peripheral blood and lymph node lymphocytes were isolated as described,[6, 7] put through a Ficoll-Hypaque gradient and the concentration adjusted to 5×10^5 cells/0.05 ml. Rosettes were formed by adding 0.05 ml erythrocytes (0.4%) to the 0.05 ml lymphocyte suspension just prior to centrifugation at 1500 RPM/1 min at 4° C. Rosette inhibition of thymosin coupled sheep erythrocytes was achieved by preincubating lymphocytes with appropriate concentrations of soluble thymosin for 30 minutes at 4° C. The mixed antiglobulin reaction was performed as described.[6] Rosetting with the hapten 3-nitro-4-hydroxy-5-iodophenyl acetic acid (NIP) coupled erythrocytes was performed as described.[7]

Results and Discussion

The complete secondary antibody response *in vitro* could be carried out in defined media without the requirement of serum.[2, 9] This was particularly important when quantitative assessments were to be made on the degree of thymosin binding to cells, leading to antibody formation. The possibility existed that serum proteins in the medium could bind thymosin or otherwise compete with thymosin binding to cells. A typical secondary response is shown in Figure 1, wherein the lymph node fragments that had received a 2 hour sensitization synthesized antibody continuously for 2 to 2.5 weeks. Those fragments that were not sensitized with antigen did not undergo the secondary response *in vitro*. Although Figure 1 indicates that those fragments that were not stimulated with antigen were uniformly nonresponsive (titers (<1:10)), in a few experiments these formed antibody during a continuing primary response.

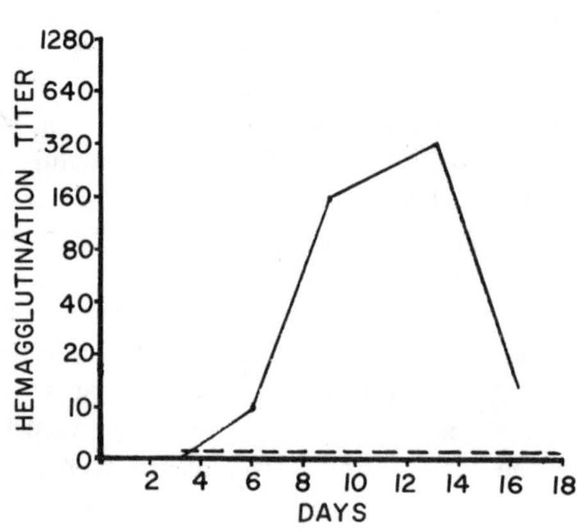

Figure 1. A typical secondary response *in vitro*. The solid line shows antibody synthesis by lymph node fragments sensitized with 5.0 units of diphtheria toxoid/ml. The broken line shows the lack of synthesis by unsensitized fragments.

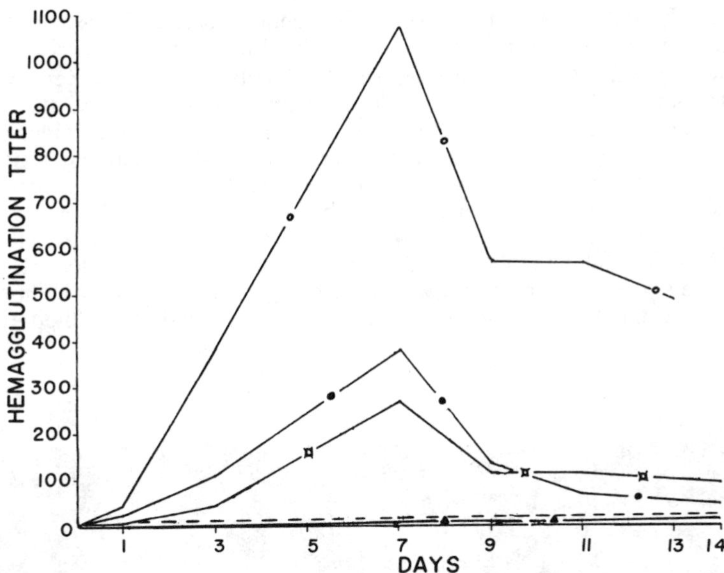

FIGURE 2. Enhancement by normal thymus, heat-killed thymus, and normal spleen. ○, secondary-sensitized lymph node plus normal thymus; ●, secondary-sensitized lymph node plus heat killed (50°/30 min) thymus; □, secondary-sensitized lymph node; - - -, secondary-sensitized lymph node plus normal spleen; ▲, primary-sensitized lymph node.

Previous work had established that the thymus would potentiate an ongoing secondary response *in vitro.*[1] It was important to determine whether the thymus would increase antibody synthesis during the secondary response initiated *in vitro.* After sensitization of the lymph node fragments with antigen, 3 fragments were co-incubated contiguously with 6 normal thymus fragments. Thymus fragments that had been heated at 56° C for 30 minutes to kill the cells were added to another set of tubes. Another control tested the effectiveness of normal spleen fragments that were added to the secondarily sensitized lymph node fragments. The results are summarized in FIGURE 2. Stimulation with thymus began at the initiation of the secondary response, peaked at about day 7, and remained higher throughout the duration of the experiment. Increased titers were observed, ranging from a 4-fold difference on day 7 to approximately 5-fold on day 11, although the overall antibody-forming capacity of the cultures was declining at this time. Heated thymus also potentiated antibody synthesis, but the titers were considerably lower than those found when untreated thymus was employed. Therefore it was assumed that living cells as well as metabolic products were important for stimulation. When this experiment was repeated, it was found that heated thymus caused greater stimulation than unheated thymus. It was therefore not possible to compare the relative potency of either effect in the present system. When the normal spleen was employed, antibody synthesis was suppressed in every instance. The reason for this is not known, but it might be explained by the observation of Lapresle and Webb [10] that the spleen contains proteases responsible for antigen degradation, and therefore a critical level of antigen was necessary.

Since heated thymus was active, soluble (humoral) products were considered to play a role. A parabiotic culture assembly was devised so that when the thymic fragments were cultured in one chamber and the lymph node fragments in the other, the exchange of culture fluids containing metabolic products from each organ through a cell impermeable filter could be effectively maintained. FIGURE 3 illustrates the parabiotic chamber, actually a 16×125 mm roller tube cut in half. The two halves are separated by a polyethylene sleeve with a Millipore filter (0.45 μ porosity) inserted between each tube. Inside the sleeve are threads into which the two glass cylinders may be inserted. A millipore flat O ring between the lip of the tube and the millipore filter protects the filter from tearing and leaking. FIGURE 4 illustrates the results obtained in parabiotic chambers. It was noted that the lymph node fragments per se did not synthesize as much antibody in parabiotic chambers. But when the thymus was added to the system, antibody synthesis was consistently enhanced.

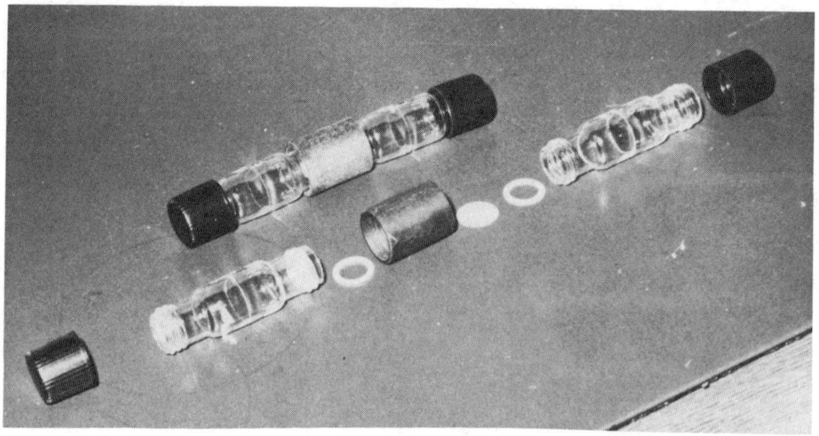

FIGURE 3. The parabiotic chamber, containing 2 glass tubes, 2 polyethylene flat O rings, 1 polyethylene sleeve to join the tubes, and 1 Millipore filter, porosity 0.45 μ.

Although the alternative at this point was to try to purify active rabbit thymic humoral factors, we chose instead to assay the well characterized thymosin. Thymosin Fraction 3 was added to the culture fluid in concentrations of 10 μg/ml, 1 μg/ml, and 0.1 μg/ml. FIGURE 5 illustrates the data in one experiment. The peak of antibody synthesis was reached on day 10 in all the tubes. In the control tubes, in which the lymph node fragments were secondarily-sensitized with antigen but to which no thymosin was added, the

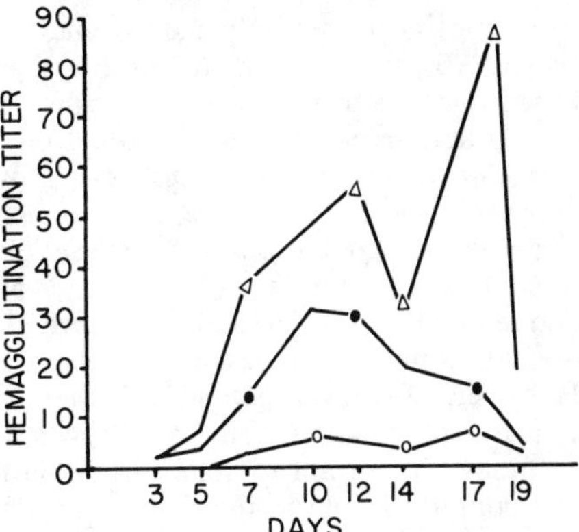

FIGURE 4. Thymus stimulation in the parabiotic chamber. △, secondary-sensitized lymph node plus normal thymus in separate chambers; ●, secondary-sensitized lymph node but no thymus in the other chamber; ○, primary-sensitized lymph node but no thymus in the other chamber.

mean titer on day 10 was 320. Upon the addition of thymosin an inverse relationship between thymosin concentration and enhancement of antibody synthesis was seen. Employing 10 μg/ml thymosin, the mean titer on day 10 was 1280 or about 4-fold greater than controls without thymosin. Lowering the concentration of thymosin to 1 μg/ml resulted in greater stimulation, a titer of 3676 or nearly a 12-fold increase on day 10. Still lower concentrations

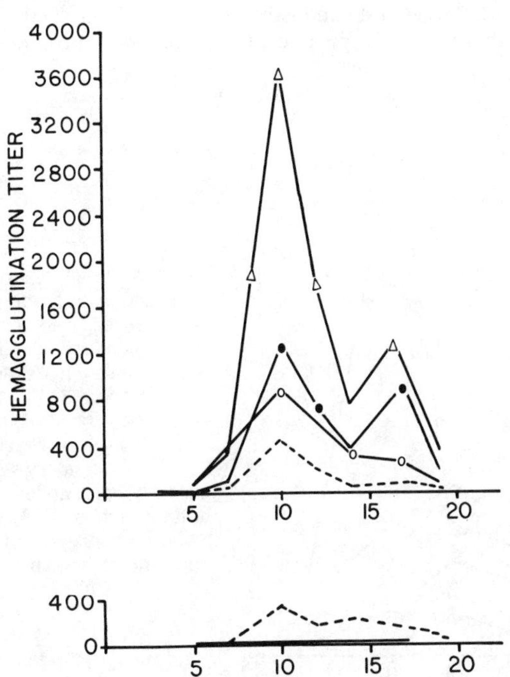

FIGURE 5. Dose-dependent thymosin stimulation. *Upper graph:* ●, thymosin, 10 μg/ml; △, thymosin, 1 μg/ml; ○, thymosin, 0.1 μg/ml; - - -, thymosin, 0.01 μg/ml. *Lower graph:* - - -, secondary-sensitized lymph node, no thymosin; —, primary-sensitized lymph node, no thymosin.

of thymosin did not enhance as much; 0.1 μg/ml thymosin resulted in a mean titer of 907 and 0.01 μg/ml led to a titer of 452, which was close to that found in the controls to which no thymosin was added.

To determine whether thymosin might have exerted its effect by containing antigenic determinant groups that cross-reacted with diphtheria toxoid, two approaches were tried. The first was hemagglutination-inhibition with thymosin in a known toxoid-antitoxoid system. Here, thymosin did not inhibit hemagglutination when an excess (100 μg/ml) of thymosin was added to tissue culture-derived antibody. In addition, several different concentrations of thymosin did not stimulate the secondary response in the absence of diphtheria toxoid. However, thymosin potentiated the anamnestic response in antigen-induced cells from the same rabbit.

It was important to determine whether the activity of the thymosin fraction was contained only in the thymus or whether an identically derived Fraction 3 from other tissues, e.g., spleen and brain, would exhibit similar activity. Therefore, in the next experiment Fraction 3 from calf thymus, calf spleen, and calf brain were examined, employing 1 μg/ml of each. As can be seen in FIGURE 6, the brain fraction showed no activity, and the spleen fraction demonstrated only a small level of activity. Thymosin, however, displayed marked activity.

The possibility was considered that thymosin stimulation depended largely on cell membrane activation without the need for inclusion of thymosin during the culture period. FIGURE 7 shows that the addition of thymosin toxoid for a 2-hour pulse, but washing them free before culture, resulted in an enhanced stimulation by thymosin. The degree of stimulation was again inversely dependent on the dose of thymosin, with the most marked effects observed generally with 1 μg/ml, less with 10 μg/ml, and still less with 100 μg/ml. An interesting observation was that when lymph node fragments that infrequently

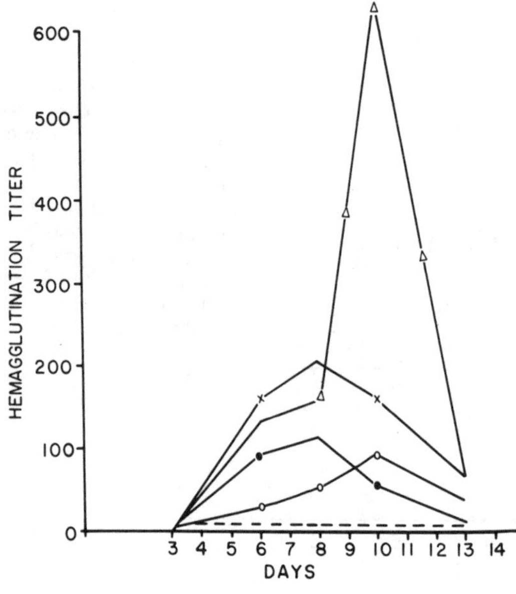

FIGURE 6. Comparison of Fraction 3 from thymus, spleen and brain. Δ, secondary-sensitized lymph node plus thymosin, Fraction 3; X, secondary-sensitized lymph node plus spleen Fraction 3; —, secondary-sensitized lymph node plus brain Fraction 3; ●, secondary-sensitized lymph node, no thymosin.

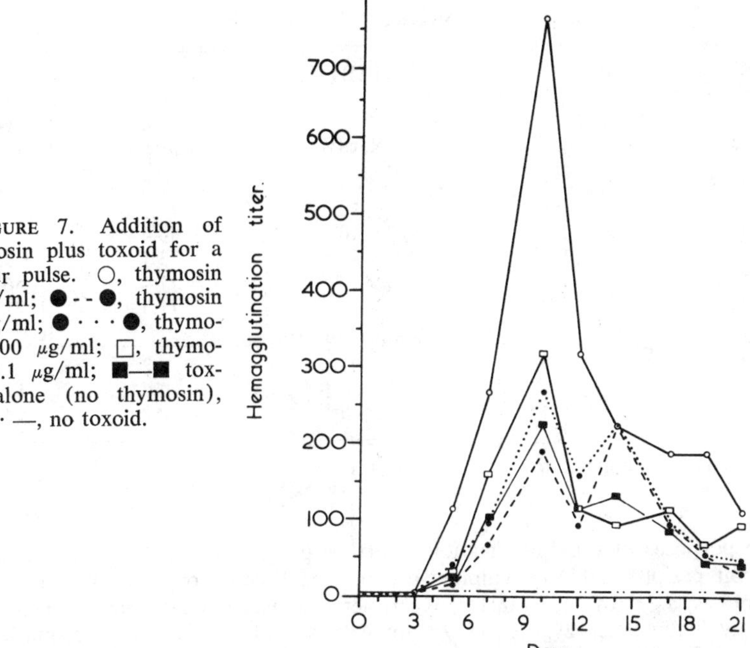

FIGURE 7. Addition of thymosin plus toxoid for a 2-hour pulse. ○, thymosin 1 μg/ml; ● - - ●, thymosin 10 μg/ml; ● · · · ●, thymosin 100 μg/ml; □, thymosin 0.1 μg/ml; ■—■ toxoid alone (no thymosin), — · · —, no toxoid.

secreted antibody in a continuing primary response *in vitro* were tested, thymosin was found not to stimulate. The reasons for this are not clear but may be related to competitive binding of thymosin and secreted antibody at the cell surface.

Because thymosin activation was thought to be mediated by its ability to bind to cell membranes, the types of cells putatively involved were investigated. However, even if the cell types were identified to which thymosin was bound, subsequent antibody synthesis might involve still other cells. Bone marrow derived (B) cells and thymus derived (T) cells were now studied.

To investigate whether thymosin would bind to B- and T-cells in general, chicken thymus and bursa cells were prepared by Dr. W. T. Weber. The T-cells came from 20 day embryonic thymus and constituted 99% of the population, while the B-cells came from a 4 week old bursa and were 100% of the population. Thymosin was linked to sheep erythrocytes via the $CrCl_3$ method and rosettes were formed by direct uptake employing centrifugation-suspension at 4° C. Pretreating the lymphoid cells at 4° C for 30 minutes with soluble thymosin was used for rosette inhibition. TABLE 1 shows that both B- and T-cells rosetted; however, the extent of rosette formation varied between T-cell and B-cell preparations. For example, another T-cell suspension showed 40% rosettes. Inhibition of rosette formation by thymosin was demonstrated in both B- and T-cells by 8.3×10^{-13} to 8.3×10^{-15} M thymosin. This would indicate a quantitative similarity of B- and T-cell receptors for thymosin.

Although there are no confirmed B- and T-cell markers in the rabbit, the immunoglobulin (Ig) bearing rabbit lymphocyte might be called a "B"-cell for

TABLE 1

BINDING OF THYMOSIN TO CHICKEN B- AND T-CELLS

Tube	Thymosin mg/ml	Thymosin molarity	Rosette * Formation (percent)	Inhibition by Thymosin (percent)
	Bursal (B) Cells			
1	—	—	40.8	—
2	10^{-2}	8.3×10^{-7}	44.5	—
3	10^{-4}	8.3×10^{-9}	40.4	—
4	10^{-6}	8.3×10^{-11}	33.1	19.3
5	10^{-8}	8.3×10^{-13}	17.4	56.4
6	10^{-10}	8.3×10^{-15}	11.3	71.5
	Thymus (T) Cells			
1	—	—	5.2	—
2	10^{-8}	8.3×10^{-13}	4.6	11.5
3	10^{-10}	8.3×10^{-15}	2.2	57.5

* Thymosin coupled to sheep erythrocytes.

the purposes of this investigation. Further proof that immunoglobulin-bearing rabbit peripheral blood lymphocytes may be B-cells comes from the work of Jones *et al.*[11] In cell transfer experiments it was noticed that the cells from allotypically heterozygous *b*5/9 animals that did not bear the *b*5 marker on the surface matured to cells in which 93–99% of the cells contained *b*9 allotype in the cytoplasm. Other more defined markers would still need be elucidated to identify B-cells. "B"-cells were obtained from the peripheral blood of a rabbit in which 86% of the cells exhibited Ig (allotype *b*4) at the surface by the mixed antiglobulin test.[6] As TABLE 2 indicates, 27.8% of these lymphocytes rosetted with thymosin coupled through $CrCl_3$ sheep erythrocytes, and the best inhibition was achieved with relatively the same levels (8.3×10^{-13} to 8.3×10^{-15} M) of soluble thymosin as was earlier shown by chicken B- and

TABLE 2

BINDING OF THYMOSIN TO RABBIT "B"-CELLS (Peripheral Blood Lymphocytes) *

Tube	Thymosin mg/ml	Thymosin molarity	Rosette † Formation (percent)	Inhibition by Thymosin (percent)
1	—	—	27.8	—
2	10^{-6}	8.3×10^{-11}	11.3	17.4
3	10^{-8}	8.3×10^{-13}	9.5	32.0
4	10^{-10}	8.3×10^{-15}	5.5	60.7
5	10^{-12}	8.3×10^{-17}	12.0	14.3

* Eighty-six percent of these lymphocytes expressed immunoglobulins on their surfaces as the *b*4 allotype.

† Thymosin coupled to sheep erythrocytes.

TABLE 3

FAILURE OF THYMOSIN TO BIND TO IMMUNOGLOBULINS OF RABBIT "B"-CELLS (Peripheral Blood Lymphocytes)

Tube	Thymosin mg/ml	Thymosin molarity	Rosette * Formation (Ig–SRBC) (percent)	Inhibition by Thymosin (percent)
1	—	—	82.6	—
2	10^{-2}	8.3×10^{-7}	73.9	10.6
3	10^{-4}	8.3×10^{-9}	75.2	7.8
4	10^{-6}	8.3×10^{-11}	80.1	3.8
5	10^{-8}	8.3×10^{-13}	77.4	6.3

* Rosettes obtained by mixed antiglobulin reaction for the *b*4 allotype.

T-cells. Presumably the thymosin receptors were similar for the chicken B- and T-cell and the rabbit "B"-cell.

It was of interest to investigate now whether thymosin binding occurred at membrane sites at or apart from immunoglobulin determinants and receptors. TABLE 3 indicates that when rosettes were formed to detect immunoglobulin at the surface of rabbit peripheral blood lymphocytes, 82% exhibited Ig. When various levels of soluble thymosin were employed in an attempt to inhibit rosette formation, essentially little to none was found, indicating no competition at Ig sites on the membrane. TABLE 4 is a follow-up of TABLE 3 in which the "B"-cell thymosin receptor was further investigated using another "B"-cell model, i.e., antihapten receptors rosetting with hapten-coupled sheep erythrocytes. The red cells were coupled with the hapten, 3-nitro-4-hydroxy-5-iodophenyl acetic acid (NIP). The lymph node cells came from a rabbit immunized 5 days previously. As was found earlier, thymosin in various concentrations failed to inhibit rosette formation, thus indicating failure to bind to specific receptors.

TABLE 4

FAILURE OF THYMOSIN TO BIND TO HAPTEN RECEPTORS OF RABBIT "B" LYMPH NODE CELLS

Tube	Thymosin mg/ml	Thymosin molarity	Rosette * Formation (NIP–SRBC) (percent)	Inhibition by Thymosin (percent)
1	—	—	4.0	—
2	10^{-6}	8.3×10^{-11}	2.9	27
3	10^{-8}	8.3×10^{-13}	3.1	22
4	10^{-10}	8.3×10^{-15}	4.7	—

* 3-iodo, 4-hydroxy, 5-nitro, phenyl acetic acid (NIP) coupled to sheep erythrocytes.

It remained to investigate whether thymosin would bind to lymphoid cells bearing specific receptors for diphtheria toxoid. In lymph node cells from rabbits that had undergone a 5 to 6 month primary response, very low levels of the cells bound toxoid-coupled sheep erythrocytes ($<1\%$), so thymosin binding could not be investigated. But more sensitive rosette assays or other surface-binding methods could be used to investigate this aspect further.

Thus thymosin binding occurred on chicken B- and T-cells and immunoglobulin containing rabbit "B"-cells. Thymosin apparently bound to membrane sites on rabbit "B"-cells not associated with immunoglobulin determinants or receptors. Whether thymosin binding leads to antibody synthesis after binding to "B"-cells remains to be investigated. The evidence however indicates that thymosin influences rabbit "B"-cells by both binding to them and stimulating antibody synthesis by them.

Summary

An *in vitro* model has been employed in which diphtheria toxoid induced a secondary response in nonsecreting, rabbit lymphoid cells in long-term memory. In this system, heated normal neonatal rabbit thymus, as well as diffusable rabbit thymus factors and thymosin caused increased stimulation over a 2 to 3 week period. Stimulation was increased proportionately as the concentration of thymosin decreased from 100 μg/ml to 10 μg/ml to 1.0 μg/ml. This was observed when thymosin plus antigen sensitized the cells during a 2-hour pulse. Using thymosin coupled to sheep erythrocytes to form rosettes, thymosin binding occurred at least on immunoglobulin-bearing "B"-lymphocytes. However, thymosin binding was seen on membrane sites apart from immunoglobulin determinants or immunoglobulin receptors. The data indicate that thymosin activation involves minimally B-cell activation to induce and maintain a secondary response.

References

1. Wolf, B. 1968. Potentiation of lymph node antibody synthesis by normal thymus *in vitro*. Immunology **14:** 235.
2. Ambrose, C. T. 1964. The requirement for hydrocortisone in antibody-forming tissue cultivated in serum-free medium. J. Exp. Med. **119:** 1027.
3. Stavitsky, A. B. & B. Wolf. 1958. Mechanisms of antibody globulin synthesis by lymphoid tissues *in vitro*. Biochim. Biophys. Acta **27:** 4.
4. Jacobsen, E. B. & G. J. Thorbecke. 1967. The proliferative and anamnestic antibody response of rabbit lymphoid cells *in vitro*. 1. Immunological memory in the lymph nodes draining and contralateral to the site of a primary antigen injection. J. Exp. Med. **130:** 287.
5. Gold, E. R. & H. H. Fudenberg. 1967. Chromic chloride: a coupling reagent for passive hemagglutination reactions. J. Immunol. **99:** 859.
6. Coombs, R. R. A., B. W. Gurner, C. A. Janeway, Jr., A. B. Wilson, P. G. H. Gell & A. S. Kelus. 1970. Immunoglobulin determinants on the lymphocytes of normal rabbits. I. Demonstration by the mixed antiglobulin reaction of determinants recognized by anti-γ, anti-μ, anti-Fab and the anti-allotype sera anti-As4 and As6. Immunology **18:** 417.
7. Bankert, R. B. & B. Wolf. 1973. Simultaneous expression of hapten-binding and antibody secretion by NIP-primed lymph node cells early in the immune response. J. Immunol. **111:** 1790.

8. An, T., K. Miyai & S. Sell. 1972. Electron microscopic localization of rabbit immunoglobulin allotype *b*4 on blood lymphocytes by an indirect ferritin immune complex labeling technique. J. Immunol. **108:** 1271.

9. Halliday, W. J. & J. S. Garvey. 1964. Some factors affecting the secondary immune response in tissue cultures containing hydrocortisone. J. Immunol. **93:** 756.

10. Lapresle, C. & T. Webb. 1960. Étude de la degradation de la sérum-albumin humaine par un extrait de rate de lapin. VII Isolement et proprietés d'un fragment d'albumine. Ann. Inst. Past. **99:** 523.

11. Jones, P. P., J. J. Cebra & L. A. Herzenberg. 1974. Restriction of gene expression in B lymphocytes and their progeny. I. Commitment to immunoglobulin allotype. J. Exp. Med. **139:** 581.

ANTIGENIC AND FUNCTIONAL EVIDENCE FOR THE *IN VITRO* INDUCTIVE ACTIVITY OF THYMOPOIETIN (THYMIN) ON THYMOCYTE PRECURSORS *

Ross S. Basch and Gideon Goldstein †

Department of Pathology and
The Irvington House Institute
New York University School of Medicine
New York, New York 10016

The isolation of two closely related polypeptides, thymopoietin I and II, from bovine thymus has been described previously.[1, 2] Originally referred to as thymin I and II and now renamed the thymopoietins,[3, 4] these purified polypeptides have been shown to induce *in vitro* the differentiation of precursor cells found in the bone marrow and spleen of adult mice.[5] Concentrations of thymopoietin as low as 20 pg/ml were effective in several test systems. The induction occurs rapidly *in vitro* and results in the appearance of cells with antigenic and functional characteristics resembling intrathymic T-cells. These effects of thymopoietin on cultures of hemopoietic cells appear highly specific since no changes could be detected in several other differentiating hemopoietic systems studied under similar conditions.

Materials and Methods

Animals

All of the mice used in these experiments were purchased from the Jackson Laboratories (Bar Harbor, Maine) except the A·TL⁻ mice which were bred at New York University from a foundation stock kindly given us by Dr. E. A. Boyse. All mice were housed eight to a cage, fed commercial high protein mouse pellets, and allowed water *ad libitum*.

Antisera, cytotoxic tests, and the cytotoxic inhibition test were prepared or performed as previously described.[5]

Thymopoietin

The isolation and bioassay of these polypeptides has been reviewed in this volume.[2] Lots GG 83BT 1 of thymopoietin I and GG 81BT II of thymopoietin II were used throughout. They were dissolved in phosphate-buffered saline

* This work was supported by United States Public Health Service Grants A1–11326 and NS–09173, a grant from the Muscular Dystrophy Associations of America, and the Sackler Research Fund. R. S. B. is a recipient of United States Public Health Service Career Development Award HD 34968.

† Present address: Memorial Sloan-Kettering Cancer Center, New York, N.Y. 10021.

containing 1 mg/ml bovine serum albumin, distributed in 1 μg aliquots, and lyophilized. For use they were diluted with tissue culture medium containing 4% adult bovine serum.

Induction of T-cell Precursors in Vitro

Bone marrow cells were obtained from the femoral marrow. These cells, or cells from spleen or thymus, were teased into single cell suspensions and washed three times in tissue culture medium RPMI 1640 supplemented with 10 mM Hepes, 1.5×10^{-5} M 2-mercaptoethanol, 100 U/ml penicillin, 100 μg/ml Streptomycin, and 4% adult bovine serum.

For induction the cells were suspended in medium at 5×10^{6}/ml and incubated with the desired concentration of thymopoietin at 37° C in plastic petri dishes in a humidified atmosphere of 5% CO_2 in air.

Cell Separation by Flotation on Bovine Serum Albumin (BSA) Gradients

Spleen and bone marrow cells were separated by flotation in discontinuous gradients of BSA as previously described.[6] The A layer was collected from the interface between 21 and 23% BSA, while the B layer was found at the 23 and 25% interface. The BSA used was purchased from Miles Laboratories as a 35% stock concentrate (Pathocyte 5) and was diluted with phosphate buffered saline (pH 7.4) for use in the gradients. The tubes were centrifuged in a Beckman model L2–65 ultracentrifuge for 30 minutes at 13,000 rpm at 4° C using a SW 50.1 rotor.

Stimulation by Mitogens

The optimal concentration of Concanavalin A (Con-A) (Pharmacia), Phytohemagglutinin (PHA) (Burroughs Wellcome) and *E. coli* lipopolysaccharide 0111-B4 (Diffico) were determined in preliminary titrations with normal spleen and thymus cells. In the experiments described the following concentrations were used: Con-A 6 μg/ml; PHA 2 μg/ml; and LPS 10 μg/ml. These were prepared as 100-fold concentrates in saline, stored at —70° C and added to 0.2 ml microtiter cultures as needed. The cells were incubated with various concentrations of thymopoietin and mitogen as indicated in the text. Tritiated thymidine ([^{3}H]TdR, 20 mCi/μM, New England Nuclear) was added at a concentration of 2.5 μC/ml for the last 2–4 hours of the culture period. The cells were lysed with distilled water and the DNA gel collected on glass fiber filters, with the aid of an automatic cell harvester. The filters were dried and, using a toluene-based scintillation fluid, the radioactivity of the precipitate was determined in a Packard model 3380 liquid scintillation spectrometer.

Erythropoietin (ESF)

Human urinary erythropoietin was obtained from the USPHS National Heart Institute pool *A-1 TaLSL*. It was procured by them from the Department of Physiology, University of the North East, Corrientes, Argentina and processed by the Hematology Research Laboratories of the Children's Hospital of Los Angeles under Research Grant HE 10880. For use it was dissolved in the tissue culture medium at a concentration of 0.4 U/ml. The effects of ESF and the influence of thymopoietin on these effects were assessed either by measuring the incorporation of [^{3}H]TdR into DNA as described above or by measuring the incorporation of ^{55}Fe into hemoglobin. When hemoglobin synthesis was being determined, transferrin (1 mg/ml) and ^{55}Fe citrate (2.5 μc/ml; Sp. Act. 20 Ci/g, Amersham Searle) were added to the culture medium at the appropriate time, and the radioactivity incorporated into TCA-precipitable material measured.

Colony-forming Cells

Spleen colony-forming cells were measured after 18 hours in culture with or without thymopoietin by the method of Till and McCulloch.[7]

Results

FIGURE 1 shows the results of a cytotoxic inhibition test using an anti-TL antiserum. The target cells were normal A/J thymocytes and the inhibitory cells were A/J bone marrow cells incubated for 18 hours with various concentrations of thymopoietin I. Cultures incubated with concentrations of thymopoietin from 2.0 to 200 ng/ml absorbed anti-TL antibodies equally well and

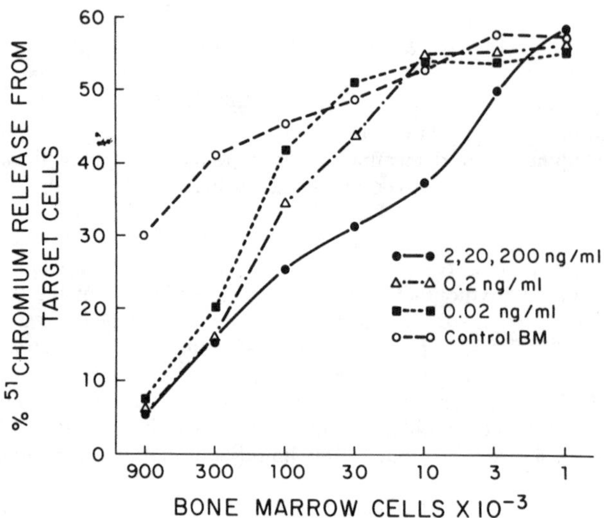

FIGURE 1. Absorption of anti-TL Antibody by mouse bone marrow cells incubated with thymopoietin I. The bone marrow cells were incubated for 18 hours before being tested for their TL content. Cells not treated with thymopoietin absorbed little or no antibody (open circles).

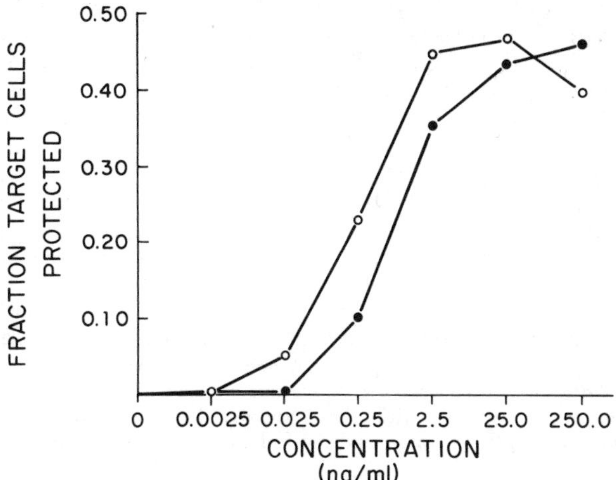

FIGURE 2. The relationship between the concentrations of thymopoietins I & II and the amount of TL antigen induced in mouse bone marrow cell cultures. The bone marrow cells were incubated for 6 hours with either thymopoietin I (open circles) or II (closed circles). The abscissa represents the fraction of the target cells protected from cytolysis by 100,000 bone marrow cells. 50,000 target cells were present in each assay, of which 25,000 were lysed in the absence of protecting bone marrow. Thus complete absorption of the anti-TL antibody is indicated by the protection of 0.5 of the target cells.

activity was apparent with concentrations as low as 0.02 μg/ml. These cells also expressed the Thy-1 (θ) antigen. Cells incubated under similar conditions in the absence of thymopoietin expressed neither TL nor Thy 1 (θ). Cells cultured at 4° C also failed to express TL. Bone marrow cells from mice of the A·TL⁻ strain expressed Thy-1 (θ) but not TL when incubated with thymopoietin.

Similar results were obtained with thymopoietin II although on a weight basis it was slightly less active than thymopoietin I in most experiments. The dose responses obtained with both polypeptides are shown in FIGURE 2. All of these results were obtained with unfractionated bone marrow cells. TL induction in spleen cells was also demonstrable by this technique, which is clearly more sensitive than the direct cytotoxic test. Thus, using the direct cytotoxic tests on unfractionated spleen or bone marrow cells, we were unable to demonstrate significant increases in either anti-TL or anti-Thy-1 (θ) sensitive cells. Inducible cells could only be demonstrated by the direct cytotoxic test when the precursors were concentrated by flotation on discontinuous bovine serum albumin gradients.[5, 6] In these studies the thymopoietin-sensitive cells were restricted to the lightest layers of the gradients (layers A and B), as described originally by Komuro and Boyse.[6] It should be noted that 80% of the cells found in the spleen are found in the denser layers. These cells never expressed the TL antigen nor did mouse fibroblasts (3T3) or TL⁻ lymphoma cells (EL4).[8, 9]

DNA synthesis (as measured by [^{3}H]TdR incorporation) in spleen cell cultures was increased by incubation of the cells with relatively high concentrations

TABLE 1

EFFECT OF THYMOPOIETIN (THYMIN) ON [^{3}H]TDR INCORPORATION BY SPLEEN CELLS *

Thymopoietin Concentration (ng/ml)	CPM/10^6 Cells ($\pm$ SD)
0	1165 $\pm$ 83
0.025	1192 $\pm$ 68
0.25	1315 $\pm$ 59
2.5	1314 $\pm$ 104
25.0	1667 $\pm$ 143
250.0	1453 $\pm$ 155

* 5 $\times$ 10^7 spleen cells from the pooled A and B layers were incubated in 10 ml of medium for 24 hours in the presence of various concentrations of thymopoietin. [^{3}H] TdR was then added to each culture for 2 hours and the cells collected on glass fiber filters, washed with distilled water, and the radioactivity incorporated counted.

of thymopoietin. The extent of this increase is shown in TABLE 1. It did not become apparent until the cells had been cultured with thymopoietin for 16 hours, but persisted for at least an additional 32 hours. These kinetics are illustrated in FIGURE 3. The biological significance of this increase in DNA synthesis remains obscure. It is possible that it represents a true mitotic effect, but antigenic stimulation or the improved survival of a small population of cells in the culture could also account for these results.

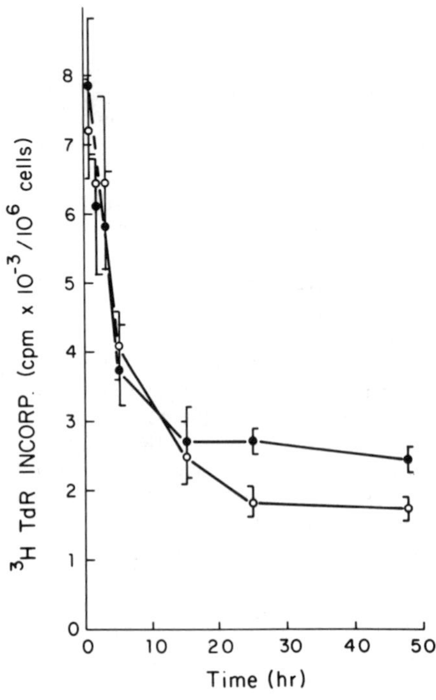

FIGURE 3. Effect of thymopoietn on the incorporation of [^{3}H]TdR by spleen cells. Spleen cells from the A and B layers of a BSA gradent were incubated at a concentration of 5$\times$ 10^6/ml in $RPMI_{1640}$ plus 4% adult bovine serum with or without 10 ng/ml thymopoietin I. [^{3}H]TdR was present for the last hour before the cells were harvested at the times indicated. The vertical lines indicate the standard error of the mean (n=6). The closed circles indicate the thymopoietin-treated cells while the open circles represent the controls.

TABLE 2

EFFECT OF THYMOPOIETIN ON MITOGEN RESPONSES
[³H]TDR INCORPORATION *

	Thymo-poietin concen-tration (ng/ml)	No Mitogen	Mitogen Con-A	PHA	LPS
Bone marrow	0	1034 ± 160	3206 ± 963	3692 ± 435	2438 ± 201
	10	1182 ± 278	3687 ± 953	3497 ± 204	2501 ± 429
Spleen	0	1747 ± 276	15,660 ± 1355	15,783 ± 1455	6705 ± 864
	10	1809 ± 302	18,984 ± 852	16,111 ± 1435	6482 ± 917
Thymus	0	207 ± 96	1220 ± 279	571 ± 380	236 ± 80
	10	234 ± 137	1187 ± 212	528 ± 67	227 ± 54

* CPM/10^6 cell ± SD. n=6. The cells were cultured for 24 hours with thymopoietin, washed, and cultured an additional 44 hours with the mitogen. [³H]TdR was present for the last 4 hours of the culture.

Lymphocytes have been characterized by their ability to respond to various mitogens.[10, 11] Unlike responses to antigens, which occur in only the limited numbers of cells bearing appropriate receptors, mitogen responses occur in large numbers of cells and have been used here as a sensitive indicator of the state of lymphoid differentiation. The effect of thymopoietin on the mitogen responses of unfractionated bone marrow, spleen, and thymus cells are shown in TABLE 2. The increase in Con-A reactivity in spleen cells is highly statistically significant ($p < 0.005$).

The effects of thymopoietin are in part obscured by the preexisting mitogen responsive population. When this population was reduced by separating the cells according to their density by flotation on BSA density gradients, the extent of the thymopoietin-induced Con-A reactivity became more evident (TABLE 3). In other experiments, the Con-A response in thymopoietin treated "B"-cell

TABLE 3

EFFECT OF THYMOPOIETIN ON THE MITOGEN RESPONSIVENESS
OF THE SPLEEN CELLS OF THE "B" * LAYER OF BSA DENSITY GRADIENT
[³H]TDR INCORPORATION †

Thymopoietin Concentration (ng/ml)	No Mitogen	PHA (2 μg/ml)	Con-A (6 μg/ml)	LPS (10 μg/ml)
0	994 ± 19	892 ± 108	1270 ± 64	1406 ± 108
10	1092 ± 26	991 ± 52	1958 ± 145	1501 ± 168

* The B layer consists of the cells formed at the interface between 23 and 25% BSA.

† Cpm/10^6 cell ± SD. n=4. The cells were cultured for 21 hours with thymopoietin, washed and cultured an additional 36 hours with mitogen. [³H]TdR was present for the last 4 hours of the culture.

TABLE 4

EFFECT OF THYMOPOIETIN ON THE PLURIPOTENTIAL STEM CELLS (CFU-S) OF THE BONE MARROW

Number of Bone Marrow Cells Injected	Number of CFU/spleen * Thymopoietin- † treated Bone Marrow	Control Bone Marrow
3.3×10^5	11.3 ± 2.6	11.6 ± 5.4
1.0×10^5	3.0 ± 1.6	2.4 ± 0.9

* Mean of 5 mice/group ± SD.

† Incubated for 18 hours in RPMI 1640 with 4% adult bovine serum containing 10 ng/ml thymopoietin I.

layers exceeded that in the controls by almost 3-fold. No change in the response to LPS (a "B"-cell mitogen[12]) was ever seen. Similar results were obtained using cultures of fractionated bone marrow, but no alterations in the responsiveness of cells taken from adult thymus have been found.

The degree of differentiation of the thymopoietin-sensitive cell has not been firmly established, but it is presumably a specifically committed thymocyte precursor (prothymocyte) and distinct from other hemopoietic cell lineages. Evidence supporting this conclusion is shown in TABLES 4 and 5. The data in TABLE 4 indicate that the totipotent stem cell (colony forming cell) found in the spleen is unaffected by thymopoietin I. Cultures incubated with 10 ng/ml for 18 hours produced the same numbers of colonies as did control cultures. Similar results were obtained with both thymopoietins using cultures of shorter duration and a variety of thymopoietin concentrations.

TABLE 5 shows the lack of effect of thymopoietin on erythropoiesis in bone marrow cell cultures. Both endogenously initiated erythropoiesis and erythropoietin-stimulated erythropoiesis in the cultures were evaluated. Neither was altered by treatment with thymopoietin.

TABLE 5

EFFECT OF THYMOPOIETIN ON HEMOGLOBIN SYNTHESIS AND ERYTHROPOIETIN (ESF) RESPONSIVENESS *

	[^{3}H]TdR Incorporation †		^{55}Fe Incorporation †	
	+ESF (0.4 U/ml)	−ESF	+ESF (0.4 U/ml)	−ESF
With Thymopoietin (10 ng ml)	1606 ± 357	1229 ± 139	26,905 ± 2813	20,598 ± 1577
Without Thymopoietin	1507 ± 138	1123 ± 166	29,725 ± 3711	22,847 ± 3711

* Bone marrow cells (10^7/ml) were cultured for 24 hours with or without thymopoietin and then for an additional 18 hours with or without ESF. During the last 6 hours of the ESF period, appropriate radioisotopic labels were present.

† CPM ± SD.

Discussion

The primary function of the thymus is to provide an appropriate microenvironment for the development of a differentiated subset of lymphocytes. In this microenvironment precursor cells (prothymocytes) acquire new surface antigens and a characteristic pattern of mitogen reactivity. These newly differentiated cells proliferate in the thymus and are then distributed to the peripheral lymphoid tissues as thymus-derived lymphocytes (T-cells). Using thymopoietin we have succeeded in reproducing the initial stages of this developmental sequence *in vitro*. Concentrations of thymopoietin as low as 3×10^{12} M are effective in the *in vitro* system. The response is detectable within two hours after exposure to thymopoietin and occurs in approximately 5% of the cells of a normal bone marrow obtained from genetically appropriate mice.[5] These cells are present in early fetal liver and the spleens of nude mice and are therefore almost certainly prethymic.[13] The rapidity of the expression of differentiated properties by these cells after exposure to thymopoietin[5, 13] suggests that the events triggered are to a large measure preprogrammed. In any event the data indicate that thymopoietin provides a specific signal for the differentiation of a committed thymocyte precursor. Other hemopoietic stem cells remain unaffected. Neither the pluripotential stem cell measured in the spleen colony assay (CFU-S) nor the erythropoietin-sensitive cell respond to thymopoietin. Similarly, no effect of thymopoietin on the maturation of bone marrow derived B-cells has been found.

Although evidence has been presented that thymopoietin is released from the thymus,[14] it is presumed that the normal or at least predominant site of the cellular interaction with these peptides is in the thymus itself where they are found in high concentrations. How the prothymocyte gets to this site has not been established.

No specific immunologic competence has yet been reported for thymopoietin-treated cells. This does not indicate that these cells are not, or do not become competent. It merely reflects the experiments that have been completed at this time. We must however note that thymocytes (i.e. the TL^+ Thy-1 $(\theta)^+$ Con-A reactive cells found in the normal thymus) have only a low level of immunologic competence in comparison with peripheral T-cells.[15, 16] These intrathymic cells, which we believe to be the *in vivo* counterpart of the thymopoietin-induced cell, undergo maturation and/or selection before they are distributed to the peripheral lymphoid tissues as immunocompetent T-cells. The influence of the thymopoietins on this further differentiation is under active investigation. The question remains; will thymopoietin-treated cells go on to become immunologically competent T-cells, with or without mitosis, or is an additional humoral signal required to initiate further development.

Summary

Thymopoietin, a polypeptide hormone isolated from bovine thymus, induced *in vitro* the differentiation of prothymocytes to cells with the antigenic and functional characteristics of intrathymic thymocytes. These changes included the acquisition of the differentiation antigens TL and Thy-1 (θ) and the ability to respond to the mitogen Con-A.

Thymopoietin appears to be highly specific in inducing the prothymocyte to thymocyte differentiation and does not affect the pluripotential stem cell measured by the colony forming assay (CFU-S), the erythropoietin-sensitive cell or B-cells.

Experiments are in progress to determine whether additional hormonal inductive signals are required to complete the differentiation of an immunologically competent T-cell.

Acknowledgments

We wish to thank Bohumila Fahmy, Shirley Carchi, Ronald King, and Miriam Siegelman for their excellent technical assistance.

References

1. Goldstein, G. 1974. Isolation of bovine thymin: a polypeptide hormone of the thymus. Nature **247:** 11–14.
2. Goldstein, G. 1975. Isolation of thymopoietin (thymin). This volume.
3. Roth, M. 1974. Matters arising. Nature **249:** 863.
4. Goldstein, G. 1974. Matters arising. Nature **249:** 863–864.
5. Basch, R. S. & G. Goldstein. 1974. Induction of T cell differentiation by thymin, a purified polypeptide hormone of the thymus. Proc. Nat. Acad. Sci. U.S. **71:** 1474–1478.
6. Komuro, K. & E. A. Boyse. 1973. *In vitro* demonstration of thymic hormone in the mouse by conversion of precursor cells into lymphocytes. Lancet **1:** 740–43.
7. Till, J. E. & E. A. McCulloch. 1961. A direct measurement of the radiation sensitivity of normal mouse bone marrow cells. Radition Research **14:** 213–22.
8. Todaro, G. J. & H. Green. 1963. Quantitative studies on the growth of mouse embryo cells in culture and the development into established lines. J. Cell Biol. **17:** 299–313.
9. Boyse, E. A., E. Stockert & L. J. Old. 1967. Modification of the antigenic structure of the cell membrane by thymus-lukemia (TL) antibody. Proc. Nat. Acad. Sci. U.S. **58:** 954–57.
10. Stobo, J. D., A. S. Rosenthal & W. E. Paul. 1972. Functional Heterogeneity of murine lymphoid cells. I. Responsiveness to and surface binding of concanavalin A and phytohemagglutinin. J. Immunol. **108:** 1–17.
11. Greaves, M. & Janossy. 1972. Elicitation of selective T and B responses by cell surface binding agents. Transplant. Rev. **11:** 87–130.
12. Andersson, B. & H. Blomgren. 1971. Evidence for thymus independent humoral antibody production in mice against polyvinylpyrrolidine and *E. coli* lipopolysaccharide. Cell Immunol. **2:** 411–424.
13. Komuro, K. & E. A. Boyse. 1973. Induction of T lymphocytes from precursor cells *in vitro* by a product of the thymus. J. Exp. Med. **138:** 479–82.
14. Goldstein, G. & W. W. Hofmann. 1969. Endocrine function of the thymus affecting neuromuscular transmission. Clin. Exp. Immunol. **4:** 181–189.
15. Takiguchi, T., W. H. Adler & R. T. Smith. 1971. Identification of mouse thymus antigen recognition function in a minor low-density, low-θ cell subpopulation Cell. Immunol. **2:** 373–80.
16. Leckband, E. & E. A. Boyse. 1971. Immunocompetent cells among mouse thymocytes, a minor population. Science **172:** 1258–60.

Discussion of the Paper

Dr. J. F. A. P. Miller: Both Dr. Scheid and Drs. Basch and Goldstein have shown the appearance of TL positive cells after incubation with thymic factors. Now TL positive cells are usually not immunocompetent cells. This is one difficulty I have in appreciating that you are inducing the differentiation pathway of immunocompetent cells; other difficulties stem from work done in Australia and in Israel that suggests that TL positive cells do not differentiate into TL negative cells. There are two different pathways of differentiation, one which leads to the formation of T-positive cells which are never competent, and another one which goes through the pathway of never forming TL but just becomes immunocompetent.

Dr. R. Basch: My answer to that is I believe it is irrelevant to the point and my paper. I do not know if these are immunologically competent cells, and we have not made the claim at this point that this is so, are these cells immunologically competent? We incubate these bone marrow cells with thymopoietin, then TL antigens appear. These are antigens which are found in the majority of cells in the normal thymus and these cells do respond to Con-A. Now whether this is an aberrant pathway of differentiation as a consequence of some physiological regulation we cannot tell. Ninety-nine percent of the cells which appear in the thymus are fated to die there as TL positive cells and never leave. Thus we are saying that we are mimicking what happens in the bone marrow; 99% of these cells are TL positive, θ-positive, and there may be a minority population which will be immunocompetent.

Dr. J. F. A. P. Miller: Did you, then, imply that thymopoietin induces competence?

Dr. R. Basch: I did not imply that. What I said is that during a period of 2 to 4 hours in culture these cells are immunocompetent. Now you are asking "what will happen to these cells later." Will they die or would they die in an animal? Would they acquire competence? We have some suggestive data that in an animal they will mature. We don't know whether that requires another factor, or whether they are already precommitted to maturation, or whether only 1% of them go on to maturity. I believe none of the data presented here on different factors that have been highly purified are incompatible with one another. We are convinced that the thymopoietins are physiological products of the thymus. We have no data that they are the only physiological product of the thymus or that they are necessary and efficient for thymocyte maturation. We are claiming, however, that they initiate it.

Dr. Cohen: I would like to comment about the model that Dr. Allan Goldstein described this morning concerning the mechanism of action of thymosin. We believe it takes a pre-T-cell, which is θ minus, and "pushes" it to a TL cell, a cell that would be highly reactive to Con-A and in the presence of antigen and thymosin would then be pushed to a T-2 cell.

Dr. R. Basch: I have no disagreement with that model. At this point I don't think there is any evidence that thymosin does both things, because everything that works in fraction three and four is called thymosin.

THYMOSIN: EFFECTS ON NORMAL HUMAN BLOOD T-CELLS *

Joseph Wybran, Alan S. Levin, and H. Hugh Fudenberg

Department of Medicine
University of California School of Medicine
San Francisco, California 94143

Allan L. Goldstein

Division of Biochemistry
University of Texas Medical Branch
Galveston, Texas 77550

Introduction

It has recently been shown that thymosin, an extract of calf thymus, can rapidly induce the appearance of specific T-cell markers on lymphoid cells of mice.[1–3] It has been postulated that thymosin produces this effect by acting on a stem T-cell to confer upon it T-cell characteristics. Thus, thymosin may be the factor responsible for the differentiation of T-cells within the thymus. In both animals and man it is assumed that the T-cells present in the peripheral blood are fully differentiated. Stem cells are probably present in the bone marrow but rarely, if at all, in normal peripheral blood.

Thymosin is not species specific; indeed, most of the extracts are prepared from calf thymus and have been assayed in mice.[1–3] Therefore, calf thymosin presumably could similarly affect human cells. The present data confirm this hypothesis.

In view of the difficulties of obtaining normal human bone marrow, we decided to investigate the action of thymosin on human peripheral blood lymphocytes through their ability to bind to normal sheep red blood cells (SRBC). Such binding produces a morphologic configuration termed a "rosette." The rosette-forming cells (RFC) so detected are T-cells.[4–7] In the present reports two techniques were used for rosette formation. (1) One, termed the "active" rosette test, requires only a short incubation time between SRBC and lymphocytes;[8–10] it detects some subpopulation(s) of T-cells. (2) The other rosette test requires a substantially longer incubation time between SRBC and lymphocytes; it probably detects all or almost all T-cells.[11]

Materials and Methods

Thymosin was extracted from calf thymus and purified fraction 5 isolated as previously described.[12, 13] Extracts of control calf organs (brain, liver and spleen) were similarly prepared. Thymosin and each of the other organ extracts was diluted in Hepes-RPMI 1640 Medium (Grand Island Biological Co.,

* This work was supported by grants from the United States Public Health Service (HD-05894-3), American Cancer Society (IM-16H), National Cancer Institute (CA-14108, CA-15419) and the John Hartford Foundation, Inc.

New York) at a final concentration of 1, 10, 100 1000 μg of protein per ml. One "unit" of transfer factor was prepared using a modification of the previously published method.[14, 15] This material was diluted in Hepes-RPMI, (1:10 to 1:10,000 dilutions).

Mononuclear cells were separated from heparinized blood by spinning over a Ficoll-Hypaque layer.[16] The cells were washed and resuspended in phosphate buffered-saline (PBS; Dulbecco's formula, pH 7.3) at a final concentration of 1×10^6 cells per 0.03 ml of Hepes RPMI. For each rosette test (in both active and total methods), 1.10^6 cells were placed in a plastic tube (13×100 mm, Falcon Plastics, Oxnard, Ca. 93030). To these cells was added 0.03 ml of thymosin or other organ extract (or Hepes-RPMI without any organ extract). The cells were incubated for one hour at 37° C in a waterbath. In some cases, duplicate tubes were incubated for two hours at 37° C in a waterbath. The cells were then washed three times in PBS and assayed for active and total T-RFC as previously described.[8, 9] Basically, in the "active" rosette test, the cells are incubated in heat inactivated fetal calf serum for 60 minutes at 37° C in a 5% CO_2 incubator. SRBC are added to the cells after the incubation; the tubes are spun for 5 minutes at 200 *g* at room temperature. The tubes are gently shaken by wrist motion to resuspend the cells, and the "active" T-RFC (TE_a) are immediately read in a hemocytometer. To measure total T-RFC, (TE_c) heat-inactivated fetal calf serum, and SRBC are added to the mononuclear cells. The tubes are spun for 5 minutes at 400 *g* at room temperature. The tubes stand at room temperature for one hour. The cells are then resuspended and RFC (TE_t) are counted.[11]

In some experiments B-lymphocytes were studied before and after thymosin incubation, using as a criterion for B-cells the detection of surface immunoglobulins with a fluorescent, anti-immunoglobulin serum. Monocytes were also studied by counting the percentage of cells phagocitizing yeast particles. In another set of experiments, mononuclear cells were separated into a T-cell-rich population and T-cell-poor population, using a method previously described.[17] The cells so obtained were incubated with and without thymosin, washed, and assayed for both "active" and "total" T-RFC.

Results

An increase in the percentage of TE_a in the peripheral blood was always noted (TABLE 1) after addition of thymosin in concentrations as low as 1 μg/ml. The increase with 10 μg/ml were greater than with 1 μg/ml. The increases with 100 μg and 1000 μg/ml were, however, not much greater than with 10 μg and a type of plateau was reached for these concentrations. When duplicate tests were run for a two-hour incubation, the values obtained were slightly higher than with a one-hour incubation. With thymosin preparations stored more than three months at —20° C, an increase was not noted with the one-hour incubation, but was noted with the two-hour incubation. Activity of the spleen extract was noted only in two experiments out of five. None of the other control extracts (brain, liver) induced any change in the percentage of TE_a or TE_t. The percentage of monocytes ingesting yeast particles was not affected by thymosin. Similarly, the percentage of B-cells did not change. In one experiment, where peripheral blood cells were incubated with thymosin at 4° C, no changes in TE_a or total T-RFC were noted.

TABLE 1

THYMOSIN AND NORMAL BLOOD HUMAN T-ROSETTES

Tests *	Thymosin concentration (μg/ml of protein)				
	0	1	10	100	1000
active T-rosettes	18.6 (7–34)	24.5 † (10–39)	30.1 † (14–40)	28.1 † (14–45)	28.3 † (10–41)
total R-rosettes	60.8 (50–74)	58.8 (52–70)	62.4 (42–79)	62.2 (51–71)	59.6 (40–72)

* The data represent the mean of the results of eight normal subjects. The results are expressed in percentage of RFC. The ranges of the values are given between parentheses.

† These values are significantly different (p at least <0.05) from the controls using the student t-test for paired data.

The incubation of thymosin with cell populations rich in, or depleted of, T-cells gave interesting results. In the T-cell-rich population the TE_a always increased, but the percentage of TE_t remained unchanged (Table 2). In contrast, thymosin produced no changes in either TE_a or TE_t in the T-cell-poor populations (Table 3). In experiments where transfer factor was used alone or in the presence of thymosin, TE_a or TE_t were not modified. Preincubation of lymphocytes with transfer factor followed by thymosin did not yield higher percentages of TE_a or TE_t than thymosin alone. Similarly, preincubation of lymphocytes with thymosin followed by transfer factor did not give higher percentages of TE_a or TE_t than thymosin alone.

Discussion

Using rosette formation with SRBC and human peripheral blood lymphocytes as a marker for T-cells, the present study demonstrates that thymosin can increase the percentage of "active" T-RFC. However, the percentage of total T-RFC remains unaffected by thymosin. In previous papers, the technical differences and the possible different functional meanings between TE_a and TE_t were stressed.[18, 19] Technically, SRBC and lymphocytes are incubated together for 5 minutes to perform the "active" rosette test, whereas a long incubation is required for measuring the total T-rosettes. We have postulated that the "active" rosette test is a good reflection of the overall T-cell competence.[18, 19] Indeed, rosette formation is dependent on active mechanisms and also requires an intact glycolytic system. Since the "active" rosette test, because of the short incubation time, represents a point in the curve of the dynamics of rosette formation, one can hypothesize that a low value reflects a defect in the dynamics of rosette formation. Therefore, the "active" test is more sensitive in detecting T-cell defects than the total T-rosette assay. Alternatively, the "active" rosette test may detect some T-cells with high affinity receptors for SRBC. The percentage of such high affinity lymphocytes may be more dependent on active mechanisms than lymphocytes with low affinity receptors. In any case, it seems logical to postulate that the "active" test measures only subpopulation(s) of total T-cells (that are measured in the total T-RFC test). In other data described in detail elsewhere, we showed that these two tests are not always directly correlated. For example, in patients with cancer and in various immunological disorders the "active" test may be low, but the total T-RFC are in the normal range.[10] Furthermore, induction of immune functions after transfer factor therapy[9, 20] or intralesional injection of BCG can increase the TE_a without affecting the TE_t.[21] These data strongly support the hypothesis that the two tests, although both measuring human T-cells, have different meanings. A recent report supports this hypothesis: patients with lupus erythematosus disseminated always had low active T-RFC, but their total T-RFC were not always decreased.[22]

In the present study, the differences between the two tests have also given various information about the mode of action of thymosin. Using normal peripheral blood lymphocytes as target cells, thymosin was found always to induce a very rapid (one hour) increase in percentage of TE_a. In contrast, the percentage of total T-rosettes was not affected. Transfer factor did not modify the TE_a or TE_t in presence or absence of thymosin. (Incidentally, thymosin also did not modify the percentage of B-cells and of monocytes.)

TABLE 2

THYMOSIN ACTION ON T-CELL-RICH POPULATIONS OF NORMAL BLOOD

Tests *	Thymosin concentration (μg/ml of protein)				
	0	1	10	100	1000
active T-rosettes	50.8 (20–77)	53.4 † (23–81)	63.0 † (25–82)	62.8 † (34–75)	66.4 † (39–85)
total R-rosettes	86.8 (72–94)	84.6 (74–90)	83.8 (63–92)	86.0 (80–92)	89.6 (81–96)

* The data represent the mean of the results of the testing of the T-cell-rich population isolated from the blood of five normal subjects. The results are expressed in percentage of RFC. The ranges of the values are between parentheses.

† The values are significantly different (p at least <0.05) from the controls using the student t-test for paired data.

TABLE 3

THYMOSIN ACTION ON T-CELL-POOR POPULATIONS OF NORMAL BLOOD

Tests *	Thymosin concentration (μg/ml of protein)				
	0	1	10	100	1000
active T-rosettes	7.2 (3–17)	7.2 † (2–15)	7.0 † (3–19)	6.4 † (3–14)	7.0 † (3–15)
total T-rosettes	26.6 (15–51)	27.4 † (11–44)	30.6 † (16–57)	29.0 † (14–47)	27.0 † (21–38)

* The data represent the mean of the results of the testing of the T-cell-poor population isolated from the blood of the same five normals subjects as in TABLE 2. The results are expressed in percentage of RFC. The ranges of the values are given between parentheses.

† None of these values are significantly different from the controls using Student's t-test for paired data.

Thus, at first analysis, these results appear analogous to the induction of specific T-cell markers by thymosin in mice. However, it has been assumed that, in mice, thymosin acts on a stem T-cell rather than on a T-cell already possessing specific T-cell markers.[1-3] This hypothesis cannot be applied to the present study. Firstly, very few, if any, stem cells are present in human peripheral blood. Secondly, even if one assumes that the blood null cells (lymphocytes lacking both T and B markers) represent stem cells, the hypothesis is still unlikely. Indeed, in some cases, thymosin increased the percentage of blood TE_a by more than 10%. The percentage of null cells in normal blood does not exceed 5%. Since thymosin did not affect the percentage of B-cells, it is clear that thymosin must act on subpopulations of blood T-cells detected in the "active" test. Furthermore, since even with increasing concentrations of thymosin a plateau of TE_a was obtained, one must conclude that only some T-cells are sensitive to thymosin. In order to verify these hypotheses directly, a T-cell-rich population and a T-cell-poor population were separated from the peripheral blood using a previously described method.[17] Thymosin quite consistently increased the percentage of TE_a in the quasi-pure T-cell population and TE_t remained unchanged. In contrast, in the T-cell-poor fraction, neither TE_a nor TE_t were affected. These observations allow the following conclusions: Firstly, it appears clear that thymosin acts on T-cells. Indeed, the population rich in T-cells is almost pure using the criterion of total T-RFC. Since the increase in TE_a was always very great in this population, one must conclude that thymosin acts on peripheral blood T-cells converting "nonactive" T-cells into "active" T-cells. When we introduced the concept of "active" T cells, it was based on the observation of the correlation obtained in some immunodeficient patients between the "active" test and their immune competence.[9, 18] The present findings strongly support this concept. Indeed, thymosin has been shown to increase lymphocyte responsiveness to phytohemagglutinin (PHA) and in mixed leukocyte cultures.[23] These observations are best explained by an activation of T-cells. One could, only by analogy, compare a "nonactive" T-cell as a T_1 cell and an "active" T cell as a T_2 cell. However, this analogy has to remain very restricted, since conversion of T_1 to T_2 requires the presence of antigen, whereas a "nonactive" T-RFC can become an "active" RFC, *in vitro,* only in presence of thymosin without antigen. The increase in blood TE_a seen, *in vivo,* in subjects receiving transfer factor or intralesional BCG into malignant melanoma nodules probably depends on other mechanisms than the one described in the present study.

The direct action of thymosin on normal human blood T-cells does not exclude the possibility that thymosin can also act on stem T-cells or perhaps on null cells.

Secondly, thymosin appears to act more selectively on certain T-cell subpopulation(s). Indeed, increasing concentrations of thymosin were not associated with an increased percentage of TE_a in unseparated blood. There was a plateau between 10 and 1000 μg/ml, suggesting that thymosin acts only on some cell populations. Furthermore, no changes in either TE_a or TE_t was noted in the T-cell-poor fraction. This is another argument for the now compelling evidence of the heterogeneity of T-lymphocytes. In previous studies, we showed the cells from the T-cell-rich fraction respond to both PHA and pokeweed mitogen (PWM).[11] Preliminary data indicate that the T-cells isolated from the T-cell-poor fraction respond better to PHA but very slowly or not at all to PWM.[24] Thus, subsets of different human T-cells show a different pattern of response to same mitogens. Other functional data (e.g. cytotoxicity) comparing these various T-cells subpopulations are not yet available. The action of thymosin on T-cells is thus selective and affects only some T-cell subpopulations. Their nature remains unclear.

The present data indicate a new target for thymosin. No attempt was made to investigate the mechanism whereby thymosin acts on the regulation of the receptors for SRBC. It appears that thymosin acts selectively on some subsets of T-cells. One can postulate that the functional analysis of these subsets might lead to the concept of specificity of action of thymosin.

Finally, one can predict with some confidence that with technical improvements the active rosette test will become useful in measuring thymosin activity. This assay system should also be of value in predicting in which clinical conditions thymosin may be beneficial.

References

1. Bach, J. F., M. Dardenne, A. L. Goldstein, A. Guha & A. White. 1971. Proc. Nat. Acad. Sci. **68:** 2734.
2. Goldstein, A. L., A. Guha, M. M. Katz, M. M. Hardy & A. White. 1972. Proc. Nat. Acad. Sci. **69:** 1800.
3. Komuro, K. & E. A. Boyse. 1973. Lancet **1:** 740.
4. Wybran, J. & H. H. Fudenberg. 1971. Trans. Assoc. Am. Phys. **84:** 239.
5. Wybran, J., M. C. Carr & H. H. Fudenberg. 1972. J. Clin. Invest. **51:** 2537.
6. Fröland, S. S. 1972. Scand. J. Immunol. **1:** 269.
7. Jondal, M., G. Holm & H. Wigzell. 1972. J. Exp. Med. **136:** 207.
8. Wybran, J., M. C. Carr & H. H. Fudenberg. 1973. Clin. Immunol. and Immunopathol. **1:** 408.
9. Wybran, J., A. S. Levin, L. E. Spitler & H. H. Fudenberg. 1973. N. Engl. J. Med. **288:** 710.
10. Wybran, J. & H. H. Fudenberg. 1973. J. Clin. Invest. **52:** 1026.
11. Wybran, J., S. Chantler & H. H. Fudenberg. 1973. Lancet **1:** 126.
12. Hooper, J. A., G. H. Cohen, A. White & A. L. Goldstein. 1973. Fed. Proceed. **32:** 489a.
13. Hooper, J. A., G. H. Cohen, G. B. Thurman, M. McDaniel & A. L. Goldstein. This volume.
14. Levin, A. S., L. E. Spitler, D. P. Stites & H. H. Fudenberg. 1970. Proc. Nat. Acad. Sci. **67:** 821.
15. Spitler, L. E., A. S. Levin & H. H. Fudenberg. 1973. Methods in Cancer Research **8:** 59.
16. Böyum, A. 1968. Scand. J. Clin. Lab. Invest. **21**(Supp. 97)**:** 1.
17. Wybran, J., S. Chantler & H. H. Fudenberg. 1973. J. Immunol. **110:** 1157.
18. Wybran, J. & H. H. Fudenberg. 1973. N. Engl. J. Med. **288:** 1072.
19. Wybran, J. & H. H. Fudenberg. 1973. *In* Primary Immunodeficiency Diseases. R. A. Good, Ed. The National Foundation. New York, N.Y.
20. Fudenberg, H. H., A. S. Levin, L. E. Spitler, J. Wybran & V. Byers. 1974. Hospital Practice **9:** 95.
21. Wybran, J., L. E. Spitler, R. Liberman & H. H. Fudenberg. 1974. Clin. Research. In press.
22. Yu, D. T., P. J. Clements, J. B. Peter, J. Levy, H. E. Paulus & E. V. Barnett. 1974. Arthritis Rheumat. **17:** 37.
23. Cohen, G., J. A. Hooper & A. L. Goldstein. This volume.
24. Belohradsky, B. H., J. Wybran & H. H. Fudenberg. In preparation.

Discussion of the Paper

Dr. M. Scheinberg (*Boston University, Boston, Massachusetts*): Are you sure that you are dealing with the same rosette formation that Coomb deals with because he cannot block his phenomenon with antiserum and I understand you can. Also, have you checked for the possibility that your preparation is contaminated with neuraminidase-like material and that is why you see an enhancement of the active T-cell.

Dr. J. Wybran: In answer to the first question, Coombs described the binding between sheep red blood cells and normal lymphocytes and he could not inhibit this binding by antiimmunoglobulin serum. But at that time he was not thinking that they would be T-cells; he said they were a subpopulation of lymphocytes. We are not using the same type of method. He showed 30 to 60% of these cells in peripheral blood and these are obviously T-cells. We have about 25% positive cells. Thus I believe that we are probably looking at the same phenomenon. Now when you refer to my earlier work where I could block rosette formation with antiimmunoglobulin serum, I just want to remind you that I was using at that time a very poor technique. We were incubating cells in PBS. I was finding only 3 to 4% rosette-forming cells. Recently there was a paper showing that some rosette-forming cells can carry surface immunoglobulins and that might explain my findings that antiimmunoglobulin serum can block rosette formation. Furthermore, as you know, activated T-cells possess F receptors.

Dr. A. Goldstein: In answer to the second question, fraction five contains no neuronimidase activity. I would like to make one other comment about fraction five that many investigators are using. It is not the totally purified thymosin, but it contains the biologically active materials. We do have some biological evidence that the purified thymosin is inactive in a number of systems. We do not have conclusive evidence that everything from fraction five to eight is contained within the same molecule. I would suspect that there is going to be a whole family of biologically active thymosins. Now obviously we are going to try and characterize chemically as well as biologically all of the thymosins that we can, and it may be very much like the prostoglandin story.

Dr. M. Schlesinger: I would like to question the use of the term "active." It seems that the rosettes one tests for in man seem to be "active." If one does a rosette test in the cold, for instance, or with various inhibitors, one does not get rosettes, unlike other types of rosettes that we know of in the mouse. Thus my question is: wouldn't it be more correct to say that there are subsets of human T-cells, maybe with a different change or with different properties, which tend more or less easily to form rosettes? One can "push" with thymosin the cell surface property towards that kind of condition which would favor the formation of rosettes. So rather than distinguish between active and nonactive fractions, one should distinguish between rosettes more susceptible to forming rosettes and those less susceptible.

Dr. J. Wybran: I can agree with you about this, but the terminology of active was really meant to imply those cells actively involved in cell-mediated immunity. They may have indeed high affinity receptors for sheep red blood cells and maybe thymosin activates such receptors.

ACTIVATION OF T-CELL ROSETTES IN IMMUNODEFICIENT PATIENTS BY THYMOSIN

D. W. Wara and A. J. Ammann

Division of Pediatric Immunology
University of California, San Francisco
San Francisco, California 94143

Introduction

The reconstitution of cellular immunity in neonatally thymectomized mice following transplantation of thymus in cell-impermeable millipore chambers [1, 2] first suggested the presence of a thymic hormone. Subsequently, Goldstein *et al.*[3] purified a substance isolated from bovine thymus, termed thymosin. Bovine thymosin fraction V was shown to have the following capabilities in neonatally thymectomized mice: it decreased the incidence of wasting disease [4] and increased the development of cell-mediated immune responses, including the capacity of host cells to elicit a normal graft-versus-host reaction [5] and to reject histoincompatible skin grafts.[6] Mice injected with thymosin were shown to develop resistance to progressive tumor growth after inoculation with Maloney Sarcoma virus.[7] Recently, Komuro and Boyse [8] succeeded in generating T-lymphocytes with specific antigenic markers by incubating mice spleen and bone marrow cells *in vitro* with thymosin.

Evidence for thymosin activity in man is limited; the hormone has not been administered *in vivo.* However, a patient with thymic hypoplasia and hypoparathyroidism (DiGeorge syndrome) had partial reconstitution of cellular immunity following transplantation of a fetal thymus in a millipore chamber.[9] Reconstitution of the patient's lymphocyte response to phytohemagglutinin was presumably mediated by a hormone. Select patients with thymic hypoplasia and immunoglobulin synthesis, treated with transfer factor and thymus transplantation, experienced reconstitution of cellular immunity within three weeks that lasted from three months to one year and was not associated with thymus cell engraftment. Clinical improvement was temporally related to improved cellular immunity.[10] As no cell chimerism occurred, it is probable that the transplanted thymus glands were supplying a hormone with a limited production.

A method for the direct quantitation of serum thymosin is not available. Until recently, the bioassay of Bach *et al.*[11] that measures the capacity of thymosin to reconstitute the ability of azathioprine sensitive mouse spleen cells to form rosettes was the single method for assessing human serum thymosin. We have modified the T-cell rosette assay (E rosettes) to identify those patients whose depressed T-cell rosettes increase following incubation with thymosin. The assay system does not involve animals and is reproducible. This assay may help to predict patient response to thymosin therapy *in vivo.*

Methods

Patient's lymphocytes were isolated by Hypaque-ficoll gradient and adjusted to 4×10^6/ml. Sheep red blood cells (SRBC) were washed three times and a 1% suspension was prepared. All washes and suspensions were in Hank's Balanced Salt solution supplemented with 10% heat-inactivated SRBC absorbed fetal calf serum. Lymphocytes, 0.25 ml, were incubated with SRBC, 0.25 ml. Bovine thymosin fraction V, supplied by Dr. A. Goldstein, was added in concentrations varying from 50 μg/ml to 500 μg/ml to the cell suspension. The suspension was incubated for five minutes at 37° C, centrifuged for 5 minutes at 200 $\times$ g, and then incubated at 4° C for 18 hours. Following incubation, the supernatant was discarded, and a wet preparation of the cell suspension prepared. In each preparation, 200 lymphocytes were counted under phase microscopy and the percentage of lymphocytes with three or more SRBC attached was determined. All preparations were performed in triplicate; the mean maximum difference between triplicate determinations was 4%. Normal T-cell rosette values in our laboratory were 56 ± 5%.

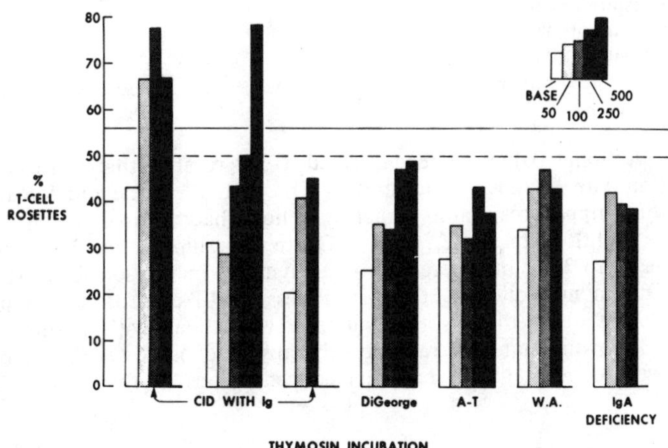

FIGURE 1. Primary immunodeficiency.

Results

Seven children with primary immunodeficiency had depressed T-cell rosettes ranging from 20% to 45%; following incubation with varying concentrations of thymosin their maximum T-cell rosettes ranged from 43% to 78% (FIGURE 1). Primary immunodeficiency diseases evaluated included cellular immunodeficiency with immunoglobulin synthesis, DiGeorge syndrome, ataxia-telangiectasia, Wiscott-Aldrich syndrome, and isolated IgA deficiency. Maximum percent increase in T-cell rosettes (% increase = final % − initial %/initial %) ranged from 38% to 152% (TABLE 1). The greatest maximum percent increase in T-cell rosettes was found in patients with cellular immunodeficiency and immunoglobulin synthesis. The increase in each patients' T-cell rosettes following incubation with varying thymosin concentrations had a dose-response relationship.

TABLE 1

MAXIMUM PERCENT INCREASE IN T-CELL ROSETTES FOLLOWING THYMOSIN INCUBATION

Primary Immunodeficiency Disease	Percent
Cellular immunodeficiency with Ig synthesis	74
Cellular immunodeficiency with Ig synthesis	152
Cellular immunodeficiency with Ig synthesis	63
Cellular immunodeficiency with Ig synthesis	125
DiGeorge syndrome	96
Ataxia-telangiectasia	59
Wiskott-Aldrich syndrome	38
IgA deficiency	58
Secondary Immunodeficiency	
Viral upper respiratory infection	118
Nasopharynx carcinoma	244
Nasopharynx carcinoma	30

Three additional patients had depressed T-cell rosettes that were activated by incubation with thymosin (FIGURE 2). The first, a 25 year old female with a severe viral upper respiratory tract infection, had normal T-cell rosettes (65%) one month prior to her illness. During her illness, her T-cell rosettes were depressed to 33% but increased with thymosin incubation to a maximum of 72%. One month following the viral illness, her T-cell rosettes were again normal (72%) without thymosin activation. Two patients with nasopharyngeal carcinoma, following standard radiation therapy, had depressed T-cell rosettes that increased to normal with maximal concentrations of thymosin.

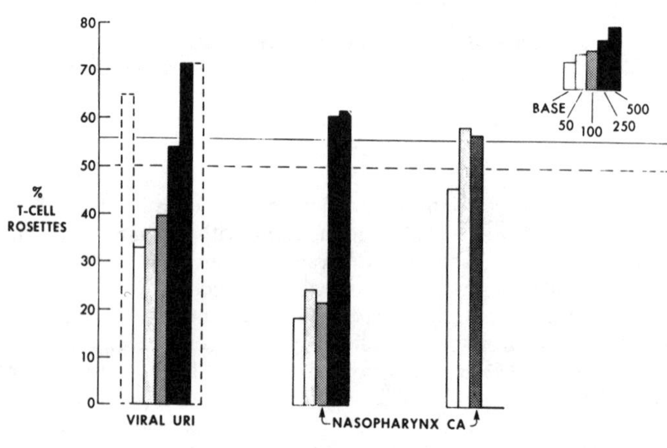

FIGURE 2. Secondary immunodeficiency.

Four patients were studied who had received fetal thymus transplants in an attempt to reconstitute their cellular immunity (FIGURE 3). The first, 6 months old with severe combined immunodeficiency, had 5% T-cell rosettes prior to transplant. One month posttransplant his T-cell rosettes had increased to 17% but did not respond further to incubation with thymosin. The child subsequently died with pseudomonas sepsis and graft-versus-host reaction. A second child with severe combined immunodeficiency was studied two years after a thymus transplantation that had resulted in successful reconstitution of cellular immunity and thymus cell engraftment detected by HL-A chimerism.[12] His T-cell rosettes were normal (56%) and did not respond significantly to incubation with thymosin. Two additional children with cellular immunodeficiency and immunoglobulin synthesis had depressed T-cell rosettes prior to transplantation, an increase to near-normal values following transplantation, and no further increase with thymosin incubation.

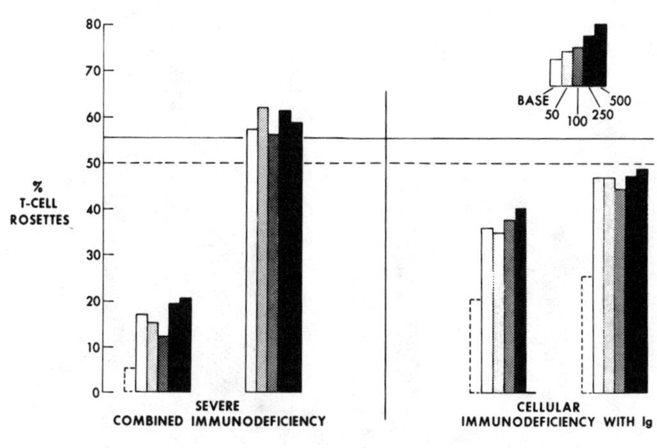

FIGURE 3. Immunodeficiency after thymus transplant.

Ten normal patients with normal T-cell rosettes did not have significant activation of rosettes following incubation with thymosin. Maximum percentage increase in T-cell rosettes ranged from 0% to 13% with a mean of 4.7%.

Bovine spleen and liver fraction 5, prepared in the same manner as thymosin fraction V by Dr. A. Goldstein, were incubated in varying doses with T-cell rosettes to evaluate the possibility of nonspecific biological activity in the thymosin preparation. An example of such a control experiment is presented in FIGURE 4. The patient had cellular immunodeficiency with immunoglobulin synthesis and T-cell rosettes of 30%. Following incubation with 25 and 100 μg/ml suspensions of thymosin, T-cell rosettes increased; there was no increase at these concentrations with either spleen or liver fractions. However, with 250 and 500 μg/ml suspensions, spleen fraction V incubation increased T-cell rosettes minimally to 35% and 37%. Liver fraction V at these concentrations activated T-cell rosettes to approximately the same extent that thymosin did.

Discussion

T-cell rosette formation is felt to quantitate the number of circulating thymus-derived lymphocytes in man.[13] However, whether the cells are precursor or mature thymic cells is unknown. In mice, Raff *et al.*[14] have hypothesized that thymosin acts on T_0 cells driving them to T_1 cells and allowing them to progress to T_2 or immunocompetent cells. If the addition of a thymic hormone to a cell suspension containing human peripheral lymphocytes and SRBC can increase the number of T-cell rosettes formed in immunodeficient patients, two possibilities exist. The hormone may be acting on bone-marrow-derived lymphocytes allowing them to form spontaneous T-cell rosettes. Although the work presented does not exclude this possibility since the simultaneous immunofluorescence of lymphocytes and T-cell rosette formation was not examined, the results favor the alternative explanation. That is, thymosin activates thymic precursor cells to become mature thymic-derived lymphocytes capable of forming T-cell rosettes. Thymosin appears necessary to maintain such a population of cells.

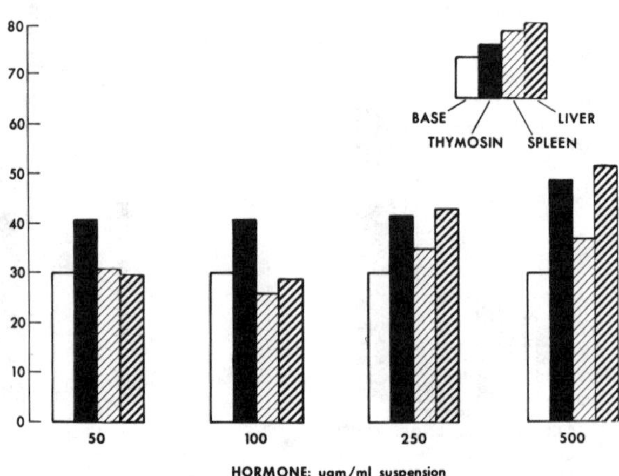

FIGURE 4. Rosette—thymosin, spleen, and liver incubation.

Patients may have a deficiency of thymic precursor cells: in this instance, addition of thymosin would not be expected to increase T-cell rosette formation. Two patients with severe combined immunodeficiency treated with thymus transplantation and transfer factor were included in this study. The first child died two months following transplant. Although his T-cell rosettes increased from 5% to 17% during this interval, the addition of thymosin did not further activate the system *in vitro*. The limiting factor for increase in T-cell rosettes following thymosin incubation was probably a markedly decreased number of thymic precursor cells.

Two children with cellular immunodeficiency and immunoglobulin synthesis were studied who had received transfer factor and fetal thymus transplants.

Neither had an increase in their T-cell rosettes following incubation with thymosin. Although children with this diagnosis probably represent a heterogeneous population,[15] we have found that repeat thymus transplantation is necessary to maintain normal cellular immunity and that cell chimerism does not occur. It is possible that in this patient population, thymus transplantation supplies thymosin *in vivo*. Maximum numbers of mature thymic-derived lymphocytes are present *in vivo* and therefore further incubation with thymosin *in vitro* does not increase the percent of T-cell rosettes. In the future, thymosin injections may substitute for repeat fetal thymus transplantation in this patient population.

Control studies in normals indicated that T-cell rosettes do not increase further following thymosin incubation. The assay system used probably quantitates all circulating mature T-cells.

In other control studies, activation of rosettes by a tenfold increase in concentration over thymosin of spleen and liver fractions was not unexpected; thymosin probably is present at lower concentrations in these tissues. The marked activation of T-cell rosettes by high concentrations of liver fraction V is interesting but unexplainable.

Since we have demonstrated that viremia in a normal person can temporarily suppress T-cell rosettes that are then activated by incubation with thymosin *in vitro,* caution must be used in interpreting an isolated study in patients with cellular immunodeficiency who have a known increased susceptibility to viral infections. However, three of the patients with cellular immunodeficiency and immunoglobulin synthesis were evaluated serially when they were clinically well; the results were consistent. The limited number of studies performed on patients with carcinoma allows only for speculation that in a subpopulation of these patients thymosin therapy *in vivo* may prove appropriate.

Summary

1. Thymosin increases T-cell rosettes in a dose response relationship in primary immunodeficiency; 2. Thymosin increases T-cell rosettes to normal in secondary immunodeficiency; 3. Thymic precursor cells are required for an increase in T-cell rosettes following thymosin incubation; 4. Normal T-cell rosettes do not increase further when incubated with thymosin; 5. Tenfold greater concentrations of liver and spleen extracts are necessary for effects comparable to thymosin; 6. Increase in T-cell rosettes following incubation with thymosin *in vitro* may predict which patients will respond to thymosin therapy *in vivo*.

References

1. Osoba, D. & J. F. A. P. Miller. 1964. J. Exp. Med. **111:** 177–194.
2. Osoba, D. 1965. J. Exp. Med. **122:** 633–650.
3. Goldstein, A. L., A. Geeha, M. M. Katz, *et al.* 1972. Proc. Nat. Acad. Sci. **69:** 1800–1803.
4. Asanuma, Y., A. L. Goldstein & A. White. 1970. Endocrinology **86:** 600–610.
5. Law, L. W., A. L. Goldstein & A. White. 1968. Nature **219:** 1391–1393.
6. Goldstein, A. L., Y. Asanuma, J. R. Battisto, *et al.* 1970. J. Immunol. **104:** 359–366.

7. ZISBLATT, M., A. L. GOLDSTEIN, F. LILLY, *et al.* 1970. Proc. Nat. Acad. Sci. **66:** 1170–1174.
8. KOMURO, K. & E. A. BOYSE. 1973. Lancet **1:** 740–743.
9. STEELE, R. W., C. LIMAS & G. B. THURMAN, *et al.* 1972. New Engl. J. Med. **287:** 787–791.
10. AMMANN, A. J., D. W. WARA & S. SALMON. 1974. Cell. Immunol. In press.
11. BACH, J. F., M. DARDENNE & A. L. GOLDSTEIN, *et al.* 1971. Proc. Nat. Acad. Sci. **68:** 2734–2738.
12. AMMANN, A. J., D. W. WARA & S. SALMON, *et al.* 1973. New Engl. J. Med. **289:** 5–9.
13. JONDAHL, M., G. HOLM & H. WIGZELL. 1972. J. Exp. Med. **136:** 207.
14. RAFF, M. C. & H. CANTOR. 1970. *In* Progress in Immunology. B. Amos, Ed. : 83. Academic Press, New York, N.Y.
15. LAWLOR, G. J., A. J. AMMANN, W. C. WRIGHT, *et al.* 1974. J. Pediat. **84:** 183–192.

DISCUSSION OF THE PAPER

DR. A. GOLDSTEIN: I wish to comment that you have a beautiful study which has good clinical application. Your last comment about using this type of assay, as well as the activated rosette assay, is probably going to be very meaningful in looking at patients considered for thymosin therapy.

DR. R. MARCUS (*Montefiore Hospital & Albert Einstein College of Medicine, Bronx, N.Y.*): We have been following a 58-year-old woman for approximately 5 to 6 years after removal of a thymoma. Four years after removal of the thymoma she developed a severe rheumatoid arthritis-like illness, agammaglobulinemia and chronic mucocutaneous candidasis. Our studies with Dr. Arthur Grazell, and Caroline Beck and with Dr. Winchester and his group have shown that she has approximately 97 percent T-cells. Her total lymphocyte count is normal. We cannot detect any immunoglobulin-bearing cells or complement receptors. My question is, have you studied any thymoma patients and have you studied any normal patients who have had thymectomies for open heart surgery or sternal splitting procedures? Why do you think we have these normal T-cells so long after removal of a thymus?

DR. D. WARA: The answer to your first question is that I have not studied anyone who has had a thymoma and a thymectomy. In answer to your second question is that we have also not studied normal patients who have had thymectomies. However, we did study a population of 25 and 30 year old individuals who underwent irradiation of the thymus as young children to see if they had any change in their cellular immunity. We were unable to detect any marked changes. I have not studied anyone similar to your patient.

DR. J. BACH: We have not studied normal people having thymectomy. I believe this is difficult technically. We have however looked at the affects of adult thymectomy in the pig, since the pig has spontaneous rosettes which do resemble very much the human phenomenon. Ten or 20 days following adult thymectomy there was no decrease in the total number of rosettes. We did not look at active vs. non-active rosettes, but I think there is, of course, a very simple explanation that this rosette phenomenon does detect long-lived T-cells, although there is no reason to think that adult thymectomy should suppress this phenomenon in a matter of days.

Dr. L. Pachman (*Children's Memorial Hospital, Chicago, Ill.*): I believe we have been seeing here a heterogeneity of responses in animal models. We have reported that we have had four children with thymic dysplasia and immunoglobulin synthesis, two of whom received thymic transplants. None of these showed a restitution of responsiveness. I believe it is important to stress here that thymic dysplasia in the human is probably not as simple a phenomenon as most believe.

Dr. D. Wara: I indicated that I thought that these patients represented a very heterogeneous population. Our success with thymus transplantation in the two patients presented and in several other patients with thymic hypoplasia suggest that this group of immunodeficiency disorders is indeed a heterogeneous group.

REGULATION OF θ-ANTIGEN EXPRESSION BY AGENTS ALTERING CYCLIC AMP LEVEL AND BY THYMIC FACTOR

Marie-Anne Bach, Catherine Fournier, and Jean-François Bach

Hôpital Necker
75730 Paris Cedex 15 France

Introduction

The maturation of thymus-derived lymphocytes is associated with variations in the expression of several "differentiation" alloantigens such as the antigens TL, θ, and Ly in the mouse. One may wonder, however, whether the expression of these antigens might not also depend on the cell metabolic activity in addition to the state of differentiation. Thus, it is known that B-cells show variations in exposition of surface immunoglobulins during the cell cycle.[1] The adenyl cyclase system has been considered recently as a possible important intermediate in antigen and mitogen-induced lymphocyte stimulation. In this context it is interesting to note that cyclic AMP inhibits the cytotoxic action of sensitized lymphocytes against their target cells (whereas cytotoxicity is increased by cyclic GMP treatment).[2] Similarly, cyclic AMP alters *in vitro* primary responses giving inhibition or stimulation according to concentrations and protocols used.[3] Cyclic AMP has also been considered as being possibly involved in the action of thymic hormones in the maturation of T-cells. This latter role for cyclic AMP was envisaged when we first reported that, like thymic extracts and circulating thymic factors, cyclic AMP and poly A-poly U induced the appearance of the θ-antigen on the θ-negative spleen rosette-forming cells (RFC) from adult thymectomized mice.[4, 5]

Two main approaches can be investigated in this line: one may look for the thymic hormone-like effect of cyclic AMP or of drugs increasing cyclic AMP level on lymphoid cells or look at the direct effect of thymic factors on the cyclic AMP level in the lymphocytes. We have undertaken the first of these approaches with the rosette assay using the thymic serum factor isolated on the basis of this assay. We have extended data obtained with RFC to lymphoid cells generally, using a direct cytotoxic assay with antiθ serum.

Material and Methods

Mice

Eight-to-twelve-week old C57 Bl/6, CBA/H were used in most experiments. Nude mice were also used in some experiments.

Thymectomies

Adult thymectomy was performed by suction after anesthesia with nembutal. Thymectomized mice were used 10–30 days after the operation. The absence of thymic remnants was always verified macroscopically when the mice were sacrificed. In some experiments, adult thymectomized mice were irradiated (850 R) and reconstituted within 4 hours with 15×10^6 normal syngeneic bone marrow cells.

Chemicals

Cyclic AMP (cAMP), dibutyryl cAMP (dibu-cAMP) and adenosine were obtained from Böhringer, theophylline, acetylcholine, and cyclic GMP (cGMP) from Sigma, and Indomethacin from Merck Sharpe and Dohme. Azathioprine was used as the sodium salt and provided by Burroughs Wellcome. Prostaglandins E_1, E_2, A_1, A_2 and $F_{2\alpha}$ were supplied by J. Pike of the Upjohn Company.

Antiθ Serum (AθS)

AθS used in most experiments was prepared by injecting AKR mice with 10×10^6 CBA thymocytes intraperitoneally weekly for 6 weeks and bleeding one week after the last injection. The specificity of the AθS was verified by cytotoxicity and rosette inhibition against thymus and spleen cells from AKR and CBA mice. In some experiments an AθS batch prepared in A mice congenic at the θ allele (given by E. Boyse) was used as a further specificity control.

Thymic Factors

The thymic factor used in most experiments was obtained from pig serum as described elsewhere.[6] In short, pig serum was dialysed and the dialysate was concentrated on UM2 Amicon membranes, filtered on a G 25 Sephadex® column and chromatographed on CM cellulose. Thymic extracts ("thymosin," fraction 3), donated by A. L. Goldstein and A. White[7] were used in other experiments. When the serum thymic factor was used *in vivo,* it was previously bound to CM cellulose in order to increase its serum half-life, as discussed elsewhere in this volume.[6]

Rosette Inhibition Tests

The techniques for rosette formation and its inhibition by azathioprine and AθS have already been reported.[8]

Cytotoxic Assay

Cytotoxic assay was performed by incubating spleen cells with AθS in the presence of complement (guinea-pig serum previously absorbed with mouse thymocytes and red cells). A suspension of spleen cells was prepared in Hank's medium (6×10^6 spleen cells/ml) and placed in hemolysis tubes (50 μl per tube). Log 2 dilutions of AθS (100 μl) were added. After 15 minutes incubation at 37° C, complement (50 μl) was added and the cell suspension incubated for 45 minutes. Trypan blue was then added in order to evaluate the percentage of dead cells.

BSA Gradients

Cells were separated on BSA gradients as described by Komuro and Boyse.[9]

Experimental Protocols

In Vitro *Experiments*

In rosette experiments, the products to be tested were added simultaneously with azathioprine or AθS to the cell suspension. In cytotoxicity experiments, the cells were first incubated with the tested products for two hours at 37° C before AθS was added. In some experiments 5% BSA or 5% fetal calf serum was added during the first incubation in order to reduce nonspecific cell death.

In Vivo *Experiments*

The various products used in these experiments were injected intraperitoneally. The thymic factor was injected subcutaneously bound to 50 mg of CM cellulose previously equilibrated with phosphate buffer (0.02 M pH 6.3).

Results

θ Induction

Induction of θ-antigen in θ-negative cells was obtained using spleen cells from nude mice, thymectomized irradiated bone-marrow-reconstituted mice, adult thymectomized mice for rosette experiments, and normal mice for cytotoxicity experiments. In the latter case, spleen cells were previously fractionated on a BSA discontinuous gradient in order to isolate a θ-negative spleen cell subpopulation. Products used to induce θ-antigen expression included thymic fractions, cyclic AMP, dibu-cAMP, theophylline, and prostaglandins PGE_1 and PGE_2.

Rosette Experiments

Theta conversion of θ-negative RFC by thymic factors, cAMP, theophylline, and prostaglandins PGE_1 and PGE_2 has already been reported in detail[4, 5] and will only be described briefly here. As shown on Figure 1, TF-containing normal mouse serum and cyclic AMP (10^{-8}M) make spleen RFC from adult thymectomized mice sensitive to AθS; in control experiments (Table 1) thy-

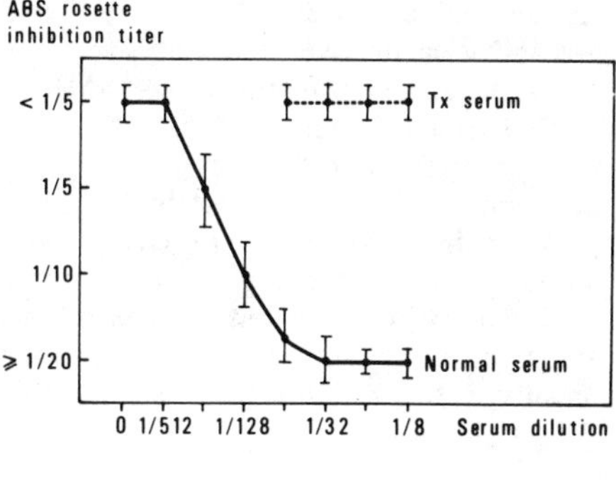

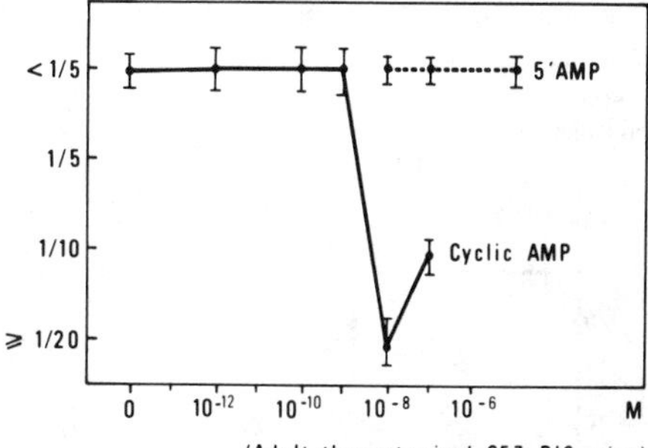

FIGURE 1. Differential effects of cyclic AMP and noncyclic 5′AMP on anti-θ serum sensitivity of spleen RFC from adult thymectomized mice. Comparison with the effects of sera from normal or thymectomized mice.

mectomized serum and *non*cyclic 5′AMP proved to be inactive. Identical results were obtained with purified pig serum thymic factor, which was active at 10 pg/ml.[6] It should be emphasized that neither TF nor cAMP modified rosette numbers when applied alone to spleen cells. Interestingly, similar effects were observed in nude mice but the active cAMP concentrations were 10^4 times higher than in adult thymectomized mice. Prostaglandins PGE_1 and PGE_2 had

TABLE 1

EFFECTS OF CYCLIC NUCLEOTIDES AND VARIOUS CONTROL COMPOUNDS ON SPLEEN RFC FROM NORMAL AND THYMECTOMIZED MICE *

	Normal Mice		Tx Mice	
	In Vitro	*In Vivo*	*In Vitro*	*In Vivo*
cAMP	+++	—	++/+++	—
Dibu-cAMP	+++	+++	++/+++	+++
Theophylline	—	+++	++	+++
PGE_1, PGE_2	—		++++	
Thymic hormone	—	—	++++	++++
cGMP, 5′ AMP	—	—	—	—
Adenosine	—	—	—	—
PGA_1, PGA_2	—	—	—	—
$PGF_{2\alpha}$	—	—	—	—
Acetylcholine	—	—	—	—

* See Bach & Bach.[5]

identical effects to cAMP at 10^{-8}M, but PGA_1, PGA_2 and $PGF_{2\alpha}$ were much less active or inactive [5] (FIGURE 2).

In *in vivo* experiments dibu-cAMP (but not cAMP) showed the same effect as that noted *in vitro* (TABLE 1). It is noteworthy that dibu-cAMP effects were reversible since maximum activity was obtained 1–2 hours after the injection and much of the effect had disappeared at 24 hours.

Both in *in vitro* and *in vivo* experiments, it was noted that all products tested except thymic factors lost their effect at highest doses.

Lastly, when very low concentrations of thymic extracts or serum TF were mixed with very low cAMP concentrations (10^{-12}M), full conversion of RFC sensitivity to azathioprine was obtained *in vitro*.[5]

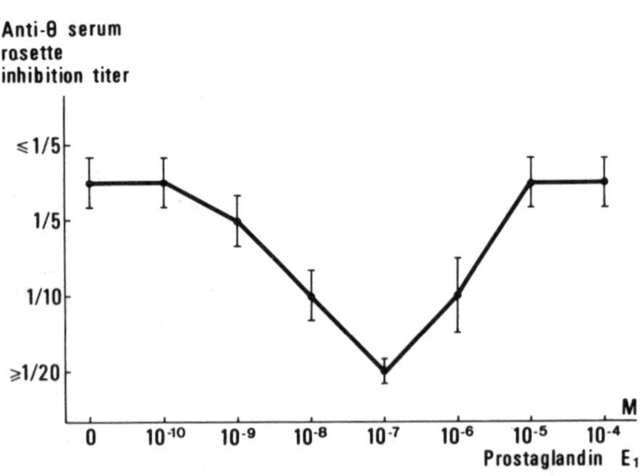

FIGURE 2. *In vitro* effects of Prostaglandin PGE_1 on anti-θ serum sensitivity of spleen RFC from adult thymectomized mice.

Cytotoxicity Experiments (FIGURES 3 and 4)

In *in vitro* experiments, normal spleen cells were separated on a BSA discontinuous gradient. Each of the layers were tested immediately after cell collection and washing. It was observed as already reported by others [9] that only a few θ-positive cells were found in the less dense cells, the majority of θ-positive cells being found in the densest cells. Cell aliquots from each layer were incubated for 120 minutes at 37° C in Hank's medium sometimes added with 5% BSA or fetal calf serum, in the presence or absence of low concentrations of purified serum TF. Twenty-six experiments were performed in total. θ conversion was regularly obtained as represented in FIGURES 3 and 4 (6/6 experiments) when the following conditions were present: (1) successful θ-positive cell depletion by the gradient (less than 10% θ-positive cells in the A layer); (2) absence of excess spontaneous cell death. This may be prevented by the addition of BSA or fetal calf serum but this was inappropriate in these experiments because these substances have been shown to inhibit TF activity by binding as previously demonstrated for the rosette assay.[6, 8] It should be emphasized that both these conditions were obtained in only 6 out of 20 experi-

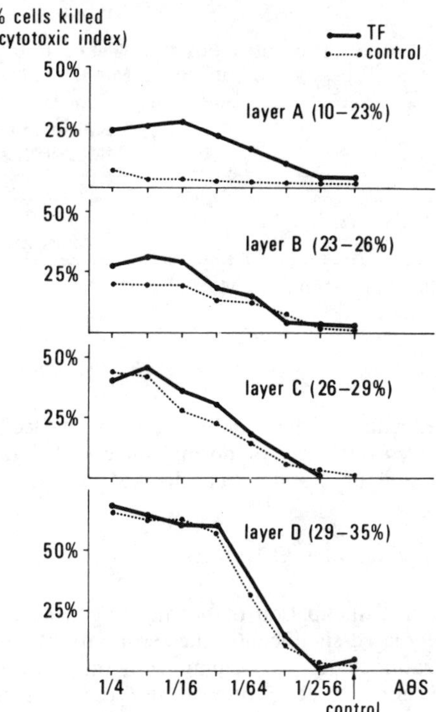

FIGURE 3. Effect of purified pig serum TF on the number of θ-positive cells among BSA separated spleen cells (Each layer is given with the corresponding BSA density). See protocol in the text.

ments. The efficacy of BSA fractionation with respect to θ-positive cell depletion was fairly variable especially when using different lots of BSA (even from the same source) and also excess cell death occurred in 8 experiments, due to the absence of the above mentioned high molecular weight proteins. This made assessment of θ conversion difficult.

In *in vivo* experiments, it was shown that nude mice or adult thymectomized mice injected with CM cellulose-bound purified TF (50–200 ng) revealed a significant increase in the number of θ-positive spleen cells when tested 24 hours later (TABLE 2).

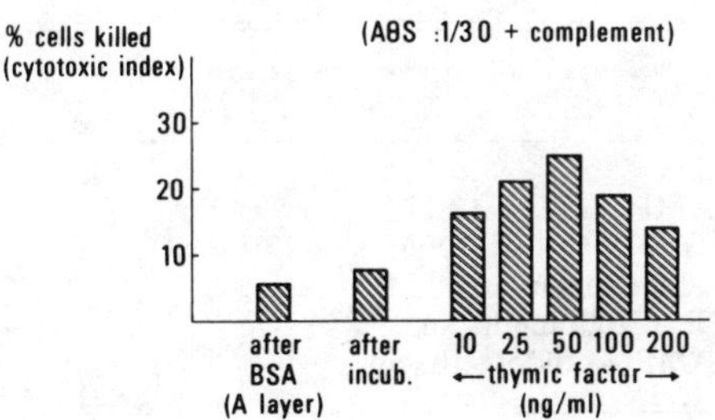

FIGURE 4. Dose effect relationship of serum TF for θ conversion of the A layer of BSA-separated normal spleen cells (Anti-θ serum, 1/16, + complement).

TABLE 2

INDUCTION OF θ-POSITIVE CELLS BY *In Vivo* TF TREATMENT OF NUDE MICE * (MEAN±SD)

	% θ-Positive Cells (Cytotoxic Assay)	AθS Rosette Inhibition Titer
No treatment	2% ± 2%	≤ 1/5
TF + CMC	18% ± 3%	1/40
CMC	3% ± 2%	≤ 1/5

* 200 ng i.p. bound to CM cellulose.

θ Reduction

Reduction in the number of θ-positive cells has been obtained by *in vivo* or *in vitro* treatment of normal mice with indomethacin (a prostaglandin synthetase inhibitor) and with cyclic AMP itself.

Rosette Experiments

In vitro incubation of normal spleen cells with indomethacin ($10^{-5}-10^{-7}$ M) decreased significantly the sensitivity of normal spleen RFC to antiθ serum and azathioprine. In keeping with this observation, indomethacin suppressed the TF effect on RFC preventing θ induction in θ-negative RFC from thymectomized mice (TABLE 3). Similar results were obtained when indomethacin was administered *in vivo* (50 μg per mouse i.p.) in normal mice. Spleen RFC lost their sensitivity to azathioprine and to AθS. The effect already significant one hour after the injection was maximum at 24 hours and had largely disappeared at 48 hours (FIGURE 5).

Reduction in θ expression could also be obtained with cyclic AMP itself. Thus, incubation of normal spleen cells with low concentrations of cAMP (10^{-6}M) induced the disappearance of RFC sensitivity to AθS as described above for indomethacin. An identical effect was obtained after i.p. injection of dibutyryl cyclic AMP (10–100 μg). Interestingly, prostaglandins and thymic factor had no effect on normal spleen RFC in *in vitro* or *in vivo* experiments.

TABLE 3

INHIBITION OF TF EFFECT ON RFC BY INDOMETHACIN

		Hormone-like Effect on RFC
TF	10^{-10}M	+
cAMP	10^{-9} M	+
PGE_1	10^{-8} M	+
Indomethacin	10^{-7} M	—
TF + Indomethacin		—
cAMP + Indomethacin		+

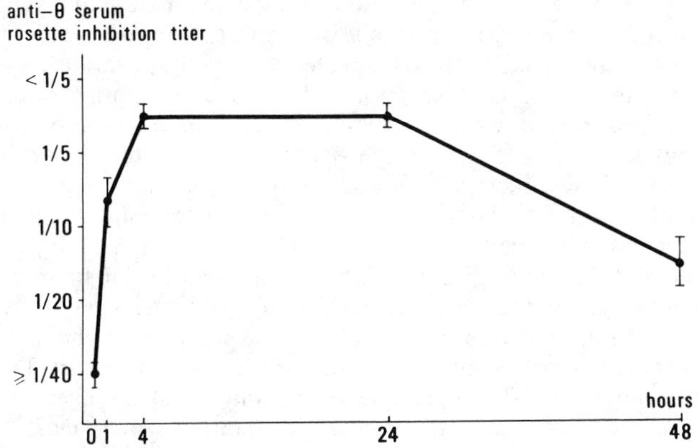

FIGURE 5. Effects of *in vivo* treatment by indomethacin (50 μg/i.p.) on normal mouse spleen RFC (anti-θ serum rosette inhibition titers).

Moreover spleen RFC made θ-negative by cAMP treatment did not recover the θ-antigen after TF treatment.

Cytotoxicity Experiments

Similar data have been obtained in cytotoxicity experiments as has been reported for rosette-forming cells. Normal mice were injected with indomethacin (50 μg i.p.) or dibutyryl cyclic AMP. One hour later a drastic reduction occurred in the number of spleen θ-positive cells (FIGURE 6). The effect persisted with indomethacin 24 hours after the injection.

The thymic factor, administered *in vivo* or used *in vitro* in the conditions described above has no effect whatsoever on θ-positive cells in normal animals.

DISCUSSION

Our data clearly demonstrate that it is possible to modify in a reversible way the expression of the θ-antigen on the surface of lymphoid cells from

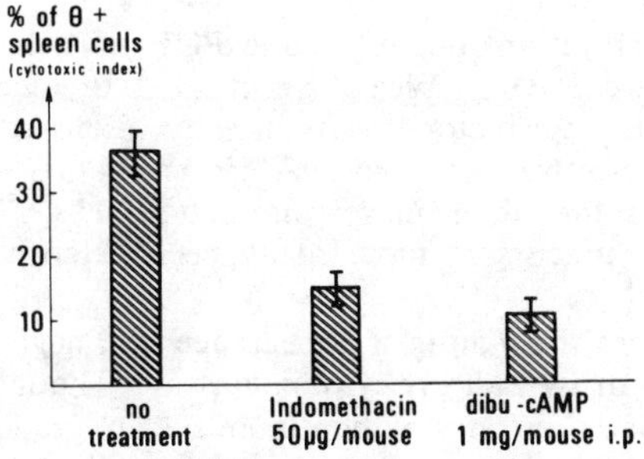

FIGURE 6. Effects of *in vivo* treatment by indomethacin (50 μg/i.p.) on normal mouse spleen cells (cytotoxicity by antiθ serum).

normal or thymectomized mice. Selection of adequate dosage and timing makes it possible to induce the appearance of θ-antigen on θ-negative cells with cyclic AMP or prostaglandins or, more unexpectedly, the disappearance of θ-antigen on θ-positive cells with cyclic AMP or indomethacin. Similar results are obtained *in vitro* and *in vivo,* whether looking at the subpopulation of lymphocytes forming spontaneous rosettes or at the overall lymphocyte populations with a cytotoxic assay. Dose effects and time influence have been established in each system. Control compounds without effect on θ expression include 5′AMP, adenosine, cyclic GMP, acetylcholine, prostaglandin A_1, A_2 and $F_{2\alpha}$ (TABLE 1).

It is impossible so far to give a definitive interpretation of these data. However, one may consider that they are compatible with the hypothesis giving to cyclic AMP an important role in controlling θ expression on the T-lymphocyte surface. Maximum θ expression as seen in normal mice in mature T-cells might depend on optimal cAMP lymphocyte level, and slight changes in this level would diminish θ expression. Thymectomized mice, which lack TF, would have a low intracellular level of cAMP, at least in T-cell precursors and thus would lose their ability to express the θ-antigen in this cell population. Cyclic AMP or products increasing its cellular level such as PGE_1[10] would induce the appearance of θ-antigen in these cells. Conversely an excessive increase in the cAMP level as obtained by low cAMP doses in normal mice, or by higher cAMP doses in thymectomized mice, would exceed the optimal cAMP level. In this scheme indomethacin would inhibit cyclic AMP synthesis by reducing prostaglandin synthesis. The latter synthesis is normally stimulated by other products including probably thymic hormones since indomethacin suppressed TF effects on RFC. Indomethacin would act by reduction of the cAMP level in the cell which opposes it to cAMP which reduces θ expression by increasing cAMP level. However, several important reservations must be made about this tentative interpretation, and direct intralymphocyte evaluation of cAMP will be needed before relating θ changes and cAMP level. These reservations are the following: (1) the drugs used may have a direct cellular effect independent of any increase of intracellular cAMP level; (2) as azathioprine is an AMP-analogue precursor, there may be competitive inhibition of AZ cell uptake or a direct extracellular or intracellular interaction of the compounds with azathioprine, thus suppressing its actions (but this does not hold for studies with AθS); (3) it is usually thought that an increase of the intracellular level of cAMP is difficult to obtain by direct incubation of living cells with cAMP. However, cAMP did work in our system and in fact, we found dibu-cAMP more active than cAMP in *in vivo* experiments. This could be suspected from the better cell penetration of the latter product. Anyhow, many studies have shown that cAMP had *in vitro* effects on living cells suggestive of a direct increase of intracellular cAMP level.

The striking need for higher concentrations of cAMP and PGE_1 to achieve the effect in nude mice and "thymus-deprived" mice than in adult thymectomized mice has also been found for thymic factor.[6, 8] As already discussed in this latter context, this suggests a selective action of cAMP and PGE_1 on already differentiated cell precursors rather than on very immature cells. The origin of spleen T-RFC and of their precursors has already been extensively discussed and will not be reconsidered here.

The thymic factor efficiently induces the θ-antigen appearance in θ-negative cells either assessed by a rosette assay or by a direct cytotoxic assay. The latter assay required a preliminary cell separation on a discontinuous BSA gradient to pick up the hormone target cells. Some difficulties have been encountered with this gradient especially in our experimental conditions without proteins in the medium made necessary by TF binding (or lysis) by large molecular weight proteins. However, Komuro and Boyse [9] results have been confirmed here using our purified TF. An exact comparison of active TF concentrations with other preparations is made difficult by differences in optimal conditions for each of these preparations.

TF synergism with cyclic AMP as well as direct cAMP experiments suggest that TF might act through cAMP synthesis stimulation as with many other polypeptidic hormones. Indirect data obtained with prostaglandins and with indomethacin would indicate that prostaglandin might eventually be an intermediate between TF receptors and ultimate cyclic AMP stimulation as also discussed for other hormones.[11] The blocking of TF effect by indomethacin would then be explained. This hypothesis needs however a direct demonstration. The recent findings by Kook and Trainin [12] are encouraging in that context, since these authors have shown that dialysed extracts of thymic tissue stimulated adenylcyclase in thymocytes and in spleen cells. Confirmation of these results is however needed with more purified products since cyclic AMP synthesis may be induced in a nonspecific way by various products, such as isoproterenol, or even serum fractions obtained from thymectomized mice (our unpublished observation).

If our data cast some light on the mode of action of TF, they pose also the problem of the θ assay used for the study of thymic hormones and more generally of the use of AθS in certain experimental conditions. In our experiments the difference in the effects of thymectomized mouse serum and of normal serum is reassuring but other biological assays must be performed before claiming the T-cell maturing effect of a thymic factor. We have such evidence for the purified serum TF which has been shown to induce *in vitro* responsiveness to Concanavalin A and enables thymectomized, irradiated, bone marrow reconstituted mice to reject MSV-Moloney virus-induced sarcomas.[6]

Summary

Thymic factor, cyclic AMP, and products increasing its cellular level, such as Prostaglandin E_1, induce the appearance of the θ-antigen on T-cell precursors whether assessed by a rosette-inhibition assay or a cytotoxic assay after cell fractionation on BSA discontinuous gradient. Synergism has been demonstrated between cyclic AMP and TF for that effect. Conversely, decrease of θ expression has been obtained by altering cyclic AMP level in θ-positive cells either increasing it by dibutyryl cAMP treatment or decreasing it by indomethacin treatment. Finally, these data suggest the involvement of cyclic AMP in the regulation of θ expression under thymic hormone control.

References

1. Kerbel, M. & M. Doenhoff. Nature. In press.
2. Strom, T. B., C. B. Carpenter, M. R. Garovoy, F. K. Austen, J. P. Merrill & M. Kaliner. 1973. The modulating influence of cyclic nucleotides upon lymphocyte-mediated cytotoxicity. J. Exp. Med. **138:** 381–383.

3. BRAUN, W. & M. ISHIZUKA. 1971. Antibody formation reduced responses after administration of excessive amounts of non-specific stimulators. Proc. Nat. Acad. Sci. U.S. **68:** 1114–1116.
4. BACH, M. A. & J. F. BACH. 1972. Effects de l'AMP cylique sur les cellules formant des rosettes spontanées. Compt. Rend. Acad. Sci. **275:** 2783.
5. BACH, M. A. & J. F. BACH. 1973. Studies on thymus products. VI. The effects of cyclic nucleotides and prostaglandins on rosette forming cells. Interactions with thymic factor. Eur. J. Immunol. **3:** 778–783.
6. BACH, J. F., M. DARDENNE, J. M. PLEAU & M. A. BACH. 1975. Biochemical characteristics and biological activity of a serum factor produced by the mouse and the human thymus. This volume.
7. GOLDSTEIN, A. L., A. GUHA, M. M. ZATZ, M. A. HARDY & A. WHITE. 1972. Purification and biological activity of thymosin, a hormone of the thymus gland. Proc. Nat. Acad. Sci. U.S. **69:** 1800–1803.
8. BACH, J. F. & M. DARDENNE. 1973. Demonstration and characterization of a circulating thymic hormone. Immunology **25:** 353–366.
9. KOMURO, O. & E. A. BOYSE. 1973. *In vitro* demonstration of thymic hormone in the mouse by conversion of precursor cell into T lymphocytes. Lancet **1:** 740–743.
10. HENNEY, C. S., H. R. BOURNE & L. M. LICHSTENSTEIN. 1972. The role of cyclic 3′5′ adenosine monophosphate in the specific cytolytic activity of lymphocytes. J. Immunol. **108:** 1526–1534.
11. KUEHL, F. A. *In* Les Prostaglandines. : 55. INSERM. Paris, France.
12. KOOK, A. & N. TRAININ. 1974. Hormone-like activity of a thymus humoral factor on the induction of immune competence in lymphoid cells. J. Exp. Med. **139:** 193–207.

DISCUSSION OF THE PAPER

DR. A. WHITE: To help clarify a point, the words "decreasing and increasing" are a little confusing with regard to the appearance or disappearance of θ-positive cells. Does dibutyryl cyclic AMP increase or decrease the amount of θ-antigen on the cells or the splenic responses?

DR. M. BACH: It decreases θ expression in normal spleen cells.

DR. A. WHITE: If it decreases it in normal spleen cells, does it increase it in cells of thymectomized mice?

DR. M. BACH: Yes, in a certain range of concentrations.

DR. A. WHITE: Obviously, the reason I ask is because you could block rosette formation and azathioprine sensitivity with antiθ serum and it was not clear therefore how you were invoking cyclic AMP if at the same time you produced a decrease of θ-antigen on the cell surface.

DR. SCHWARTZ (*National Institutes of Health*): Have you looked at stimulators of adenyl cyclase, such as isoproterenol or blockers of phosphodiesterase?

DR. M. BACH: I have not looked yet, but we should very shortly.

DR. J. F. A. P. MILLER: Dr. Bach, have you or any of your colleagues looked at other T-cell functions, such as helper, suppressor, or memory functions?

DR. M. BACH: This has been discussed before by Dr. J. Bach, but I can say we have tested our product for antitumor immunity and the ability of rosette-forming cells to form caps, as well as the presence of receptors for steroids.

DR. H. MILLER: But have you studied humoral immunity?

DR. M. BACH: No.

DR. LIEF (*Miami, Florida*): I noticed people are still using discontinuous-density gradients, presumably made with hypertonic BSA, because the densities you have are extremely high. There is no reason to believe that the distribution one obtains with these arbitrary four steps have any great sense of reality. I would suggest that these data could only be verified by using linear gradients, either by my technique or Shortman's technique.

T-LYMPHOCYTE MATURATION AND ANTITUMORAL EFFECT OF A THYMIC EXTRACT OBTAINED FROM A STIMULATED MODEL

B. Serrou, T. Reme, R. Senelar, B. Delor, J. B. Dubois, and C. Thierry

Department of Clinical and Experimental Immunology
Centre Paul Lamarque Hôpital St-Eloi
34059 Montpellier, France

Although the role of the thymus in T-lymphocyte maturation cannot be denied,[1] the mechanism of thymus function is still poorly known. Certain authors [2–5] have suggested that a factor secreted by thymic epithelial cells might allow the transformation of bone-marrow lymphocytes (Bo) to T-lymphocytes or the transformation of T_1-lymphocytes to T_2-lymphocytes. Nevertheless, this factor and its mode of action remains poorly characterized. In addition, the work done up until now does not allow any formal conclusions to be drawn on the epithelial origin of such a factor.

In this paper, we supply proofs for the probably epithelial origin of such a factor that we extracted from the thymus of animals stimulated either by sheep red blood cells (SRBC) or by skin allografts. Results demonstrated that such a factor permitted the transformation of Bo to T-lymphocytes stimulable by phytohemagglutinin (PHA), the transformation of T-lymphocytes precursors (in nude mice) into effector lymphocytes, and finally an increase in antitumor activity of mice with a transplanted Lewis tumor.

Materials and Methods

Removing the Thymuses for Histological Study

We did skin grafts between New Zealand and Fauve de Bourgogne rabbits according to a technique previously described.[6] We examined the morphological modifications of the thymuses from the animals after coloration with hematein-eosin, periodic acid Schiff reagent (PAS), and methylpyronine green. They were removed on the fourth and eleventh days and on the day of complete rejection.

Preparation Technique for the Stimulated Thymuses

All thymic extractions were from animals stimulated by either SRBC (0.25 ml of a 50% solution given iv) or by skin allografts. Removals of all thymuses were done between the fourth and sixth day after the graft or after the injection of SRBC.

Preparation Technique for Thymic and Renal Extracts

When the animals were sacrificed, all the thymuses were taken out at +4° C while making sure that the parathymic lymph nodes were not included. The thymuses were washed in PBS, then crushed and homogenized at +4° C. The homogenate was centrifuged at 105,000 × *g* and the supernatant was taken off and dialyzed for 48 hours at +4° C. The dialysis was followed by an ultrafiltration that retained only those molecules with a molecular weight equal or inferior to 1,000. The ultrafiltrate was then lyophilized and the amount, in milligrams, of protein was evaluated by Lowry's method.[7] The same technique was used to obtain an identical kidney extract from the same animals.

Bone Marrow Lymphocyte Blastic Stimulation

Lymphocytes were removed from the bone marrow of C57Bl/6 × DBA2F1 mice. They were counted, and viability was evaluated by trypan blue exclusion. All the manipulations were done at +4° C. The lymphocytes were brought to a concentration of 2×10^5 cells per milliliter. Stimulation was done on 3040 microplates in RPMI medium with antibiotics. The microplate cultures were then incubated for 3 days at +37° C in the presence of 5% CO_2 and 95% air. RPMI (200 μl) was put into each well along with 10 μg/ml of PHA (PHA P. DIFCO), and 0.2 μCi of tritiated methyl-thymidine was added four hours before harvesting the cells. Harvesting was done in a semiautomatic apparatus ("MASH 1"). After harvesting the lymphocytes on membranes, the count was done in a liquid scintillator (Intertechnique). The results are expressed in d.p.m. The thymic extracts to be tested were added to each well at a dose of 100 μg of protein per milliliter.

Plaque-forming Cells Technique [8]

In this technique we used nu/nu homozygote (CNRS-ORLEANS-LA-SOURCE) nude mice. The thymic extract was injected intraperitoneally twice a day for a week at a dose of 0.5 mg of protein. SRBC were injected intraperitoneally (0.25 ml of 50% solution).

Tumor System

We used Lewis tumors in 2 month old C57Bl/6 × DBA2F1 mice. We evaluated the survival time of the mice, the time of appearance, the weight, the surface, and the number of pulmonary metastases of the tumor. The thymic extract was injected according to the following protocol: at day 0, that is, the day of tumor implantation, and at day + 14, that is, 14 days after tumor implantation. Two protocols, both with controls, were used: either thymic extract injection alone, or thymic extract injection in animals thymectomized 2 weeks previous to injection (injections either on day 0 or the 14th day after tumor implantation).

Thymectomy

Thymectomies were done in two month old C57Bl/6 × DBA2F1 mice using the suction technique and Nembutal anesthesia. We systematically eliminated at the time of autopsy all those animals that had persisting thymic fragments.

Thymic Extract and Kidney Extract Injection

Injection of the extracts was always done intravenously at a dose of 0.5 mg of protein twice a day for a week. In each *in vivo* and *in vitro* technique an identical kidney extract served as control.

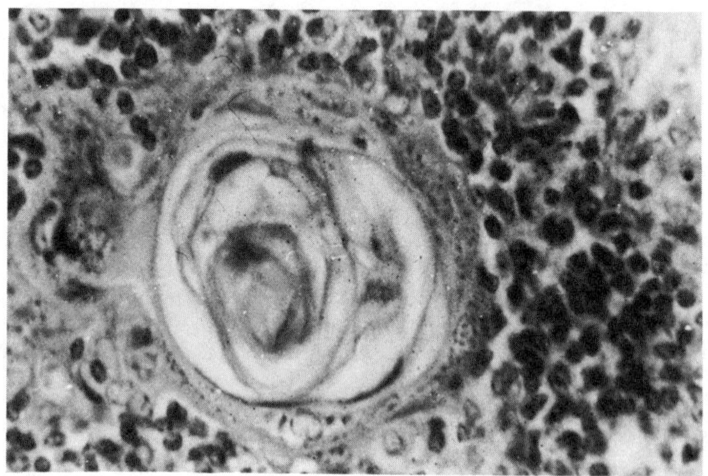

FIGURE 1. Thymus of skin allografted rabbits, showing the appearance of extremely numerous grains of RNA, colored by methyl-pyronine green, in the epithelial cells of the thymic medullary. Stuck to these RNA grains was a substance that colored with PAS (× 735)

RESULTS

Histological studies (FIGURE 1) showed the appearance of extremely numerous grains of RNA, colored by methyl-pyronine green, in the epithelial cells of the thymic medullary. Stuck to these RNA grains was a substance that colored with PAS, that is, a glycoprotein-like substance.

Bone marrow lymphocytes, in the presence of PHA, were stimulated very little; the same thing happened after previous incubation with 100 μg/ml of kidney extract. However, bone marrow lymphocytes previously incubated with the thymic factor at a dose of 100 μg/ml showed a stimulation ratio four times greater than the controls (FIGURE 2).

The number of PFC per spleen in nude mice (TABLE 1) treated with thymic extract doubled and this as compared to the controls or the same

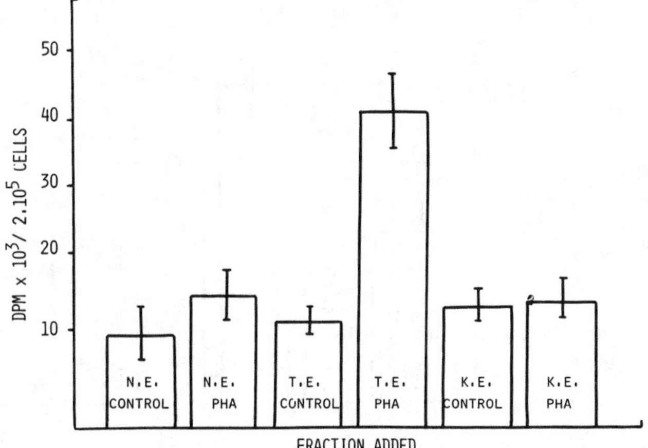

FIGURE 2. Bone marrow lymphocytes previously incubated with the thymic factor at a dose of 100 μg/ml showed a stimulation ratio four times greater than the controls. The response of the cultures to mitogenic stimulation was recorded as follows: deintegration/min/(dpm)/culture of 2.10^5 viable cells.

animals treated with an identical kidney extract. The doses of the extracts were the same in both cases.

By using a tumor system we were able to demonstrate a prolonged survival time in animals treated with the thymic extract the day of tumor implantation, day 0, as compared with the controls and thymectomized animals (FIGURE 3). The difference is statistically significant ($p < 0.01$). However, for animals treated with the thymic extract on day +14, we found no significant difference with the controls. In addition, we were able to show a prolongation of survival time that was slightly longer for thymectomized and thymic extract treated animals. Nevertheless, this difference is not significant. Also, tumor appearance time (FIGURE 4) was significantly delayed in animals treated with thymic extract on day 0 whether or not they had been previously thymectomized, as compared with the controls and untreated thymectomized animals. However,

TABLE 1

NUMBER OF PFC IN THE SPLEEN OF NUDE MICE INJECTED WITH THYMIC EXTRACT *

	Number of Animals	PFC/Spleen	PFC/10^6 Lys.
Control	5	6.100	39.8
Kidney extract	5	6.354	40.2
Thymic extract	5	10.285	62.3

* PFC: Plaque forming cells (SRBC: 0.25 ml at 50%). Kidney extract: 0.5 mg protein intraperitoneally 2 times a day for 1 week. Thymic extract: 0.5 mg protein intraperitoneally 2 times a day for 1 week.

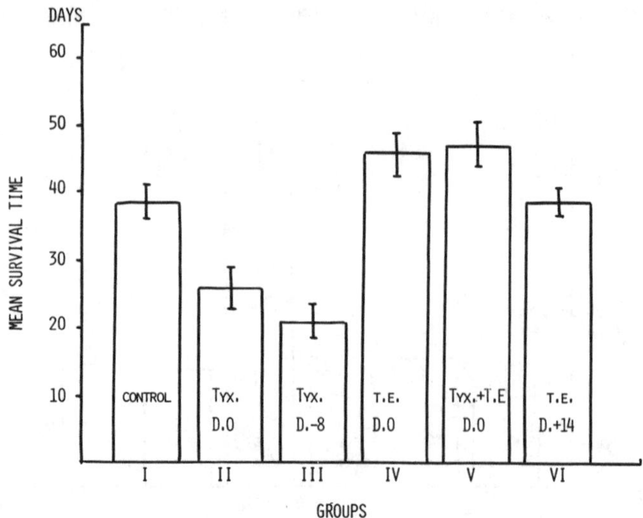

FIGURE 3. Prolonged survival time in animals treated with the thymic extract the day of tumor implantation (D.0.). *Group I:* Control 38.5 days ± 3.1. *Group II:* Thymectomy the day of tumor implantation (TyX. D.0.), 25.8 days ± 2.75. *Group III:* Thymectomy 8 days before tumor implantation (TyX. D. −8), 21 days ± 1.63). *Group IV:* Thymic Extract given the day of tumor implantation (T.E.D. 0), 45.7 days ± 3.12. *Group V:* Thymectomy performed and Thymic Extract given the day of tumor implantation (TyX. + T.E.D. 0), 47.2 days ± 3.21. *Group VI:* Thymic Extract given 14 days after tumor implantation (T.E.D. +14), 38 days ± 2.75.

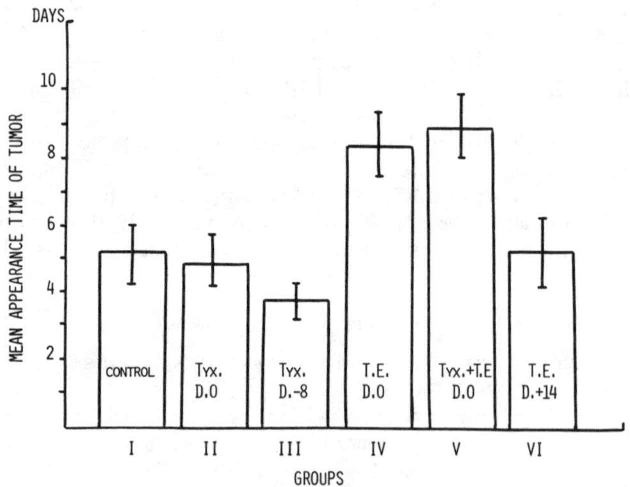

FIGURE 4. Significantly delayed tumor appearance time in animals treated with thymic extract on day 0. *Group I:* Control 5.16 days ± 0.92. *Group II:* Thymectomy performed the day of tumor implantation (TyX. D.0.), 4.92 days ±0.86. *Group III:* Thymectomy performed 8 days before tumor implantation (TyX. D. −8), 3.84 days ± 0.54. *Group IV:* Thymic extract given the day of tumor implantation (T.E. D.0.), 8.32 days ± 1.04. *Group V:* Thymectomy performed and thymic extract given the day of tumor implantation (TyX. + T.E. D.0.), 8.86 days ± 1.02. *Group VI:* Thymic extract given 14 days after tumor implantation, 5.21 days ± 1.

this difference was not found in animals treated with thymic extract on the 14th day after tumor implantation. Tumor surface (FIGURE 5) was significantly ($p < 0.01$) smaller in those animals treated with thymic extract on the day of tumor implantation regardless of whether the animal was thymectomized or not. This difference is no longer significant if the animals are treated on the 14th day after tumor implantation. We observed no significant influence of treatment with the extract on pulmonary metastases. The number of pulmonary metastases was apparently the same in all series, except the thymectomy series in which we noticed a significantly greater number of pulmonary metastases.

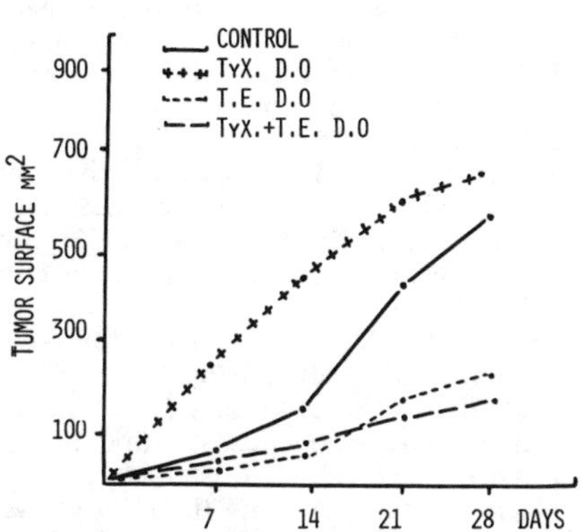

FIGURE 5. This figure shows a smaller tumor surface in animals treated with thymic extract on the day of tumor implantation. This difference is no longer significant if the animals are treated on the 14th day after tumor implantation.

DISCUSSION

Evidence shows that there exist considerable modifications of the epithelial cells in the thymus medullary during skin allografts as well as during injection of large doses of SRBC. These modifications are essentially the appearance of RNA grains stuck to a glycoprotein. Such a substance, already studied by certain authors,[9] observed by us in stimulated thymuses, might correspond to a thymic factor for the maturation of T-lymphocytes.

For this reason, we did the thymic extract from thymuses of animals stimulated by SRBC or by skin allografts. The results that we are presenting show that such an extract is effective. On this point, our results concur with those of Trainin,[2, 10] Goldstein,[3] and Bach.[4, 11]

The extract that we prepared is effective on the maturation of Bo lymphocytes to T-lymphocytes giving a clear response in PHA blastic stimulation after incubation with this extract. This same extract might not only act at this level but, also, at the level of certain T-lymphocyte precursors in nude mice.[12] In fact, it might be that this same extract acts at different stages of T-lymphocyte maturation, the target varying according to the quantity of thymic extract used.[4]

In addition, the fact that this extract increases the animal's protection against tumor development reinforces the notion that its essential role is in the production of effector mature and active T-lymphocytes. This effect may perhaps be greater if the animal has been previously thymectomized. The results corroborate those presented by Goldstein.[13]

The relation existing between such an active thymic extract and those obtained by different workers [2–5] is still to be established. In effect, the extract is prepared from the thymus of stimulated animals but, it has not yet been purified. This is the work we are presently pursuing. This approach strongly emphasizes the major role that the epithelial cells of thymic medullary might have in T-lymphocyte maturation and, therefore, in the immune response.

References

1. Osoba, D. & J. F. A. P. Miller. 1963. Evidence for a humoral thymus factor responsible for the maturation of immunological faculty. Nature **199:** 359.
2. Trainin, N. & M. Linker-Israeli. 1967. Restoration of immunologic reactivity of thymectomized mice by calf thymus extracts. Cancer Res. **27:** 309.
3. Goldstein, A. L., A. Guha, M. M. Zatz, M. A. Hardy & A. White. 1972. Purification and Biological Activity of thymosin, a hormone of the thymus gland. Proc. Nat. Acad. Sci. U.S. **69:** 1800.
4. Bach, J. F. & M. Dardenne. 1973. Studies on thymus products. II. Demonstration and characterization of a circulating thymic hormone. Immunology **25:** 353.
5. Goldstein, G. 1974. Isolation of bovine thymus: a polypeptide hormone of the thymus. Nature **247:** 11.
6. Serrou, B., Cl. Solassol, H. Joyeux, H. Pujol & Cl. Romieu. 1972. Immunosuppressive effect of Rifampicin. Transplantation **14:** 654.
7. Lowry, O. H., N. G. Rosenbrough, A. L. Farr & R. J. Randall. 1951. Protein measurement with the folin phenol reagent. J. Biol. Chem. **193:** 265.
8. Jerne, N. K. & A. A. Nordin. 1963. Plaque formation in agar by single antibody-producing cells. Science **140:** 405.
9. Clark, S. L. 1966. Cytological evidences of secretion in the thymus. *In* Thymus —Experimental and Clinical Studies. G. E. W. Wolstenholme & R. Porter, Eds. **:** 3. J. & A. Churchill, Ltd. London, England.
10. Rotter, V., A. Globerson, I. Nakamura & N. Trainin. 1973. Studies on characterization of the lymphoid target cell for activity of a thymus hormonal factor. J. Exp. Med. **138:** 130.
11. Dardenne, M. & J. F. Bach. 1973. Studies on thymus products. I. Modification of rosette-forming-cells by thymic extracts. Determination of the target RFC sub-population. Immunology **25:** 343.
12. Wortis, H. H., S. Nehlsen & J. J. Owen. 1971. A tumoral development of the thymus in nude mice. J. Exp. Med. **134:** 681.
13. Zisblatt, M., A. L. Goldstein, F. Lilly & R. White. 1970. Acceleration by thymosin of the development of resistance to murine sarcoma virus-induced tumor in mice. Proc. Nat. Acad. Sci. U.S. **66:** 1170.

EFFECT OF THYMIC FACTORS ON THE DIFFERENTIATION OF HUMAN MARROW CELLS INTO T-LYMPHOCYTES *IN VITRO* IN NORMALS AND PATIENTS WITH IMMUNODEFICIENCIES *

J. L. Touraine,† F. Touraine, G. S. Incefy, and R. A. Good

Memorial Sloan-Kettering Cancer Center
New York, New York 10021

Introduction

Immune functions can be restored by thymus grafting in neonatally thymectomized animals, nude mice, and in patients with DiGeorge syndrome.[1–4] In these situations, unlike in stem-cell deficiencies, the newly developed T-lymphocytes usually bear markers of the recipient,[5, 6] thus suggesting that the reconstitution has not involved a proliferation of the donor's thymocytes but rather the "induction" of differentiation into T-lymphocytes from the recipient's precursor cells. That such an effect was in part under the dependence of diffusible humoral factors, has been suggested by the restoration of some immunological functions when the thymus graft was placed in a Millipore® diffusion chamber[7] or when injection of acellular extracts was performed instead of the organ graft.[8] Although some controversy still exists on that matter,[9] the investigation of the *in vivo* and *in vitro* effects of thymic extracts or factors has been extensively carried out over the past years. Recent studies in the mouse have shown that a fraction of spleen or bone marrow cells can acquire T-lymphocyte characteristics *in vitro* after a short incubation with thymic extracts[10, 11] or with a serum factor of thymic origin.[12] We have obtained similar results in man,[13] thus providing a means for the study of differentiation of human lymphocytes and for the analysis of various immunodeficiency diseases.[14, 15]

Materials and Methods

The protocol for the entire experimental procedure is shown in Figure 1.

Fractionation of Bone Marrow Cells

Bone marrow was obtained by small aspirations (0.5 to 0.7 ml) with an heparinized syringe, from various points of the iliac crest or the proximal

* We acknowledge support from grants by the National Institutes of Health, The National Cancer Institute (CA–08748–08S1), The National Foundation—March of Dimes, The American Cancer Society, The French DGRST and Foreign Office.

† Present address and correspondence: Dr. J. L. Touraine, Transplantation and Immunobiology Unit, Clinic of Nephrology, Hôpital Ed. Herriot, 69003 Lyon, France.

portion of the tibia in cadavers, patients in irreversible coma, volunteer donors, or patients with immunodeficiencies. After centrifugation at $200 \times g$ for 5 minutes, the buffy coat was aspirated and subjected to the density gradient fractionation technique of Dicke *et al.*[16] Marrow cells were resuspended in 17% bovine serum albumin (BSA Pentex, 35% solution, Miles Laboratories, Inc., Kankakee, Ill.) prepared in tissue culture medium RPMI-1640 containing 50 u/ml of penicillin and 50 μg/ml of streptomycin (Grand Island Biological Company, Grand Island, N.Y.). This cell suspension was carefully layered on top of the discontinuous density gradient made of the following dilutions of BSA in RPMI-1640: 19%, 21%, 23%, 25% and 27%. Following centrifugation ($750 \times g$ for 30 minutes) the cell layers were removed and labeled: I (at the 17–19% interface), II (19–21%), III (21–23%), IV (23–25%) and V (25–27%). The yield of cells recovered in layer III was between 1 and 10% of the total number of nucleated cells in the starting suspension. Cells from each layer were washed in Hanks' balanced salt solution and the suspensions adjusted to a concentration of 2×10^6 cells/ml. Viability, checked by trypan blue exclusion, was found to be above 95%.

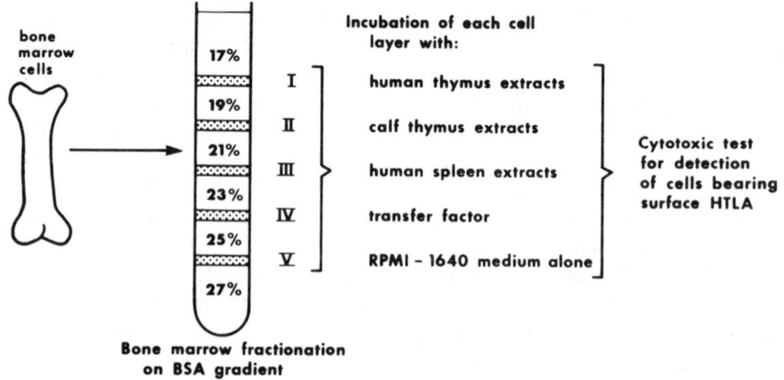

FIGURE 1. Experimental protocol.

Incubation with Tissue Extracts

Human thymuses were obtained from young children undergoing cardiac surgery. Spleens were removed at autopsy immediately after accidental death. Frozen calf thymuses were purchased from a local slaughter house. Extracts were prepared using the procedure of A. Goldstein *et al.*[17] Tissues were homogenized in 0.15 M NaCl and sonicated for 10 seconds at 4° C. The homogenate was filtered and purified by several centrifugations. The supernatant solution obtained was heated for 15 minutes at 80° C, centrifuged again and filtered through a 0.45 μ millipore membrane (fraction 2). The acetone insoluble precipitate was redissolved in 0.1 M phosphate buffer, pH 7.2 (fraction 3). Protein content was determined by the method of Lowry *et al.*[18] using bovine albumin as a standard. All tissue extracts were used at a final protein concentration between 0.6 and 3.6 mg/ml.

Transfer factor was prepared by the method of Lawrence [19] and was shown to transfer delayed hypersensitivity to several antigens *in vivo*.[20] Ten milliliters of transfer factor solution were prepared from 6×10^9 peripheral blood leukocytes of normal donors and this was used undiluted.

Equal volumes of bone marrow cell suspension (2×10^6 cells/ml) from each layer and tissue extract, or transfer factor solution, were mixed together and incubated for 2 hours at 37° C, in a humidified atmosphere of 5% CO_2-95% air. Cells were washed in Hanks' balanced salt solution and each suspension was adjusted to a concentration of 2×10^6 cells/ml. Viability was usually above 95%, always above 90%.

Detection of Cells with Surface Characteristics of T-lymphocytes

These cells were recognized by a heterologous specific anti-human T-cell serum (ATCS), using a two-stage microlymphocytotoxicity method. The preparation, absorption, and T-lymphocyte specificity of the antiserum have been previously described.[21, 22] The antigenic markers detected on lymphocyte surface by this procedure have been called human specific T-lymphocyte antigens (HTLA).

The suspension of bone marrow cells (2×10^6 cells/ml) was incubated with the antiserum in the well of a microtest tissue culture plate (Falcon Plastics 3034, Los Angeles, California), then washed and rabbit complement added. The number of dead cells was determined after staining with trypan blue. Three hundred cells were examined in each well and every test was done in duplicate. Controls were performed with normal rabbit serum (NRS) and complement. The cytotoxic index (or percentage of cells with $HTLA^+$ phenotype) was given by the formula:

$$\text{cytotoxic index} = 100\left(\frac{\%\text{ alive with NRS} - \%\text{ alive with ATCS}}{\%\text{ alive with NRS}}\right)$$

Other Techniques

Human thymus-dependent E-rosette-forming cells (RFC) were quantified with a technique comparable to that of J. F. Bach,[23] using sheep erythrocytes (SRBC) in the presence of SRBC-absorbed fetal calf serum. Lymphocyte cultures in the presence of phytohemagglutinin (PHA), concanavalin A (Con-A) or mitomycin-treated allogeneic cells were performed as previously described.[13] [^{3}H]thymidine was added 24 hours before the harvest. Incorporation of the radioactive label was measured on the 3rd day after mitogen addition and on the 6th day of the mixed leukocyte cultures.

Results

Normal Donors

As shown in Table 1, each bone marrow layer contained a small percentage of $HTLA^+$ cells, which might be the equivalent of the postthymic or T_1 cells of the mouse. This percentage was unaffected by a 2-hour incubation in tissue culture medium. In all normal bone marrow experiments and regardless of the layer, it was always found to be between 1 and 12%. After incubation with spleen extracts, the number of HTLA⁺ cells was sometimes slightly increased but was never above 15% (10% as shown in TABLE 1). By contrast, the presence of thymic extracts during incubation of marrow cells from layer III significantly increased the proportion of cells bearing surface HTLA. Calf thymus extracts were nearly as effective as human thymus extracts, and no major difference could be detected using fraction 2 from the slightly more purified fraction 3. To a lesser degree, this conversion from $HTLA^-$ to $HTLA^+$ phenotype was occasionally observed in a few cells from layer II or IV. Assuming the absence of proliferation of a cell population during this short incubation, it could be calculated that thymic extracts induced between 16 and 38% of cells from layer III to become $HTLA^+$.[13]

TABLE 1

PERCENTAGE OF T-LYMPHOCYTES ($HTLA^+$ CELLS) AFTER *in Vitro* INCUBATION OF HUMAN BONE MARROW CELLS WITH TISSUE EXTRACTS OR TRANSFER FACTOR *

	Cytotoxic Index After Incubation with Extracts							
Bone marrow cells	Human Thymus F2 †	Human Thymus F3	Calf Thymus F2	Calf Thymus F3	Human Spleen F2	Human Spleen F3	Transfer Factor	Medium RPMI–1640
Normal donor								
Layer I	—	10	—	7	—	5	—	6
Layer II	—	8	—	8	—	5	—	4
Layer III	29	30	19	27	10	7	—	4
Layer IV	—	8	—	7	—	8	—	6
Layer V	—	4	—	3	—	3	—	4
Partial DiGeorge syndrome								
Layer I		—	14	2			—	8
Layer II		10	15	11			7	8
Layer III		29	30	30			4	3
Layer IV		3	6	3			1	3
Layer V		—	4	6			—	3

* Bone marrow cells from each layer were incubated at 37° C for 2 hours with tissue extracts or transfer factor; the presence of HTLA on cell surface was then determined in a cytotoxicity test with ATCS and rabbit complement.

† F2 and F3 = successive fractions 2 and 3 of tissue extracts.

To eliminate the possibility of a passive absorption of HTLA at the cell surface, the absence of free HTLA in the thymic extracts was verified by absorption experiments: the anti-T-lymphocyte activity of ATCS was not altered by prior incubation of this antiserum with the extracts.

The percentage of RFC among cells from layer III was also slightly increased by a 2-hour incubation with thymic extracts (from 1–2% to 4–7%). A longer incubation period (24 hours) sometimes induced the capacity to form rosettes in a relatively more significant number of cells but it was never as manifest and important as the induction of $HTLA^+$ phenotype. Again the effect was more restricted in the other layers.

Layer III thus contains the larger proportion of T-cell precursors able to express specific surface characteristics after incubation with thymic extracts. In this layer, there is also an enrichment in cells able to form granulopoietic colonies (P. L'Espérance and reference 14).

When thymic extracts were added alone to cultures of bone marrow cells, it was observed that some extracts had no effect (or were even inhibitory on the spontaneous proliferation) whereas others induced some degree of stimulation. However, this effect on proliferation was not correlated to the capacity to induce the acquisition of surface markers specific of the T-cell population. When the bone marrow cells were incubated for 24 hours with thymic extracts alone or associated with transfer factor, and then assayed for their ability to respond to mitogens or allogeneic cells, no significant increase was observed as compared with the controls. Only a minimal and questionable effect was occasionally observed when cells from layer III were used and response to allogeneic cells or Con-A was investigated.

Patient with Partial DiGeorge Syndrome

The clinical case report of this infant and the results of immunological studies are reported elsewhere.[15] In brief, no thymus was detected macroscopically and only systematic sections of mediastinum at autopsy revealed a very small piece of tissue 7 × 3 mm identifiable as a thymus. Histology showed the presence of Hassall's corpuscles and thymocytes.[15] The percentage of peripheral blood T-lymphocytes was relatively low (46–50% $HTLA^+$ cells and 24–28% RFC), whereas the proportion of B-cells with a high density of surface immunoglobulin was increased (44–38%).

In this patient, as in every normal individual so far tested, a substantial number of bone marrow cells from layer III were converted from $HTLA^-$ to $HTLA^+$ phenotype after incubation with extracts from calf or human thymuses (TABLE 1). Appearance of surface characteristics of T-lymphocytes was noted in a much smaller percentage of cells from other layers. Incubation with transfer factor in place of thymic extracts did not induce conversion to $HTLA^+$ phenotype.

Patient with Severe Congenital Combined Immunodeficiency (SCID)

This 2 month old male infant whose sister had died of SCID presented a severe deficit in numbers and functions of the T- and B-cell populations.[14] The amount of adenosine deaminase in erythrocytes was normal.

Incubation of bone marrow cells from each layer in the presence of thymic extracts did not increase the number of $HTLA^+$ cells (TABLE 2). Even tissue extracts concentrated four times were inefficient on cells of layer III. Similarly, the number of RFC among the patient's bone marrow cells remained below 1.5% after a 2-hour incubation with thymic extracts. By contrast, the formation of granulopoietic colonies from precursor cells of layer III was significant.[14]

Patient with Common Variable Immunodeficiency

This 36 year old male patient presented both an agammaglobulinemia and a severe functional deficit of T-lymphocytes.[14]

After incubation of bone marrow cells with thymic extracts, the number of HTLA+ cells increased significantly in layer III (TABLE 2). The increase was slightly less prominent than in a normal donor but this may be due to the presence of T-cell precursors, not only in layer III but apparently also in layers II and IV. The same incubation increased slightly the number of RFC, from less than 1.5% up to 3% among layer III cells.

TABLE 2

PERCENTAGE OF T-LYMPHOCYTES (HTLA+ CELLS) AFTER *in Vitro* INCUBATION OF HUMAN BONE MARROW CELLS WITH TISSUE EXTRACTS *

	Cytotoxic Index After Incubation with Extracts						
	Human Thymus		Calf Thymus		Human Spleen		Medium
Bone marrow cells	F2	F3	F2	F3	F2	F3	RPMI–1640
Patient A †							
Layer I	—	4	—	—	—	—	3
Layer II	—	4	—	4	—	4	3
Layer III	6	6	5	5	—	5	5
Layer IV	—	3	—	2	—	2	3
Layer V	—	6	—	3	—	4	4
Patient B							
Layer I	—	6	—	—	—	—	—
Layer II	—	11	—	—	—	—	7
Layer III	—	20	—	14	—	6	7
Layer IV	—	11	—	11	—	5	4

* Same procedure as TABLE 1.

† *Patient A*=Severe congenital combined immunodeficiency. *Patient B*=Common variable immunodeficiency with agammaglobulinemia and severe functional deficit of T-lymphocytes.

DISCUSSION

Significant modifications are observed in a fraction of normal human bone marrow cells after incubation with thymic extracts. These modifications are not attributable to a proliferation of the small T-lymphocyte population present in bone marrow. There is no correlation between the (moderate and inconstant) proliferative effect of the extracts and their ability to induce the appearance of T-cell surface markers. Furthermore, this proliferative effect, when noted, is only apparent after some days and cannot be significant in two hours. A different explanation that has not been excluded is a possibly direct alteration of the cell surface, but it would not be a mere fixation of antigens because thymic extracts were shown to lack free HTLA. A more likely hypothesis is that we have induced some degree of T-lymphocyte differentiation, whether the underlying mechanism involves derepression or activation of the T-cell precursors. This hypothesis would also be in agreement with the results of Komuro and Boyse [11] who showed that mouse spleen cells incubated with thymic extracts express only the Thy-1 or TL phenotype for which they are genetically determined. Such derepression or activation could also be induced by a variety of agents such as endotoxin and poly A:U.[24] How the thymic factors exert their effect on the precursor cells remains to be determined. Recent results indicate that cyclic AMP may play a role.[24–26]

The differences observed in the induction of the various characteristics of the T-lymphocyte population may have several explanations, the more likely being that they are related to successive stages of differentiation. Appearance of antigenic markers would be an early event, followed by the capacity to form "T-rosettes." Later the changes would occur that make it possible to respond to allogeneic cells and to mitogens.

Studies on human T-lymphocyte differentiation under the influence of thymic extracts not only provide insight on fundamental issues and ontogeny. They also permit analyses of immunodeficiencies with a new approach, namely the investigation of bone marrow T-lymphocyte precursors. In the partial DiGeorge syndrome that we explored, these precursor cells were present and able to differentiate into T-lymphocytes. This finding is in agreement with similar observations in the experimental counterpart, the nude mice.[27]

Bone marrow studies in the two patients with severe deficits of both T- and B-lymphocyte functions led to different results. In the infant with SCID, no T-cell differentiation could be induced, which suggests the absence of stem cells or T-lymphocyte precursors or else the nonsusceptibility to thymic factors. In the common variable immunodeficiency, T-lymphocyte differentiation was induced *in vitro* and the suggestion is that of a block in a more advanced stage of maturation of both T- and B-cell populations.

Thus the study of human T-lymphocyte differentiation from bone marrow cells of some immunodeficient patients has given some information on the basic defect. This may have therapeutic implications, especially as far as cellular engineering is concerned. It is hoped that comparable analysis of other immunodeficiencies as well as improvement of the *in vitro* and *in vivo* monitoring of T- and B-cell differentiation will provide much more knowledge on human lymphoid system, its diseases and their treatment. Toward this end, thymic factors are expected to play a significant role.

Summary

Extracts of human or calf thymus influence the differentiation of human bone marrow cells *in vitro*. Incubation of a stem cell-enriched fraction of normal marrow with extracts of human or calf thymus led to the appearance of lymphocytes with surface antigens recognized by a highly specific anti-human T-cell serum. To a lesser degree, development of lymphocytes having the capacity to form rosettes with sheep erythrocytes was observed, but the induction of the capacity to respond to allogeneic cells or to mitogens was weaker and inconstant. This procedure was later utilized for the study of 3 patients. Inability of marrow cells to differentiate into T-lymphocytes under the influence of thymic factors was noted in a patient with severe congenital combined immunodeficiency. By contrast, some precursor cells able to differentiate into T-lymphocytes were observed in common variable immunodeficiency and partial DiGeorge syndrome.

Acknowledgments

We are grateful to Professor P. A. Ebert of the Department of Surgery, New York Hospital and Dr. Y. M. Rho of the Institute for Forensic Medicine for their generous gifts of tissues; to Dr. R. Gilly for referring one of the patients to us; and to Mrs. R. Anninipot and Miss O. Voute for skilled technical assistance.

References

1. Stutman, O., E. J. Yunis & R. A. Good. 1969. Transplant. Proc. **1:** 614.
2. Wortis, H. H., S. Nehlsen & J. J. Owen. 1971. J. Exp. Med. **134:** 681.
3. August, C. S., F. S. Rosen, R. M. Filler, C. A. Janeway, B. Markowski & H. E. M. Kay. 1968. Lancet **ii:** 1210.
4. Cleveland, W. W., B. J. Fogel, W. T. Brown & H. E. M. Kay. 1968. Lancet **ii:** 1211.
5. Pritchard, H. & H. S. Micklem. 1973. Clin. Exp. Immunol. **14:** 597.
6. Loor, F. & B. Kindred. 1973. J. Exp. Med. **138:** 1044.
7. Osoba, D. & J. F. A. P. Miller. 1964. J. Exp. Med. **119:** 177.
8. Trainin, N. & M. Small. 1970. J. Exp. Med. **132:** 885.
9. Stutman, O. 1974. Fed. Proc. **33:** 736 Abstract.
10. Bach, J. F., M. Dardenne, A. L. Goldstein, A. Guha & A. White. 1971. Proc. Nat. Acad. Sci. U.S. **68:** 2734.
11. Komuro, K. & E. A. Boyse. 1973. Lancet **i:** 740.
12. Bach, J. F. & M. Dardenne. 1973. Immunology **25:** 353.
13. Touraine, J. L., G. S. Incefy, F. Touraine, Y. M. Rho & R. A. Good. 1974. Clin. Exp. Immunol. **17:** 151.
14. Touraine, J. L., G. S. Incefy, F. Touraine, P. L'Espérance, F. P. Siegal & R. A. Good. 1974. Clin. Immunol. Immunopathol. In press.
15. Touraine, J. L., F. Touraine, J. Dutruge, J. Gilly, S. Colon & R. Gilly. 1975. Clin. Exp. Immunol. In press.
16. Dicke, K. A., P. H. C. Lina & D. W. Van Bekkum. 1970. Rev. Eur. Etud. Clin. Biol. **15:** 305.
17. Goldstein, A. L., A. Guha, M. M. Katz, M. A. Hardy & A. White. 1972. Proc. Nat. Acad. Sci. U.S. **69:** 1800.
18. Lowry, O. H., N. J. Rosenbrough, A. L. Farr & R. J. Randall. 1951. J. Biol. Chem. **193:** 265.
19. Lawrence, H. S. 1969. Advan. Immunol. **11:** 195.
20. Griscelli, C., J. P. Revillard, H. Betuel, C. Herzog & J. L. Touraine. 1973. Biomedicine **18:** 220.
21. Touraine, J. L., D. F. Kiszkiss, Y. S. Choi & R. A. Good. 1973. Fed. Proc. **32:** 975. Abstract.
22. Touraine, J. L., F. Touraine, D. F. Kiszkiss, Y. S. Choi & R. A. Good. 1974. Clin. Exp. Immunol. **16:** 503.
23. Bach, J. F. 1973. Transplant. Rev. **16:** 196.
24. Sheid, M. P., M. K. Hoffman, K. Komuro, U. Hammerling, J. Abbott, E. A. Boyse, G. H. Cohen, J. A. Hooper, R. S. Schulof & A. L. Goldstein. 1973. J. Exp. Med. **138:** 1027.
25. Bach, M. A. & J. F. Bach. 1972. C. R. Acad. Sci. (Paris) **275:** 2783.
26. Hadden, J. W. Personal communication.
27. Komuro, K. & E. A. Boyse. 1973. J. Exp. Med. **138:** 479.

PART V. *In Vivo* EFFECTS OF THYMUS EXTRACTS

INFLUENCE OF THYMUS EXTRACTS ON THE MATURATION OF THE IMMUNE RESPONSE IN NEONATAL MICE

W. S. Ceglowski and G. U. LaBadie

Department of Microbiology
Pennsylvania State University
University Park, Pennsylvania 16802

It has been observed in a number of laboratories that neonatal animals do not develop the capacity to form antibodies to sheep erythrocytes or bacterial antigens until several days or weeks after birth.[1–7] The capacity of rodents to develop immune competence is related to a number of factors. One of the more important factors appears to be an intact thymus.[8–11] It has been clearly demonstrated that thymectomy of newborn mice drastically reduces their immunocompetence to sheep erythrocytes.

The mechanism by which the thymus exerts its effect on immune competence has been an area of intense contemporary investigation. For many years experimental biologists have studied the effects of administering homologous and heterologous extracts of thymus on a number of biological parameters. Some of these extracts and their activities were reviewed by White and Goldstein in 1968.[12] Since that time the number of investigations into the effect of thymic extracts or factors on a variety of immunologic processes has increased.[13–17]

Our studies in this area represent an extension of the study by Hand, Caster, and Luckey.[18] In these studies[19–22] we have administered extracts of calf thymus to newborn mice and subsequently assessed their level of immune competence to sheep erythrocytes compared to that of a group of appropriate controls.

The experimental protocol can be briefly described in the following manner.

For most of our materials we have started with kilogram quantities of calf thymus, and have utilized the fractionation scheme described by Hand *et al.*[20] We have harvested gram quantities of a crude saline extract, and obtained milligram quantities of a methanol precipitate fraction. In an earlier study[20] we then isolated microgram quantities of acrylamide gel purified fractions. Following electrophoresis, two of these fractions were used for the biologic studies. The first fraction, designated "B-C," was previously found to contain a lymphoid cell stimulator. The second fraction, with less rapid mobility in the electrophoretic field, was designated fraction "D-E" and had been previously found to contain an inhibitory material for lymphocytopoesis.[18] We used the same fractionation scheme for calf serum, calf kidney, calf liver, and calf spleen in order to determine if the effects were specific for calf thymus or if they could be mediated by extracts of these tissues. In general, yields of partially purified extracts from these tissues were much less than those of calf thymus.

As an assay system for biologic activity, we have utilized the newborn mouse. In all our studies, newborn mice, either random-bred Swiss (ICR) or inbred BALB/c, have been injected within 12 hours of birth with solutions of the crude thymus extract, the methanol precipitate extract, or the purified protein in microgram quantities. In earlier work each value was the average of three separate pooled litters. All litters of newborn mice were standardized to contain no more than eight mice. At varying time intervals thereafter, we immunized these animals by intraperitoneal inoculation of 0.1 ml of 50% sheep erythrocytes. The test animals along with the appropriate control mice were then assayed for their ability to respond to the antigen. The immune response was assessed in two ways. The first was by performing hemagglutination assays. In brief, individual mice 2 weeks or older were bled from the retro-orbital venous plexus. Younger animals were decapitated, and blood was pooled from mice. Serum was separated from all blood specimens by clotting at room temperature and was stored at —20 C until used. For serologic assay, 0.025-ml dilutions of each serum sample were prepared in microtiter plates. To each dilution cup was added 0.025 ml of an 0.5% suspension of washed sheep erythrocytes. The plates were then agitated on a vibrating platform and incubated for 2 hours at 37 C and overnight in the cold. Serum titers were recorded as the reciprocal of the highest dilution resulting in complete hemagglutination of the added sheep red blood cells.

The second assay utilized was the antibody plaque-forming cell technique in agar gel. In brief, 0.1 ml of a freshly prepared mouse spleen cell suspension in Hank's solution was rapidly mixed with 2.0 ml of melted 0.9% Noble agar containing 0.1% dextran and SRBC. This mixture was then carefully poured onto the surface of a previously prepared Petri plate containing 10 ml solidified 1% Noble agar. These plates were incubated at 37 C for 1 hour and then treated with 2.0 ml of a 1:20 dilution of guinea pig complement. Plates were incubated for an additional 30 minutes at 37 C. The resulting zones of hemolysis were regarded as being due to high efficiency 19S hemolysins (IgM) secreted by individual antibody-forming cells. The total number of plaques per spleen, as well as the number of plaques per 10^6 leukocytes, was calculated. Usually two to three concentrations of leukocytes were plated in triplicate. Total leukocyte counts were determined with a hemocytometer with the use of acetic acid-methylene blue diluent, and viability was assessed by means of the Trypan blue dye exclusion technique.

A number of studies in our laboratory with crude saline extracts of calf thymus have consistently showed a lack of any marked (greater than 50%) increase in the immune competence of either neonatal or adult animals.[20] In subsequent studies these materials have been tested at concentrations from 10 μg up to 1 mg. This failure to observe activity may be a concentration effect, since the active material is believed to be present in extremely low concentrations.[21]

A methanol-precipitated mixture of proteins derived from the crude saline extract has also been tested for an effect on the immunologic maturation of newborn mice.[20–22] In these studies, inoculation of the methanol-precipitate fraction in microgram quantities at birth did enhance the immune response to sheep erythrocytes of these animals when they were immunized at one or two weeks of age.[21, 22] The studies presented in TABLE 1 demonstrated that this material had essentially no effect on immune competence in adult BALB/c mice either at doses equal to those utilized in neonates or at doses equivalent (based on μg extract per g body weight) to those found to be active in neonatal mice. Doses of methanol-precipitated protein ten times that of the equivalent dose were also ineffective in adult mice.

Extracts of other bovine tissues such as calf spleen kidney or serum have

TABLE 1

EFFECT OF THYMUS EXTRACTS ON THE IMMUNE COMPETENCE OF ADULT BALB/c MICE

Treatment Group	Immune Response * 4 Days After Immunization
Methanol Precipitate	
equal to neonate dose	1.3
equivalent to neonate dose	1.4
10× equivalent neonate dose	0.9
Purified Protein	
equal to neonate dose	1.1
equivalent to neonate dose	0.8

* Ratio—splenic PFC treated immunized/splenic PFC control immunized.

never demonstrated stimulating activity equal to those of calf thymus.[21, 22] These collective studies lead us to conclude that extracts of calf thymus partially purified by methanol precipitation possess the ability to enhance immunologic maturation as measured by the antibody plaque-forming cell response to sheep erythrocytes. The activity appeared to be thymus-specific since similar activities were not noted with extracts of other tissues.

A single protein was purified from the methanol precipitate mixture by Robey *et al.*[23] This material was studied by Luckey *et al.*[24] and has been shown to enhance the immune competence of neonatal mice. We have studied this material[23] and have demonstrated that microgram quantities of this purified material can enhance the immune response of neonatal mice to sheep erythrocytes. The result of a series of studies with the most active preparation of this purified material we have used to date is presented in TABLE 2. The data demonstrate that concentrations of the purified thymic proteins in the range of 0.05–1.0 μg appear to enhance immunologic maturation markedly. The effect appears to be time and dose dependent. It should be pointed out that

TABLE 2

EFFECT OF PURIFIED THYMUS PROTEIN ON THE IMMUNE COMPETENCE OF NEONATAL MICE (PFC/Spleen; Four Days After Immunization; Treated Immunized/Control Immunized *)

Treatment at birth	Age at Assay (Days) 8	18	25
3.9 μg	NT	1.2	1.5
1.0 μg	6.9	12.6	1.1
0.2 μg	37.9	8.0	2.2
0.05 μg	NT	10.0	NT

* Ratio of PFC Treated Immunized Group/PFC Control Immunized Group from TABLE 3.

other preparations of the same material had much less activity and that some preparations were completely devoid of activity when tested in a wide range of concentrations. An additional consideration in evaluating these extracts is the assay system utilized. TABLE 3 presents information concerning the process of immunologic maturation in normal ICR mice. It is clear that between birth and 28 days of age the neonatal mouse is rapidly acquiring immunologic competence. We have observed considerable variation between the immunologic competence of animals from the same litter as well as between litters. This is the rationale for utilizing an average PFC value derived from a large number of observations instead of utilizing a single age-matched litter as the control. We would summarize our collective experiments in the following manner. Under appropriate experimental conditions, both a partially purified thymus extract and a purified protein of thymic origin can substantially enhance the process of immunologic maturation in neonatal mice. The mechanism of action and the relationship of these thymic materials to those utilized by other investigators are at present not known.

TABLE 3

IMMUNE RESPONSE TO SHEEP ERYTHROCYTES AT 4 DAYS AFTER IMMUNIZATION

Age at Assay	Average PFC *	± SEM
4 days	5	4
8 days	51	8
9 days	110	15
12 days	700	110
18 days	7,200	800
26 days	53,300	8,400
32 days	74,180	11,517

* The average number of plaque-forming cells per spleen of ICR mice based on individual determinations in groups of 50 to 168 mice.

References

1. ROWLEY, D. A. & F. W. FITCH. 1965. The Mechanism of Tolerance Produced in Rats to Sheep Erythrocytes. I. Plaque-forming Cell and Antibody Response to Single and Multiple Injections of Antigens. J. Exp. Med. **121:** 671–681.
2. STERZL, J. 1967. Factors Determining the Differentiation Pathways of Immunocompetent Cells. Cold Spring Harbor Symp. Quant. Biol. **32:** 493.
3. FRIEDMAN, H. 1966. Immunological Tolerance to Microbial Antigens. II. Suppressed Antibody Plaque Formation to *Shigella* Antigens by Spleen Cells from Tolerant Mice. J. Bacteriol. **92:** 820–827.
4. HECHTEL, M., T. DISHON & W. BRAUN. 1965. Hemolysin Formation in Newborn Mice of Different Strains. Proc. Soc. Exp. Biol. Med. **120:** 728–732.
5. HECHTEL, M., T. DISHON & W. BRAUN. 1965. Influence of Oligodeoxyribonucleotides on the Immune Response of Newborn AKR Mice. Proc. Soc. Exp. Biol. Med. **119:** 991–993.
6. CHENG, V. & J. J. TRENTIN. 1967. Enteric Bacteria as a Possible Cause of Hemolytic Antibody-Forming Cells in Normal Mouse Spleens. Proc. Soc. Exp. Biol. Med. **126:** 467–470.

7. Nordin, A. A. 1967. The Occurrence of Plaque Forming Cells in Normal and Immunized Conventional and Germfree Mice. Proc. Soc. Exp. Biol. Med. **129:** 57–62.
8. Miller, J. F. A. P. & D. Osoba. 1967. Current Concepts of the Immunological Functions of the Thymus. Physiol. Rev. **47:** 437–520.
9. Metcalf, D. 1966. Recent Results in Cancer Research. The Thymus. Springer-Verlag. New York, N.Y.
10. Hess, M. W. 1968. Experimental Thymectomy. Springer-Verlag. New York, N.Y.
11. Good, R. A. & B. W. Papermaster. 1964. Ontogeny and Phylogeny of Adoptive Immunity. Adv. Immunol. **4:** 1–115.
12. White, A. & A. L. Goldstein. 1968. Is the thymus an endocrine gland. Old problem, new data. Perspect. Biol. Med. **11:** 475–484.
13. Carpenter, C. B., A. W. Boylston, II & J. P. Merrill. 1971. Immunosuppressive alpha globulin from bovine thymus. I. Preparation and assay. Cell. Immunol. **2:** 425–434.
14. Doria, G., G. Agarossi & S. DiPietro. 1972. Enhancing activity of Thymocyte culture cell-free medium on the *in vitro* immune response of spleen cells from neonatally thymectomized mice to sheep RBC. J. Immunol. **108:** 268–270.
15. Kiger, N., I. Florentine & G. Mathe. 1972. Some effects of a partially purified lymphocyte-inhibiting factor from calf thymus. Transplantation **14:** 448–454.
16. Schimpl, A. & E. Wecker. 1972. Replacement of T-cell function by a T-cell product. Nature New Biol. **237:** 15–17.
17. Garaci, E. & W. Djaczenko. 1973. Diffusible factor of thymus is responsible for the recovery from some effects of heterologous anti-lymphocyte serum. Experientia **29:** 337–338.
18. Hand, T., P. Caster & T. D. Luckey. 1967. Isolation of a thymus hormone, LSH. Biochem. Biophys. Res. Commun. **26:** 18–23.
19. Hand, T., W. S. Ceglowski & H. Friedman. 1970. Calf thymus fractions: Enhancement and suppression of immunocompetent cells in neonatal mice. Experientia **26:** 653–655.
20. Hand, T. L., W. S. Ceglowski, D. Damrongsak & H. Friedman. 1970. Development of antibody forming cells in neonatal mice: Stimulation and inhibition by calf thymus fractions. J. Immunol. **105:** 442–450.
21. Robey, W. G., W. S. Ceglowski, T. D. Luckey & H. Friedman. 1973. Thymus Factors and Immunity: Enhancement of immunologic maturation by a purified calf thymus extract. : 295–300. *In* Microenvironmental Aspects of Immunity. B. D. Jankovic & K. Isakovic, Eds. Plenum Press. New York, N.Y.
22. Ceglowski, W. S., T. L. Hand & H. Friedman. 1973. Biologic Activity of Thymic Proteins in the Maturation of the Immune Response. : 185–192. *In* Thymic Hormones. T. D. Luckey, Ed. University Park Press. Baltimore, Md.
23. Robey, W. G., B. J. Campbell & T. D. Luckey. 1972. Isolation and characterization of a thymic hormone. Infect. Immunity **6:** 682–688.
24. Luckey, T. D., W. G. Robey & B. J. Campbell. 1973. LSH, a Lymphocyte-Stimulating Hormone. : 167–183. *In* Thymic Hormones. T. D. Luckey, Ed. University Park Press. Baltimore, Md.

Discussion of the Paper

Dr. N. Rose: I understand that you tested for antibody four days after immunization. This is the maximum when IgM antibody plaques occur. Did you look at IgG antibody plaques? What is the target cell of action of your factor? Do you believe it might be a macrophage, since macrophages seem to be deficient in young mice?

DR. W. CEGLOWSKI: The answer to the first question is that we have not looked at IgG plaque-forming cells. We really don't have any good idea as to the target cell. However, I wonder whether other people working with various extracts have mentioned the variability in activity? If every preparation were active, sequential experiments would be relatively straight forward. Unfortunately, the next batch that might be prepared often showed less activity, another batch might show no activity. I must qualify my statements by saying we have been looking at microgram quantities. When we find a batch with low activity, we increase the dose to 2, 3, 4, 5, or even 10 micrograms. Again, based on information we have been hearing here at the conference, perhaps we might have done better to look at lower concentrations.

THE NATURE AND MECHANISM OF STIMULATION OF IMMUNE RESPONSIVENESS BY THYMUS EXTRACTS *

Nathan Trainin, Abraham I. Kook, Tehila Umiel, and Maurizio Albala

Department of Cell Biology
The Weizmann Institute of Science
Rehovot, Israel

Introduction

A humoral factor isolated from the thymus of mice or calves (THF) has been shown to restore the ability of mouse spleen cells from neonatally thymectomized (NTx) mice to react in an *in vitro* graft-versus-host (GVH) assay.[1, 2] THF is obtained following homogenization of thymus tissue; the homogenate is spun at $105.000 \times g$ for 5 hours and the supernatant is then dialyzed. THF passes through the dialysis bag.[2] It appears to be a polypeptide of $5000 > MW > 700$ as demonstrated by gel filtration on Sephadex® G-25, paper chromatography, paper electrophoresis and ion exchange chromatography on DEAE Sephadex. The activity of the preparation is lost upon treatment with proteolytic enzymes (Kook and Trainin, unpublished data). Results previously obtained in our laboratory[3] demonstrated that dibutyryl cAMP (D-B cAMP) or substances which increase intracellular levels of cAMP in lymphoid cells such as poly (A:U),[4] theophylline or PGE_2[5, 6] were shown to mimic the effect of THF and confer reactivity in an *in vitro* GvH response to spleen cells from NTx mice. Flufenamic acid, an antagonist to PGE_2,[7] was shown to inhibit the induction of competence by this substance. It was found that THF induces competence by increasing membranal adenyl cyclase activity, which leads to a rise in intracellular cAMP in thymus-derived cells only.[3] These biochemical changes occur prior to antigenic stimulation and are unrelated to antigenic challenge.[3] These findings indicate that THF exerts its effect via an obligatory rise in intracellular cAMP and are in agreement with the concepts that permit the classification of THF as a thymus hormone.[8] Our working hypothesis is that THF exerts its effect on nonimmunocompetent spleen cells by inducing them to differentiate into mature immunocompetent cells and that differentiation is initiated by a rise in cellular cAMP levels. The present experiments were aimed at further investigating the biochemical events leading to acquisition of immunocompetence that follow the rise in cAMP induced by THF.

Results and Discussion

Biochemical Events Induced in Lymphoid Cells by THF

It has been shown that among the effects of cAMP on cellular metabolism it can also stimulate the expression of genetic information and induce protein

* This work was supported by a grant from the Talisman Foundation, Inc., New York, New York and by the National Institutes of Health, under agreement NCI-G-72-3890.

synthesis in certain cases.[9] Moreover, differentiation processes are often expressed by *de novo* protein synthesis.[10, 11] We therefore attempted to find out whether the increase in cellular cAMP is followed by a step of protein synthesis in the chain of events leading to the differentiation of spleen cells from NTx mice by THF.

We decided to use in these studies cycloheximide as an inhibitor of protein synthesis because of its reversible effect depending upon its continuous presence in the system tested.[12] As seen in TABLE 1 the effect of cycloheximide on protein synthesis in muscle and lymphoid cells was tested during 1 hour of incubation of cells in the presence of [1-^{14}C]leucine. Muscle cells were obtained from Lewis rats and grown as primary cultures. When tested, the cells were in their growth phase. A concentration of 20 μg per ml of cycloheximide was used, since it was found to produce maximal inhibition of protein synthesis without causing cell death in our system. Cycloheximide inhibited over 90% of the protein synthesis in muscle cells, as measured either by total ^{14}C incorporation or by specific activity. Under the same conditions, cycloheximide exerted a very mild inhibitory effect on spleen cells from intact mice (15–16% inhibition). On the other hand, a stronger inhibition of protein synthesis was observed in spleen cells from NTx mice (40–42%). These observations suggest that spleen cells from NTx mice are more sensitive to cycloheximide than spleen cells of intact mice, probably reflecting the presence of a younger and less mature cell population in the spleens of NTx mice.[13]

We then proceeded to investigate the effect of cycloheximide on the induction of immunocompetence in spleen cells from NTx mice by THF. The *in vitro* GvH assay was used. In this assay, the relative enlargement of an F_1 newborn spleen explant by parental spleen cells, compared to a paired explant challenged by spleen cells of the same F_1 origin 4 days after challenge reflects the degree of immunological competence of the grafted cells.[14] Parental spleen cells from NTx mice are not competent to react in this assay unless THF is added to the culture medium.[1, 2] We have also demonstrated previously that preincubation of spleen cells from NTx mice for 1 hour with THF restores the capacity of these cells to react in the *in vitro* GvH assay thus indicating that antigenic stimulation is not required for the induction of immunological competence by THF.[1] These findings permitted us to study the effect of cycloheximide on the processes leading to induction of competence by THF during the preincubation period. Spleen cells from intact or NTx mice were incubated for 1 hour at 37° C in Eagle's medium (EM) in the presence or absence of THF. Cycloheximide was added 15 minutes before addition of THF, simultaneously with THF, or 15 minutes after the addition of THF. Following incubation the cells were washed twice and tested in the GvH assay. Results of such experiments are shown in TABLE 2. It can be noted that preincubation of spleen cells from intact mice with cycloheximide did not abolish their ability to induce GvH response. In contrast the administration of cycloheximide abolished the inductive effect of THF on spleen cells from NTx mice during preincubation. These results suggest that protein synthesis is involved in the process of acquisition of immunocompetence induced by THF in spleen cells from NTx mice. Such a step is not required by the mature and competent spleen cells from intact mice under the experimental conditions used.

At this stage of the investigation, it was felt that certain controls were required to further clarify this point. It was essential to demonstrate that cycloheximide is indeed removed from the cells following the period of preincubation

TABLE 1

THE EFFECT OF CYCLOHEXIMIDE ON PROTEIN SYNTHESIS IN MUSCLE AND LYMPHOID CELLS *

					Cycloheximide (20 μg/ml)				
								Inhibition (%)	
Experiment	Cell Type	[^{14}C]CPM	Protein (mg)	[^{14}C]CPM/ mg Protein	[^{14}C]CPM	Protein (mg)	[^{14}C]CPM/ mg Protein	[^{14}C]CPM	[^{14}C]CPM/ mg Protein
I	Muscle	39952	0.79	50587	3262	0.76	4303	92	92
II	Spleen cells of intact mice	12732	2.90	4390	10822	2.85	3797	15	14
III	Spleen cells of intact mice	15895	—	—	13352	—	—	16	—
IV	Spleen cells of NTx mice	10563	—	—	6138	—	—	42	—
V	Spleen cells of NTx mice	12339	—	—	7359	—	—	40	—
VI	Spleen cells of NTx mice	15667	4.34	3615	9260	4.15	2234	41	38

* Each experiment was done in triplicates. 20×10^6 spleen cells from normal or NTx C57BL/6 mice and 2×10^6 muscle cells from normal rats were incubated for 1 hour at 37° C in 1 ml EM with 2 μCi [1-^{14}C]Leucine in the presence or absence of 20 μg cycloheximide. The results shown are averages.

TABLE 2

THE INDUCTION OF GVH RESPONSE IN SPLEEN CELLS OBTAINED FROM INTACT OR NTX C57BL/6 MICE FOLLOWING PREINCUBATION IN PRESENCE OF THF AND CYCLOHEXIMIDE *

Substance Tested (concentration)	Source of Spleen Cells	Time of Cyclohexi-mide Addition Following Start of Incubation (minutes)	Incidence of Reactive Cultures			Culture Response (%)
—	intact	—	4/5	4/5	4/5	80
Cycloheximide (20 μg/ml)	intact	0	5/5	5/5	4/5	93
—	NTx	—	0/5	0/5	0/5	0
THF (20 μg protein/ml)	NTx	—	4/5	3/5	4/5	73
Cycloheximide (20 μg/ml)	NTx	0	0/5	0/5	0/5	0
THF (20 μg protein/ml) + cycloheximide (20 μg/ml)	NTx	−15	0/5	1/5	0/5	6
THF (20 μg protein/ml) + cycloheximide (20 μg/ml)	NTx	0	0/5	0/5	0/5	0
THF (20 μg protein/ml) + cycloheximide (20 μg/ml)	NTx	+15	0/5	0/5	0/5	0

* 20×10^6 cells per ml were incubated for 1 hour at 37° C in EM in the presence or absence of THF. Cycloheximide was added 15 minutes prior to addition of THF, with THF, or 15 minutes after addition of THF. Following incubation the cells were washed twice in OCM and 1×10^6 live cells tested in the GvH assay.

before the lymphoid cells were applied to the *in vitro* GvH test, and that the effect of cycloheximide on spleen cells from NTx mice reflects its interference with the metabolic pathway that leads to the differentiation of cells by THF. The effect of the continuous presence of cycloheximide during the 4-day GvH assay was therefore tested. It was shown that cycloheximide completely inhibited the response of both spleen cells from intact mice or of spleen cells from NTx mice stimulated by THF. We proceeded then to investigate the reversibility of the blocking effect by cycloheximide. Cells were incubated for 1 hour with or without cycloheximide. The cells were then thoroughly washed and incubated in presence or absence of THF. Following this, the cells were tested for their ability to induce GvH response. We observed that spleen cells from intact mice and spleen cells from NTx mice incubated with THF regained their ability to induce GvH response following the removal of cycloheximide. Thus the continuous presence of cycloheximide during the 4 day GvH assay blocked the reactivity of normal spleen cells as well as of spleen cells from NTx mice in the presence of THF. On the other hand, the removal of cycloheximide restored the ability of normal cells to react in the *in vitro* GvH, and also enabled spleen cells from NTx mice to differentiate into competent cells in the presence of THF. These results led us to conclude that (1) the presence of THF during the 1-hour period of preincubation initiated a protein synthesis step that is required for the induction of competence in spleen cells of NTx mice and (2) the presence of cycloheximide during this period prevented this event.

As stated previously, we have suggested that the first biochemical event in the induction of immunocompetence by THF is an immediate and rapid increase in the activity of membranal adenyl cyclase which leads to a rise in cellular cAMP levels.[3] Cycloheximide prevents spleen cells from NTx mice from gaining competence even when added 15 minutes after the addition of THF (TABLE 2). This observation strongly suggests that protein synthesis which is required for acquisition of immunocompetence by spleen cells from NTx mice in presence of THF is an event that follows the increase in adenyl cyclase activity and is probably induced by the rise in cellular levels of cAMP. To rule out the possibility that the inhibitory effect of cycloheximide on protein synthesis was a reflection of inhibition of adenyl cyclase activation by THF, we investigated the effect of THF on adenyl cyclase activity in presence of cycloheximide. In this assay, the activation of membranal adenyl cyclase is measured by its ability to convert exogenous [^{3}H]ATP to [^{3}H]cAMP.[15] The results are shown in FIGURE 1. It can be seen that THF induced within 5 minutes a rapid increase in adenyl cyclase activity in spleen cells from NTx mice. It can also be noted that cycloheximide did not abolish the activation of adenyl cyclase by THF. In these experiments, cycloheximide was added 15 minutes prior to addition of THF and adenyl cyclase activity was measured 15 minutes following the addition of THF in presence of cycloheximide. Thus, the activation of adenyl cyclase by THF was not affected by cycloheximide. These experiments support the concept that the effect of cycloheximide on spleen cells from NTx

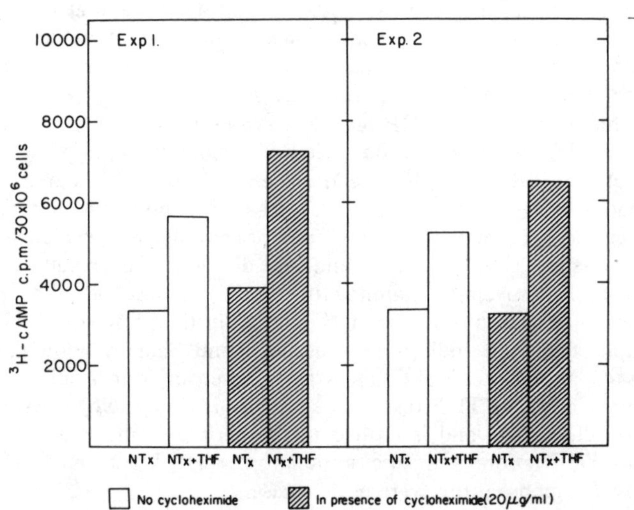

FIGURE 1. The effect of THF on adenyl cyclase activity in spleen cells from NTx C57BL/6 mice in presence or absence of cycloheximide. Cells were incubated in the presence of 20 μg protein/ml of THF for 5 minutes at 37° C in EM. When used, cycloheximide at a concentration of 20 μg/ml was added 15 minutes prior to addition of THF, and the effect of THF on adenyl cyclase activity was measured 15 minutes after addition of THF.

mice induced by THF is due to inhibition of a protein synthesis step that follows the increase in adenyl cyclase activity in the chain of events leading to the differentiation of these cells. They also suggest that the activation of adenyl cyclase by THF involves structural changes of the cell membrane rather than new synthesis of adenyl cyclase. We have previously demonstrated that THF induced a rise in cellular levels of cAMP in thymocytes as well as an increase in adenyl cyclase activity in spleen cells from either normal or NTx mice. These levels were higher than control levels and persisted during the incubation period with THF.[3] There is evidence that cAMP exerts a basic regulatory function on cell growth and differentiation.[16–18] It has been demonstrated that cAMP inhibits the growth of fibroblasts and that slowly growing cells have high endogenous levels of cAMP, whereas rapidly growing transformed cells have low cAMP levels.[19] Other results indicate that there is a cAMP-sensitive interval in the G_1 phase of human fibroblasts during which events necessary for the cells to enter into S phase are inhibited by high intracellular levels of cAMP.[20] A rapid arrest of DNA synthesis by D-B cAMP in cultured hepatoma cells has also been shown.[21] Furthermore, the addition of dibutyryl cAMP to cultures of human lymphoid cells that were synchronized in S phase resulted in a delay of mitotic activity of these cells.[22] It thus became of interest to investigate the effect of THF on DNA synthesis in thymocytes and in spleen cells from intact or NTx mice. The uptake of [^{3}H]thymidine into acid-precipitable material was used to measure the rate of DNA synthesis and therefore the proliferative activity in cell suspensions.[23] Cells were incubated in EM in presence or absence of 20 μg protein per ml of THF. In some experiments 20 μg protein per ml of calf spleen extract (SE) prepared in a similar way to THF was used as control. A pulse of 2 μCi of [^{3}H]thymidine was given before each time point determination. It can be seen in FIGURE 2 and TABLE 3 that the presence of THF during the incubation period strongly suppressed the incorporation of [^{3}H]thymidine into DNA in both thymocytes and spleen cells from NTx or intact mice. Spleen extract did not affect DNA synthesis.

The inhibitory effect of THF on DNA synthesis brought up the question of whether this effect is limited to the period of preincubation in presence of THF and is related to the steps which lead spleen cells from NTx mice to acquire immunocompetence. This concept was tested by preincubating spleen cells from intact and NTx mice in the presence of mitomycin-C, which is known to inhibit irreversibly DNA synthesis and cell division. The results can be seen in TABLE 4. Mitomycin-C inhibited the GvH response of both spleen cells from intact mice and spleen cells of NTx mice in the presence of THF. These results support similar findings by Auerbach and Shalaby[24] on the effect of mitomycin-C in the *in vitro* GvH assay. Moreover, our results suggest that the inhibitory effect of THF on DNA synthesis is a physiological step allowing the cell to differentiate and is limited to the period during which the cells are exposed to THF before antigenic stimulation. THF would have inhibited the *in vitro* GvH response if this were not the case.

Several lines of evidence indicate that increased levels of cellular cAMP changes cell morphology,[25–27] and leads to increase in cell volume.[25] It was thus of interest to test whether incubation of thymocytes in the presence of THF modifies some of the physical properties of these cells. Thymus cells were incubated for 1 hour with THF and submitted to a bovine serum albumin gradient.[28] Following centrifugation 4 layers of cells were obtained. The layers

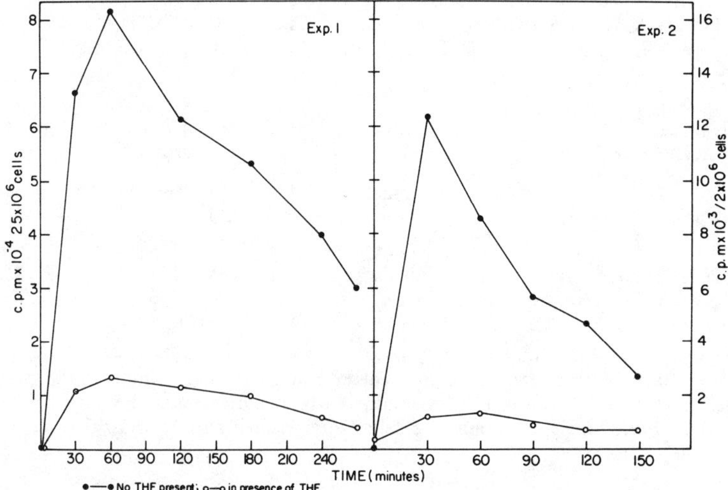

FIGURE 2. The effect of THF on the incorporation of [^{3}H]thymidine into DNA of thymocytes (Exp. 1) and of spleen cells from NTx C57BL/6 mice (Exp. 2). Cells were collected on ice and incubated in 1 ml EM at 37° C in presence of 20 μg protein per ml of THF. A 30-minute pulse of 2 μCi[^{3}H]thymidine was given before each time-point determination.

TABLE 3

THE EFFECT OF THF AND OF SPLEEN EXTRACT (SE) ON THE INCORPORATION OF [^{3}H]THYMIDINE INTO DNA OF LYMPHOID CELLS FROM C57BL/6 MICE

Cell Type	Substance Tested *	[^{3}H]CPM/10 × 10^6 Cells
	—	25958
Thymocytes	SE	23915
	THF	2069
	—	9672
Spleen cells from NTx mice	SE	9995
	THF	2176
	—	5579
Spleen cells from intact mice	SE	5544
	THF	1675

* Cells were incubated in 1 ml EM for 1 hour at 37° C in the presence of 20 μg protein of spleen extract (SE) or 20 μg protein in THF. A 30-minute pulse of 2 μCi[^{3}H]thymidine was given before incubation was ended. The results shown are averages of two such experiments showing a close pattern.

TABLE 4

THE EFFECT OF MITOMYCIN-C ON THE ABILITY OF SPLEEN CELLS FROM INTACT C57BL/6 MICE OR OF SPLEEN CELLS FROM NTx C57BL/6 MICE IN THE PRESENCE OF THF TO INDUCE *in Vitro* GvH RESPONSE *

Substance Tested (concentration)	Source of Spleen Cells	Incidence of Reactive Cultures				Culture Response (%)
—	intact	4/5	4/5			80
Mitomycin-C (25 μg/ml)	intact	0/5	1/5			10
—	NTx	1/5	0/5	0/5	0/5	5
THF (20 μg protein/ml)	NTx	4/5	4/5	3/5	3/5	70
THF (20 μg protein/ml) +mitomycin=C (25 μg/ml)	NTx	1/5	0/5	0/5	0/5	5

* 20 $\times$ 10^6 cells were incubated in 1 ml EM at 37° C for 1 hour in the presence or absence of THF. Mitomycin-C was added where indicated at the start of incubation period. Following incubation, the cells were washed and 1 $\times$ 10^6 live cells were tested in the GvH assay.

were as follows: A (at the 10–23% interface), B (23–26%), C (26–29%) and D (29–35%).[28]

Controls consisted of thymic cells exposed to spleen extract or incubated with no addition. The results of these experiments are presented in FIGURE 3. It can be seen that exposure of the cells to THF increased the proportion of cells in the top layer thus reflecting a change in cell density, whereas this effect was not observed in the controls. These preliminary findings indicate that THF

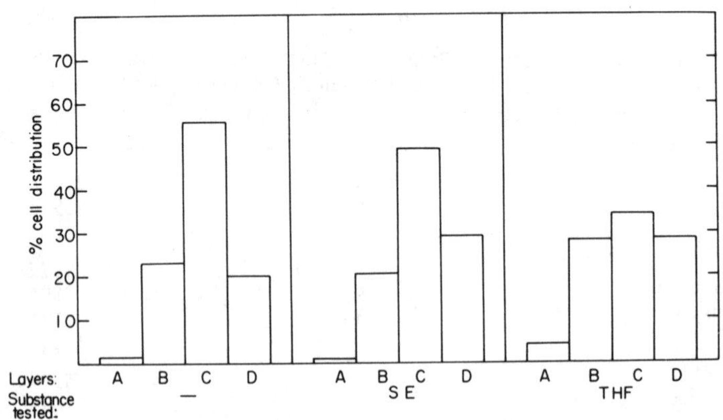

FIGURE 3. The effect of THF and of spleen extract (SE) on the distribution pattern of thymus cells from C57BL/6 mice by equilibrium density centrifugation. Cells were incubated for 1 hour at 37° C in EM in the presence of 50 μg protein per ml of THF or spleen extract. Following incubation 130 $\times$ 10^6 cells were applied to the gradient. Recovery in all samples was greater than 90%. The results shown are typical of three such experiments all showing the same pattern.

modifies cellular morphology during the events leading to acquisition of immunocompetence by lymphoid cells.

The Effect of THF on Lymphoid Cell Reactivity in MLC

The observation that DNA synthesis in lymphoid cells is inhibited in the presence of THF led us to assume that immunological reactions that involve intensive and repeated cell divisions should be inhibited by the presence of THF during the assay. Indeed it has been demonstrated that agents that activate adenyl cyclase strongly inhibited the response of lymphoid cells in immunological reactions.[5, 6, 29, 30] Our hypothesis on the mechanism of THF activity was therefore tested in a one way MLC assay.[31] This model was preferred since by pretreatment of the stimulator cells by mitomycin-C the effect measured refers only to the degree of immunological competence of the effector cells. TABLE 5 summarizes the results of one-way MLC assay in which effector spleen cells from intact mice were exposed to THF during the MLC reaction or by 1-hour preincubation with THF. It was found that the presence of THF during the MLC reaction significantly decreased the response of the effector cells in the assay. On the contrary, preincubation with THF raised the response of these cells over and above that seen in the controls. These results are in line with the concepts previously stated on the mechanism of cellular activation by THF. Similarly PGE_2 which we have shown to increase cellular cAMP levels[3]

TABLE 5

MIXED LEUKOCYTE CULTURE (MLC) BY SPLEEN CELLS PREINCUBATED OR IN THE PRESENCE OF THF

Experiment	Cell Mixture *	THF †	CPM±S.E.	Stimulation Index
Incubation ‡	ab → abm	−	4,099±1,558	
	ab → abm	+	7,317±889	
	a → abm	−	68,075±8,212	16.6
	a → abm	+	30,172±5,176	4.12
Incubation	ab → abm	−	2,865±542	
	ab → abm	+	4,068±248	
	a → abm	−	18,465±3,083	6.4
	a → abm	+	12,984±2,690	3.1
Preincubation §	ab → abm	−	1,530±60	
	ab → abm	+	1,742±64	
	a → abm	−	17,707±462	11.5
	a → abm	+	27,609±684	15.8

* a=10^6 C57BL/6 spleen cells; ab=10^6 (C3H/eb × C57BL/6)F_1 spleen cells; m=mitomycin-C 25 μg/ml cell suspension.

† 20 μg protein/ml.

‡ THF present in the culture medium during the MLC assay.

§ Preincubation for 1 hour at 37° C before exposure to MLC.

TABLE 6

EFFECT OF PROSTAGLANDIN E_2 (PGE_2) ON MLC BY SPLEEN CELLS

Cell Mixture *	PGE_2 †	CPM±S.E.	Stimulation Index
ab → abm	—	3,568±818	
ab → abm	+ ‡	1,915±149	
ab → abm	+ §	2,560±225	
a → abm	—	16,993±2,805	4.7
a → abm	+ ‡	4,379±405	2.2
a → abm	+ §	17,259±1,423	6.7

* a=10^6 C57BL/6 spleen cells; ab=10^6 (C3H/eb × C57BL/6)F_1 spleen cells; m=mitomycin-C 25 μg/ml cell suspension.

† 5 μg PGE_2/ml.

‡ PGE_2 present in the culture medium during the MLC assay.

§ Preincubation in PGE_2 for 1 hour at 37° C before exposure to MLC.

was tested in the same MLC model and found to mimic the effect of THF as seen in TABLE 6. The results presented point to the fact that preincubation with THF markedly increased the reactivity of spleen cells from intact mice in the MLC assay. This suggests that the spleen of normal mice contains cells that could still be activated by THF. This effect of THF on spleen cells from intact mice could not be measured in the *in vitro* GvH response, which by nature is an all or nothing type of response.

The last point in this series of experiments was to test whether the above described effect is preferentially exerted on a certain lymphoid cell population. For this purpose, cells of various origins were preincubated in THF and then subjected to one way MLC assay. The results are presented in TABLE 7. It can be appreciated that THF increased the response of thymus cells. On the other hand, bone marrow derived spleen cells were not affected by THF in this assay. These results are in line with our previous observations that THF activates adenyl cyclase in thymus-derived cells only.[3]

CONCLUSIONS

The present experiments demonstrate that THF restores the immunocompetence of spleen cells from NTx mice to induce an *in vitro* GvH response. This acquisition of immunocompetence is mediated as a first step by an obligatory rapid increase in adenyl cyclase activity and in intracellular levels of cAMP in lymphoid cells. Protein synthesis occurs as a further step in events leading to induction of immunocompetence by THF. This event could be blocked by cycloheximide which has no effect on normal cells.

The acquisition of competence by THF is accompanied by a reduction in DNA synthesis. When the effect of THF was assayed in a one way MLC it was found that preincubation of effector cells significantly increased their reactivity in the assay. On the contrary, the presence of THF during the MLC reaction seems to suppress the proliferation of the effector cells as a result of

TABLE 7

EFFECT OF THF ON MLC REACTIVITY BY LYMPHOID CELLS OF VARIOUS SOURCES

Source	Cell Mixture *	THF †	CPM±S.E.	Stimulation Index
B spleen ‡	a → am	−	2,557±389	
	a → am	+	3,189±268	
	a → amb	−	4,437±968	1.7
	a → amb	+	5,320±200	1.6
Lymph nodes §	ab → abm	−	918±267	
	ab → abm	+	3,530±1,100	
	a → abm	−	5,533±838	6.0
	a → abm	+	13,763±1,220	4.0
Thymus ¶	ab → abm	−	3,668±530	
	ab → abm	+	3,271±1,268	
	a → abm	−	6,300±1,620	1.7
	a → abm	+	6,352±1,256	1.9
Thymus **	ab → abm	−	1,647±197	
	ab → abm	+	1,558±117	
	a → abm	−	3,516±367	2.1
	a → abm	+	12,836±1,325	8.2

* a=10^6 C57BL/6 lymphoid cells; ab=10^6 (C3H/eb × C57BL/6)F_1 spleen cells; m=mitomycin-C 25 μg/ml cell suspension.

† Preincubation for 1 hour at 37° C in THF 20 μg protein/ml before exposure to MLC.

‡ 10^6 Cells recovered from spleens of thymectomized irradiated mice reconstituted with BM cells.

§ 10^6 Cells recovered from pools of peripheral lymph nodes.

¶ 10^6 Thymus cells.

** 2×10^6 Thymus cells.

the above observed reduction in DNA synthesis. The MLC assay enabled us to confirm that the target cells of THF activity are thymus-derived cells.

REFERENCES

1. TRAININ, N., M. SMALL & A. GLOBERSON. 1969. Immunocompetence of spleen cells from neonatally thymectomized mice conferred *in vitro* by a syngeneic thymus extract. J. Exp. Med. **130:** 765–775.
2. TRAININ, N. & M. SMALL. 1970. Studies on some physiochemical properties of a thymus humoral factor conferring immunocompetence on lymphoid cells. J. Exp. Med. **132:** 885–897.
3. KOOK, A. I. & N. TRAININ. 1974. Hormone-like activity of a thymus humoral factor on the induction of immune competence in lymphoid cells. J. Exp. Med. **139:** 193–207.
4. WINCHURCH, R., M. WHIZUKA, D. WEBB & W. BRAUN. 1971. Adenyl cyclase activity of spleen cells exposed to immunoenhancing synthetic oligo and polynucleotides. J. Immunol. **106:** 1399–1400.

5. Henny, C. S. & L. M. Lichtenstein. 1971. The role of cyclic AMP in the cytolytic activity of lymphocytes. J. Immunol. **107:** 610–612.
6. Henny, C. S., H. E. Bourne & L. M. Lichtenstein. 1972. The role of cyclic 3′,5′-adenosine monophosphate in the specific cytolytic activity of lymphocytes. J. Immunol. **108:** 1526–1534.
7. Collier, H. O. J. & W. J. F. Seatman. 1968. Antagonism by fenamates of prostaglandin $F_{\alpha 2}$ and of slow reacting substances on human bronchial muscle. Nature **219:** 864–865.
8. Sutherland, E. W. 1972. Studies on the mechanism of hormone action. Science **177:** 401–408.
9. Pastan, I. 1972. Cyclic AMP. Scientific American **227:** 97–105.
10. Shainberg, A., G. Yagil & D. Yaffe. 1971. Alteration of enzymatic activities during muscle differentiation *in vitro*. Develop. Biol. **25:** 1–29.
11. Yaffe, D. & H. Dym. 1973. Gene expression during differentiation of contractile muscle fibers. Cold Spring Harbor Symp. Quant. Biol. **XXXVII:** 543–547.
12. Gale, E. F., E. Cundlife, P. E. Reynolds, M. H. Richmond & M. J. Waring. 1972. *In* The Molecular Basis of Antibiotic Action. : 358–360. John Wiley & Sons, Inc. New York, N.Y.
13. Raff, M. C. & H. Cantor. 1972. Subpopulation of thymus cells and thymus-derived cells. *In* First International Congress of Immunology. Progress in Immunology. B. Amos, Ed. : 83–98. Academic Press. New York, N.Y.
14. Auerbach, R. & A. Globerson. 1966. *In vitro* induction of the graft-versus-host reaction. Exp. Cell Res. **42:** 31–41.
15. Krishna, G., B. Weiss & B. B. Brodie. 1968. A simple sensitive method for the assay of adenyl cyclase. J. Pharm. Exp. Therap. **163:** 379–385.
16. Sheppard, R. J. 1972. Difference in the cyclic adenosine 3′,5′-monophosphate levels in normal and transformed cells. Nature New Biol. **236:** 14–16.
17. Prasad, K. N. & A. W. Hsie. 1971. Morphologic differentiation of mouse neuroblastoma cells induced *in vitro* by Dibutyryl adenosine 3′,5′-cyclic monophosphate. Nature **233:** 141–142.
18. Burger, M. M., B. M. Bombik, B. McL. Breckenridge & J. R. Sheppard. 1972. Growth control and cyclic alteration of cyclic AMP in the cell cycle. Nature New Biol. **239:** 161–163.
19. Otten, J., G. S. Johnson & I. Pastan. 1971. Cyclic AMP levels in fibroblasts: Relationship to growth rate and contact inhibition of growth. Biochem. Biophys. Res. Commun. **44:** 1192–1198.
20. Froehlich, J. E. & M. Rachmeler. 1974. Inhibition of cell growth in the G_1 phase by adenosine 3′,5′-cyclic monophosphate. J. Cell. Biol. **60:** 249–257.
21. Van Wijk, R., W. D. Wicks, M. M. Bevers & J. Van Rijm. 1973. Rapid arrest of DNA synthesis by $N^6,O^{2'}$-dibutyryl cyclic adenosine 3′,5′-monophosphate in cultured hepatoma cells. Cancer Res. **33:** 1331–1338.
22. Millis, A. J. T., G. Forrest & D. A. Pious. 1972. Cyclic AMP in cultured human lymphoid cells: Relationship to mitosis. Biochem. Biophys. Res. Commun. **49:** 1645–1649.
23. Froehlich, J. E. & M. Rachmeler. 1972. Effect of adenosine 3′,5′-cyclic monophosphate on cell proliferations. J. Cell. Biol. **55:** 19–31.
24. Auerbach, R. & M. R. Shalaby. 1973. Graft-versus-host reaction in tissue culture. J. Exp. Med. **138:** 1506–1520.
25. Curtis, G. L., J. A. Elliott, R. B. Wilson & W. L. Ryan. 1973. Cyclic adenosine 3′,5′-monophosphate and cell volume. Cancer Res. **33:** 3273–3276.
26. Johnson, G. S., R. M. Friedman & I. Pastan. 1971. Restoration of several morphological characteristics of normal fibroblasts in sarcoma cells treated with adenosine 3′,5′-cyclic monophosphate and its derivatives. Proc. Nat. Acad. Sci. U.S. **68:** 425–429.
27. Kreider, J. W., M. Rosenthal & N. Lengle. 1973. Cyclic adenosine 3′,5′-monophosphate in the control of melanoma cell replication and differentiation. J. Nat. Cancer Inst. **50:** 555–558.

28. Komuro, K. & E. A. Boyse. 1973. *In vitro* demonstration of thymic hormone in the mouse by conversion of precursor cells into lymphocytes. Lancet. April **7:** 740–743.
29. Strom, T. B., A. Deisseroth, J. Morganroth, C. B. Carpenter & J. P. Merrill. 1972. Alteration of the cytotoxic action of sensitized lymphocytes by cholinergic agents and activators of adenyl cyclase. Proc. Nat. Acad. Sci. U.S. **69:** 2995–2999.
30. Hadden, J. W., E. M. Hadden, M. K. Haddox & N. D. Goldberg. 1972. Guanosine 3′,5′-cyclic monophosphate: A possible intracellular mediator of mitogenic influence in lymphocytes. Proc. Nat. Acad. Sci. U.S. **69:** 3024–3027.
31. Bach, F. H. & K. Voynow. 1966. One way stimulation in mixed leukocyte cultures. Science **153:** 545–547.

Discussion of the Paper

Dr. A. Goldstein: Dr. Trainin, that was a beautiful lecture and I think it was appropriate that from the Land of the Bible has come all of this information, rediscovering that it says in the Talmud that the thymus is good for the health; you certainly have shown that. We have shown and have been able to confirm your earlier suggestions that thymosin also acts at the level of T-1 cells in addition to the stem cell. And we have seen essentially what you've reported here; that is if you add thymosin to T-cells you enhance the MLR responsiveness. The questions that I have deal with two chemistry questions. Have you looked at the nature of your extract? Have you looked for the presence of cyclic nucleotides in your preparation? We have found that unless we use means to get rid of cyclic nucleotides they certainly are present in thymic extracts. If so, they could complicate some of the interpretations that we are all seeing. The second question, do you still feel that THF is heat labile now that Gideon Goldstein has found that his factor, like thymosin, is heat stable and so have several other investigators? I'd like to know whether you've repeated your heat stability studies? Thirdly, how long do you incubate your cells with THF? Do you keep THF in medium or is it possible to wash THF away from the cells? What is the time involved?

Dr. N. Trainin: The answer to the first question is that there is no cyclic AMP whatsoever in our preparations. As far as other nucleotides are concerned, we thought initially that there was some contamination with RNA, but we have been able to treat these preparations with RNAase and DNAase. No inhibition occurs. The only enzyme which destroys the activity of our preparations is pronase or other protelytic enzymes. Our very early reports mentioned heat instability of the material. Lately we have used a preparation which is most certainly a polypeptide and this polypeptide is not unstable. We think today that it is heat stable. For the final question, we incubated incompetent cells for as little as 20 minutes. We have not done enough experiments to say that 20 minutes is a critical time. We usually do an incubation of one hour. After one hour of incubation we wash the THF away. We can wash three times and the cells will recover their competence.

Dr. B. Waksman: I believe that Dr. Trainin has introduced a literary note which is very welcome in our otherwise rather heavy proceedings. But I think it is only proper to remark that the word thymus is a Greek word that means "the soul." And, of course, in the New Testament it is used repeatedly.

EARLY CELLULAR EVENTS IN THE RESPONSE OF MICE TO SHEEP RED BLOOD CELLS REFLECTED BY CHANGES IN THE SPLEEN LEVEL OF CYCLIC AMP *

Otto J. Plescia, Itaru Yamamoto, Tadakatsu Shimamura, and Carl Feit

Waksman Institute of Microbiology
Rutgers University, The State University of New Jersey
New Brunswick, New Jersey 08903

Our approach to the question of the role of thymus-derived cells and thymus factors in immunity has been to inject antigen into normal immunologically competent animals and subsequently to follow the course of the immune response occurring under physiological conditions by isolating and characterizing antigen-activated functional cells in the early stages. Using sheep red blood cells (SRBC) as an antigenic source, we have been able to isolate from the spleen functional antigen-carrying cells that bear θ antigen and are presumably T-cells.[1,2]

The next step was to examine the spleen of immunized mice for changes in cAMP associated with the appearance of antigen-carrying T-cells and antibody-producing B-cells, based on the established fact that cAMP mediates hormonal activity by serving as a second messenger in regulating cellular interactions and processes[3–9] and on reports that addition of stimulators of endogenous cAMP and of exogenous dibutyrl cAMP influences the outcome of the immune response.[10–15] The latter provide indirect evidence for a role of cAMP in immunity and lead to the prediction that immune lymphocytes, on reaction with antigen or products of antigen-activated lymphocytes, would undergo changes in cAMP. This expectation has been verified directly by quantitating the cAMP in the spleen of mice during the course of their response to SRBC, as documented in this report.

MATERIALS AND METHODS

Experimental Design

The experimental approach we adopted is both straightforward and relatively simple. Groups of mice of an inbred strain were given an immunogenic dose of SRBC and at defined times thereafter, for a period of 7 days that covers the early cellular events in the immune response and the proliferation of antibody-forming cells, individual groups of mice were sacrificed, their spleens were excised and were assayed for cAMP and protein. The time of sampling proved to be a critical factor because of the speed with which the initial cellular events occur, resulting in changes in the spleen level of cAMP. Also important was the dose of SRBC administered and the route used.

* Supported by United States Public Health Service Grant AI-11006.

Preparation of Spleen Samples for Assay

Female C57Bl/6J strain mice 6 to 7 weeks-old were used throughout. At time of sampling the mice were sacrificed by cervical dislocation, their spleens were excised instantly and immediately homogenized in ice-cold 5% TCA. The homogenate was transferred to a centrifuge tube and kept in an ice-water bath for 20 to 30 minutes, after which time a 0.5 ml aliquot was removed for protein assay and the remainder of the homogenate was centrifuged at $12{,}800 \times g$ for 10 minutes. One ml portions of the supernate were added to glass test tubes containing 100 μl of 1.0 M HCl and mixed, after which the TCA was removed by 5 successive extractions each with 2 ml of water-saturated ether. The remaining aqueous phase was lyophilized and kept in this form until time for cAMP assay, at which time it was dissolved in 300 μl of 50 mM acetate buffer (pH 4.5).

Assay Procedures

The assay for cAMP was essentially the method of Gilman [16] except for some minor modifications.[17] The binding reaction was carried out at 4° C for 50 minutes in a total volume of 135 μl consisting of 90 μl of 50 mM sodium acetate buffer (pH 4.5), 0.54 pmole of cyclic-[^{3}H]AMP, 1.3 μg of beef heart binding protein (Sigma Chemical Co.), 8 μg of protein kinase inhibitor (histone from Sigma Chemical Co.), and 20 μl of test sample or of standard solution containing 2 to 18 pmole of cAMP. The reaction was terminated by adding 100 μl of a suspension of hydroxylapatite (12.5 mg in 10 mM phosphate buffer, pH 6.0) and mixing for 5 minutes, after which the hydroxylapatite was separated and washed twice with 10 mM phosphate buffer (pH 6). To the washed hydroxylapatite was added 100 μl of 3 M HCl to dissolve the hydroxylapatite. The resulting solution was transferred quantitatively to a counting vial, using 200 μl of water to wash the tube. After adding 5.0 ml of Aquasol (New England Nuclear), the radioactivity was counted in a scintillation counter.

The content of protein in the TCA-precipitated fraction was determined according to the method of Lowry *et al.*,[18] using the Folin phenol reagent and bovine serum albumin as a reference standard.

The outcome of the immune response to SRBC was monitored by assaying the spleen of immunized mice for antibody-forming cells according to the hemolytic plaque assay of Jerne *et al.*[19]

Results

Changes in cAMP in Response to Antigen

To determine whether or not the level of cAMP changes in the spleen during the course of the immune response to SRBC, groups of mice were sacrificed at times ranging from 2 minutes to 7 days after being given 3×10^8 SRBC, and their spleens were excised and assayed for cAMP and protein. At critical times, when significant changes in the cAMP level were found to occur, individual spleens were assayed. In all instances the results are expressed as pmoles cAMP/mg protein and are shown in Figure 1. Compared to control mice that received physiological saline instead of SRBC, the experimental mice showed significant changes in the spleen level of cAMP. These changes occurred at two distinct time periods, one within minutes after injecting SRBC and the second at 3 to 4 days. The early change was a marked increase, the level of cAMP increasing 2 to 3-fold over base level, and it was short-lived. In contrast, the later change in cAMP level was a relatively small decrease that extended over a period of some 3 days rather than minutes.

Because of the large increase in the cAMP level observed at 2 minutes, attention was focused on this time phase which is associated with early events in the immune response. As was expected, the magnitude of the change in cAMP level at 2 minutes was a function of the number of SRBC injected. This is evident from the results shown in FIGURE 2. The increase in cAMP reaches a

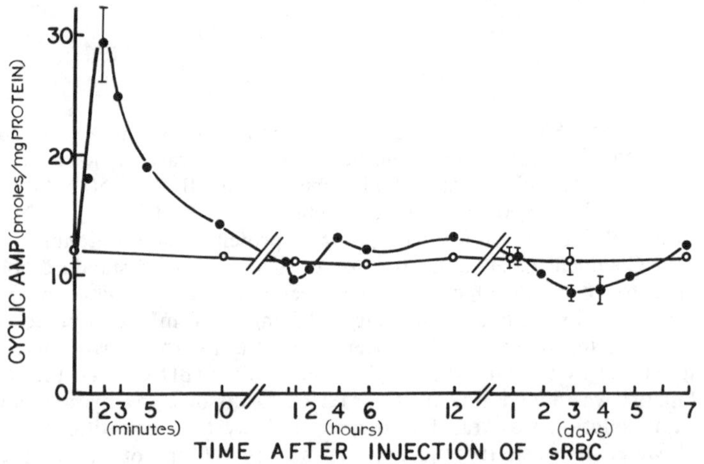

FIGURE 1. Changes in the level of cAMP in the spleen of C57Bl/6J mice during the course of their immune response to SRBC. At times indicated, experimental mice given 3×10^8 SRBC i.v. (●) and control mice given physiological saline (○) were sacrificed and their spleens were assayed for cAMP and protein. The values are the mean of 5 replicate analyses of pools of 5 spleens or the mean of analyses of 5 individual spleens ± S.E.

plateau at about 10^9 SRBC. The point of inflection in the dose-response curve is at 3×10^8 SRBC, and for this reason this number of SRBC was adopted as standard in subsequent experiments designed to characterize the interaction of SRBC with host cells resulting in elevation of cAMP in the spleen.

Specificity of Antigen-stimulated Cells

To investigate the specificity of the change in spleen level of cAMP in response to SRBC, groups of mice were given SRBC or mouse RBC of syngeneic or allogeneic origin. Control mice, as before, were given physiological saline. At 2 minutes, all mice were sacrificed and their spleens were assayed for cAMP

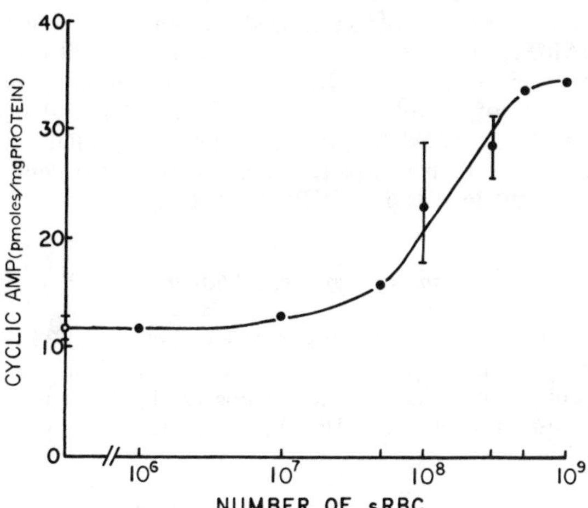

FIGURE 2. Change in the level of cAMP in the spleen of C57Bl/6J mice 2 minutes after being given SRBC i.v., as a function of the number of SRBC injected. The values for experimental mice given SRBC (●) and control mice given physiological saline (○) are the mean of analyses of 10 to 12 individual spleens ± S.E. or the mean of analyses of 5 replicate samples of pools of 5 spleens.

and protein. The results are shown in TABLE 1. Clearly, no significant elevation in cAMP is induced by mouse RBC, including allogeneic RBC, in contrast to SRBC. Apparently, the change in spleen level of cAMP results from the reaction of host cells with foreign substances, the extent of change being a function of the degree of foreignness or antigenicity relative to the host.

The relatively large increase in cAMP in response to SRBC indicates: (1) either a few cells, specific for SRBC, undergo phenomenal changes in cAMP or (2) a large number of cells, nonspecific in the sense that they can not discriminate among "non-self" substances but can distinguish between "self" and "non-self," undergo a modest and realistic change in cAMP.

TABLE 1

SPECIFICITY OF THE CHANGE IN THE LEVEL OF CYCLIC AMP IN SPLEENS OF C57Bl/6J MICE IN RESPONSE TO SHEEP RED BLOOD CELLS (SRBC) *

Mice/Group	Species of RBC	cAMP (pmoles/mg protein) 2 Minutes After Injection of RBC
5	sheep	26.5
5	mouse (C57Bl/6J)	13.4
5	mouse (DBA)	13.7
5	mouse (Balb/c)	13.2
5	saline control	12.1

* Groups of 5 animals each were given (i.v.) 10^8 RBC of sheep or mouse origin, and a group of 5 control animals was given physiological saline. Two minutes later all animals were sacrificed and their spleens were excised for cyclic AMP assay. The value for each group is the mean of 5 aliquots of a pool of the spleens in the group.

To decide between these alternatives, chicken RBC were tested competitively with SRBC in inducing a change in spleen level of cAMP. The number of each species of RBC used was optimal in giving maximal stimulation of cAMP. From the results, shown in TABLE 2, it is clear that there is competition between SRBC and CRBC. The stimulation in response to a mixture of the two is not additive, and in fact it is equal to that observed with SRBC alone. The fact that SRBC produce a greater stimulation of cAMP than CRBC indicates less than complete cross-reactivity between them, the SRBC being able to stimulate cells that CRBC cannot.

Properties of Cells Showing cAMP Response to Antigen

This finding of cross-reactivity between SRBC and CRBC, both of them being immunogenic in the test mice, raised the question whether immunogenicity might be a critical property of a foreign substance in inducing changes in spleen level of cAMP. Accordingly, carbon particles that are rapidly cleared

TABLE 2

COMPETITION BETWEEN SHEEP AND CHICKEN RED BLOOD CELLS IN INDUCING CHANGES IN SPLEEN LEVEL OF cAMP

Mice/Group	Antigen	cAMP (pmoles/mg protein) *
5	—(saline control)	9.3
5	SRBC (10^9)	34.6
5	SRBC (2×10^9)	36.7
5	CRBC (10^9)	23.1
5	CRBC (2×10^9)	23.5
5	SRBC (10^9)+CRBC (10^9)	32.3

* Mice (C57Bl/6J) were sacrificed 2 minutes after being given antigen and their spleens assayed for cAMP.

from the circulation by phagocytic cells, were tested for their ability to alter the spleen level of cAMP. No significant change was observed in conjunction with carbon clearance, as shown in TABLE 3. We also have evidence that carbon particles do not compete with SRBC in stimulating cAMP.

Role of cAMP in the Immune Response

From the foregoing results, we may conclude that the early increase in spleen level of cAMP in response to heterologous RBC reflects early events in the immune response that involve processing of antigen by cells other than phagocytic cells that clear nonantigenic foreign particles such as carbon. If, in fact, an increase in endogenous cAMP is essential for activation and function of antigen-reactive cells in the initial step of the immune response, it follows that agents, such as poly A:U that stimulate endogenous cAMP, should be most effective as adjuvants if given together with the antigen. Moreover, these agents should be immunosuppressive if administered at a time when the spleen

TABLE 3

EFFECT OF CARBON CLEARANCE *in Vivo* ON THE CYCLIC AMP LEVEL IN SPLEENS OF C57Bl/6J MICE

Treatment of Mice	Time (min) *	Assay of Cyclic AMP pmoles/mg Protein
saline	2	11.7
SRBC (10^8)	2	20.0
carbon (0.1 ml) †	2	10.8
carbon (0.1 ml)	5	10.8
carbon (0.1 ml)	10	11.0
carbon (0.1 ml)	30	11.2
carbon (0.1 ml) ‡	2	11.0

* Groups of 5 mice were sacrificed at times indicated, their spleens were excised and immediately assayed for cyclic AMP. Each value is the mean of 5 aliquots of a pool of the spleens of animals in each group.

† Composition of carbon mixture injected i.v. was 1.5 ml pelikan ink (c 11/1431 a, Gunther Wagner), 3.0 ml saline and 0.5 ml of gelatine (6%) in saline.

‡ The concentration of carbon was increased 2-fold, keeping the medium unchanged.

level of cAMP is decreasing during the normal course of the immune response. This is indeed the case, as is evident from the results shown in TABLE 4. There is maximal stimulation in terms of antibody-forming cells by poly A:U at 0 time and maximal suppression at 2 days, at a time when antibody-forming cells are proliferating. The time course of appearance of antibody-forming cells in the spleen following administration of SRBC is shown in FIGURE 3. It is important to note that the maximal decrease in the spleen level of cAMP occurs at a time when the number of antibody-forming cells is at its peak. This is presumptive evidence that decrease in cAMP following activation by processed antigen and/or helper cells is a signal for cell proliferation.

TABLE 4

TIME OF ADMINISTRATION OF POLY A:U AS A FACTOR IN MODIFYING THE IMMUNE RESPONSE OF C57Bl/6J MICE TO SHEEP RED BLOOD CELLS *

Mice/Group	Poly A:U Given at Time Indicated	PFC/10^8 Spleen Cells (day 14)
5	(control)	2051
5	0 hours	3440
5	4 hours	2802
5	24 hours	1692
5	48 hours	1500
5	96 hours	2494

* All mice, including control group, were given 10^8 SRBC i.v. at 0 time, and at times thereafter as indicated groups of mice were given 300 μg Poly A:U i.v. On day 14 all mice were sacrificed and their spleens assayed for antibody-forming cells as plaque-forming cells (PFC).

Discussion

Following the administration of SRBC into immunologically competent hosts significant and characteristic changes in the spleen level of cAMP occur over a time period ranging from initiation of the immune response to proliferation of antibody-forming cells. The early initiation period, from 2 to 10 minutes, is marked by a 2 to 3-fold increase in cAMP level, whereas the later cell proliferation period, from 2 to 5 days, is characterized by a relatively small but significant decrease in cAMP. These changes in spleen level of cAMP occur only in response to foreign substances that are immunogenic, such as heterologous RBC, and not to antigenically inert carbon particles, and these cAMP changes are dose-dependent. The cells undergoing early changes in cAMP seem incapable of fine discrimination among different antigens because of the competition between SRBC and CRBC for these cells. Also, poly A:U, which stimulates endogenous cAMP, is immunoenhancing if it is given together with antigen and immunosuppressive if it is given at the beginning of antibody-cell proliferation. Together these data provide direct evidence for the role of cAMP in differentiation and proliferation of immunocompetent cells activated by antigen, and they provide a rational basis for using substances, such as poly A:U, that stimulate cAMP as both immunoenhancing and immunosuppressive agents.

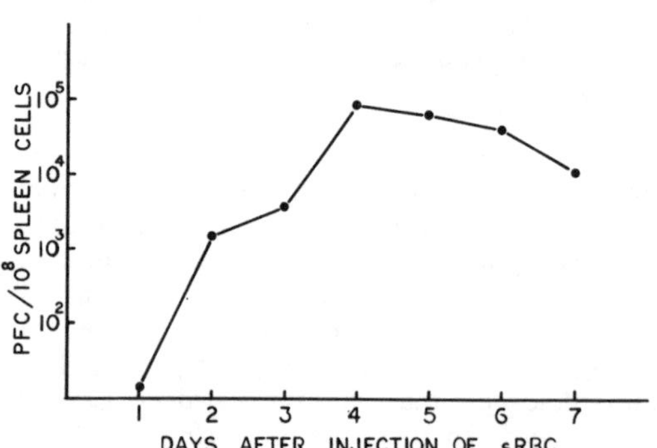

FIGURE 3. Kinetics of the immune response of C57Bl/6J mice to 3×10^8 SRBC given i.v. in terms of plaque-forming cells (PFC) in the spleen. Groups of 4 mice were sacrificed at times indicated, their spleens were pooled, and replicate samples assayed for PFC per 10^8 viable spleen cells.

References

1. Plescia, O. J. & J. S. Hirsch. 1973. Ann. N. Y. Acad Sci. **207:** 49.
2. Hirsch, J. S. & O. J. Plescia. 1972. Immunol. Commun. **1:** 199.
3. Robison, G. A., R. W. Butcher & E. W. Sutherland. 1971. *In* Cyclic AMP. Academic Press, Inc. New York, N.Y.
4. Robison, G. A., G. G. Nahas & L. Trimer. 1971. Ann. N.Y. Acad. Sci. **185:** 1.
5. Rasmussen, H. 1970. Science **180:** 404.
6. Varmus, H. E., R. L. Perlman & I. Pastan. 1970. J. Biol. Chem. **245:** 2259.
7. Zubay, G., D. Schwartz & J. Beckwith. 1970. Proc. Nat. Acad. Sci. U.S. **66:** 104.
8. Pastan, I. & R. L. Perlman. 1970. Science **169:** 339.

9. Dokas, L. A. & L. J. Kleinsmith. 1971. Science **172:** 1237.
10. Ishizuka, M., M. Gafni & W. Braun. 1970. Proc. Soc. Exp. Biol. Med. **134:** 963.
11. Braun, W., M. Ishizuka, R. Winchurch & D. Webb. 1971. Ann. N.Y. Acad. Sci **181:** 289.
12. Braun, W., M. Ishizuka, R. Winchurch & D. Webb. 1971. Ann. N.Y. Acad. Sci. **195:** 417.
13. Braun, W. & M. Ishizuka. 1971. Proc. Nat. Acad. Sci. U.S. **68:** 1114.
14. Ishizuka, M., W. Braun & T. Matsumoto. 1971. J. Immunol. **107:** 1027.
15. Braun, W. & M. Ishizuka. 1971. J. Immunol. **107:** 1036.
16. Gilman, A. J. 1970. Proc. Nat. Acad. Sci. U.S. **67:** 305.
17. Brostrom, C. & C. Kon. 1974. Anal. Biochem. **58:** 459.
18. Lowry, O. H., N. J. Rosebrough, A. L. Farr & R. J. Randall. 1951. J. Biol. Chem. **193:** 265.
19. Jerne, N. J., A. A. Nordin & C. Henry. 1963. *In* Cell Bound Antibodies. B. Amos & H. Koprowski, Eds. : 109. Wistar Institute Press. Philadelphia, Pa.

Discussion of the Paper

Dr. M. P. Scheid: Did you have the chance to see any difference between T-cell dependent and T-cell independent antigens in your systems?

Dr. O. J. Plescia: No, I think we have used only T-cell dependent antigens. We have also looked at the response to soluble protein antigens and we see a similar increase in cAMP levels in the spleen of animals injected with those soluble antigens. But the magnitude of change that one sees is considerably less than that which we get with erythrocytes.

Dr. M. P. Scheid: The second point is that I want to caution that one might, in these complex T- and B-cell systems *in vivo,* have some difficulties to locate the cAMP to one target cell. It would be probably favorable to do this study in *in vitro* culture systems and use antiglobulin serum for B-cell markers.

Dr. O. J. Plescia: I agree with you, but I have taken the position that I want to be sure that these events occur under physiologic conditions *in vivo* and when I have confidence I will then test the same events in defined or closed systems. We will be proceeding to the *in vitro* system as soon as we have completed all that we can do effectively *in vivo.* I believe that I'm correct in saying that what we have done is to convince ourselves that the observed cAMP changes are relevant and we are shortly going to go to *in vitro* work.

THE MITOGENIC ACTIVITY OF POLYADENYLIC-POLYURIDYLIC ACID COMPLEXES

Ihn H. Han and Arthur G. Johnson

Department of Microbiology
University of Michigan Medical School
Ann Arbor, Michigan 48104

The capacity of synthetic polyadenylic and polyuridylic acid complexes (poly A:U) to increase antibody synthesis to a number of different antigens given via several different routes has been characterized.[1,2] The adjuvant activity was most readily apparent when immunity was partially depressed, as for example by thymectomy,[3] or when the antigenicity of the material was low.[1] The functional activities of several different cell types, including lymphocytes, macrophages, stem cells, and memory cells,[4] as well as the immunologically unrelated cells found in the parotid and pancreas,[5] have been shown to be enhanced. The mode of action of the polynucleotides is unknown, but their ability to activate 10^4 T-cells to a state functionally similar to that expressed by 10^6 T-cells not exposed to poly A:U is impressive, and suggests that this adjuvant may amplify the number of T-cells.[3] In addition, poly-A:U-treated mice were found to be susceptible to the antimitotic drug vinblastine some 6 hours earlier than controls, suggesting that cells were stimulated into division more rapidly under the stimulus of poly A:U.[6] To test this hypothesis, the effect of poly A:U on the division of thymocytes, spleen and bone marrow cells, *in vitro* and *in vivo,* was measured and the results are presented herein.

Materials and Methods

Animals

Balb/Aj mice either 4–5 weeks or 10–13 weeks in age were inbred in our laboratory and used throughout the study. They were supplied with Purina rat chow and water *ad libitum.*

Antigen

Sheep red blood cells (SRBC) were obtained from the Colorado Serum Company, Denver, Colorado. The cells were stored at 4° C in modified Alsever's solution, washed 3 times and resuspended in phosphate buffered saline (PBS), pH 7.2, for injection. For *in vivo* experiments 2×10^7 SRBC were injected intravenously, whereas 1×10^6 SRBC was added to each culture dish for experiments *in vitro.*

Homoribopolynucleotides

Polyadenylic acid (poly A), potassium salt (10t 69) and polyuridylic acid (poly U), ammonium salt (lot 77) were purchased from Miles Laboratories,

Elkhart, Indiana. Polymers were complexed *in vitro* to form poly A:U by mixing equal amounts of polynucleotides before use, as previously described.[1]

Cortisone Administration

In experiments aimed at studying the responsiveness of cortisone-resistant spleen cells, 2.5 mg of hydrocortisone sodium succinate [7] were injected intraperitoneally 48 hours prior to the injection of antigen, or poly A:U and antigen. The control mice received appropriate amounts of saline in lieu of cortisone.

In Vitro *Cell Culture*

Spleens and mesenteric lymph nodes from normal, adult Balb mice or thymuses from 4-week-old Balb mice were removed aseptically. Single-cell suspensions were prepared in the following way. Intact organs were washed 2 times with Hank's balanced salt solution (HBSS) containing 100 units of penicillin and 100 μg streptomycin/ml, gently teased, and kept in an ice bath for 10 minutes to permit large fragments to settle by gravity. Suspensions of bone marrow cells were prepared by flushing the marrow from femurs and tibia with a syringe and 26 gauge needle containing cold Eagle's basal medium. The extruded plugs were dispersed by aspiration with a 21 gauge needle and syringe. The fragment-free supernatant was then centrifuged in the cold for 10 minutes at 1,000 rpm. The cell pellet was washed with HBSS and finally suspended into a culture medium containing 100 units of penicillin and 100 μg streptomycin per ml of medium. The concentration of the cell suspension was adjusted to 5×10^6 per ml.

Culture Medium

The culture medium used here consisted of: Aqua dist. water, 85 ml; Hank's MEM 10x, 10 ml; Vitamins 100x, 1 ml; Essential amino acid 50x, 2 ml; Non-essential amino acid 100x, 1 ml; L-glutamine 100x, 1 ml; Pyruvate 100x, 1 ml; Na_2HCO_3 (7.5%), 3.9 ml; and Fetal calf serum, 10 ml.

Incorporation of [^{3}H]Thymidine

Tritiated thymidine (methyl-^{3}H, Code TRK 120 Batch 70, specific activity 18.9 Ci/mM, Amersham/Searle) was used in all *in vivo* experiments at 0.5 μci per gram body weight. For *in vitro* work, 4–6 μci of [^{3}H]thymidine was added to the culture fluid per dish. In early *in vitro* experiments, a labeling period of 24 hours was adopted, whereas in later experiments an incorporation time of 2 hours was used.

Determination of Radioactivity

At the time of sacrifice, mice were killed by cervical dislocation, and the spleen was removed and homogenized with a Harlbrook hand homogenizer in

5 ml of PBS at pH 7.2. One hundred, 200 or 500 μl of homogenate was put on a Millipore® or glass-fiber filter paper, and washed with 10 ml saline, 10 ml of ice cold 10% TCA, 2 ml of 95% ethanol, and 2 ml of absolute ethanol. Following this, the filter paper was transferred to a scintillation vial and 10 ml of scintillation fluid (15 g of PPO and 0.4 g POPOP per gallon of toluene) was added to the sample. The samples were counted in a Packard Tri-Carb liquid scintillation spectrometer, model 3320. In light of the variation in total counts among different experiments, results were expressed as percentage of control values ± standard deviations.

Results

Thymus Lymphocytes

Single-cell suspensions of thymus tissue could not be stimulated into division with poly A:U alone under our conditions. Thus, titration of the dose of adjuvant from 1×10^{-4} to 20 μg did not significantly increase the uptake of tritiated thymidine added to separate cultures at either 0, 3, 6, 12, 18, 24, or 48 hours. However, slight, but consistent stimulation was achieved by 5×10^{-2} to 5×10^{-3} μg poly A:U, but only when SRBC was added as antigen (125–130% of controls receiving SRBC alone).

Peripheral T-lymphocytes

Inasmuch as thymocytes per se appeared unable to respond to poly A:U under our culture conditions, the mitogenic effect of poly A:U on the division

TABLE 1

KINETICS OF MITOGENIC EFFECTS OF POLY A:U AND/OR SRBC ON MOUSE SPLEEN CELLS *in Vitro*

Spleen Cells * Incubated with: SRBC	Poly A:U	[³H]thymidine Incorporation After Culture for Cpm±SD (% cpm) † 6 hours	12 hours	24 hours	48 hours
–	–	5,600±270 (100±5)	2,700±550 (100±20)	1,580±234 (100±14)	2,000±360 (100±18)
+	–	5,300±700 (93±13)	2,400±150 (88±6)	2,180±192 (138±8)	2,480±225 (124±9)
–	+	4,500±380 (79±8)	3,500±500 (128±14)	1,960±124 (124±6)	2,560±500 (128±5)
+	+	4,300±640 (75±14)	3,300±640 (119±19)	2,400±490 (150±20)	2,440±290 (122±12)

* 5×10^6 spleen cells in 0.5 ml MEM were incubated with 30 μl of 0.1% SRBC (1×10^6) and/or 1 μg poly A:U for different time intervals, followed by the addition of 6 μci [³H]thymidine into the culture fluid and an additional 6 hours incubation.

† (Cpm exp. group/cpm control group) × 100 ± standard deviation.

TABLE 2

In Vitro INCORPORATION OF [^{3}H]THYMIDINE BY NORMAL SPLEEN CELLS IN SERUM-FREE MEDIUM

Spleen Cells * Incubated with: SRBC	Poly A:U	[^{3}H]Thymidine Incorporation for Cpm (% cpm) † ±SD	
−	−	11,600±60	(100±0.5)
+	−	14,900±1200	(130±8)
−	1.5 μg	18,000±800	(155±5)
−	4.5 μg	20,800±960	(180±4)
+	1.5 μg	22,700±4200	(195±18)
+	4.5 μg	26,300±500	(226±2)

* 5 × 10^6 spleen cells in 1 ml MEM were incubated with 30 μl of 0.1% SRBC (1 × 10^6) and/or 1.5 μg–4.5 μg poly A:U for 48 hours, followed by 4 μci of [^{3}H] thymidine added into the culture fluid and an additional 18 hours incubation.

† (Cpm exp. group/cpm control group) × 100 ± standard deviation.

of peripheral T-lymphocytes in the spleen was tested. Thus, 5 × 10^6 spleen cells were cultured for varying periods of time with or without SRBC and/or 1 μg poly A:U/dish. TABLE 1 records the results of one experiment representative of the 6 performed. Beginning at 12 hours of culture, there was an increase in [^{3}H]thymidine incorporation in tissues containing poly A:U both in the presence and absence of SRBC. However, the increase at this time was variable and statistically insignificant. By 24 hours the cells given antigen alone showed a 38% increase in [^{3}H]thymidine incorporation, whereas poly A:U alone produced a 24% increase. Under the combined stimulation of poly A:U and antigen, incorporation increased to 150% of the control value. After 48 hours of culture, incorporation was greater than the control in all experimental combinations, i.e. those containing either the antigen alone, poly A:U alone, or antigen plus poly A:U. However, no significant differences were noted among the 3 experimental groups.

Similar results were obtained when the same experiments were performed without the addition of calf serum. As shown in TABLE 2, the thymidine incorporation by spleen cells in the presence of 4.5 μg poly A:U with or without SRBC was 226% and 180% of the control, respectively. A significant point to be noted was that poly A:U alone, in the absence of serum or antigen, was as mitogenic as SRBC.

In Vivo *Effects of Poly A:U*

In order to place in perspective the results gained in the *in vitro* experiments performed above, the mitogenic effect of poly A:U on spleen cells was tested by giving poly A:U intravenously to mice on day 0 with or without a concomitant injection of SRBC. At 2 hours prior to sacrifice, [^{3}H]thymidine was injected. Results from a representative experiment are recorded in TABLE 3. No significant effect was evident 18 hours after poly A:U administration;

however, 2 days after poly A:U was given, 260% stimulation was observed. Similar values were obtained in animals receiving poly A:U plus SRBC, and the stimulatory effects were still observable on days 3 and 4 following injection. No effect was measurable on thymus cells.

Effect of Poly A:U on Cortison-resistant Spleen Cells

Inasmuch as poly A:U had not affected B-cells under our previously published experimental conditions, the above effect was hypothesized to be exerted on T-cells peripheralized to the spleen. To test whether poly A:U might be affecting selectively the peripheral T-cell population resistant to corticosteroids,[7] mice were given cortisone 2 days prior to the injection of poly A:U and/or SRBC. The results of 5 experiments are given in TABLE 4. In control mice receiving saline, poly A:U alone had a greater degree of mitogenic effect than the antigen (235% vs. 160% of the control value), whereas SRBC plus poly A:U gave an additive effect, approximately 330% of the control value. Mice that were given cortisone showed similar results, SRBC alone increasing [^{3}H]-thymidine uptake to 175% of the control, whereas poly A:U and poly A:U plus the antigen, showed 213% and 291% of the control results, respectively. Thus elimination of cortisone-sensitive lymphocytes did not reduce or modify the mitogenic effects of poly A:U, indicating an effect on other than the T_0-cells.

Effect on DNA Synthesis by Cortisone-resistant Spleen Cells In Vitro

To test whether or not the *in vivo* effects observed in the preceding experiments might be mediated through differences in homeostatic factors related to cortisone treatment, the following *in vitro* experiments were done. Spleen cells from mice treated with 2.5 mg cortisone 2 days prior to sacrifice were cultured;

TABLE 3

KINETICS OF MITOGENIC EFFECTS OF POLY A:U AND/OR SRBC ON MOUSE SPLEEN CELLS *in Vivo*

Mice * Injected with: SRBC	Poly A:U	[^{3}H]Thymidine Incorporation Cpm (% cpm) † 18 hours	2 days	3 days	4 days
—	—	4,460±670 (100±14)	1,800±210 (100±11)	2,600±20 (100±8)	1,380±400 (100±30)
—	+	3,420±1000 (77±21)	4,700±850 (260±47)	5,200±440 (200±16)	3,560±740 (260±52)
+	+	2,850±280 (63±6)	6,000±1150 (300±66)	5,250±800 (200±30)	3,350±400 (250±30)

* Mice were injected with 2 × 10^7 SRBC and/or 300 μg poly A:U intravenously 18 hours, 2, 3, or 4 days prior to the injection of [^{3}H]thymidine, which lasted for 2 hours.

† (Cpm exp. group/cpm control group) × 100 ± standard deviation.

TABLE 4

MITOGENIC EFFECTS OF POLY A:U AND/OR SRBC ON CORTISONE-RESISTANT SPLEEN CELLS *in Vivo* *

Mice † Injected with: First	Second	[³H]Thymidine Incorporation Cpm (% cpm) ‡ 86 §	87	88	89	93	Average % of cpm±SD
saline	saline	500 (100)	220 (100)	1265 (100)	545 (100)	250 (100)	100
saline	SRBC	680 (136)	250 (114)	2570 (200)	870 (160)	450 (180)	160±50
saline	poly A:U	935 (187)	600 (270)	3060 (240)	1160 (200)	740 (280)	235±41
saline	SRBC and poly A:U	1100 (220)	650 (300)	4450 (350)	2040 (374)	1050 (420)	330±76
cortisone	saline		310 (100)	1300 (100)	630 (100)	225 (100)	100
cortisone	SRBC		400 (129)	2850 (219)	1170 (185)	380 (169)	175±37
cortisone	poly A:U		860 (277)	2290 (176)	910 (144)	575 (256)	213±63
cortisone	SRBC and poly A:U		1020 (329)	4380 (337)	1400 (222)	625 (278)	291±53

* Spleens were removed 2 days after the 2nd injection, preceded by 2 hrs. [³H] thymidine pulse labeling.

† Mice were injected intraperitoneally with saline or 2.5 mg Hydrocortisone sodium succinate 2 days prior to second injection of 300μ poly A:U and/or 2 $\times$ 10^7 SRBC intravenously.

‡ (Cpm exp group/cpm control group) $\times$ 100 $\pm$ standard deviation.

§ Refers to experimental numbers.

10^6 SRBC and/or 4.5 μg poly A:U each was added to the culture medium containing 5 $\times$ 10^6 spleen cells, and the cells subsequently incubated for 48 hours, at which time 6 μci of [³H]thymidine/culture dish were added. Following an additional 18-hour culture period, cells were harvested and prepared for scintillation counting. TABLE 5 summarizes results from one of the typical experiments in this series. It may be noted that once again poly A:U increased the stimulatory effect somewhat. In cortisone-treated animals, an even greater level of DNA synthesis, was stimulated.

Effects of Poly A:U on Bone Marrow Cells

To determine whether the above described effects indeed were restricted to peripheralized T-cells in the spleen, bone marrow cells were incubated for 24 hours with 1 or 5 μg poly A:U in the presence or absence of SRBC. A 180% increase in [³H]thymidine incorporation was observed 18 hours after addition of 4 μci of the latter, irrespective of the dose level of poly A:U or the presence or absence of the antigen. These figures were clearly greater than the values for SRBC alone, which produced only 135% of the control (TABLE 6).

DISCUSSION

The results obtained from the present investigation render additional support to preliminary data showing that mitogenic activity by poly A:U can be demonstrated in mouse spleen cells.[6, 8] Furthermore, it shows clearly that such stimulatory effects of poly A:U on [^{3}H]thymidine incorporation can be elicited in the absence of injected antigen (TABLE 3). Repeated experiments with cells obtained 2 days after the adjuvant and/or the antigen injection show that the combination of the two produces an additive effect (TABLE 4). The possibility that the mitogenic effect *in vivo* is induced within 6 hours has been raised by Cone and Johnson[6] who were able to suppress up to 90% of the immune response against SRBC with a single injection of vinblastine given 6 hours after the antigen plus poly A:U. Although similar enhancement effects were observed under *in vitro* conditions, the mitogenic effect of poly A:U under culture conditions was more consistent in the presence of antigen. This conclusion was supported also by Jaroslow and Ortiz-Ortiz[9] in their study of the effect of oligonucleotides on antibody synthesis *in vitro.*

Assuming that the surviving spleen cells following cortisone treatment are T-cells,[7] the observations made from both *in vivo* and *in vitro* experiments dealing with cortisone-treated animals (TABLES 4 and 5) indicate that cortisone-resistant T-cells may be responsible for the enhanced incorporation of [^{3}H]-thymidine. Indeed, the cells from cortisone-treated animals have shown a greater amount of [^{3}H]thymidine incorporation, particularly under *in vitro* conditions. Whether all of the B-cell population are killed by a single injection

TABLE 5

In Vitro INCORPORATION OF [^{3}H]THYMIDINE BY CORTISONE-RESISTANT SPLEEN CELLS

Substances Added into Culture: Spleen Cells * from:	SRBC	Poly A:U	[^{3}H]Thymidine Incorporation: Cpm±SD	(% cpm±SD) †
normal	—	—	6,310±158	(100±3)
normal	+	—	10,240±700	(160±10)
normal	—	+	10,240±125	(160±3)
normal	+	+	13,510±4260	(210±7)
cortisone †	—	—	7,880±390	(100±5)
cortisone	+	—	13,100±146	(166±1)
cortisone	—	+	14,400±100	(183±0.7)
cortisone	+	+	23,000±2500	(292±11)

* Mice were injected intraperitoneally with saline or 2.5 mg hydrocortisone sodium succinate 2 days prior to sacrifice. 5 × 10^6 spleen cells in 0.5 ml MEM were incubated with 30 μl of 0.1% SRBC (1 × 10^6) and/or 0.5 μg poly A:U for 48 hours, followed by 6 μci of [^{3}H]thymidine added into the culture fluid and an additional 18 hours incubation.

† (Cpm exp. group/cpm control group) × 100 ± standard deviation.

TABLE 6

MITOGENIC EFFECTS OF POLY A:U ON MOUSE BONE MARROW CELLS *in Vitro*

Bone Marrow Cells * Incubated with:			[³H]thymidine Incorporation	
SRBC	Poly A:U	LPS	Cpm±SD	(% cpm±SD) †
—	—	—	83,470±8,900	100±10
+	—	—	112,870±5,800	135±5
—	1 μg	—	152,870±12,900	180±8
—	5 μg	—	141,900±14,800	170±10
+	1 μg	—	152,300±22,400	180±15
+	5 μg	—	159,500±4,590	190±2
—	—	10^{-2} μg	197,000±41,700	235±21

* 5 × 10^6 bone marrow cells from normal mice were incubated with 30 μl of 0.1% SRBC (1 × 10^6) and/or 1–5 μg poly A:U or 10^{-2} μg LPS for 24 hrs., followed by 4 μci of [³H]thymidine added into the culture fluid and an additional 18 hours incubation.

† (Cpm exp. group/cpm control group) × 100 ± SD.

of 2.5 mg cortisone at 2 days prior to poly A:U administration has not been determined, and thus this conclusion must be tentative. This is particularly pertinent in view of the fact that all our efforts at inducing mitogenicity in cells from the thymus and lymph nodes with poly A:U alone have produced negative results. However, T-cells in the circulation have different properties when compared to the T-cells present in the thymus.[10] Further fractionation and characterization of T-cell subpopulations are underway to resolve this issue.

The results of the *in vitro* experiments in which bone marrow cells were stimulated by poly A:U may not necessarily mean that poly A:U has the capacity to stimulate B-cells, in light of the recent data of Claman.[11] He has reported the presence of T-cells in mouse bone marrow as suggested by the positive response of the bone marrow cells towards specific T-cell mitogens such as phytohemagglutinin and concanavalin-A.

SUMMARY

Polyadenylic-polyuridylic acid complexes (poly A:U) at the 1–5 μg level, were mitogenic for spleen cells when given intravenously to normal Balb or cortisone-treated mice. Similarly, mitogenicity was evident when poly A:U was added to tissue culture fluids containing spleen cells from normal or cortisone-treated mice, or bone marrow cells from normal mice. Under these conditions, this adjuvant was not mitogenic for thymus cells or mesenteric lymph node cells, either *in vivo* or *in vitro*.

REFERENCES

1. SCHMIDTKE, J. R. & A. G. JOHNSON. 1971. Regulation of the immune system by synthetic polynucleotides. I. Characteristics of adjuvant action on antibody synthesis. J. Immunol. **106:** 1191–1200.

2. HAN, I. H., A. G. JOHNSON, J. COOK & S. S. HAN. 1973. Comparative biological activity of endotoxin and synthetic polyribonucleotides. J. Infec. Dis. **128:** S232–S237.
3. CONE, R. E. & A. G. JOHNSON. 1971. Regulation of the immune system by synthetic polynucleotides. III. Action on antigen reactive cells of thymic origin. J. Exp. Med. **133:** 665–676.
4. JOHNSON, A. G. 1973. The adjuvant action of polynucleotides. J. Reticuloendothel. Soc. **14:** 441–448.
5. KIM, Y. G. & S. S. HAN. 1973. Effects of polynucleotides on normal and hypoxie pancreas of rats. Unpublished observation.
6. CONE, R. E. & A. G. JOHNSON. 1972. Regulation of the immune sytsem by synthetic polynucleotides. IV. Amplification of proliferation of thymus influenced lymphocytes. Cell. Immunol. **3:** 283–293.
7. COHEN, J. J. & H. N. CLAMAN. 1971. Thymus-marrow immunocompetence. V. Hydrocortisone-resistant cells and processes in the hemolytic antibody response of mice. J. Exp. Med. **133:** 1026–1034.
8. JOHNSON, A. G. & I. H. HAN. 1972. Mitogenic activity of polynucleotides on thymus influenced lymphocytes. *In* Conference on cyclic nucleotides, immune responses and tumor growth. W. Braun, L. Lichtenstein & C. Parker, Eds. Springer-Verlag. New York, N.Y.
9. JAROSLOW, B. N. & L. ORTIZ-ORTIZ. 1972. Influence of poly A-poly U on early events in the immune response *in vitro*. Cell. Immunol. **3:** 123–132.
10. CANTOR, H. & R. ASOFSKY. 1972. Synergy among lymphoid cells mediating the graft-versus host response. III. Evidence for interaction between two types of thymus-derived cells. J. Exp. Med. **135:** 764–779.
11. CLAMAN, H. N. 1974. Bone Marrow T-cells. I. Response to the T-cell mitogens, phytohemagglutinin and Concanavalin A. J. Immunol. **112:** 960–964.

DISCUSSION OF THE PAPER

DR. A. WHITE: Have you looked in the supernatants for cAMP? I ask this question because since the Bible has been mentioned I rise as a sinner. The fact that cAMP does not readily enter cells is well known. However, I should like to call attention to observations made in several laboratories that have indicated that, *in vitro,* certain lines of cells in culture export up to as much as three to five times as much cAMP as is synthesized during such an incubation period. I believe, therefore, that in any *in vitro* study one should be aware of this.

DR. A. G. JOHNSON: Although we are students of the Bible we have not yet gotten to Revelations and we hope that we can find out what the substance is. It is entirely possible, of course, that it might be a cAMP derivative. It does not negate the results.

DR. J. F. A. P. MILLER: I wish to ask if you have looked at the effects of poly A:U on the response to an antigen like polysaccharide or an antigen that is T-cell independent?

DR. A. G. JOHNSON: We did preliminary experiments along this line, and it showed no effect on thymus-independent antigens.

DR. J. F. A. P. MILLER: As second question, there is some suggestion that cellular resistance to infection by intracellular parasites is negated by T-cells acting on macrophages. Is there any effect of poly A:U on the resistance of nude mice to some of these intracellular parasites?

DR. A. G. JOHNSON: We have not tested for that.

DR. G. MÖLLER: Do you believe that poly A:U works on T-cells in culture and is that the interpretation?

DR. A. G. JOHNSON: Yes, although we have not yet ruled out that we can use B-cells alone plus the T-cell factor and then determine whether the poly A:U acts on these cells.

STIMULATION OF ANTIBODY FORMATION THROUGH POLYPEPTIDE THYMIC FRACTION (TP) IN IRRADIATED ANIMALS

S. M. Milcu, Isabela Potop, Vera Boeru, and N. Olinici

Academia de Stiinte Medicale
Institutul de Endocrinologie
Bucharest, Romania

During the last decades, thanks to a large number of works by outstanding thymus specialists, an ever increasing importance has been given to the thymus in the development of the immunologic system and in regeneration of the lymphoid tissue after x-ray irradiation.

After the works of Miller,[29] Osoba,[31] Small and Trainin,[41] and others, and after the success obtained in isolating and characterizing chemically and biologically, the various factors of the thymus, scientists have reached the conclusion that the thymus secretes one or more factors necessary for immunologic maturation of the lymphoid tissue.

Experiments have shown, on the one hand, that x-irradiation causes important biochemical, immunological, and biological alteration at the level of the thymus, and on the other hand, that this gland plays an important part in the regeneration of the immunological processes. Among other things, it was discovered that lymphocytes migrate from the bone marrow into the thymus in the mouse after x-irradiation. Gibertini *et al.*[18] showed the relationships between the lymphocyte population in the thymus and the lymphatic ganglia of the mouse after partial and total x-irradiation, thereby underlining the implication of the thymus in their regeneration.

But the alterations of the thymus caused by irradiation were disclosed by changes in other parameters as well. Thus, the biochemical parameters, for example, suffer important perturbations; it was noticed that there were (1) an alteration in the synthesis of DNA contained in the thymic nuclei or cells;[21] and (2) changes in the enzymatic activity including alkaline phosphatase[10] inhibition of cytomonoxidase and succin-dehydrogenase[14] effects on the bound water,[20] ATP synthesis, and especially inhibition of the P/O implied in the conductor mechanism in the phase previous to death.[5]

Protection of the organism after its exposure to radiation was provided by extracts of organs, by cellular constituents, nucleoproteins, proteins, nucleic acids, etc.[38] Maisin *et al.*[24] reported the action of certain radioprotecting mixtures noting that after administration of dimethyl-sulfoxide and cysteamine, survival of the irradiated mouse was higher.

The glands with internal secretion play an important part in the irradiation process. The role of the thymus in protecting the organism from radiation is now being studied with interest. Thus, Frigo[16] demonstrated that if a rabbit is irradiated and then treated with thymic extracts there is stimulation of antibody formation. An increase in the white cells of lymphoid type was found in the blood of rabbits and rats. Goldstein *et al.*,[17] studying the action of thymosin in irradiated and thymectomized mice, supported the idea of the endocrine role of the thymus. They suggest that the control by the thymus of the cells involved in immunity lies mainly in an endocrine function of the gland concerned with maturation of the peripheral cells, which takes place through thymosin. The immune response was studied by means of skin grafts and by the ability to form humoral antibodies.

According to Williams *et al.*[41] the cells that differentiate in the thymus and go to the peripheral lymphoid organs play a major role in the response to humoral antigens since they are associated with the immunocompetence. On the other hand, grafts of medullar cells associated with lymphoid or thymic cells have been applied to the lethally irradiated mouse, and it was found that combined administration does not cause an accumulation of lymphoid cells in the marrow.[13] It has also been demonstrated that recovery of the cellular population attacked by irradiation is accomplished by means of the thymus and the lymphatic ganglia;[40] it was found that the bone marrow in the irradiated rat is also made through the thymus gland.[15] Bortin[6] obtained survival of the lethally irradiated animal by treatment with hepatic cells and fetal thymus combined allogeneically. The mice also survived after transplantation of hematopoietic fetal, neonatal, or adult cells syngenically combined.

Hanzel *et al.*[19] demonstrated the role of the thymus and the bone marrow cells of immunized donors in the recovery of the ability to form antibodies by the irradiated mouse. Sudo *et al.*[42] have pointed out a specific radioprotecting activity of a purified thymus extract as compared to a control extract.

In the research reported herein, the influence of the polypeptide thymic extract, TP, on humoral antibody formation in x-rayed animals immunized with the Salmonella TH 901 antigen was studied.

Materials and Methods

Male adult Chinchilla rabbits weighing 1800–2200 g were treated during a period of 14 days with TP thymus extract by the subcutaneous administration of 5 ml of extract at an interval of 2 days (1 ml extract corresponds to 0.5 g crude thymus). After this preliminary treatment, the animals were completely irradiated with x-rays: 180 R, 7′, at a distance of 145 cm. Fifteen minutes after irradiation each animal was injected with 5 ml of TP thymus extract. The treatment with TP was continued all during the experiment. Immunization was produced by i.v. administration of the Salmonella TH 901 antigen in four doses during a 3-week period, as follows: 0.2 ml, 0.5 ml, 1 ml, and 1.5 ml. The antigen was prepared from a 6-hour culture at 37° C and then inactivated with 4% formalin.

Blood samples for antibody assay were drawn 2, 3 and 4 weeks after antigen administration. Three lots of animals were made up: immunized animals (lot 1), irradiated and immunized animals (lot 2), and irradiated animals immunized and treated with TP (lot 3). The thymic extract utilized in this research was calf thymic extract prepared according to a method reported by I. Milcu elsewhere.[34] The results are given in the tables and figures below.

Results

It may be seen that the titer of Salmonella antiflagellar agglutinines, after the second administration of antigen, differs in each of the three lots (TABLE 1). Thus, the control lot, irradiated and immunized, shows at this stage a slight

TABLE 1

AGGLUTININ TITERS AFTER THE SECOND ADMINISTRATION OF SALMONELLA TH 901 ANTIGEN

Lot	Titer 1/400	1/800	1/1600	1/3200	1/6400	1/12800	1/16000	1/32000
1. Immunized	—	—	18.18%	45.45%	36.36%	—	—	—
2. Irradiated and immunized	—	18.18%	18.18%	54.54%	9.09%	—	—	—
3. Irradiated, immunized, and treated with TP	—	—	—	30.70%	38.46%	15.30%	—	—

TABLE 3

AGGLUTININ TITERS AFTER THE FOURTH ADMINISTRATION OF SALMONELLA TH 901

Lot	Titer 1/4000	1/8000	1/16000	1/32000	1/64000	1/128000	1/256000
1. Immunized	—	—	—	80%	10%	10%	—
2. Irradiated and immunized	—	—	40%	60%	—	—	—
3. Irradiated, immunized, and treated with TP	—	—	—	38.61%	30.30%	23.30%	7.69%

decrease in the antibody titer, whereas in the treated animals the antibody titer is slightly increased as compared with the immunized but nonirradiated controls. The agglutinin titer after the third antigen administration shows differences both under the influence of irradiation and under the influence of TP (TABLE 2). It may be observed that irradiation produces a great lowering of the antibody level as compared with the immunized but nonirradiated controls. Thus, while in the irradiated and immunized lot the sera can be diluted to a titer of 1/8000, in the immunized but nonirradiated controls the antibody titer rises to 1/32 000. Under the influence of the TP extract, the antibody titers return in a higher percent, to the values obtained in nonirradiated controls.

The results obtained after the fourth immunization show that whereas in the immunized controls the antibody titer is clearly elevated as compared to the values obtained in the previous titers (the titration limits being between 1/32 000 and 1/128 000), in the irradiated and immunized animals the antibody level remains low (1/16 000–1/32 000) as compared with the immunized but nonirradiated animals.

Administration of thymic extract increases the antibody titer above the values in the immunized controls, so that it reaches a proportion of 1/256 000 (TABLE 3).

TABLE 2

AGGLUTININ TITERS AFTER THE THIRD ADMINISTRATION OF SALMONELLA TH 901 ANTIGEN

Lot	Titer 1/4000	1/8000	1/16000	1/32000	1/64000
1. Immunized	18.18%	45.45%	27.27%	9.09%	—
2. Irradiated and immunized	36.36%	63.63%	—	—	—
3. Irradiated, immunized, and treated with TP	7.69%	15.30%	23.07%	53.84%	—

Discussion

The results obtained in our experiments show on the one hand that x-irradiation lowers the serum antibody level in the rabbit immunized with TH 901 Salmonella, and on the other hand, that administration of TP thymic extract produces a stimulation of antibody formation in this animal. Our results are concordant with those obtained by other authors who demonstrated a decrease of antibody genesis in irradiated animals and regeneration of the immunological process by the thymus.

The radioprotection offered by the thymus and recovery of the immune response have been achieved by various means such as, thymus or thymic tissue grafts in diffusion chambers,[2, 22, 31, 41] thymic cells that react synergically with the bone marrow cells,[7, 11, 30] administration of thymic extracts [1, 43] by transplantation of bone marrow and thymic tissue under the renal capsule or intraperitoneally in a diffusion chamber.[39] Some authors [12] have studied the response to bacterial antigens i.e. Salmonella flagellar antigen and the polysaccharide from the pneumococcus, and demonstrated that animals with thymic cell deficiencies are incapable of producing antibodies. In our experiments the antibody genesis, reduced after irradiation, is stimulated after administration of the TP fraction. This phenomenon was observed both after the first and after the second antigen administration. The action of the TP thymic extract is that of stimulating antibody genesis after irradiation, thereby demonstrating a protective action on the organism in this process.

The results of our experiments evidenced that the immunological capacity, reduced through irradiation, was restored by administration of the TP polypeptide extract prepared in our laboratory. The important stimulatory effect of TP extract in immunological processes is shown by its ability to restore the immunological capacity damaged by irradiation. Our results confirm that the resistance of the organism to irradiation increased when the TP polypeptide extract was administered, either before or after irradiation. In the treated animals there is no decrease in the level of antibodies after irradiation and the final values are higher than in the immunized but nonirradiated controls. The results corroborated those of other authors dealing with this problem, and they show that when immunological competence has been abolished by irradiation, it can be restored by grafts of thymic tissue or by administration of thymic extracts. These processes of an immunological nature, might suggest that the radioprotective action of the thymus occurs at the moment when the precursors nonresponsive to antigens become immunocompetent cells.[32]

In a recent work Milcu *et al.*[26] reported the influence of the TP fraction on antibody formation in the rat immunized with the A_2 influenza antigen. The results showed that administration of the TP fraction to immunized and irradiated rats stimulates the development of antibodies by comparison with immunized, irradiated and nontreated controls. At the same time, there is an increase in the number of serum lymphocytes and alterations of some enzymatic actions. Studying the effect of the thymic extracts (TP polypeptide and B lipid) on the kinetics of serum and cellular hemolitic antibodies in the spleen of rats immunized by sheep red blood cells, Babeş *et al.*[4] found that stimulation of the thymus occurs at the level of the immunocompetent cellular precursors. These results are confirmed by our experiment reported herein.

The biological and metabolic aspects of the protective effect of the thymus in irradiated animals was reported by Potop *et al.* in some previous work. Studying the metabolism of nucleic acids and the activity of β-glucuronidase in x-irradiated mice, they found that the activity of this enzyme in the thymus decreased after irradiation but that its value returned to normal after administration of TP thymic extract.[35] We have also pointed out that the thymus plays an important part in irradiation and neoplastic processes by inhibiting tumoral development in the rat treated with the thymic fraction.[25, 36]

In our investigation, we were also interested in the effect of the thymus on serum lymphocytes and leukocytes. The action of a thymic fraction in animals with irradiated thymuses was reported as early as 1951 by Potop and Boeru;[33] later, Potop *et al.*[37] reported an important increase in the number of leukocytes under the influence of the thymic extract. Babeş *et al.*[3] utilizing the TP fraction prepared by us demonstrated the influence of the thymic extracts on the development of serum antibodies to mumps virus and antibodies to influenza virus.

The influence of the TP fraction on rabbits immunized with bacterial antigens has been reported by Milcu *et al.* (1973, unpublished data). Milcu *et al.*[27] have also demonstrated the stimulating role of the TP fraction on antibody formation in the rabbit immunized with Salmonella para-AH 1015 and para-BH_3 antigens.

Another problem discussed in the literature is that of relieving the morphological and functional alterations produced by irradiation on the endocrine system. Different hormones influence the survival period of the irradiated animal differently. Comsa[8, 9] has demonstrated that the pituitary growth hormone, deoxycorticosterone, and the thymic hormone prepared by the author prolongs the life of the irradiated animal and that adrenalin shortens it.

Despite all the experiments in this field, the mechanism by which the thymus provides radioprotection is not yet clear. According to some authors, the thymus has a granulo- and erythropoietic trophic function (Miller, Osoba[28]) or a pharmacologic role (Miller[29]), etc. A number of the works mentioned in this paper have been included in the monographic work, "The Thymic Hormones."[23] It is worth pointing out that our results, corroborated by other literature, demonstrate the protective action of thymic extract after X-irradiation, as shown by the elevation of the humoral antibody level.

The works dealing with the role of the thymus in immunological processes are in progress, and the results are encouraging as far as their utilization in clinics is concerned. Today a number of substances with established chemical identity have proved their competence in producing antibodies. Among these are the hormones isolated by Luckey *et al.* (LSHh, LSHr), Comsa (HTH), and Trainin (THT).[23]

Conclusions

Total sublethal irradiation with x-rays of the rabbits immunized with the Salmonella TH 901 antigen induces a decrease in the serum antibody level as compared with nonirradiated controls.

Administration of the TP extract to rabbits immunized with antigen and x-rayed in similar conditions produces a stimulation of antibody formation in these animals as compared to the nontreated controls. The level of antibodies is altered in the animals irradiated, and treatment with the TP extract shows that it has a protective effect on the organism.

References

1. Aisenberg, A. 1967. J. Exp. Med. **125:** 833.
2. Aisenberg, A. & C. Devis. 1968. J. Exp. Med. **128:** 1327.
3. Babes, V. & G. Rutter. 1968. Stud. Cercet. Inframicrobiol. **19:** 169.
4. Babes, V., D. Badescu, G. Mreana, A. Petrescu & I. Potop. 1971. Rev. Roum. Endocrinol. **8:** 457.
5. Betel, I. 1967. Int. J. Radiat. Biol. **12:** 459.
6. Bortin, M. & E. Saletein. 1969. Science **164:** 316.
7. Braun, H. 1968. Experentia **29:** 1145.
8. Comsa, J. 1965. Strahlentherapie **126:** 366.
9. Comsa, J. 1965. Strahlentherapie **126:** 541.
10. Le Dak, L. & A. Kuzin. 1972. Radiobiologhia **12:** 171.
11. Davis, W. & L. Cole. 1969. Proc. Soc. Exp. Biol. Med. **130:** 1336.
12. Davis, A. & R. Carter. 1970. Immunology **19:** 6.
13. Delbez, M. & J. Hoat. 1969. C. R. Soc. Biol. **162:** 2038.
14. Demetyeva, T., G. Dokshina & V. Pegel. 1969. Vop. Med. Khimii **15:** 535.

15. Fedotova, M. & O. Belousova. 1972. Biul. Exp. Biol. Med. **73:** 101.
16. Frigo, G. 1970. Minerva Medica **61:** 3787.
17. Goldstein, A., J. Asanuma & J. Battisto. 1970. J. Immunol. **104:** 359.
18. Gibertini, G., N. Catalini & S. Filoni. 1972. Acta Embriol. Exp. **107:** 1.
19. Handzel, Z. & A. Fiensdorff. 1972. Immunology **23:** 651.
20. Kawamura, F., J. Kolayashi, S. Kawano. 1969. J. Exp. Med. **16:** 33.
21. Kostadinov, D. 1971. Vestn. Akad. Med. Nauk SSSR **26:** 93.
22. Krsak, J., K. Nonzi, V. Kolas & G. Mathe. 1968. Rev. Fr. Etud. Clin. Biol. **13:** 887.
23. Luckey, T. 1973. Thymic Hormones. University Park Press. Baltimore, Md.
24. Maisin, J., G. Mattelin, A. Fridman-Handuzio & E. Parre. 1968. Radiat. Res. **35:** 26.
25. Milcu, S. M. & I. Potop. 1970. Farmacodinamia substanţelor hormonal asemănătoare din timus. Ed. Acad. RSR. Bucharest, Romania.
26. Milcu, S. M., V. Boeru, V. Babes, G. Panaitiu & I. Potop. 1973. Stud. Cercet. Endocrinol. **24:** 483.
27. Milcu, S. M., I. Potop, N. Olenici, G. Panaitiu & V. Boeru. 1973. Stud. Cercet. Endocrinol. **24:** 85.
28. Miller, J. F. A. P. & D. Osoba. 1967. Physiol. Rev. **47:** 437.
29. Miller, J. F. A. P. 1969. Rev. Fr. Etud. Clin. Biol. **4:** 614.
30. Nettesheim, P., S. William & A. Hammon. 1969. J. Immunol. **103:** 505.
31. Osoba, D. 1965. J. Exp. Med. **122:** 633.
32. Osoba, D. 1968. Proc. Soc. Exp. Biol. Med. **127:** 418.
33. Potop, I. & V. Boeru. 1951. Comun. Acad. Repub. Pop. Rom. **1:** 641.
34. Potop, I., V. Boeru & G. Mreana. 1966. Biochem. J. **101:** 454.
35. Potop, I., E. Juvina, J. Biener & G. Mreana. 1967. Stud. Cercet. Endocrinol. **18:** 411.
36. Potop, I., E. Juvina, G. Mreana & I. Ispas. 1967. Rev. Roum. Endocrinol. **6:** 133.
37. Potop, I., V. Boeru, V. Babes, E. Juvina, G. Mreana, M. Stoian & D. Badescu. 1970. Rev. Roum. Endocrinol. **7:** 331.
38. Pullman, I., N. Blumenthal & E. Handeler-Bernich. 1971. Radiat. Res. **45:** 476.
39. Rosenthal, M. 1969. Strahlentherapie **137:** 596.
40. Shikko, S. & S. Mastoshi. 1969. Radiat. Res. **38:** 204.
41. Small, M. & N. Trainin. 1967. Nature **216:** 379.
42. Sudo, F., S. Fumakoshi & H. Manita. 1970. Radiat. Res. **50:** 136.
43. Trainin, N. & M. Linker-Israeli. 1967. Cancer Res. **27:** 309.
44. Williams, A., A. Ghanana, E. Cronsite & B. Waksman. 1971. J. Immunol. **106:** 1143.

INFLUENCE OF THE THYMUS-CORTICOTROPIN-GROWTH HORMONE INTERACTION ON THE REJECTION OF SKIN ALLOGRAFTS IN THE RAT *

J. Comsa, H. Leonhardt, and J. A. Schwarz

Universitätskliniken im Landeskrankenhaus
665 Homburg (Saar), Federal Republic of Germany

The primary role of the thymus in immunological functions is unanimously recognized. It is also admitted that this influence is mediated by humoral factors secreted by the thymus. Preparation of an *in extenso* bibliography of this subject would approach the limit of human capability. We can indicate some reviews,[1-5] however. It is also known that the adenohypophysis influences antibody production. Hypophysectomized mice produced no antibodies and daily injections of growth hormone restored antibody production in these animals.[6] Daily injections of growth hormone enhanced hemolysin production of normal rats injected with sheep erythrocytes [7] and counteracted the immunosuppressive influence of simultaneously injected corticotropin (both in enormous doses [8]) in rats immunized with a soluble protein antigen of *Pasteurella pestis*. The well-known immunological deficiency of Snell-Bag dwarf mice [9-11, et al.] was explained as a consequence of the primary [12] deficient state of their hypophysis, especially of their deficient growth hormone production,[13, 14] since these mice produced antibodies normally when injected with growth hormone.[15-17] Still, divergent results were observed. Rats hypophysectomized at 21 days of age and injected with sheep erythrocytes 21 days later produced hemagglutinins and hemolysin normally when tested 5 days after the antigen injection.[18] Rats hypophysectomized at 60 days of age both produced hemagglutinins against sheep erythrocytes and rejected skin allografts normally. However, their immunological recovery was found to be delayed when they were subjected to x-rays (500 R) 10 days after hypophysectomy.[19]

Corticotropin is generally known to be immunosuppressive. This will be discussed below (see Discussion).

Our previous work has shown us an intricate interaction between the thymus and hypophyseal hormones: (1) The growth induced with daily growth hormone injections in thymectomized and hypophysectomized rats was slower than in those hypophysectomized only. Daily injections of 2 I.U. of growth hormone resulted in a weight increase of 34 g/15 days in hypophysectomized rats and 11 g/15 days in hypophysectomized-thymectomized rats. The normal response to growth hormone could be restored in thymectomized-hypophysectomized rats [20] by simultaneous injections of the thymic extract of Bezssonoff and Comsa.[21] (2) In thymectomized and hypophysectomized rats the stimulation of the adrenal cortex (expressed by the decrease of the ascorbic acid content) could be induced with corticotropin doses whose effect was negligible in those hypophysectomized only; 300 milliunits of corticotropin

* The contribution of a grant from the Saarland Scientific Society (Wissenschaftliche Gesellschaft des Saarlandes) to the preparation of this paper is gratefully acknowledged.

decreased the ascorbic acid content of the adrenal: from 3.68/1000 to 1.71/1000 in thymectomized-hypophysectomized rats and from 3.90/1000 to 3.79/1000 in only hypophysectomized rats.

Previous injection of 120 units of the Bezssonoff-Comsa thymic extract resulted in a complete suppression of the increased sensitivity of thymectomized-hypophysectomized rats towards corticotropin.[22]

It was concluded that circulating thymic hormone is a synergist to circulating hypophyseal growth hormone, whereas it antagonizes circulating corticotropin.

These observations could be confirmed [23] with the homogenous, presumably pure, thymic preparation of Bernardi and Comsa.[24]

The synergism between growth hormone and thymic hormone can be observed through an immunological test.[25] The production of precipitating antibodies against human serum albumin was found on the lower limit of the measurable range in thymectomized and hypophysectomized rats that were: (1) untreated; or (2) injected daily with *either* growth hormone *or* thymic hormone (Bernardi-Comsa). It was found to be fully restored to normal range in thymectomized-hypophysectomized rats injected with both compounds. We intend to enlarge those observations by verifying them with other immunological tests.

The rejection of skin allografts as a test for antibody production was proposed first by Medawar,[26] and to our knowledge its use for testing hormonal influences on immunological functions was first proposed by Morgan [27] and by Billingham, Kohn, and Medawar.[28]

Method

The rejection of skin allografts was investigated in male rats, which were: (1) Normal; (2) Thymectomized; (3) Hypophysectomized; (4) Hypophysectomized, injected daily with 10 I.U. of hypophyseal growth hormone; (5) Hypophysectomized and thymectomized; (6) Hypophysectomized and thymectomized, injected daily with 10 I.U. of hypophyseal growth hormone; (7) Hypophysectomized and thymectomized, injected daily with 120 units of a thymic hormone preparation; (8) Hypophysectomized and thymectomized, injected daily with growth hormone and thymic hormone; (9) Hypophysectomized and thymectomized, injected daily with 300 milliunits of hypophyseal corticotropin; (10) Hypophysectomized, injected daily with 300 milliunits of hypophyseal corticotropin; or (11) Hypophysectomized and thymectomized, injected daily with 300 milliunits of corticotropin and 120 units of thymic hormone.

The Animals

Normal and thymectomized rats were Sprague-Dawleys bred in our laboratory. Hypophysectomized rats were of the same strain, purchased from a commercial breeder (Charles River, France). They were operated on at the age of one month and they arrived in our laboratory 7 days later. They were housed in individual cages at 29 ± 0.5° C. They had full access to commercial rat food and 1% glucose solution in tap water.

The skin graft donors were male rats of the gray inbred DA strain of the Central Breeding Institute in Hannover, bred in our laboratory.

All animals were SPF.

The Hormones

Hypophyseal growth hormone and corticotropin were donated by the Choay Laboratories in Paris. The thymic hormone preparation was prepared in our laboratory by the Bernardi-Comsa method,[24] which yields a homogenous, presumably pure, compound that is fully substitutive in thymectomized guinea pigs [29, 30] and rats [23] and secreted.[31]

The hormone injections were begun 24 hours after the skin grafting and continued daily until the rejection of the allografts.

The Operation

Thymectomy was performed under ether anesthesia by the Segaloff technique (see Reference 32).

For skin grafting the rats were anesthetized with Nembutal. The hair on the backs of donors and recipients was clipped, and depilation completed with a commercial depilatory paste. For partial disinfection the skin was rubbed with Merfene tincture. Two (right and left) approximately circular skin fragments 15 mm in diameter were excised from the back on the level of the 12th rib with a semiautomatic device. An autograft was replaced on the left and the allograft on the right side of the recipients. The grafts were previously dipped in ice-cooled saline and carefully dissected free from subcutaneous tissue with scissors. The borders of the grafts were carefully adapted to those of the graft-bed and bordered in this position with a surgical skin adhesive (Histoacryl, Braun-Melsungen). The grafts were shielded with a wire-net square fixed to the animal with Leucoplast disposed to allow introduction of one finger for palpation of the grafts without removal of the wire-net.

Rejection was expressed by hardening and a dirty brown coloration of the allograft. Its borders detached from those of the graft-bed. In this stage the grafts could be removed by just a touch. Their deep surface was covered with a necrotic membrane. The surface of the graft-bed was intensely hyperemic. Autografts were never rejected. The time elapsed between the operation and the rejection of the allografts was expressed in days.

Results

Figure 1 summarizes our observations, which were as follows: (1) *In normal rats* the skin allografts were rejected in 7.1 ± 1.5 days. This agrees approximately with the observations made by others. (2) *Thymectomy* seemed to result in a slight delay of the rejection. This is at the limit of significance. (3) *Hypophysectomy* was followed by a significant delay. (4) In hypophysectomized animals, thymectomy showed no significant additional influence. (5) In hypophysectomized rats, daily injections of hypophyseal growth hormone resulted in a rejection of the allograft within the interval observed in normal rats.

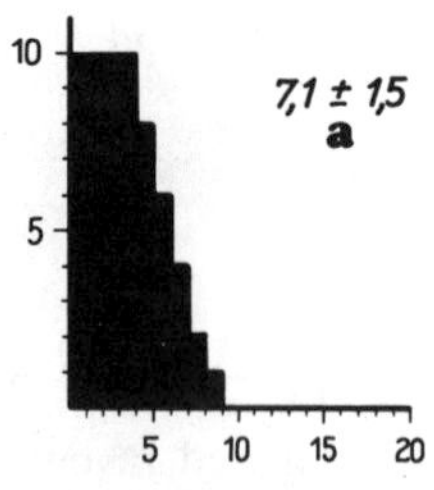
7,1 ± 1,5
a

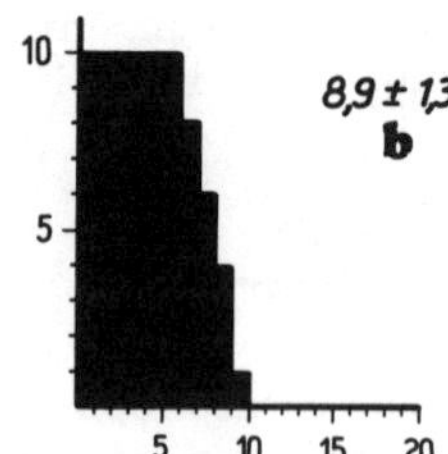
8,9 ± 1,3
b

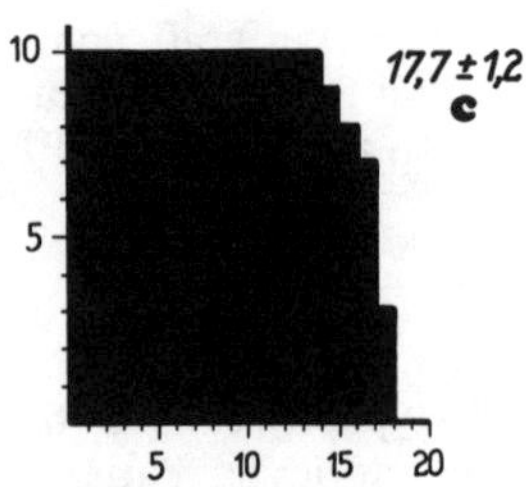
17,7 ± 1,2
c

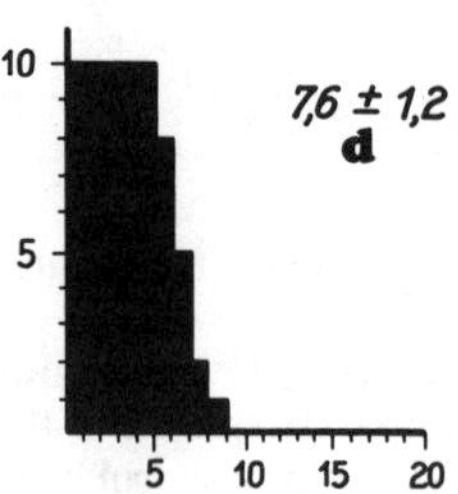
7,6 ± 1,2
d

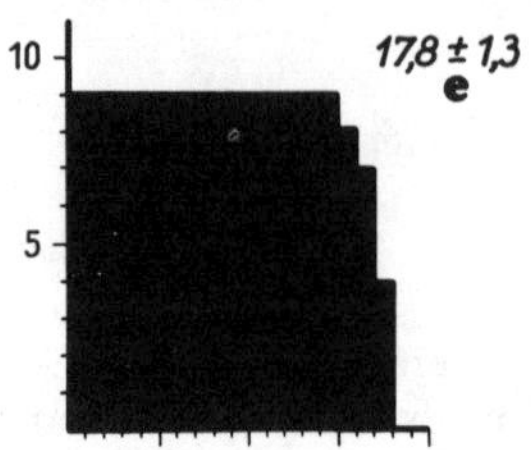
17,8 ± 1,3
e

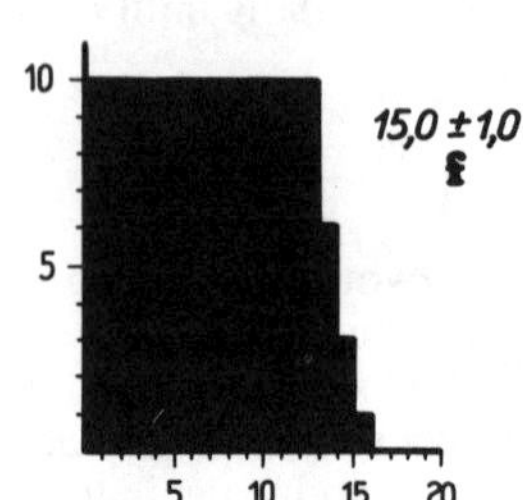
15,0 ± 1,0
f

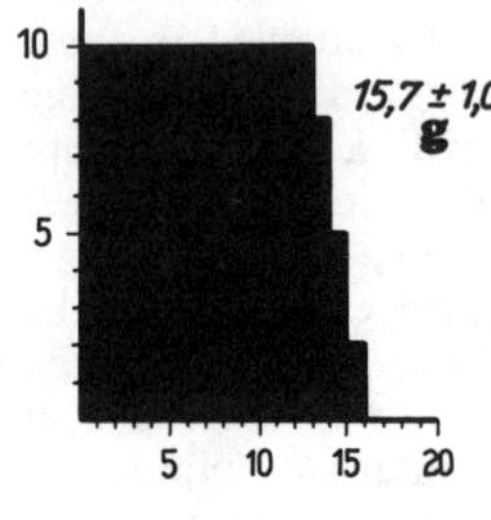
15,7 ± 1,0
g

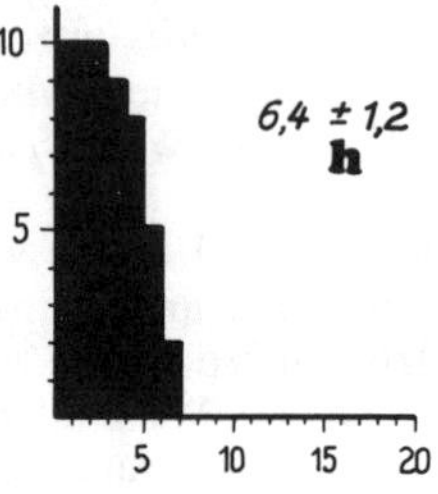
6,4 ± 1,2
h

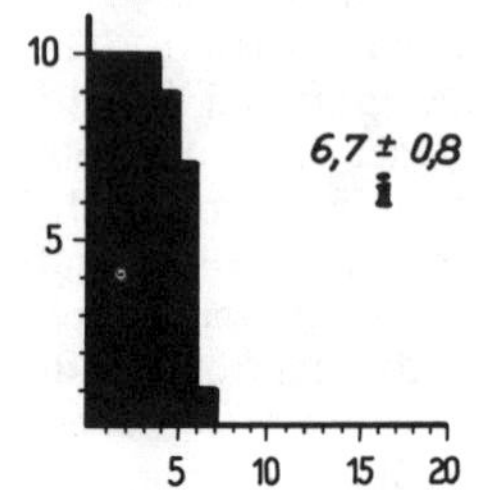
6,7 ± 0,8
i

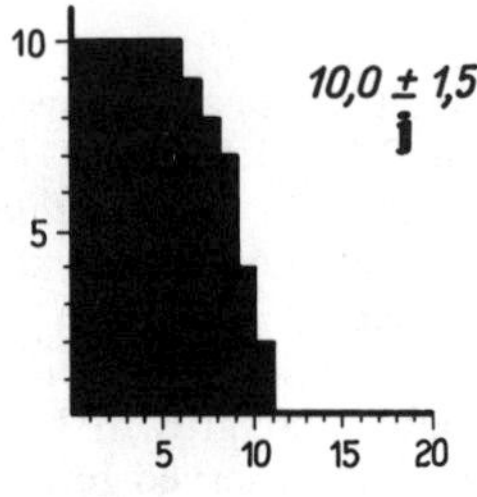
10,0 ± 1,5
j

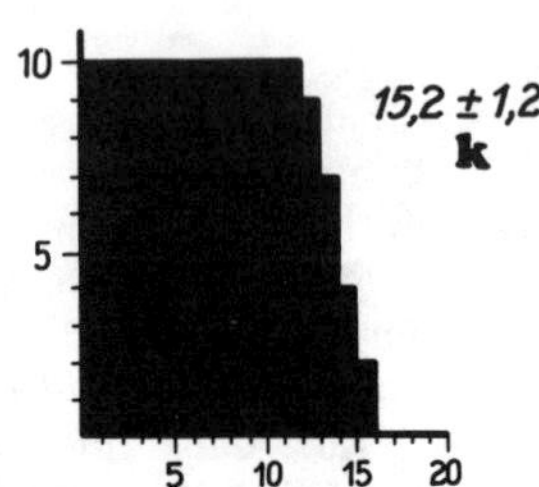
15,2 ± 1,2
k

(6) This was not the case in hypophysectomized and thymectomized rats. In these, the acceleration of the rejection under the influence of growth hormone was hardly significant and this is valid (7) for the influence of thymic hormone as well. (8) In hypophysectomized-thymectomized rats a rejection within normal intervals could be observed if the animals were injected with both growth hormone and thymic hormone. (9) Daily injections of 300 milliunits of corticotropin in thymectomized and hypophysectomized rats were followed by the rejection of allografts almost within the interval observed in normal rats. (10) By comparison with these animals, a slight delay of the rejection was observed in those that were hypophysectomized only and injected with 300 milliunits of corticotropin. (11) Thymectomized-hypophysectomized rats injected with 300 milliunits of corticotropin and 120 units of thymus rejected allografts like those injected with thymus only. (The influence of corticotropin was undetectable.)

Discussion

The experiments described above demonstrate that two adenohypophyseal hormones accelerated the rejection of skin allografts in rats: growth hormone and corticotropin (work is being done on the possible influence of other hypophyseal hormones). In other words, the adenohypophysis appears to stimulate antibody production in at least two ways.

The influence of the thymus on skin allograft rejection depended largely upon the hypophyseal hormone by which the graft rejection was stimulated. The thymus appeared as a synergist to hypophyseal growth hormone and an antagonist to corticotropin. Our previous observations are thus confirmed with an immunological test. We can represent this schematically by a sketch (Figure 2).

An interaction between the thymus and adenohypophysis has been known since Smith [33] described thymus atrophy following hypophysectomy and since it became known [34] that injection of growth-promoting hypophyseal extracts were followed by thymus hypertrophy. The thymus has been defined several times as the effector organ of growth hormone.[35, 36] Bioassay of the thymus in hypophysectomized rats has indeed shown that the hormone content was decreased and that it could be increased to the normal range with injections of growth hormone or corticotropin.[37] Still the results related above cannot be

---

Figure 1. Rejection of skin allografts in the rat: (a) Normal; (b) Thymectomized; (c) Hypophysectomized; (d) Hypophysectomized, injected daily with 10 I.U. of growth hormone; (e) Hypophysectomized and thymectomized; (f) Hypophysectomized and thymectomized, injected daily with 10 I.U. of growth hormone; (g) Hypophysectomized and thymectomized, injected daily with 120 units of thymic hormone; (h) Hypophysectomized and thymectomized, injected daily with 10 units of growth hormone and 120 units of thymic hormone; (i) Hypophysectomized and thymectomized, injected daily with 300 milliunits of corticotropin; (j) Hypophysectomized, injected daily wth 300 milliunts of corticotropin; (k) Hypophysectomized and thymectomized, injected daily with 300 milliunits of corticotropin and 120 units of thymic hormone.

The black columns represent the number of animals which still bear the skin allograft. Abscissa: time in days. Mean interval of the allograft survival ± standard deviation.

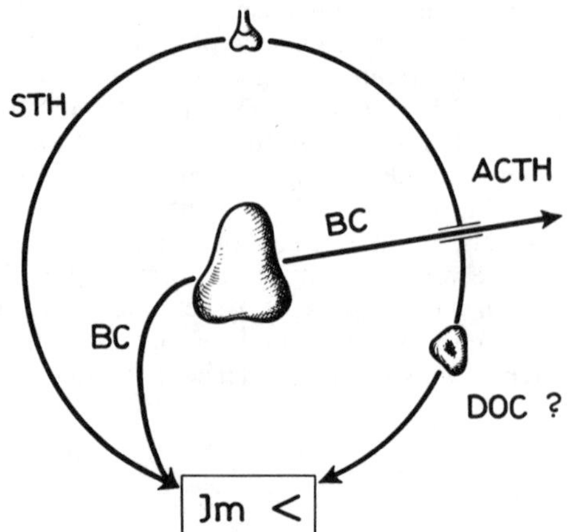

FIGURE 2. Schematic representation of the thymus-corticotropin-growth hormone interaction, as tested with the skin allograft rejection test.

TABLE 1

INFLUENCE OF CORTICOTROPIN ON ALLOGRAFT REJECTION

Reference	Subject	Corticotropin Dose	Time	Result
38	man, severe burns	infusion, not indicated (1 mg/hour)	?	homograft "takes"
39	guinea pig; intact pig	4 to 125 mg/kg daily 8 to 17 mg/kg daily	until rejection	no delay
40	rabbit, intact	25 mg daily	until rejection	no delay
41	macaca, intact	25 to 30 I.U. daily	until rejection	no delay
42	mouse, intact	0.5 to 1.0 mg daily	until rejection	rejection slightly delayed
43	guinea pig, intact	12 or 25 mg daily	until rejection	rejection delayed
44	dog, intact kidney grafted	100 mg daily "several days;" 300 mg daily later	until rejection	no delay
45	mouse, adrenalectomized	—	—	rejection sooner than in controls (difference not significant)

interpreted in these terms. To understand them we simply *must* presume a direct interaction between thymic hormone, corticotropin, and growth hormone in their circulating forms.

From an immunological point of view, the synergism between growth hormone and the thymus seems unequivocal. The case of corticotropin deserves a somewhat more thorough comment. Corticotropin is generally considered as immunosuppressive (see TABLES 1 and 2). Still, all authors who observed these effects emphasize the necessity to administer it in large amounts. Small amounts are unanimously considered as inefficient (that is, not immunosuppressive). Newson and Darrach [54] attempted to quantitate somehow the limits of the immunosuppressive range of corticotropin doses, but generally an arbitrary choice of the doses administered was made. A classification of these works from the standpoint of the corticotropin doses used is difficult because corticotropin doses were expressed in milligrams nearly from the start, regardless of the impurity of the first preparation and of the progressive purification meanwhile occurring. Moreover, so far as I know, immunological experiments with corticotropin were never performed in hypophysectomized animals. It is a commonplace in endocrinology that experiments on the action of a hormone must be made in animals deprived of the corresponding gland. That is even more true for the adenohypophysis, on account of the intricate mutual interaction between the different hypophyseal hormones:

A corticotropin injection is known to enhance the growth hormone secretion,[65-67] and circumstantial evidence permits the supposition that a thyreotropin injection enhances the corticotropin secretion.[68] It is difficult to say exactly which hormone was observed acting after injection of one of the adenohypophyseal hormones in an intact animal. These sources of error (experiments on intact animals, with preparations of a very variable activity in doses supposed exceedingly above physiological range) help us understand why the results of the experiments with corticotropin in immunological tests appear controversial on close examination.

The amount of 300 milliunits daily (our dosage) was chosen, because in previous experiments [22] it was the dose that has shown the most conspicuous difference between the reaction of thymectomized-hypophysectomized and only hypophysectomized rats. It is not small, when compared to doses found still efficient in freshly hypophysectomized rats, but it is well known that sensitivity towards corticotropin decreases in hypophysectomized rats with the time elapsed since the operation and our rats were hypophysectomized 9 days before the first corticotropin injections. Thus: (1) use of hypophysectomized animals and (2) relatively small doses of corticotropin are conditions not fulfilled by any previous author and thus it can be said that no previous observation is properly conflicting with ours. In our experiments corticotropin accelerated the rejection of skin allografts; i.e., it stimulated the immune response.

The objection may be made that corticotropin was observed apparently to increase the antibody content of the serum only through its deleterious effects on lymphocytes (mediated by the adrenal cortex). The additional antibodies found in the serum were only released from the lysed lymphocytes.[69, 70] This was not always observed.[62-64, et al.] But be that as it may, in these experiments corticotropin was administered to previously immunized animals. The explanation does not apply to our rats, which received the first corticotropin injection only 24 hours after the skin graft. A stimulating influence of corticotropin on the immune response is demonstrated by our observations.

TABLE 2

INFLUENCE OF CORTICOTROPIN ON PRODUCTION OF CIRCULATING ANTIBODIES

Reference	Subject	Antigen	Corticotropin Dose	Result
46	human (patients)	pneumonia	100 mg 1st day, 20 mg later until recovery	antipneumococci antibodies appear within normal intervals
47	human (patients)	Pneumococcus polysaccharids	not indicated	antibodies appear sooner than without corticotropin
48	human hemolytic anemia	—	100 mg 1st day, 40 later	hemolyse ceased "hot agglutinins disappeared"
49	rabbit, intact	Pneumococcus vaccine	0.5 to 1.0 mg daily for 28 days	γ-globulin increase in serum partly inhibited
50	—	—	—	antibody titer lower than in controls
51	rat, intact	sheep erythrocytes	1 injection 4 mg	antibody titer higher than in controls
	rat, adrenalectomy	—	—	antibody titer lower than in controls
52	mouse, intact	horse serum	"graded amounts"	no antibodies. Antibodies produced if antigen dose increased
53	rabbit, intact	TAB vaccine, 2 injections at 20-day interval	5 mg daily, from 12th to 28th day	agglutinin titers increased less than normal after the 2nd injection
54	mouse, intact	sheep erythrocytes daily for 6 days	twice daily: 2×1 mg 2×4 mg 4×4 mg	 hemolytic titer normal hemolytic titer reduced by ⅓ hemolytic titer near zero
55	rabbit, intact	human γ-globulin	30 units daily	antibody titer slightly lower than in controls
56	guinea pig intact	heat killed Tbc bacilli	2 mg every 8 hrs 60 days later	antibody titer equal to controls
57	rabbit, intact	bovine serum albumin	9 mg daily in 2 injections	precipitin titer lower than in controls
58	mouse, intact	horse serum 1 single dose	2 injections before the antigens 0.5 mg 1.0 mg 2.0 mg	4 days later antibodies 0 12 days later: antibodies ++ in 50% antibodies + in 50% antibodies 0

TABLE 2 (Continued)

Reference	Subject	Antigen	Corticotropin Dose	Result
59	rabbit, intact	ovalbumin	4 mg daily during immunization	precipitin titer reduced by ⅓
8	rat, intact	protein antigen of *Pasteurella pestii*	daily, sufficient to stop growth (enormous)	precipitins not produced
60	rabbit, intact	horse serum	20 mg daily from the antigen injection	precipitins slightly less than in controls
61	mouse, intact	sheep erythrocytes every 30 days for 98 days	one single injection 35 days later	before corticotropin antibodies 0 few hours after ++ (released from killed lymphocytes)
62	rabbit	ovalbumin	25 mg 3 months later	antibody titer 0 before and after corticotropin
63	rabbit, intact	ovalbumin	one single injection 25 units 90 days later	6 hours, 12 hours, and 48 hours later no antibody titer increase
64	rabbit, intact	ovalbumin 4 times weekly during 4 weeks, one month interruption, repeated 2 more times	one single injection 50 units	4 hours, 9 hours, 24 hours, and 48 hours later antibody titer decreased

How does this stimulation work?

(1) Actions of corticotropin not mediated by the adrenal were observed. Added to the medium, corticotropin increased the glucose uptake of the incubated epididymal fat pad [71] and of the thymus [72] of the rat, an influence opposed to that of all corticosteroids known thus far.

(2) Corticosteroids are known as immunosuppressants. This knowledge resulted in the paradoxical situation, noted by several reviewers,[63, 73, et al.] that Addison's disease is characterized by immunological deficiency, and corticoids are known as immunosuppressants.

Although a review of the enormous bibliography on this topic would be out of place here, we will indicate some reviews.[73-77] It is unanimously stated that corticoids must be given in large amounts for immunosuppressive effects. In these doses they have well-characterized deleterious effects. They kill lymphocytes in masses (see Reference 76), and it could be validly asserted that they are immunosuppressive inasmuch as they kill the lymphocytes.[78, 79] The parallel between corticoid effect and Addison's disease (see above) may suggest that in an intermediate range (between zero and the lower limit of the immunosuppressive dose) corticoids may be immunostimulants. This supposition has received little experimental support thus far. Corticoids were shown to enhance the immune response, but under peculiar conditions (in fish and frogs[80]) or using adrenocortical extracts.[81-83, et al.] Robinson, Mason and Smith[84] observed a beneficial influence of small doses of cortisone (from 0.5 to 2.0 mg daily) on the experimental pneumonia in rats, whereas doses from 3 to 10 mg aggravated the disease, but this may not express an influence on the immune response only (see Reference 46). To my knowledge, one experiment gives convincing evidence of an immunostimulant influence of cortisol in small doses. Added to the medium in amounts from one to 100 ng per ml cortisol permitted lymph nodes from sensitized rabbits to produce antibodies when incubated in the presence of antigen in a serum-free medium. Either serum or cortisol was required for the immune response.[85] It is interesting to confront this observation with two others: added to the medium in concentrations of 320 μg per ml cortisol suppressed antibody production in incubated spleen fragments;[86] and at 70 μg per ml it was without influence.[87] Does this suggest a dose-response curve?

Moreover, metopirone was found to inhibit the graft-versus-host reaction.[88] Experiments in adrenalectomized animals receiving graded doses of different corticoids could be of interest.

(3) One corticoid, deoxycorticosterone, is known to enhance antibody production even if administered in milligram doses.[89-92, et al.] We recall that deoxycorticosterone is not lympholytic.[78] It has been questioned whether deoxycorticosterone is a hormone or not.[93] Still, it has been found in the perfusion fluid of the isolated beef adrenal[94] in the venous blood of the adrenal in the dog[95] and in human blood plasma.[96, et al.] We have no reason to exclude deoxycorticosterone secretion in the rat; however it has not yet been demonstrated as far as I know.

Thus: (a) a possible influence of corticotropin not mediated by the adrenal; (b) the possible immunostimulant effect of corticoids in small doses; and (c) the possible secretion of deoxycorticosterone; are possible hypotheses for an approach to the problem of corticotropin experiments. We intend to test these hypotheses.

The thymus-corticotropin interaction seems somewhat surprising at a (very superficial) first look. In this experiment the thymus seemed to inhibit antibody production. This is by no means our conclusion. We interpret this observation just in terms of the antagonism between corticotropin and the thymus.

What happens in the normal animal, where all these hormones are supposed to act simultaneously? The problem must be considered from two angles.

(1) In the absence of growth hormone, corticotropin, and thymus, skin allografts are still rejected; it just takes more time. This indicates that under these conditions antibodies are still produced, only at a lower rate than in normal animals. The question as to whether antibodies are produced or not is thus answered by the immunocompetent cells and by these only (at least from present standards).

(2) The adenohypophysis and the thymus contribute to determine how quickly skin allografts are rejected, in other words, how many antibodies are produced. This indicates that in the normal animal the immunocompetent cells receive constant stimulation from the adenohypophysis and the thymus.

It could be supposed that in our opinion the interaction between the thymus and the hypophysis provides an exhaustive explanation of the role of the thymus in immunology. We don't think so. A direct chemotactic influence of the thymic hormone on lymphocytes could be demonstrated *in vivo*.[97, 98] Tissue-culture experiments may be useful in delimiting the different aspects of the influence of the thymus.

Summary

Skin allograft rejection was noticeably delayed in rats following hypophysectomy. Daily injections of hypophyseal growth hormone restored the normal reaction.

Additional thymectomy had no influence on the rejection of hypophysectomized rats. In these animals growth hormone by itself had no significant influence on the graft rejection. It only restored a normal reaction when given together with thymic hormone.

Corticotropin injections accelerated the allograft rejection. On this action of corticotropin thymic hormone has shown a significant inhibitory influence.

The thymus was thus proved to be a synergist to growth hormone and an antagonist to corticotropin. Previous observations made with usual endocrinological tests are thus confirmed with an immunological test.

Acknowledgment

We wish to thank Laboratories Choay (Paris, France) for the hypophyseal hormones we used.

References

1. Hess, M. W. 1968. Experimental thymectomy, possibilities and limitations. Springer-Verlag. Berlin, Federal Republic of Germany.
2. Good, R. A. & A. E. Gabrielsen. 1964. The thymus in immunobiology. Harper & Row. New York, N.Y.
3. Comsa, J. 1971. The thymic hormones. Hormones **2:** 226.
4. Goldstein, A. L. & A. White. 1970. The thymus as an endocrine gland. *In* Biochemical action of hormones. G. Litwac, Ed. Academic Press. New York, N.Y.
5. Luckey, T. D., Ed. 1973. Thymic hormones. University Park Press. Baltimore, Md.
6. Gisler, R. H. & L. Schenkel-Huliger. 1971. Hormonal regulation of the immune response. II. Influence of pituitary and adrenal activity on immune response *in vitro*. Cell. Immunol. **2:** 534.
7. Hoene, R., T. H. Ridani & G. Heuser. 1954. Influence of somatotrophic hormone and hydrocortisone acetate on the production of hemolytic antibodies in the rat. Am. J. Physiol. **177:** 19.
8. Hayashida, T. & Ch.-H. Li. 1957. Influence of adrenocorticotropic and growth hormone on antibody formation. J. Exp. Med. **105:** 93.
9. Baroni, C. 1967. Thymus, peripheral lymph nodes and immunological responsiveness of the pituitary dwarf mouse. Experientia **23:** 282.
10. Baroni, C., N. Fabris & G. Bertoli. 1967. Dependence of the pituitary immune response in the hereditary pituitary dwarf and normal Snell-Bagg mouse. Experientia **23:** 1059.

11. Duquesnoy, R. J., P. K. Kalpaktsoglu & R. A. Good. 1970. Immunological studies on the Snell-Bagg pituitary dwarf mouse. Proc. Soc. Exp. Biol. Med. **133:** 201.
12. Carsner, R. L. & E. G. Rennels. 1960. Primary site of gene action in dwarf mice. Science **131:** 829.
13. Lewis, W. J. 1967. Growth hormone of normal and dwarf mice. Mem. Soc. Endocrinol. **15:** 179.
14. Lewis, W. J., E. Cheever & W. D. Vanderlaan. 1965. Growth hormone in normal and dwarf mice. Endocrinology **76:** 40.
15. Pierpaoli, W., C. Baroni, N. Fabris & E. Sorkin. 1969. Reconstitution of antibody production in hormonally deficient mice by growth hormone, thyrotropin and thyroxin. Immunology **16:** 217.
16. Pierpaoli, W., N. Fabris & E. Sorkin. 1970. *In* Cellular interaction in immune response N. R. Rose, Ed. : 25. Karger. Basel, Switzerland.
17. Pierpaoli, W. & E. Sorkin. 1967. Relationship between thymus and hypophyse. Nature **215:** 834.
18. Kalden, J. R., M. M. Evans & W. J. Irvine. 1970. Effect of hypophysectomy on immune response. Immunology **18:** 671.
19. Duquesnoy, R. J., T. Mariani & R. A. Good. 1969. Effect of hypophysectomy on immunologic recovery after sublethal irradiation in adult rats. Proc. Soc. Exp. Biol. Med. **131:** 1076.
20. Comsa, J. 1958. Influence of the thymus on the reaction of the rat to anterior pituitary growth hormone. Nature **182:** 728.
21. Bezssonoff, N. A. & J. Comsa. 1958. Préparation d'un extrait purifié de thymus. Ann. Endocrinol. **19:** 222.
22. Comsa, J. 1958. Influence of the thymus on the reaction of rats to adrenocorticotropic hormone. Nature **182:** 57.
23. Comsa, J. 1965. Influence de l'hormone thymique sur l'action des hormones hypophysaires chez le rat. Ann. Endocrinol. **26:** 525.
24. Bernardi, G. & J. Comsa. 1965. Purification chromatographique d'une préparation de thymus douée d'activité hormonale. Experientia **21:** 416.
25. Comsa, J., J. A. Schwarz & H. Neu. Influence of the thymus-growth hormone interaction on the production of precipitating antibodies in the rat. In press.
26. Medawar, P. B. 1944. Behaviour and fate of skin autografts and homografts in rabbits. J. Anat. **78:** 176.
27. Morgan, J. A. 1951. Influence of cortisone on the survival of skin homografts. Surgery **30:** 506.
28. Billingham, R. E., P. L. Krohn & P. B. Medawar. 1951. Effect of cortisone on survival of skin homografts in rabbits. Brit. Med. J. **1:** 1157.
29. Comsa, J. 1965. Action of the purified thymic hormone in thymectomized guinea pigs. Am. J. Med. Sci. **250:** 79.
30. Comsa, J. & G. Filipp. 1966. Influence de l'hormone thymique sur la production d'anticorps chez le cobaye thymiprive. Ann. Inst. Pasteur **110:** 365.
31. Comsa, J. & E. M. Philipp. 1971. Essai de démonstration de la secrétion de l'hormone thymique. J. Physiol. **63:** 193a.
32. Segaloff, N. 1949. *In* The rat in laboratory investigation. E. J. Farris & J. Griffith, Eds. Hafner. New York, N.Y.
33. Smith, P. E. 1930. Effect of hypophysectomy upon the involution of the thymus in the rat. Anat. Rec. **47:** 119.
34. Benedict, E. B., T. J. Putnam & H. M. Teel. 1930. Early changes produced in dogs by injections of sterile active extract from anterior lobe of hypophyse. Am. J. Med. Sci. **179:** 489.
35. Bomskov, C. 1940. Der Thymus als immunsekretorisches Organ. Deut. Med. Wochenschr. **66:** 589.
36. Pierpaoli, W. & E. Sorkin. 1967. Relationship between thymus and hypophyse. Nature **215:** 834.

37. Comsa, J. 1959. Influence de l'hypophyse sur la teneur du thymus du rat en principe actif. Ann. Endocrinol. **20:** 795.
38. Whitelaw, M. J. 1951. Physiological reaction to pituitary adrenocorticotropic hormone in severe burns. J. Am. Med. Ass. **195:** 85.
39. Ellison, E. H., B. C. Martin, R. D. Williams, H. W. Clatworthy, G. Hanewi & R. M. Zollinger. 1951. Adrenal cortical hormone and homografting. Ann. Surg. **134:** 495.
40. Krohn, P. L. 1954. Effect of steroid hormones on survival of skin grafts in the rabbit. J. Endocrinol. **11:** 78.
41. Krohn, P. L. 1954. Effect of steroid hormones on the survival of skin grafts. J. Endocrinol. **12:** 78.
42. Medawar, P. P. & E. M. Sparrow. 1956. Effect of adrenocortical hormones, adrenocorticotropic hormone and pregnancy on skin transplantation immunity. J. Endocrinol. **14:** 240.
43. Sparrow, E. M. 1954. Effect of cortisone alcohol and ACTH on skin homografts in guinea pigs. J. Endocrinol. **11:** 57.
44. Perky, L. & S. Jacob. 1951. Effect of ACTH and cortisone on homologous kidney transplant. Proc. Soc. Exp. Biol. Med. **77:** 66.
45. Graffe, R. J., M. A. Lappe & G. D. Snell. 1969. Influence of gonad and adrenal on immune response to skin graft. Transplantation **7:** 105.
46. Kass, E. H., S. H. Ingbar & M. Friedland. 1950. Effect of ACTH in pneumonia. Ann. Intern. Med. **33:** 1081.
47. Mirick, G. S. 1950. Effect of ACTH and cortisone on antibody production in humans. J. Clin. Invest. **29:** 836.
48. Dameshek, W., M. C. Rosenthal & L. Schwartz. 1950. Treatment of acquired hemolyitc anemia with ACTH. N. Engl. J. Med. **244:** 117.
49. Bjoernboe, M. 1943. Serum protein during immunization. Acta Path. Microbiol. Scand. **20:** 221.
50. Bjoernboe, M., E. E. Fischel & H. C. Stoerk. 1951. Effect of ACTH and cortisone on concentration of circulating antibodies. J. Exp. Med. **93:** 37.
51. Roberts, S. & A. White. 1951. Influence of adrenal cortex on antibody production *in vitro*. Endocrinology **48:** 741.
52. Hayes, S. P. & T. F. Dougherty. 1952. Effect of ACTH and cortisone on antibody synthesis and rate of disappearance of antigen. Fed. Proc. **11:** 67.
53. Moeschlin, S., R. Baguerra & T. Baguerra. 1953. Influence of ACTH and cortisone on experimental antibody production in rabbits. Bull. Schweiz. Akad. Med. Wiss. **8:** 153.
54. Newson, S. E. & M. Darrach. 1954. Effect of corticotropine and corticosterone on the production of hemolytic antibodies in the mouse. Can. J. Biochem. Physiol. **32:** 372; **33:** 374.
55. Kass, E. H., M. L. Kendrick & M. Finland. 1955. Effect of corticosterone, hydrocortisone and corticotropin on the production of antibodies in rabbits. J. Exp. Med. **102:** 767.
56. Osgood, C. K. & C. B. Favour. 1951. Effect of ACTH on inflammation due to tuberculin hypersensitivity. J. Exp. Med. **94:** 415.
57. Malkiel, S. & B. J. Hargis. 1952. Effect of ACTH and cortisone on the quantitative precipitin reaction. J. Immunol. **69:** 217.
58. Dougherty, T. F. 1952. Studies on antiphlogistic and antibody-suppressive functions of pituitary and adrenocortical secretion. Recent Progr. Horm. Res. **7:** 307.
59. Germuth, E. G., T. Oyama & B. Ottinger. 1951. Mechanism of action of 17-hydroxy-11-dehydrocorticosterone and of adrenocorticotrophic hormone in experimental hypersensitivity in rabbits. J. Exp. Med. **94:** 139.
60. Beithrong, M., A. R. Rich & P. C. Griffith. 1950. Effect of ACTH upon experimental cardiovascular lesions produced by anaphylactic hypersensitivity. Bull. Johns Hopkins Hosp. **86:** 131.

61. Dougherty, T. F., J. H. Chase & A. White. 1945. Pituitary-adrenocortical control of antibody release from lymphocytes. Proc. Soc. Exp. Biol. Med. **58:** 135.
62. Fischel, E. E., M. LeMay & E. A. Kabat. 1949. Effect of adrenocorticotrophic hormones and X-rays on the amount of circulating antibody. J. Immunol. **61:** 89.
63. Fischel, E. E. 1950. Relationship of adrenal cortical activity to immune response. Bull. N.Y. Acad. Med. **26:** 255.
64. De Vries, J. A. 1950. Effect of ACTH on circulating antibody levels. J. Immunol. **65:** 1.
65. Neri, V., A. Bartonelli, B. Ambrosi, F. Beck, P. Pecoz & G. Foglia. 1970. Effect of corticotropin on plasma growth hormone. Lancet **1:** 1287.
66. Zahnd, G. R., A. Nadeau & K. E. Von Muhlendahl. 1969. Effect of corticotropin on plasma growth hormone. Lancet **1:** 1287.
67. Strauch, G., P. Pandos, J. P. Luton & H. Bricaire. 1971. Stimulation de la secrétion d'hormone de croissance par la β 1–24 corticotropine. Ann. Endocrinol. **32:** 526.
68. Eartly, H. & P. C. Leblond. 1954. Identification of the thyroxine effects mediated by the hypophyse. Endocrinology **84:** 949.
69. Dougherty, T. F. & A. White. 1943. Effect of pituitary adrenocorticotropic hormone on lymphoid tissue. Proc. Soc. Exp. Biol. Med. **53:** 132.
70. Dougherty, T. F., A. White & J. H. Chase. 1944. Relationship of the effect of adrenal cortical secretion on lymphoid tissue and antibody titer. Proc. Soc. Exp. Biol. Med. **56:** 28.
71. Glenn, J. P., W. C. Miller & C. A. Schlagel. 1963. Metabolic effects of adrenocortical steroids *in vivo* and *in vitro*. Rec. Progr. Horm. Res. **19:** 107.
72. Deschaux, P., A. Portier & R. Fontanges. 1971. Influence de l'hormone corticotrope sur la consommation d'oxygène et de glucose du rat. C. R. Soc. Biol. **165:** 2123.
73. Kass, E. H. & M. Finland. 1953. Adrenocortical hormones in infection and immunity. Ann. Rev. Microbiol. **7:** 361.
74. McMaster, P. D. & R. B. Franzl. 1961. Effect of adrenocortical steroids on antibody formation. Metabolism **10:** 990.
75. Germuth, F. G. 1956. Role of adrenocortical steroids in infection. Pharmacol. Rev. **8:** 1.
76. Dougherty, T. F. 1952. Effects of hormones on lymphatic tissue. Physiol. Rev. **32:** 379.
77. Gabrielsen, A. E. & R. A. Good. 1967. Chemical suppression of adaptive immunity. Adv. Immunol. **6:** 90.
78. Dougherty, T. F., M. Z. Berliner, G. Schnebeli & D. Berliner. 1963. Hormonal control of lymphatic structure and function. Ann. N.Y. Acad. Sci. **113:** 825.
79. Harris, T. N., S. Harris & M. B. Faber. 1954. J. Immunol. **72:** 161.
80. Bisset, K. A. 1949. Influence of adrenal cortical hormones on immunity in cold-blooded vertebrates. J. Endocrinol. **6:** 94.
81. Dougherty, T. F., A. White & J. H. Chase. 1944. Relationship of the effect of adrenal cortical secretion on lymphatic tissue and antibody titer. Proc. Soc. Exp. Biol. Med. **88:** 28.
82. Chase, J. H., A. White & T. F. Dougherty. 1946. Enhancement of circulating antibody concentration by adrenal cortical hormones. J. Immunol. **52:** 101.
83. Clark, W. G. & E. Jacobs. 1950. Experimental nonthrombocytopenic vascular purpura. Blood **5:** 320.
84. Robinson, H. J., P. C. Mason & A. L. Smith. 1953. Beneficial effects of cortisone on survival of rats injected with D. pneumoniae. Proc. Soc. Exp. Biol. Med. **84:** 712.

85. Ambrose, C. T. 1964. Requirement for hydrocortisone in antibody forming tissue cultivated in serum-free medium. J. Exp. Med. **119:** 1027.
86. Fagraeus, A. 1952. Role of ACTH and cortisone in resistance and immunity. Acta Pathol. Microbiol. Scand. Suppl. **93:** 20.
87. Mountain, I. M. 1955. Antibody production *in vitro*. J. Immunol. **74:** 270.
88. Abe, T. & M. Nomura. 1970. Amelioration of runt disease in rats by metopirone. J. Nat. Cancer Inst. **45:** 597.
89. Chebotarov, V. F. 1965. Characteristics of the titers of serum antibodies in immunization with the use of hydrocortisone and desoxycorticosterone. Fiziol. Zh. Akad. Nauk USSR **11:** 819.
90. Chebotarov, V. F. 1968. Comparative study of the effect of desoxycorticosterone acetate on the level of antibodies in seurm and lymph node extracts in rats. Vop. Immunol. **3:** 35.
91. Meshalova, A. N. & I. B. Fryazinova. 1960. Effect of cortisone on immunogenesis. IV. Comparative study of the body reactivity under the effect of various steroid hormones. Zh. Mikrobiol. Epidemiol. Immunobiol. **31:** 23.
92. Uchitel, I. Ya. & E. L. Khasman. 1968. Effect of substances of catabolic and anabolic action on the formation of antibdies. **4:** 44.
93. Soffer, L. J., R. I. Dorfman & J. L. Gabrilove. 1961. The human adrenal gland. Lea & Febiger. Philadelphia, Pa.
94. Hechter, O., A. Zaffaroni, R. P. Jacobsen, H. Levy, R. W. Jeanloz, W. Schenker & G. Pincus. 1951. Nature and biogenesis of the adrenal secretory product. Rec. Progr. Horm. Res. **6:** 215.
95. Farrel, G. L., E. W. Rauschkolb, Pc. Royce & H. Hirschmann. 1954. Isolation of DOC from adrenal venous blood of the dog. Proc. Soc. Exp. Biol. Med. **87:** 587.
96. Loras, B., A. Daford, H. Roux & J. Bertrand. 1969. Variations des taux de production du cortisol de la corticosterone de l'aldosterone et de la désoxycorticosterone. Ann. Endocrinol. **30:** 677.
97. Comsa, J. 1950. Recherches sur la mécanisme déterminant de l'afflux des lymphocytes vers le thymus. C. R. Acad. Sci. **230:** 2337.
98. Comsa, J. & R. Schweisfurth. 1972. Nouvelles recherches sur l'action chimiotactique de l'hormone thymique sur la lymphocytes. Pathol. Biol. **20:** 639.

EXTRACTION, FRACTIONATION, AND TESTING OF A HOMOGENOUS THYMIC HORMONE PREPARATION

J. Comsa

Universitätskliniken im Landeskrankenhaus
665 Homburg (Saar), Federal Republic of Germany

The first thymic extract that was proved to be substitutive was prepared by D. Asher[1] in 1933 by the following method: (1) extraction of the ground thymus with acetone, supernatant discarded; (2) extraction of the residue with ether, supernatant discarded; (3) extraction of the residue with water, residue discarded; (4) aqueous extract acidified with "a few drops" of acetic acid and boiled for one or two seconds, precipitate discarded; and (5) supernatant saturated with ammonium sulphate, the precipitate is active.

The chronologically next method (Bezssonoff and Comsa[2]) was inspired by the Asher method in two points: (1) the saturation with ammonium sulphate; and (2) Asher's observation that a solution of her extract became turbid when brought to about pH 6. She concluded: ". . . the extract is not yet pure, because it still contains protein." It was inconceivable in the early 1930's, that a protein could be a hormone.

The Bezssonoff and Comsa method is as follows: (1) extraction of the ground thymus with M sulphuric acid (0.8 ml per gram of thymus) is performed; (2) neutralization with ammonia and increase of the ammonium sulphate concentration to 17% and then filtration are accomplished. With the residue, steps (1) and (2) are repeated twice, and the filtrates united. (3) The filtrate is saturated with ammonium sulphate. The precipitate is active. (4) The precipitate is dissolved in just enough HCl 0.03 M, pH is brought to 7.0 with ethanolic ammonia (bromcresol purple) and ethanol concentration brought to 20%. A precipitate falls out. Centrifugation at 3000 rpm is performed. (5) The supernatant is acidified, pH is brought to 6.2 with ethanolic ammonia and ethanol concentration is brought to 60%. The precipitate is active. Steps (3) and (4) are repeated six times; each time the previous precipitate from the previous point (4) is dissolved in the supernatant of the following point (3). Thus, the crude preparation obtained by saturation with ammonium sulphate is exhausted and the ammonium sulphate is discarded.

The total activity of a Bezssonoff-Comsa (BC) extract (units per gram of thymus) is about ten times greater than that of an Asher extract. This extract was fractionated by Bernardi and Comsa as follows.[3]

BC is dissolved in 0.001 M potassium phosphate buffer (pH 6.8) and filtered on a Sephadex®-G 25 column. It is readily eluted in one batch. The eluate is charged on a hydroxyapatite column and eluted with potassium phosphate buffer in a molarity gradient. Three fractions are obtained of which the third is active (at the end of the corresponding peak the buffer is molar). This eluate is desalted on Sephadex-G 25 and lyophilized. This fraction is homogenous (ultracentrifugation). When divided into 4 arbitrary subfractions during the elution, its activity was found to be constant.

Asher's extract was found to be substitutive in thymectomized guinea pigs (Comsa[4]). BC and the homogenous compound of Bernardi and Comsa could also suppress the consequences of thymectomy: (1) *In guinea pigs:* on survival, growth, lymphatic tissue, adenohypophyse, thyroid, adrenal, gonads (Comsa [5]) and antibody production (Comsa and Filipp [7]). (2) *In rats:* on lymphatic tissue, adenohypophyse, thyroid, adrenal (Comsa, unpublished), reactivity towards adenohypophyseal hormones (Comsa [6]), and the production of precipitating antibodies (Comsa, Schwarz and Neu, in press). Some additional observations were reported at this conference.

Thymus, lymph nodes, and spleen of rats of graded ages were extracted with these methods (BC extraction and Bernardi-Comsa fractionation; Comsa and Philipp [8]). Previous bioassays have shown that these organs only possess a thymus-like activity (see Luckey [9]). The fraction corresponding to the active fraction of Bernardi and Comsa was found in all these organs and nowhere else (FIGURE 1 of the previous paper).

These preparations from rats were found to be active (Comsa and Philipp, unpublished). The peak corresponding to this active fraction disappeared from the lymph nodes and the spleen of thymectomized rats as early as less than 3 days after the operation.

It was concluded, that the homogenous, fully substitutive compound obtained by the Bernardi-Comsa method corresponds to a chemical entity (1) whose loss results in the thymoprivic condition in rats and in guinea pigs; and (2) which is secreted by the thymus only and only stored in organs rich in lymphocytes. The term "thymic hormone" would suffice to summarize those two conclusions.

REFERENCES

1. ASHER, D. 1933. Weitere Isolierung des wachstumsfördernden Thymocrescins. Biochem. Z. **257:** 209–12.
2. BEZSSONOFF, N. A. & J. COMSA. 1958. Préparation d'un extrait purifié de thymus, application a l'urine humaine. Ann. Endocrinol. **19:** 222–27.
3. BERNARDI, G. & J. COMSA. 1965. Purification chromatographique d'une preparation de thymus douée d'activité hormonale. Experientia **21:** 416–17.
4. COMSA, J. 1940. Action de l'extrait de thymus chez le cobaye thymiprive. C. R. Soc. Biol. **133:** 24.
5. COMSA, J. 1965. Action of the purified thymus hormone in thymectomized guinea pigs. Am. J. Med. Sci. **250:** 79–85.
6. COMSA, J. 1965. Influence de l'hormone thymique sur l'action des hormones hypophysaires. Ann. Endocrinol. **26:** 525–34.
7. COMSA, J. & G. FILIPP. 1966. Influence de l'hormone thymique sur la production d'anticorps chez le cobaye thymiprive. Ann. Inst. Pasteur **110:** 365–72.
8. COMSA, J. & E.-M. PHILIPP. 1971. Essai de demonstration de la secrétion de l'hormone thymique. J. Physiol. **63:** 193a.
9. LUCKEY, T. D., Ed. 1973. Thymic hormones. University Park Press, Baltimore, Md.

INVOLVEMENT OF T- AND B- LYMPHOCYTES IN THE IMMUNE RESPONSE TO THE PROTEIN EXOTOXIN AND THE LIPOPOLYSACCHARIDE ANTIGENS OF *VIBRIO CHOLERAE* *

John R. Kateley,† Chandu B. Patel, and Herman Friedman

Department of Microbiology
Albert Einstein Medical Center
Philadelphia, Pennsylvania 19141

Although bone marrow (B) lymphocytes are directly involved in antibody formation, it is widely known that the collaboration of thymus-derived (T) lymphocytes is often necessary for humoral immunity.[1–5] In this regard, the interaction between T- and B-lymphocytes for antibody formation has become the center of much attention in recent years. Numerous studies utilizing a variety of thymus-dependent and thymus-independent antigens have shown that collaboration between T- and B-lymphocytes, both *in vivo* and *in vitro,* is often necessary for a normal humoral immune response. Initial studies of this type were concerned with the formation of antibodies to erythrocyte antigens.[1–3] More recent studies utilizing serum protein, synthetic polypeptides, chemical hapten, etc. have confirmed and extended the earlier findings that B-cells need the "help" of T-cells for antibody formation. In contrast, it is now widely accepted that certain antigens, especially the lipopolysaccharide (LPS) somatic antigens from Gram-negative bacteria, can stimulate antibody formation without the apparent collaboration of T-cells.[4, 5] Thus the immune response to such bacterial antigens is thought to be "thymus independent."

Earlier studies in this laboratory have been concerned with the nature and mechanism of the immune response to somatic antigens derived from *Vibrio cholerae,* a Gram-negative enteric pathogen.[6, 7] Antibody-forming cells to these bacteria appear rapidly in the spleen and lymph nodes of mice immunized with vibrios and are readily recognized by the direct vibriolytic plaque assay in agar gel analogous to the localized hemolytic plaque assay with erythrocytes. Immunization of mice with the vibrio bacteria, either a cellular extract or heat-killed bacilli, results in the rapid appearance of antibody plaque-forming cells (PFC). However, the kinetics of appearance of such cells are markedly different than that observed in mice immunized with other antigens such as sheep erythrocytes (SRBC) or *E. coli* LPS. Instead of a peak antibody PFC response 4–6 days after immunization, there is an extended lag period of several days before the appearance of antibody forming cells, with a peak response 12–15 days after primary immunization. Furthermore, no antibody PFC are present to the vibrio antigens in nonimmunized mice. Such results have suggested that

* Supported in part by grants from The United States National Science Foundation and The National Institute of Allergy and Infectious Diseases, National Institutes of Health.

† Present address: Marmoset Research Center, Oak Ridge Associated Universities, Box 117, Oak Ridge, Tennessee 37830.

the response of mice to an initial injection of vibrios is a "true" primary response.[6, 7]

After secondary immunization there is a much more rapid rise in antibody-forming cells; both IgM and IgG PFC appear equally rapidly.[8] Many more IgG-secreting immunocytes appear in the spleen of primed mice as compared to IgM PFC during the height of the secondary response. In contrast, no IgG PFC appear after primary or secondary immunization of mice with *E. coli* or *Shigella* LPS. It has been assumed that the absence of an IgG response to *E. coli* and other enterobacteriaceae may be due to the absence of involvement of T-cells. Thus, since IgG PFC are readily induced to cholera antigens, it seemed of value to determine whether T-cells are involved in the immune response to this microbial antigen. Furthermore, other recent studies in this laboratory[9] with a purified exotoxin derived from cholera bacilli revealed that the kinetics of the antibody response to this extracellular antigen differs markedly from the response to the somatic antigen, i.e. there is a shorter lag period before the first appearance of antitoxin PFC and the peak of the response is much earlier (day 7 after immunization). Since the exotoxin is a protein antigen and the somatic antigen is a lipopolysaccharide, it also seemed likely that different cell populations might be involved in the primary and secondary responses to these different antigens derived from one microorganism.

Therefore, for the experiments presented here, the involvement of B- and T-lymphocytes in the immune response to the somatic and toxin antigens derived from cholera bacilli was studied at the level of individual immunocytes using an adoptive cell transfer system. Collaboration between these lymphocytes was found to be necessary for the immune response to the exotoxin antigen, whereas B-lymphocytes were found capable of responding to the somatic antigen almost as well without T-lymphocytes as in their presence.

Methods and Materials

For these experiments, young adult $C3BF_1$ male mice were used. They were housed in groups of 6–10 in plastic mouse cages and fed Purina mouse food and water *ad libitum.* Cholera antigens were obtained from Inaba 569B vibrios. An LPS extract was prepared as described by Webster *et al.*[10] Except where noted, 50 μg LPS in sterile saline were used for immunization. Cholera exotoxin (CT), also prepared from Inaba 569B vibrios, was generously supplied by Dr. R. A. Finkelstein, Southwestern Medical School, Dallas, Texas. Finkelstein has fully described the procedures necessary to purify this exotoxin from culture filtrates and has reported the biochemical nature and biophysical characteristics of this vibrio component.[11] For immunization, 0.5 μg of CT or 5.0 μg of heat-inactivated (1 hour at 100° C) toxin was used, except where noted.

The thymus dependency of the immune response to the cholera antigens was examined by injecting groups of x-irradiated (850 R) mice with isologous lymphoid cell suspensions 24 hours before inoculation with the respective antigens. Lethally irradiated mice were infused with bone marrow cells (2×10^7), thymus cells (4×10^7), thymus-marrow cell combinations, spleen cells (5×10^7), or spleen cells incubated with AKR anti-C3H thymocyte serum (anti-θ sera) and complement prior to injection. Preparation of cell suspensions and removal of θ-positive spleen cells were done according to well documented techniques.[12] Following cell transfer, mice were inoculated with cholera antigens, sheep erythrocytes (considered a T-dependent antigen) or *E. coli* LPS (considered a T-independent antigen). At varying times after antigen challenge, primary immune responses to bacterial and erythrocyte antigens were determined at the level of individual antibody plaque forming cells (PFC). Vibriolytic PFC [6, 7] were determined for mice immunized with cholera LPS whereas antitoxic PFC [8] were determined for mice inoculated with exotoxin or toxoid. The hemolytic PFC assay as initially described by Jerne *et al.*[13] was used to enumerate immunocytes releasing antibody to SRBC. Plaque-forming cells stimulated by *E. coli* LPS were assessed according to the method of Friedman *et al.*[14]

Results

Several methods can be used to determine the requirements for thymus or thymus-derived cells in producing a primary immune response after a single immunization with antigen. In the present study, the thymus dependency of the immune response to cholera LPS and CT was determined by injecting groups of irradiated mice with various isologous lymphoid cell populations shortly before challenge immunization. Each group of repopulated mice included animals injected with SRBC, a known thymus-dependent antigen, or *E. coli* LPS, a thymus-independent antigen.

As seen in Figure 1, *V. cholerae* LPS, like *E. coli* LPS, stimulated vibriolytic PFC responses in irradiated mice repopulated with 50×10^6 spleen cells or spleen cells treated with anti-θ serum and complement before injection. Initial

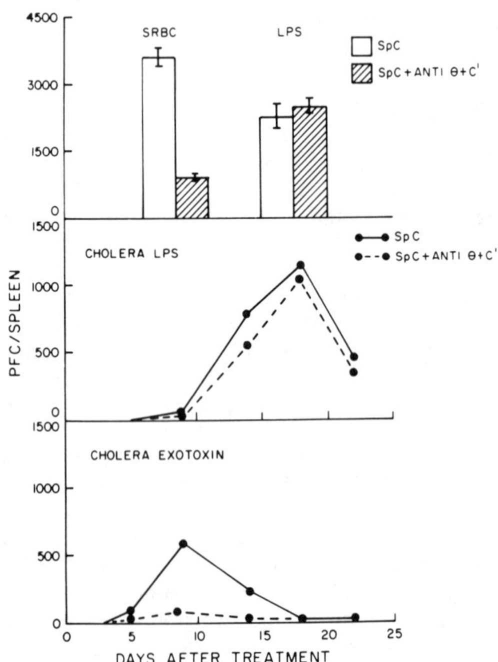

Figure 1. The antibody PFC response to SRBC, *E. coli* LPS, cholera LPS, or cholera exotoxin in spleens of x-irradiated mice repopulated either with untreated isologous spleen cells or spleen cells pretreated with anti-θ serum and complement. Each bar in the upper segment indicates the average PFC response to SRBC or LPS in spleens of 6–8 irradiated mice repopulated with either untreated or T-cell-depleted spleen cells and challenged with SRBC (4×10^8) or 25 μg *E. coli* LPS 9 days before assay. Each point in the lower two segments indicates the average PFC response per spleen, either anti-vibrio LPS or antitoxin PFC, for 10–12 mice on the day indicated after transfer of indicated cells and challenge with either LPS or exotoxin.

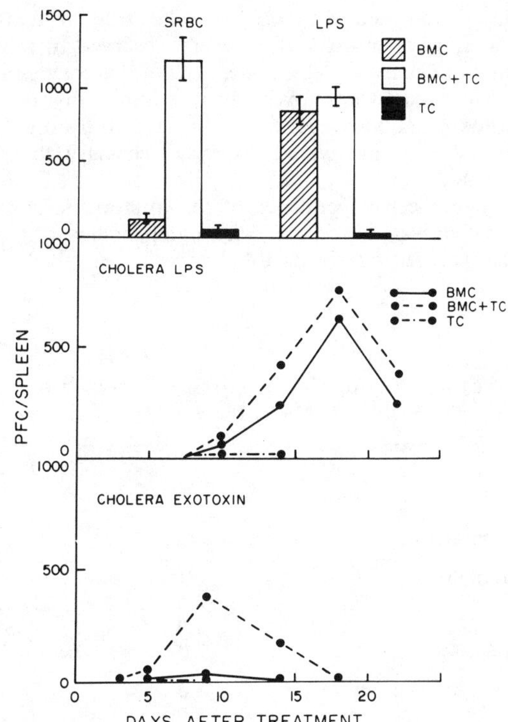

FIGURE 2. The PFC response to either SRBC, *E. coli* LPS, cholera LPS, or cholera exotoxin in spleens of x-irradiated mice repopulated with either bone marrow cells, thymus cells, or thymus-marrow cell mixtures after challenge with the indicated antigen. Each bar in the upper segment indicates the average PFC response, either to SRBC or LPS, in spleens of 6–8 mice 9 days after challenge immunization with indicated antigen. Each point in the lower two segments indicate the average PFC response, either to cholera LPS or exotoxin, in spleens of 10–12 repopulated mice.

vibriolysin-secreting immunocytes were observed on day 9 after antigen challenge, with peak responses occurring on day 18. In contrast, CT required thymus-derived, θ-positive splenocytes for production of antitoxin PFC. Approximately 8–10 times the number of antitoxin PFC were detected on day 9 in mice given untreated spleen cells as compared with mice injected with T-cell depleted splenocyte suspensions. Antitoxin PFC responses for mice repopulated with spleen cells treated with anti-θ serum alone, or complement alone, were similar to responses observed for mice injected with untreated spleen cells (data not shown).

It is noteworthy that maximum immune responses to LPS and CT were markedly different. Peak antitoxic PFC responses were detected on day 9, at least a week earlier than peak vibriolytic responses of repopulated mice injected with the cholera somatic antigen.

The T-cell dependence for the immune response to the cholera exotoxin and the T-cell independence for the response to the cholera LPS was also indicated from the results of experiments using irradiated mice repopulated with 2×10^7 marrow cells, 40×10^6 thymocytes, or marrow-thymus cell combinations. As seen in FIGURE 2, addition of thymus cells to bone marrow inocula did not significantly increase the response of mice to either vibrio or *E. coli* LPS. Similar antibacterial PFC were observed for mice repopulated with bone marrow cells only before previous immunization with these bacterial somatic antigens. In contrast, partial restoration of the antitoxin PFC response was observed in mice immunized with CT after infusion of marrow-thymus cell suspensions. Few, if any, antitoxin PFC were observed in the spleens of mice repopulated with bone marrow cells alone, or with thymocytes alone.

Heat-inactivated toxin also required thymus cells for stimulation of the antitoxin antibody. However, as seen in TABLE 1, approximately 10 times the dose of heat-inactivated CT was necessary to stimulate a response equal to unheated CT.

The T-cell dependence of the immune response to CT, either untreated or heat-inactivated, and the T-cell independence of the response to the cholera LPS was observed over a 20-fold range in antigen dose. Although more vibriolytic

TABLE 1

EFFECT OF DOSE OF CHOLERA IMMUNOGENS ON THE NUMBER OF ANTICHOLERA PFC IN IRRADIATED MICE REPOPULATED WITH ISOLOGOUS LYMPHOID CELLS

Immunogen *	Dose (μg)	PFC/spleen in x-Irradiated Mice After Repopulation † Bone Marrow	PFC/spleen in x-Irradiated Mice After Repopulation † Bone Marrow and Thymus
Exotoxin	0.1	0	48 ± 12
	0.5	15 ± 5	386 ± 58
	1.0	32 ± 14	652 ± 120
	2.0	all died	all died
Exotoxin (heated)	1.0	0	68 ± 15
	5.0	25 ± 13	420 ± 34
	10.0	64 ± 21	748 ± 152
	20.0	72 ± 30	1202 ± 246
LPS	10.0	60 ± 17	48 ± 20
	50.0	994 ± 215	1116 ± 330
	200.0	1450 ± 380	1622 ± 410

* Groups of 6–10 mice injected i.v. with indicated antigen.

† Average peak PFC response, either vibriolytic or antitoxin (± standard deviation), for x-irradiated mice given either marrow or marrow plus thymus cells and challenged wth indicated antigen.

or antitoxin PFC was observed when the dose of antigen increased, immune responsiveness to cholera LPS did not appear to be dependent on the presence of thymus cells whereas the exotoxin antigen required thymus cells for stimulation of a significant antitoxin antibody response.

Discussion

Few infectious diseases of man are more feared than cholera, which in past centuries has decimated whole populations. The current pandemic of cholera infection that is spreading westward from the Far East to the Mideast has stimulated renewed interest in prophylatic immunization against the vibrio bacilli that cause the disease. Significant advances in our knowledge concerning biochemical events during cholera infections has been achieved since the purification of cholera exotoxin, the vibrio component which causes the outpouring of fluid in the gut of experimental animals and presumably man.[11] Although cholera is best prevented by modern sanitation and clean water supplies, improved vaccines may be a more readily obtainable means of reducing the incidence of cholera in underdeveloped areas of the world. Accumulating evidence indicates that the immunologic mechanisms effective in the prevention or termination of a cholera infection may be either antibacterial, antitoxic, or associated with either specific or nonspecific (nonimmune) reduction of absorption of vibrios to the intestinal mucosal surface.[11, 15] Examples of each have been demonstrated either in clinical disease or experimental models of cholera, but data from such studies conflict and are thus difficult to interpret. It seems necessary, however, to restrict the immunologic events in cholera to the intestinal lumen or to the mucosal surface since it has been observed that vibrios do not penetrate the intestinal tract and that cholera exotoxin cannot be demonstrated in the vessels that collect intestinal lymph or blood.[11]

In terms of immunologic responsiveness, extensive investigations in recent years have shown that more than one cell type is required for the production of antibody. While immunoglobulins with specific antibody activity are synthesized by bone marrow-derived (B) cells, thymus-derived (T) cells are often necessary for production of antibody to most cellular and protein antigens.[3–5] Such antigens have been designated "thymus dependent" antigens. Recently, however, efficient antibody responses to some antigens have been stimulated *in vivo,* as well as *in vitro,* in the absence of thymocytes or thymus-derived cells. Such antigens have been designated "thymus independent" antigens and include polymerized flagellin, E. coli LPS, pneumococcal polysaccharide type S III, and polyvinylpyrollidine (PVP). However, before investigating the gut as an immunocompetent lymphoid organ with respect to cholera antigens and the mechanism of anticholera immunity, it seemed important to determine what lymphoid cells are necessary for an immune response to this microorganism.

For this purpose, initial experiments were performed to assess the role of T- and B-lymphocytes in the spleens of mice immunized with either the somatic antigen extracted from whole cholera bacilli or the purified exotoxin derived from supernatants of the microorganisms growing in culture medium.

It was anticipated that analysis of the role of T- and B-lymphocytes in the spleen of cholera-immunized mice would permit further studies of the role of these cell types in gut-associated lymphoid tissue, including the Peyer's patches and the mesenteric nodes. Thus, in the experiments described here, attempts were made to determine the cell types involved in the immune response to the two distinct antigens derived from *V. cholerae.* Earlier studies had shown that the kinetics of the immune response to the somatic antigen of the cholera organisms is quite unique in terms of the absolute absence of preexisting antibody forming cells in lymphoid tissues of unimmunized mice and the slow rate at which the first antibody forming cells appear after immunization.[6, 7] Furthermore, the peak of the immune response to the cholera somatic antigen occurs much later than the peak response to other antigens such as SRBC or *E. coli* LPS. These and other considerations suggested that mice respond to a single injection of cholera somatic antigen as a true primary immune response.

The present study concerning the role of B- and T-lymphocytes during the immune response to the somatic antigen of cholera organisms indicates that

B-cells alone are apparently capable of furnishing the cell type needed for antibody formation to the LPS moiety of the bacteria. As is the case with the response to *E. coli* LPS, antibody-forming cells were readily detected in spleens of irradiated mice repopulated with thymus-deprived spleen cells treated *in vitro* with anti-θ serum plus complement. Under these conditions the antibody responses to both *E. coli* and *V. cholerae* LPS were generally alike, i.e. similar numbers of PFC appeared in recipients of either untreated splenocytes or splenocytes depleted of T-cells when challenged with either LPS preparation. As is widely known, spleens of similar irradiated mice repopulated with T-cell-deficient splenocytes did not respond normally to sheep erythrocytes, considered a T-cell-dependent antigen. It seems noteworthy, however, that the number of vibriolytic PFC, but not anti-*E. coli* PFC, in the spleens of irradiated mice repopulated with untreated splenocytes was consistently higher by 10 to 15 percent than the number in mice given spleen cells treated with anti-θ antigens.

Similar to the results of experiments with T-cell-deprived anti-θ treated spleen cells, it was observed that the spleens of irradiated mice repopulated with bone marrow cells alone, as compared to those repopulated with marrow plus thymus cells, responded almost as well to cholera LPS as the spleens of mice repopulated with splenocytes. Thus it appeared that bone marrow cells alone can repopulate the spleens of irradiated mice with cells, presumably B-lymphocytes, capable of responding to the cholera LPS. However, as with the other experiments, there were usually 10 to 15 percent more PFC in the spleens of mice repopulated with both bone marrow and thymus cells as compared to those given bone marrow cells alone. This increased response was minimal compared to that which occurred when irradiated mice were given bone marrow and thymus cells and then challenged with sheep erythrocytes, as compared to the hemolytic PFC response in mice given bone marrow cells alone.

In contrast to the results with cholera LPS, a role for both B- and T-cells in the immune response to cholera exotoxin was readily demonstrable by similar repopulation studies. Analysis of the response to CT, as measured by the indirect hemolytic plaque assay with CT-coated sheep erythrocytes, showed that the peak response to this antigen occurred approximately one week earlier than the peak response to the somatic antigen. The same occurred in irradiated mice given normal spleen cells, i.e. peak antitoxin responses occur much earlier than peak anti-LPS responses. However, the magnitude of the antitoxin PFC response was generally much lower than the anti-LPS response. The repopulation studies indicated that both thymus and bone marrow cells were necessary for the response to this protein toxin. When spleen cells were treated with the anti-θ serum plus complement prior to injection into irradiated animals, there was essentially no response to the cholera exotoxin, as compared to the rapid PFC response to the CT in the same irradiated recipients given untreated spleen cells. Furthermore, when bone marrow and thymus cells from normal mice were transfused into irradiated animals a significant anti-CT plaque response occurred. However, mice given bone marrow cells or thymus cells alone showed essentially no response. These results clearly indicate that the immune response to the cholera toxin requires the active collaboration of both B- and T-lymphocytes, similar to the collaboration noted for sheep erythrocytes.

Since active cholera infection results in a localized disease in the intestine, with intestinal mucosal cells being mainly affected, it seems necessary to determine whether both B- and T-cells are involved in intestinal immune responses. If B-cells are present in large numbers in the intestinal tract, then it could be assumed that an anticholera somatic antigen immune response could be readily stimulated locally. However, it would be necessary to have T-cells present in the intestinal lumen to mount an effective antitoxin immune response, at least in terms of IgM PFC.

It should be noted, however, that many investigators feel that IgA antibody may be more important for local immunity, especially that involved in gut immune responses.[11, 15] Furthermore, IgG antibody to protein antigens, especially those requiring the collaboration of T-lymphocytes, probably requires both T- and B-lymphocytes. The role of the cell types in the immune response to cholera LPS and toxin antigen in either the spleen or the gut has not yet been examined. Repopulation studies similar to those described here are obviously needed to determine the role of these cell types in the anticholera response mediated by IgG or IgA antibody.

Both experimental and clinical studies indicate that anti-cholera immunity is quite weak, either after active infection or immunization. It seems plausible that this may be due not so much to the ineffectiveness of the immunogens derived from the cholera bacilli but to the absence of certain cell types necessary for an effective immune response in the intestinal tract. Further studies concerning the intestine as a lymphoid organ, both in terms of responsiveness to different cholera antigens and the source of effector cells which can collaborate in producing an immune response, awaits further investigation. Furthermore, the mechanism whereby T- and B-cells collaborate in terms of an effective anticholera toxin immune response and the apparent absence of the need for T-cells in the immune response to cholera LPS also awaits further study. Nevertheless, it seems likely that continued investigation at both the clinical and experimental level with antigens derived from cholera bacilli may be a useful model, since at least in the murine system there is an absence of preexisting antibody-forming cells that could interfere with the detection of the earlier events during immune responses to this organism at the cellular level.

Summary

The immune response at the level of individual immunocytes to the somatic lipopolysaccharide antigen derived from whole *Vibrio cholerae* and to the purified protein exotoxin from this organism were studied in terms of the role of T- and B-lymphocytes. By adoptive cell transfer studies with irradiated recipient mice, it was shown that normal spleen cells from normal syngeneic mice could readily transfer the capability of responding to both types of cholera antigens. However, when the spleen cells were depleted of T-cells with anti-θ serum and complement, antibody responsiveness to the LPS antigen, but not the exotoxin, could be achieved in recipients. Furthermore, by appropriate transfer of either bone marrow, thymus, or thymus-marrow cell mixtures to irradiated mice, it was shown that the response to the cholera somatic antigen was relatively independent of thymus cells, whereas the response to exotoxin required "helper" T-cells. The role of thymus and bone marrow cells in the intestinal tract in immune responses to the somatic and toxic antigens of cholera vibrios requires further investigation. Further studies should also provide additional information not only concerning the mechanism of the immune response to these antigens in terms of basic mechanisms of antibody formation, but also should provide valuable information in terms of anticholera immunity per se.

References

1. Miller, J. F. A. P. & G. F. Mitchell. 1969. Transplant. Rev. **1:** 3.
2. Clamen, H. N. & E. A. Chaperon. 1969. Transplant. Rev. **1:** 92.
3. Katz, D. H. & B. Benacerraf. 1972. Advan. Immunol. **15:** 1.
4. Gershon, R. K. 1973. *In* Contemporary Topics in Immunobiology. M. G. Hanna, Jr., Ed. : 1–40. Plenum Press. New York, N.Y.
5. Mitchell, G. F. 1973. *In* Contemporary Topics in Immunobiology. M. G. Hanna, Jr., Ed. : 97–116. Plenum Press. New York, N.Y.
6. Cerny, J., R. F. McAlack, M. A. Sajid, J. Fronton & H. Friedman. 1971. J. Immunol. **106:** 1371.
7. McAlack, R. F., J. Cerny & H. Friedman. 1971. J. Immunol. **107:** 1752.
8. Kateley, J. R., C. Patel & H. Friedman. 1974. J. Immunol. **113:** 1815.
9. Finkelstein, R. A. 1973. Chemical Rubber Company, Crit. Rev. Micro. **2:** 553.
10. Webster, M. E., J. F. Sagin, M. Landy & A. G. Johnson. 1955. J. Immunol. **74:** 455.
11. Finkelstein, R. A. 1973. CRC, Crit. Rev. Microbiol. **2:** 553.
12. Moller, G. & J. G. Michael. 1971. Cell Immunol. **2:** 309.
13. Jerne, N. K., A. A. Nordin & C. Henry. 1963. *In* Cell Bound Antibodies. B. Amos & H. Koprowski, Eds. : 109–116. Wistar Inst. Press. Philadelphia, Pa.
14. Friedman, H., J. Allen & J. Rosenzweig. 1969. Proc. Soc. Exp. Biol. Med. **131:** 353.
15. Fubara, E. S. & R. Freter. 1972. Infect. Immun. **6:** 965.

STIMULATION OF cAMP LEVELS AND MODULATION OF ANTIBODY FORMATION IN MICE IMMUNIZED WITH CHOLERA TOXIN *

John R. Kateley † and Herman Friedman

Department of Microbiology
Albert Einstein Medical Center
Philadelphia, Pennsylvania 19141

Stimulation of antibody formation involves a complex series of cellular and molecular events in which several cell classes of the immune response system take part. Many substances that influence the metabolic activity of lymphoid cells can markedly alter immune responsiveness. Both biological and chemical agents have been shown to either enhance or depress immune responsiveness, usually by affecting the metabolic activities of the various cell types involved in the immune response mechanism. Bacterial products, including endotoxins derived from the cell wall of Gram-negative microorganisms and exotoxins secreted by Gram-positive bacteria, are known modifiers of immune activity.[1–6] However, relatively little information is available concerning the target cells of these bacterial components or products and the cellular mechanisms involved.

Recently, an exotoxin was purified from *Vibrio cholerae,* which mediates the symptoms of cholera in laboratory animals and presumably in man.[7–9] Although this toxin exerts its pathologic actions on intestinal mucosal cells by stimulation of adenylate cyclase, this bacterial product also is known to stimulate the same enzyme activity in all tissues thus far studied.[7–9] Adenylate cyclase is the enzyme which catalyzes the degradation of adenosine triphosphate (ATP) to cyclic 3′,5′ adenosine monophosphate (cAMP) and inorganic pyrophosphate (PP). Since cAMP is a known regulator of cellular metabolism,[10] it seems plausible that the cholera exotoxin (CT) might directly affect lymphoid cells involved in antibody formation. Previous studies have indicated that CT may depress effector cells from the lymphoid tissues of sensitized animals.[11–13] In the present study CT was found to both depress and enhance the antibody plaque-forming-cell (PFC) response of mice to a thymus-dependent and thymus-independent antigen, depending upon the dose and time of CT injection relative to antigenic challenge. Furthermore, analysis of cAMP concentrations in the spleen of CT injected mice indicated that the level of this cyclic nucleotide in lymphoid tissue may be associated with the altered immune responsiveness to antigenic challenge, using both sheep erythrocytes (SRBC) or E. coli lipopolysaccharide (LPS) as the immunogenic stimulant.

* Supported in part by grants from The United States National Science Foundation and The National Institute of Allergy and Infectious Diseases, National Institutes of Health.

† Present address: Marmoset Research Center, Oak Ridge Associated Universities Box 117, Oak Ridge, Tennessee 37830.

Methods and Materials

Adult Balb/c mice were used for these studies. They were obtained from Cumberland View Farms Clinton, Tennessee and were housed in groups of 5–10 in plastic mouse cages. They were fed Purina mouse food and water *ad libitum.* To investigate the influence of CT on antibody formation, the exotoxin was given intravenously (i.v.) at various times before, simultaneously with, or after injection with SRBC (4×10^8) or *E. coli* LPS (25 μg). The cholera exotoxin was generously supplied by Dr. R. A. Finkelstein, Southwestern Medical School, Dallas, Texas. Primary and secondary immune responses to the erythrocyte and bacterial antigens were determined at the level of individual antibody PFC. For the response to SRBC, the hemolytic PFC assay in agar gel as described by Jerne and Nordin [14] was used. Plaque-forming cells to the bacterial endotoxin were determined according to the method first described by Schwarz and Braun [15] and used by Friedman *et al.*[16] In some experiments the immune response to CT was determined by a passive hemolytic immunoplaque technique with sheep erythrocytes sensitized with CT.[17] For all PFC assays spleens from test mice were dispersed into single-cell suspensions and adjusted to 10^7 nucleated cells per ml. Immune responses to the various antigens were calculated as PFC per 10^6 splenocytes or per spleen. All PFC detected after a single incubation in agar with complement were considered due to 19S IgM antibody. Indirect (IgG) PFC to SRBC were determined by the facilitation assay to detect low efficiency 7S antibody-secreting immunocytes essentially as described by Sterzl and Riha [18] and by Dresser and Wortis [19] using an enhancing antiserum in the agar plates.

The concentration of cAMP in the spleens of normal and CT-injected mice were determined by the competitive binding assay described by Gilman.[20] The reagents necessary for determination of cAMP were purchased from Nuclear Dynamic, Inc., El Monte, California. Cyclic AMP concentrations were determined individually for the spleens of at least 4–6 mice at each assay time. Concentrations of this cyclic nucleotide were calculated as picomoles (pmol) per mg spleen weight.

Cellular reconstitution experiments were performed to determine which cell population(s) involved in antibody formation was affected by the cholera toxin. For such experiments, $C3BF_1$ mice were x-irradiated (800/R) and repopulated with 2×10^7 isologous bone marrow cells, 4×10^7 thymus cells, or marrow-thymus cell combinations. Sheep erythrocytes or *E. coli* LPS was added to each lymphoid cell inoculum immediately before injection. Some irradiated mice were also given CT with antigen at the time of cell transfer. Hemolytic and anti-LPS PFC responses in the spleen were determined on the 9th day after treatment.

Results

Effect of Toxin on Primary Hemolytic PFC Response

Injection of CT simultaneously with SRBC markedly altered the hemolytic PFC response in the mouse spleen. As shown in Table 1, anti-SRBC PFC in the spleens of mice challenged with erythrocytes only increased above background levels within 2–3 days and reached a peak level of about 330 PFC/10^6

splenocytes on day 5. The hemolytic PFC response decreased during the second week after injection and by day 11, only 20 IgM PFC/10^6 splenocytes were present. For mice injected simultaneously with 1.0 μg CT and SRBC, a delay in the appearance of hemolytic PFC was observed on days 3 and 4 after injection; approximately half the number of IgM PFC were observed in spleens of CT-injected mice as compared to animals given SRBC only. On days 5–11 however, there were markedly enhanced PFC responses in spleens of these mice. Two to three times as many IgM PFC/10^6 splenocytes were present in CT-treated mice at this time.

The indirect (IgG) hemolytic PFC responses for mice given SRBC or SRBC and CT also differed markedly during the primary immune response. Immunocytes secreting 7S IgG anti-SRBC antibody were readily detected in spleens of control mice within the first week following injection with the red blood cells.

TABLE 1

CYTOKINETICS OF PRIMARY HEMOLYSIN PFC RESPONSE FOR BALB/c MICE GIVEN SRBC OR SRBC AND CT *†

Day After Immunization	PFC/10^6 Splenocytes Tested: 19S (IgM) SRBC	19S (IgM) SRBC+CT	7S (IgG) SRBC	7S (IgG) SRBC+CT
1	2 ± 1	1 ± 0.2	—	—
2	3 ± 1	1 ± 0.4	—	—
3	53 ± 15	25 ± 11	—	—
4	259 ± 22	135 ± 30	—	—
5	332 ± 67	821 ± 146	285 ± 50	1251 ± 266
6	235 ± 57	682 ± 102	890 ± 181	3515 ± 452
7	184 ± 43	427 ± 87	1200 ± 249	4880 ± 598
8	87 ± 21	310 ± 66	597 ± 88	5797 ± 765
9	40 ± 10	211 ± 35	321 ± 46	2527 ± 392
11	21 ± 6	71 ± 32	245 ± 39	1215 ± 212

* Mice injected i.v. with 4×10^8 SRBC alone or SRBC mixed with 1.0 μg CT.
† Average PFC response for 8–12 mice ± standard deviation per day tested.

Maximal IgG PFC responses were evident on day 7 for mice immunized with SRBC only, two days after the peak IgM PFC response. In contrast, peak IgG PFC responses in the spleens of the CT-injected mice occurred on day 8. At this time there were approximately 4–10 times as many IgG-secreting immunocytes in the spleens of mice given CT and SRBC simultaneously as compared with untreated mice given SRBC only. Furthermore, the number of IgG PFC, although declining during the following few days in CT-treated mice, was still markedly higher than the number present in the control mice.

Effect of Dosage and Time of CT Injection on Peak PFC Response

Although simultaneous injection of CT with SRBC stimulated an enhanced hemolytic response on day 5, the time of CT injection markedly influenced this peak immune response. Suppression or enhancement of the peak primary

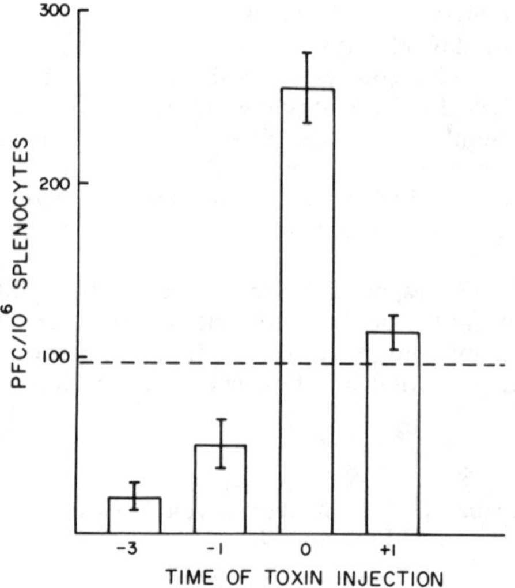

FIGURE 1. The effect of injection of cholera exotoxin (1.0 μg) at varying times before, simultaneously with, or after immunization of mice with sheep erythrocytes, (4×10^8 RBC i.v.). Each bar represents the average hemolytic PFC response per million splenocytes in spleens of 6 to 10 mice injected five days earlier with sheep erythrocytes and treated with cholera toxin on the day indicated relative to the days of immunization.

PFC response was observed depending upon the time interval between toxin injection and SRBC challenge. As shown in FIGURE 1, marked suppression of the peak immune response occurred when CT was injected 1–3 days prior to SRBC challenge, whereas enhanced PFC responses occurred when mice were injected with CT and SRBC together. Injection of CT 24 hours after SRBC did not significantly alter the peak hemolytic response. Results in FIGURE 1 also show that the dose of CT given influenced the extent of suppression or

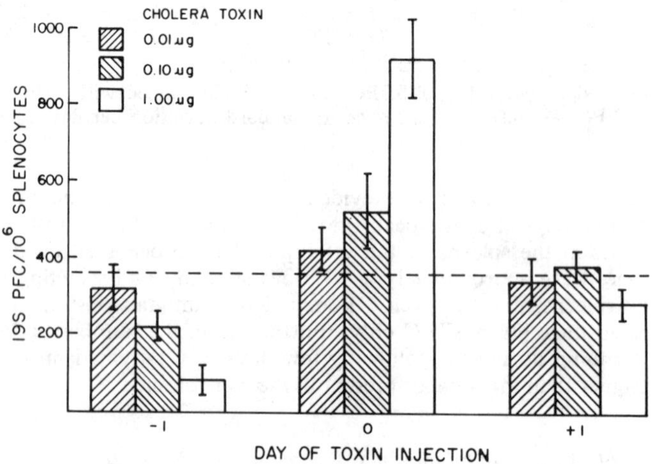

FIGURE 2. The effect of cholera toxin dose and the day of toxin injection relative to the day of immunization on the hemolytic PFC response in spleens. Each bar represents the average PFC response per million splenocytes for 6–8 mice per group 5 days after challenge immunization with 4×10^8 SRBC.

enhancement. One microgram quantities gave maximal effects. Increasing the dose to 2.0 μg killed approximately 40% of the mice before day 5, while 4–5 μg doses of CT were uniformly lethal. Heat inactivated CT, however, neither enhanced nor suppressed the SRBC response (data not shown).

As shown in FIGURE 2, similar patterns of immune reactivity were observed with spleens of mice given *E. coli* LPS and CT. Suppressed LPS responses occurred when CT was given before the challenge injection of endotoxin whereas enhanced immune activity occurred when CT was given simultaneously with the LPS.

TABLE 2

CYTOKINETICS OF THE SECONDARY HEMOLYSIN PFC RESPONSE FOR MICE PRIMED WITH SRBC AND BOOSTERED WITH SRBC OR SRBC AND CT * †

Day After Second Injection	PFC/10^6 Splenocytes 19S (IgM) SRBC	SRBC+CT	7S (IgG) SRBC	SRBC+CT
3	699 ± 174	166 ± 42	1125 ± 378	446 ± 96
4	410 ± 131	447 ± 102	4464 ± 890	1820 ± 414
5	270 ± 88	1065 ± 315	2935 ± 641	4680 ± 990
7	183 ± 69	828 ± 226	2116 ± 672	7700 ± 1470
9	102 ± 31	525 ± 110	876 ± 240	5086 ± 1520
11	88 ± 36	379 ± 91	591 ± 176	2870 ± 747

* Mice primed i.v. with 4×10^8 SRBC 30–35 days prior to a second injection with the same dose of SRBC or SRBC plus 1.0 μg CT.

† Average PFC response ± standard deviation for 10 mice per day tested.

Effect of Toxin on Secondary Hemolytic PFC Response

The effects of CT on the secondary immune response were generally similar to those observed after primary immunization. Mice given SRBC 4–5 weeks earlier showed a characteristic anamnestic PFC response when injected with SRBC for a second time (TABLE 2). There was, however, a marked delay in the direct (19S IgM) and the indirect (7S IgG) PFC responses in SRBC-primed mice given 1.0 μg CT on the same day as secondary immunization with SRBC. On day 3 after injection, CT-treated mice had many fewer IgM and IgG PFC (approximately 30–40% of control spleen values) than did untreated mice. On day 5, however, a sharp increase in the number of IgM and IgG PFC in the CT-treated mice occurred, with elevated numbers of PFC present from days 5 to 11, similar to the results obtained during the primary response for mice given CT and SRBC simultaneously.

Effect of Toxin on Primary Hemolytic PFC Response in CT-Primed Mice

For mice immunized with CT one week before simultaneous injection of 1.0 μg CT and SRBC, enhanced PFC responses were significantly inhibited.

Less than a 2-fold increase in the number of direct PFC was observed on day 5 in CT-primed mice compared with a 3-fold enhancement observed in unprimed mice injected simultaneously with 1.0 μg CT and SRBC (TABLE 3). Presumably, CT was partially neutralized *in vivo* since anti-CT antibody and anti-CT PFC were detected in the sera and spleen, respectively, in CT-primed mice.

TABLE 3

HEMOLYSIN PFC RESPONSE IN TOXIN-PRIMED MICE AND NORMAL MICE INJECTED WITH SRBC AND CT SIMULTANEOUSLY

Mouse Group	Treatment	19S PFC/10^6 Splenocytes *
Normal	SRBC	466 ± 61
	SRBC+CT (1.0 μg)	1422 ± 355
	SRBC+CT (0.1 μg)	781 ± 202
CT-primed †	SRBC	409 ± 43
	SRBC+CT (1.0 μg)	738 ± 167
	SRBC+CT (0.1 μg)	434 ± 69

* Average PFC response ± standard deviation for 10 mice per group 5 days after challenge immunization.

† Balb/c mice injected with 1.0 μg CT seven days prior to injection with 4×10^8 SRBC or SRBC and CT; an average of 60 antitoxic PFC/10^6 splenocytes and an antitoxic serum titer of 1:320 were present in CT-primed mice on the day of SRBC challenge.

Cyclic AMP Levels in Spleens of Mice Given CT

The results presented in TABLE 4 show that cholera toxin elevated the level of cAMP in spleens of mice shortly after injection. In addition, the concentration of intracellular cAMP was related to the dose of CT given. Maximal increases (60–70%) in the concentration of this cyclic nucleotide were observed within 6–8 hours after i.v. administration of a 1.0 μg dose of CT. After 18–24 hours, however, the concentration of cAMP returned to control levels. Similar results were observed during the initial 24 hours in spleens of mice injected simultaneously with SRBC and CT. In contrast, cAMP levels in spleens of mice injected with SRBC only were slightly less than control levels during the 24 hour assay period. Simultaneous injection of 1.0 μg CT and SRBC into CT-primed mice elevated cAMP levels only 10–15% within 6–8 hours following injection, whereas no increase in cAMP levels was observed in the spleens of mice primed with CT and then reinjected with 0.1 μg CT and SRBC.

Cell Populations Affected by Exotoxin

Cell transfer experiments were performed to determine which cell population(s) involved in antibody formation was affected by CT. As is evident in TABLE 5, lethally irradiated mice repopulated with bone marrow cells alone

TABLE 4

cAMP CONCENTRATIONS IN SPLEENS OF NORMAL AND CT-PRIMED MICE GIVEN SRBC, CT, OR SRBC AND CT *

Mouse Group	Treatment	0 hr.	cAMP Concentrations (pmol/mg spleen) 2–3 hrs.	6–8 hrs.	18–24 hrs.
Normal	None	.87			
	SRBC–4 × 10^8		.79	.63	.70
	CT 1.0 μg		.91	1.37	.79
	0.1 μg		.84	1.02	.83
	CT 1.0 μg + SRBC		.85	1.26	.74
	CT 0.1 μg + SRBC		.76	.96	.81
CT-primed †	None	.65			
	SRBC 4 × 10^8		.68	.52	.59
	CT 1.0 μg		.71	.80	.60
	CT 1.0 μg + SRBC		.62	.75	.66
	CT 0.1 μg + SRBC		.68	.64	.69

* Average cAMP concentrations for 5–7 mice; all injections i.v.
† Mice injected 7 days earlier with 1.0 μg CT.

TABLE 5

HEMOLYTIC AND ANTI-LPS PFC RESPONSES IN IRRADIATED MICE REPOPULATED WITH SYNGENEIC LYMPHOID CELLS AND IMMUNIZED WITH SRBC OR *E. coli* LPS, WITH OR WITHOUT CT

Treatment	SRBC	*E. coli*	CT *	PFC/Spleen †
800 R	+			20 ± 7
	+		+	12 ± 3
800 R + 2 × 10^7 BM	+			203 ± 46
	+		+	230 ± 56
800 R + 4 × 10^7 Thy	+			14 ± 6
	+		+	10 ± 4
800 R + 2 × 10^7 BM + 10^7 Thy	+			1540 ± 270
	+		+	5210 ± 640
800 R + 2 × 10^7 BM + 4 × 10^7 Thy	+			4220 ± 696
800 R		+		12 ± 4
		+	+	16 ± 8
800 R + 2 × 10^7 BM		+		1329 ± 420
		+	+	2326 ± 550
800 R + 2 × 10^7 BM + 10^7 Thy		+		1425 ± 670
		+	+	2672 ± 372

* Mice injected with 1.0 μg CT at time of cell transfer and challenge immunization.
† Average PFC ± standard deviation for 8–12 mice 9 days after cell transfer and challenge immunization with 4 × 10^8 SRBC or 25 μg LPS.

responded poorly to SRBC. Only 200 hemolytic PFC were detected on day 9 in spleens of mice given marrow cells only and SRBC on the day of irradiation. Partial restoration of the hemolytic PFC response (1540 PFC per spleen) occurred when mice were repopulated with marrow cells supplemented with 10^7 thymocytes, whereas a 20-fold increase in the anti-SRBC PFC response (4200 PFC per spleen) occurred when 4×10^7 thymocytes were added to the marrow inocula. Cholera toxin did not stimulate the number of hemolytic PFC in the spleens of mice repopulated with marrow cells only; however, when 10^7 thymocytes were added to the marrow inocula, enhanced responses were observed. In this experiment, approximately 5200 hemolytic PFC per spleen were observed from mice immunized with SRBC and CT, a 3 to 4-fold increase above the response observed for the mice repopulated similarly and immunized with SRBC alone.

For irradiated mice challenged with a thymus-independent antigen (LPS) at the time of marrow cell infusion, approximately twice the number of anti-LPS PFC were observed in the spleens of mice given CT together with LPS as compared to mice given LPS alone (TABLE 5).

DISCUSSION

Recent studies have focused attention on the protein exotoxin secreted by vibrio bacilli as the mediator of the devastating diarrhea associated with cholera infection.[7–9] Numerous earlier studies have been concerned with the immune response to the intact bacteria, per se. However, more recent studies have been concerned with antitoxin immune responses and the role of such immunity in protection from the disease.[9] In addition, several studies show that cholera exotoxin itself influences the immune responses to other antigens.[11–13, 21] Recent studies have indicated that cholera toxin affects the effector cells involved in inflammation and cellular immunity.[21] The results of the experiments described here indicate that CT can also affect the number of antibody-producing cells, either enhancing or suppressing the immune response to both a T-dependent and a T-independent antigen, depending upon the dose and the time of CT-injection relative to antigen challenge. Simultaneous injection of CT with antigen resulted in enhanced immunocyte responses whereas immune suppression occurred when CT was injected 1–3 days prior to antigen challenge.

As indicated before, several reports have shown that CT stimulates adenylate cyclase activity, the enzyme which catalyzes the conversion of ATP to cAMP and PP.[7–10] Cyclic AMP, in turn, regulates many biologic functions by activating kinases that influence the transcription of nucleic acid information and perhaps DNA replication itself.[10] Hence, it is not surprising that several investigators have shown that elevated levels of cAMP in lymphoid cells may be associated with altered immune responsiveness.[21] Furthermore, the antibody response to SRBC can be stimulated *in vivo* and *in vitro* when mice or mouse spleen cell cultures are treated simultaneously with erythrocytes and theophylline, a substance which stabilizes cAMP levels by inhibiting phosphodiesterase activity, or alternatively, with cAMP itself.[22, 23]

Additional studies have shown that polyadenylic-polyuridylic acid (poly A:U), a synthetic polynucleotide, also stimulates humoral immune responses.[24] Like CT, enhanced hemolytic PFC responses occur when poly A:U is given together with SRBC, whereas immunosuppression was reported when this synthetic agent was given 24 hours prior to erythrocyte challenge.[25] Although poly A:U and theophylline can elevate humoral immune responses, excessive stimulation or accumulation of cAMP is immunosuppressive.[23–25] Moreover, others have demonstrated that excessive levels of intracellular cAMP can inhibit lymphocyte transformation and mitosis.[26] Sultzer and Craig[27] have recently reported that DNA, RNA, and protein synthesis, events all necessary for antibody formation, are inhibited in mouse spleen cells exposed to cholera enterotoxin for 1–3 days in culture.[27]

Enhanced PFC responses that occur with simultaneous injection of CT and antigen most likely depend upon the elevated levels of cAMP stimulated by CT, whereas the immune suppression that occurs when CT is injected prior to the antigen perhaps reflects an alteration in cellular metabolism following stimulation of excessive levels of intracellular cAMP. It is noteworthy that enhanced PFC responses were not as pronounced for CT-primed mice injected a second time with CT and SRBC. Moreover, cAMP levels for mice primed with CT and reinjected with CT and SRBC were significantly less than cAMP concentrations for unprimed mice treated similarly. Presumably, CT was neutralized *in vivo* by antitoxin in the serum before it could react with the immunocompetent cells in the spleen.

Since the most pronounced changes in immune responsiveness occurred when CT was injected 24 hours before or at the same time as antigen challenge, the cells that participate in the early events required for antibody formation are seemingly most affected by changes in endogenous cAMP. However, since the pattern of immune responsiveness was similar for CT-injected mice challenged with a T-dependent antigen (SRBC), as well as a T-independent antigen (LPS), it is reasonable to suspect that changes in cAMP concentrations for macrophages and/or B-lymphocytes are responsible for the modulation of immune activity. However, the cell transfer experiments suggested that T-cells also are influenced by enterotoxin. In addition, the enhanced number of IgG-secreting immunocytes in the spleen of mice given CT and SRBC simultaneously suggests that T-cell activity is influenced by CT since recent studies have indicated that thymus cells are necessary for the switch-over from 19S to 7S antibody secretion.[28] That all cell types involved in antibody formation are influenced by CT is reasonable since synthetic polynucleotides and other modifiers of cAMP modify functions of macrophages, B-lymphocytes, and T-lymphocytes.[29]

Available evidence indicates that CT, like other cAMP stimulators, also influences the effector component of the cell-mediated immune response. Henney and colleagues have recently reported that elevated cAMP concentrations decreased the capacity of spleen cells to elicit cell-mediated cytotoxic immune reactions *in vivo* and *in vitro*.[11, 12] These investigators reported that splenic cAMP concentrations for C57B1/6 mice injected intraperitoneally increased by 70–80% following injection of 1.0 μg CT; however, maximal concentrations of cAMP were observed 24–48 hours after injection of CT. Similar increases in cAMP concentrations were observed in the present study, though peak concentrations were observed 6–8 hours after injection of CT. Presumably, the different routes of administration account for the temporal difference in the concentration of this cyclic nucleotide assayed in these two studies.

It is interesting to note that a considerable delay in the appearance of splenic PFC occurred in SRBC-primed mice rechallenged after several weeks with SRBC mixed with cholera toxin. Others have previously reported[29] that the immune response of activated immunocompetent cells, principally T-lymphocytes, to a second challenge with specific antigen in the presence of cAMP or stimulators of endogenous cAMP results in an inhibition of the release of mediators or effector substances. Thus, while modifiers of endogenous cAMP levels either enhance or inhibit the activation of previously unstimulated immunocompetent cells, they may only retard or inhibit functions in already fully activated cells.

This observation would seem to be particularly relevant to the disease-inducing properties of cholera exotoxin. While an individual may indeed be immunized with cholera vaccine, be it either a cellular or a toxoid preparation, this immune state may be of little value if reinfection occurs since secretion of exotoxin into the gut may delay or prevent anticholera immunity for a period sufficient to permit the outpouring of fluid characteristic of cholera. Hence, the model system described in this report should be of value for a further analysis of the cellular and biochemical aspects of the immune response in general and mechanisms of effective cholera immunity in actively infected individuals.

Summary

Injection of mice with 1.0 μg of a purified exotoxin derived from *Vibrio cholerae* together with a challenge injection of sheep erythrocytes (SRBC) or *E. coli* LPS markedly influenced the immune response to these antigens. Simultaneous injection of the toxin with antigen resulted in a delayed appearance of antibody-forming cells during the first few days after immunization, followed by a marked enhancement of the peak numbers of antibody-forming cells. In the case of the immune response to SRBC, both 19S and 7S plaque-forming cells (PFC) were enhanced on the peak day of response after simultaneous immunization of toxin-injected mice. The secondary immune response to SRBC was also similarly affected when cholera toxin was given along with a second injection of erythrocytes; i.e. a delay in appearance of the first antibody-forming cells followed by a marked enhancement of the peak 19S and 7S PFC response. Injection of cholera toxin 1–3 days prior to SRBC or LPS was immunosuppressive. The effect of cholera toxin on the level of splenic cyclic AMP appeared related to the effects on antibody formation.

References

1. Johnson, A. G., S. Gains & M. Landy. 1956. J. Exp. Med. **103:** 225.
2. Bradley, S. G. & D. W. Watson. 1964. Proc. Soc. Exp. Biol. Med. **117:** 570.
3. Franzl, R. E. & P. D. McMaster. 1968. J. Exp. Med. **127:** 1087.
4. Malakian, A. H. & J. H. Schwab. 1971. J. Exp. Med. **134:** 1253.
5. Miller, G. A. & R. W. Jackson. 1973. J. Immunol. **110:** 148.
6. Graig, J. P. 1970. *In* Microbial Toxins. S. Ajl, T. Montie & S. Kadis, Eds. **2a:** 189–212. Academic Press. New York, N.Y.
7. Pierce, N. F., W. B. Greenough & C. C. J. Carpenter. 1971. Bacteriol. Rev. **35:** 1.
8. Carpenter, C. C. J. 1972. J. Infec. Dis. **126:** 551.
9. Finkelstein, R. A. 1973. Chemical Rubber Company, Crit. Rev. Micro. **2:** 553.

10. Robison, G. A., R. W. Butcher & E. W. Sutherland. 1971. Cyclic AMP. Academic Press. New York, N.Y.
11. Lichtenstein, L. M., C. S. Henney, H. R. Bourne & W. B. Greenough. 1973. J. Clin. Invest. **52:** 691.
12. Henney, C. S., L. M. Lichtenstein, E. Gillespie & R. T. Rolley. 1973. J. Clin. Invest. **52:** 2853.
13. Melmon, K. L., H. R. Bourne, Y. Weinstein, G. M. Shearer, S. Bauminger & J. Kram. 1973. J. Clin. Invest. **53:** 13.
14. Jerne, N. K. & A. A. Nordin. 1963. Science **140:** 405.
15. Schwarz, S. A. & W. Braun. 1965. Science **149:** 200.
16. Friedman, H., J. Allen & J. Rosenzweig. 1969. Proc. Soc. Exp. Biol. Med. **131:** 353.
17. Kateley, J. R., S. Lyons & H. Friedman. 1974. J. Immunol. **112:** 1452.
18. Sterzl, J. & I. Riha. 1965. Nature **208:** 858.
19. Dresser, D. W. & H. H. Wortis. 1965. Nature **208:** 859.
20. Gilman, A. G. 1970. Proc. Nat. Acad. Sci. U.S. **67:** 305.
21. Bourne, H. R., L. M. Lichtenstein, K. L. Melmon, C. S. Henney, Y. Weinstein & G. M. Shearer. 1974. Science **184:** 19.
22. Winchurch, R., M. Ishizuka, D. Webb & W. Braun. 1971. J. Immunol. **106:** 1399.
23. Ishizuka, M., W. Braun & T. Matsumoto. 1971. J. Immunol. **107:** 1027.
24. Braun, W. & M. Ishizuka. 1971. Proc. Nat. Acad. Sci. U.S. **68:** 1114.
25. Johnson, A. G., R. E. Cone, H. M. Friedman, I. H. Han, I. G. Johnson, J. R. Schmidtke & R. D. Stout. 1971. *In* Biological Effects of Polynucleotides. R. F. Beers & W. Braun, Eds. Springer-Verlag. New York, N.Y.
26. Smith, J. N., A. L. Steiner & C. L. Parker. 1971. J. Clin. Invest. **50:** 442.
27. Sultzer, B. & J. P. Craig. 1973. Nature New Biol. **244:** 178.
28. Gershon, R. F. 1973. *In* Contemporary Topics in Immunobiology. M. G. Hanna, Jr., Ed. : 1–40. Plenum Press. New York, N.Y.
29. Braun, W. 1973. *In* Virus Tumorigenesis and Immunogenesis. W. S. Ceglowski & H. Friedman, Eds. : 31–50. Academic Press. New York, N.Y.

ROLE OF T-CELL IMMUNOGLOBULIN IN CELL COOPERATION, T-CELL SUPPRESSION, AND ANTIGENIC COMPETITION

Marc Feldmann, Sirkka Kontiainen,* M. F. Greaves, Nancy Hogg, and Arthur Boylston

ICRF Tumor Immunology Unit, Department of Zoology University College, London, and St. Mary's Hospital Paddington London, England

Introduction

Cell cooperation between T- and B-cells is now well recognized as a process of major importance in the induction of antibody responses (reviewed in ref. 1), *in vivo* as well as more recently *in vitro*.[2] The studies of Claman and his colleagues (reviewed in ref. 3), and Miller and collaborators (reviewed in ref. 4) emphasized the helper role of T-cells in the production of antibody by B-cells in the response to sheep red blood cells (SRBC) in irradiated mice. However, detailed concepts of how T-cells influence antibody production were not postulated until Mitchison, Rajewsky and Taylor[5] sought to explain the reasons for the obligatory molecular linkage of "carrier" and "haptenic" determinants. They proposed that the hapten-protein antigen links receptors on carrier-reactive (T) cells and hapten reactive (B) cells. As shown in Figure 1, two different mechanisms of receptor linkage are possible, either directly, by direct T-B contact with an antigen bridge, or indirectly, with T-cell receptors shed, and receptor-antigen linkage occurring on the membrane of another cell. To differentiate between these two, and other possible models of T-B cooperation, a study of cell cooperation in responses to hapten protein conjugates *in vitro* was begun in collaboration with Tony Basten. Some insight into the molecular mechanism of cooperation and its regulation has been obtained. Since most of these results have been published[e.g. 6–8] this communication will only pick out certain features and highlight more recent, and less understood, findings and concepts.

A Three Cell Model of T-B Interaction

Initial studies were undertaken to clarify which of the mechanisms represented in Figure 1 was correct. These experiments were performed in Marbrook type tissue culture flasks containing two chambers.[6] No difference in cooperation was found if T-cells activated to a protein, KLH, were placed in the same compartment as hapten (DNP) primed B-cell populations, or were separated from them by a cell impermeable nucleopore membrane of 0.2 μ to 1 μ pore size (Figure 2), even if limiting numbers of T-cells were used. With these

* Present address: Department of Bacteriology and Serology, University of Helsinki, Helsinki 29, Finland.

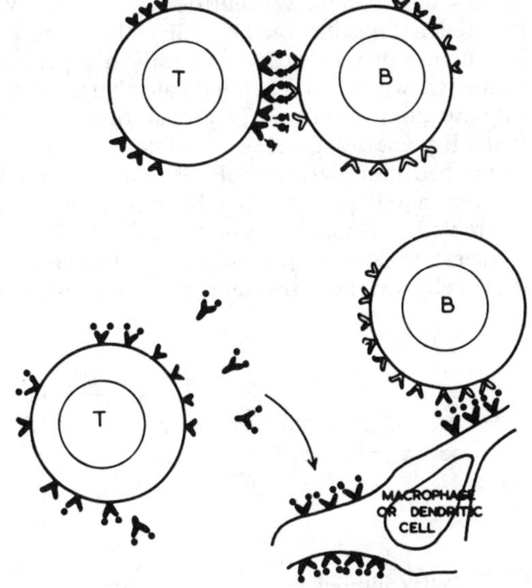

FIGURE 1. Two postulated mechanisms of T-B cooperation involving linked recognition of T- and B-cell receptors. The lower section of the figure shows interaction via IgT antigen bound to macrophages. (From M. Feldmann. 1973. Transplant. Proc. **5:** 43–48. By permission of the publisher.)

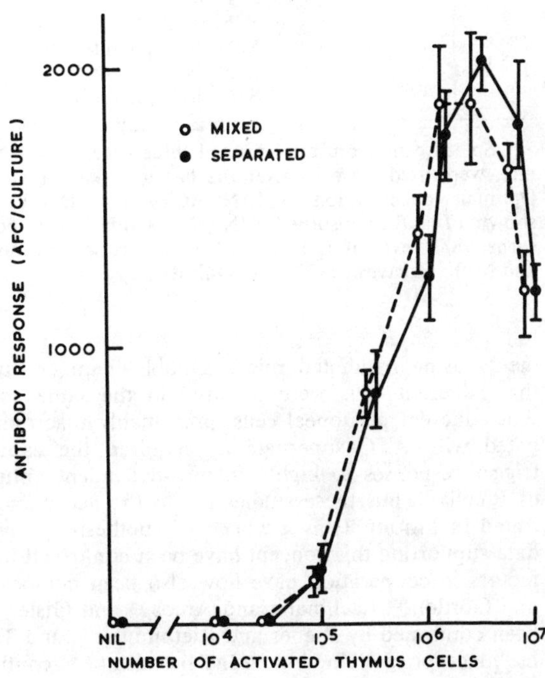

FIGURE 2. Cooperation between T- and B-cells across a 1μ nucleopore filter ATC_{KLH} in upper compartment, DNP-Flagella-primed spleen cells in lower compartment and 1 μg/ml DNP KLH as antigen. Anti-DNP response at day 4. Arithmetic means and standard errors of 3 cultures shown. (From M. Feldmann & A. Basten. 1973. J. Exp. Med. **136:** 49–66. By permission of the publisher.)

studies and specificity controls as a basis, we argued that activated T-cells released a "specific factor" (SF) that was required for specific cooperation. The nature of this "specific factor" in supernatants of ATC was analyzed. The results shown in TABLE 1 indicate that specific cooperative activity is removed by absorption with anti-Ig preparations conjugated to Sepharose® beads, and that SF possesses Ig, K, and μ-like antigenic determinants. Since other experiments had indicated that SF also contained antigen, it was thus concluded that SF was a complex of T-cell-released Ig, "IgT" and antigen,[28] and that IgT resembled in some ways 8 S IgM.[8, 9] The *in vitro* analysis of specific T-B cooperation also emphasized the importance of adherent cells,[8] which, since these cells are radio resistant, could not have been realized from *in vivo* experi-

TABLE 1

IMMUNOGLOBULIN NATURE OF COOPERATIVE FACTOR *

Cells Cultured	Stimulus	Response (AFC/Culture ±SE) Anti-DNP IgM	IgG
TNP- KLH-primed spleen	nil	110±86	0
TNP KLH-primed spleen	TNP KLH	3820±271	2670±361
Anti-T-treated TNP-KLH-primed spleen	nil	50±32	0
↓	TNP KLH	175±54	0
	S/N of $ATC_{F\gamma G}$+DNP FγG	1625±285	1920±392
	S/N abs Seph-anti-MIg	210±122	0
	S/N abs Seph-anti-K	160±86	115±85
	S/N abs Seph-anti-μ	365±205	85±37

* Spleen cells from mice primed three times with TNP KLH adsorbed onto bentonite, were used 6 weeks after the last injection. TNP KLH was used at 10^{-2} μg/ml Optimal concentration of S/N $ACT_{F\gamma G}$ + DNFG FγG used. Similar dilution shown of anti-Ig-absorbed S/N. No significant responses were obtained with absorbed S/N even if used at 100 greater concentrations. (Data from M. Feldmann and M. F. Greaves. 1973. Unpublished)

ments using irradiated mice. Double-chamber culture experiments indicated that adherent cells were required in the same compartment as B-cells[8] and that adherent peritoneal cells, presumably macrophages, which had been incubated with ATC supernatants, acquired the capacity to "cooperate" i.e. to trigger responses to highly thymus-dependent antigens in purified populations of B-cells. Thus these studies led to the acceptance of the 3-cell model, illustrated in FIGURE 1, as a working hypothesis of *specific* T-B cooperation. The data supporting this concept have been confirmed in other laboratories. Specific factors in cooperation have now also been demonstrated, by, for example, Yu and Gordon,[12] Lachmann and Amos,[13] and Gisler *et al.*[10] Their Ig nature has been confirmed by Rieber and Riethmuller[11] and Tada *et al.*[14] The importance of "macrophages" in binding IgT has also been confirmed.[10, 11]

However, details of this 3-cell model still await clarification. For example, the nature of the third cell has not been studied. It is known to be adherent, and present in spleen and peritoneum,[2, 8] but the precise nature of this cell and its origin are not yet known. It could be a dendritic reticular cell [15] rather than a typical macrophage. Identification of the nature of this cell is of importance, as it may indicate the anatomical site where T-B cooperation takes place *in vivo*. Speculations on this point range from the follicles of germinal centers,[16] to the red pulp of the spleen.[11]

The exact role of the third cell is also not clear. The diagramatic representation in FIGURE 1 suggests that surface-bound IgT-antigen complexes may form matrices of antigenic determinants that closely resemble the antigenic surface of thymus-independent antigens and permit the simplifying hypothesis that there is a final common pathway for the triggering of B-cells, via a matrix of determinants. However, it is not yet proven that such matrices are formed. Autoradiographic studies of the binding of [^{125}I]IgT [18] do indicate a patchy localization, as do some functional studies.[19] The elegance of this unifying concept of B-cell triggering has been diminished by recent studies indicating that there is heterogeneity in the B-cell antibody-forming cell precursors responding to thymus-independent or thymus-dependent antigens.[20, 21] Whether macrophage-like cells have merely a passive role in antigen presentation, or a more active role in cooperation, e.g. in producing mediators that facilitate or augment triggering,[22, 23] is not yet clear for IgM responses. For IgG responses an active role seems highly likely.[24]

Other influences on cell cooperation, such as the role of nonspecific "T-cell" factors, have been ignored as they will be amply dealt with by other papers in this volume. It should suffice to emphasize that the studies described above do not investigate these factors and thus do not rule out the participation of the factors, produced by either T-cells or macrophages in T-B cell cooperation.[25–27, et al.]

Currently it seems reasonable to suggest that specific and nonspecific T-cell factors act in unison in the triggering of B-cell responses (discussed more fully in ref. 2).

Regulation of the Cooperative Antibody Response

Specific T-cell Suppression

The cooperative capacity of T-cell supernatants is not expressed in the absence of macrophages.[2, 8] Thus it was of interest to know whether the lack of response was due to lack of stimulation or to tolerance. Preincubation experiments were thus performed, which indicated that a state of partial tolerance, of either T- or B-cells was induced.[28] In TABLE 2, an experiment is shown that was performed with supraimmunogenic doses of T-cell supernatants. Analogous results are reported elsewhere, using immunogenic doses of supernatants, but either in the absence of macrophages, or in the presence of antimacrophage serum.[29]

The nature of the suppressive factor in ATC supernatants was investigated by the use of anti-Ig sera, or anti-K or anti-μ antibodies coupled to Sepharose beads. Incubation of ATC supernatants with these beads abrogated their suppressing potential, as indicated in TABLE 3. Other resemblances between T-cell suppressive and cooperative factors were noted: both were specific, required hapten and carrier to be linked (on the same molecule) for effective suppression of hapten reactive cells, and were absorbed out by macrophages.[29]

The mechanism of specific T-cell suppression is not yet understood in detail. Basically, since IgT is divalent, suppression by IgT-antigen complexes should resemble complexes of humoral antibody and antigen, which if formed in the right proportions induce "antibody mediated tolerance" induced *in vitro* (reviewed in ref. 30) or "blocking antibodies" *in vivo* (e.g. ref. 31). However, the mechanism, after binding of these complexes to the cell surface, is unclear. For example it is not known if these cells rapidly recover responsiveness, or are irreversibly deleted. It is also not clear whether the specific factors responsible for both these cooperative: suppressive actions are identical, i.e. whether

TABLE 2

INDUCTION OF TOLERANCE BY T-CELL SUPERNATANTS *

Supernatant	Challenge	Anti-DNP Response IgM	IgG
nil	nil	110	0
nil	TNP KLH	2255	1560
nil	DNP POL	1640	815
ATC_{KLH}+KLH	nil	210	0
↓	TNP KLH	640	0
	DNP POL	1820	610
	TNP KLH+PE	510	0
ATC_{KLH}+DNP KLH	nil	355	0
↓	TNP KLH	565	0
	DNP POL	350	0
	TNP KLH+PE	305	0

* Spleen cells from mice primed with TNP KLH, last injection 8 weeks previously. Response at day 5. Antigen—1 μg/ml TNP KLH, 10 μg/ml DNP POL. PE—2×10^6 anti-θ-treated peritoneal exudate cells. Supernatants used—500 μl, derived from about 5×10^6 ATC, containing 10^{-1} μg/ml of antigen.

the same IgT molecule expresses both functions, and suppression is caused by "excess help."

Several examples of T-cell-mediated tolerance and suppression have been reported *in vivo*.[32–35] Whether these are also due to "excess help" is not clear, although preliminary results are suggestive.[33–35] Against this possibility are the results of Tada *et al.*[4] who have biochemically separated rat specific helper and suppressive factors for the IgE response from T-cells. The helper factor was Ig, but the suppressor factor had a lower MW and was not absorbed onto anti-Ig Sepharose, in contrast to our results in the mouse (TABLE 3).

Antigenic Competition

The literature so abounds in diverse experimental models and contrasting theories of the mechanism of antigenic competition (see reviews in refs. 36–38)

TABLE 3

IMMUNOGLOBULIN NATURE OF T-CELL SUPPRESSION *

Cells Cultured	Supernatant	Challenge	Anti-DNP Response (AFC/Culture ± SE) IgM	IgG
TNP KLH spleen depleted	—	TNP KLH	255±20	0
of adherent cells	—	nil	50±40	0
↓	—	DNP POL	950±155	610±410
↓	S/N of $ATC_{F\gamma G}$+DNP FγG	↓	110±80	0
↓	S/N abs Seph-anti-MIg	↓	1150±155	580±210
↓	S/N abs Seph-anti-K	↓	1210±210	1650±360
↓	S/N abs Seph-anti-μ	↓	995±110	910±115
↓	S/N abs Seph-anti-NRG	↓	155±100	0

* Adherent cells were removed by technique of Shortman *et al.* Challenging doses of antigen were 10 μg/ml. Response was measured at day 5. Optimal concentrations of S/N were used. Equivalent dilutions of absorbed S/N are shown here. Analogous results were obtained with higher or lower concentrations.

that generalities are difficult to formulate. However, as postulated by Taussig and Lachmann [e.g. 36] and ourselves [8, 39] on the basis of the mechanism of co-operation shown in FIGURE 1, it is evident that one possible locus of "antigenic competition" is at the surface of macrophages. This postulate has been tested using a model of antigenic competition, induced *in vivo,* but expressed *in vivo* in the same manner as *in vitro.*[39] The injection of red cells abrogated cooperative responses but not T-independent antibody production *in vitro.* Responsiveness *in vitro* could be restored by either adding purified macrophages, or by trypsinizing the spleen cell supension [39] indicating that the inhibition was indeed due to a macrophage surface block. Such a macrophage surface block may be mimicked, *in vitro,* by the sequential addition of two ATC supernatants to a single population of macrophages.[19] Responsiveness was induced to the first of ATC added, but not to the second, as shown in TABLE 4. The inducer of this

TABLE 4

IG NATURE OF HELPER AND COMPETITIVE MATERIAL FROM ATC *

Macrophages Incubated with Supernatants from:	Antibody Response (AFC/Culture) DNP	$F\gamma G$
(1) $ATC_{F\gamma G}$ & $F\gamma G$	0	445
(2) ATC_{KLH} & DNP KLH	720	0
(3) (1) and subsequently (2)	80	400
(4) (1) and (2) simultaneously	65	55
(5) (1) incubated anti-Ig beads	0	0
(6) (5) and then (2)	375	0

* 10^5 macrophages incubated 2 hours with supernatants from ATC and then with 1.5×10^7 DNP-POL-primed cells. 10^5 anti-θ-treated peritoneal exudate cells incubated 2 hours at 4° C with supernatants, washed, and then cultured with 1.5×10^7 DNP-POL-primed cells. Response at day 4.

block was also an IgT-antigen complex (TABLE 4). The same question thus presents itself, as did before with T-cell suppression, of whether the mediator of antigenic competition is the same IgT molecule that participates in specific T-B collaboration. Elution experiments, which may resolve this issue, have not yet been successful.

The precise molecular details of this mechanism of antigenic competition are not known. It seemed unlikely, *a priori,* that a T-cell supernatant *in vitro,* or a response even to a strong antigen would effectively saturate *all* the receptors for IgT. Since it was shown that a second IgT did bind to macrophages, immunogenicity must, therefore, be reduced by an alteration, by the first IgT, of the exact manner of binding of the second IgT. Such as interference is readily envisaged if it is assumed that matrices of antigen need be formed on the macrophage surface (see above), as the formation of matrices would be inhibited by multiple IgT specificities. Support for this concept is shown in the fourth line of TABLE 4, which indicates that the simultaneous addition of *two* supernatants to a single population of macrophages results in diminished responsiveness to both (TABLE 4). This observation is difficult to explain in any other way i.e. on the basis of suppressive factors released by macrophages, another suggested mechanism of antigenic competition.[39]

TABLE 5

EFFECT OF EL 4 IG *

Antigen	Ig (μg/ml)		Anti-DNP Response (AFC/Culture) IgM	IgG
TNP KLH	—		250	0
nil	—		2485	0
TNP KLH	EL4	1	310	0
↓	↓	10^{-1}	555	50
		10^{-2}	715	350
		10^{-3}	1150	1640
	MOPC 104E	10	2560	0
		1	2920	0

* Spleen cells from TNP-KLH-primed mice; response at day 4. Antigen used was 10^{-2} μg/ml TNP KLH. Ig added at initiation of culture. Data from M. Feldmann and A. Boylston. 1974. Unpublished.

Effect of "IgT" Derived from Lymphoid Tumors

Certain mouse lymphoid cell lines that possess the θ alloantigen, a marker for T-cells, also make detectable quantities of Ig. The effect of Ig purified from two such tumours, EL4 [40] and WEHI 22 [41] on the *in vitro* antibody response has been studied.[24] Two effects were noted. The first, entirely predictable on the basis of the antigenic competition results, was that thymus-dependent, but not thymus-independent IgM responses are blocked by EL4 or WEHI 22 Ig (TABLES 5 and 6).

TABLE 6

EFFECT OF W22 IG *

Antigen	Ig (μg/ml)		Anti-DNP Response (AFC/Culture) IgM	IgG
TNP KLH	—		2300	0
nil	—		115	0
TNP KLH	W22	1	455	0
↓	W22	10^{-1}	560	25
	W22	10^{-2}	855	625
	EL4	10^{-1}	810	560
	EL4	10^{-2}	1100	810
DNP POL	EL4	—	1620	0
DNP POL	W22	10^{-1}	1580	1100
DNP POL	EL4	10^{-1}	1920	865

* Spleen cells from TNP-KLH-primed mice; response at day 4. Antigen used 10^{-2} μg/ml TNP KLH. Ig added at initiation of culture. Data from M. Feldmann, A. Boylston, and N. Hogg. Unpublished.

Not so predictable was the fact that IgG responses were augmented by relatively low doses of EL4 or WEHI 22 Ig. Currently, the working hypothesis for the block of the IgM response is blockage of macrophage receptors for IgT occurs, analogous to the results shown in TABLE 4. The working hypothesis for the IgG enhancement is currently speculative, but invokes the production of a nonspecific mediator by macrophages, in response to the binding of large quantities of IgT to the cell surface. Tests of this hypothesis are currently in progress.

Cellular Source of IgT

Most of the work discussed above deals with IgT as an effector of T-cell function. In this role it is not crucial whether this effector is actually synthesized by the cells that release it. Precedents exist for this sort of phenomenon, e.g. with the neurotransmitter, noradrenaline. However, IgT is thought by some workers to have another function, as a receptor for antigen. In this instance, because of the clonal nature of T-cell function, the origin of IgT is a matter of theoretical importance. Several workers have shown, in the rat and the mouse [e.g. 42, 43] that certain T-cells may cytophilically adsorb Ig of B-cell origin, leading to suggestions that perhaps all IgT is synthesized by B-cells. These suggestions are rather premature, however, since it was not shown that the cytophilic Ig had any functional role. Indeed, the reports of cytophilic, readily detectable Ig (see above) do not readily fit in with other reports that T-cells have no readily detectable surface Ig.[44] Various studies have attempted to probe the origin of IgT. Roelants *et al.*[55] have found that antigen binding to T-cells (θ-positive cells) can be "capped" by anti-Ig, with subsequent loss of receptors and antigen binding capacity. The number of antigen binding T-cells recovered to previous levels with culture at 37° C. These studies were interpreted as supporting the synthesis by T-cells of their Ig receptors. Rieber *et al.*[45] measured surface Ig on thymus cells by a ^{125}I-labeled Fab of rabbit anti-Ig antibody. They showed that trypsinization diminished the amount of anti-Ig bound, but that these cells, cultured at 37° C recovered their surface Ig. We have used *in vitro* activated T-cells derived from purified populations of unprimed T-cells to investigate the same question. Some of the results are shown in TABLE 7. There was no correlation between the number of B-cells present during the induction of helper cells and the cooperation obtained. Lymph node cells (28% B) were no more active than cortisone-resistant thymus cells (0.2% B), or the latter purified further (TABLE 7). These results suggest, but do not prove, the T-cell synthesis of IgT, since there are very few B-cells in each culture.

CELL COOPERATION AND ITS REGULATION: AN INTEGRATED VIEW

The results presented above, [2, 6–9, 18, 19, 28, 29] make a strong case for a central role of IgT in the induction and regulation of cooperative antibody responses. Four different functions were described: (1) Induction of specific cooperation. This takes place after IgT complexes bind to adherent cells. Major unknowns in this area include the anatomical site of cooperation *in vivo,* the nature of the third party cell, details of the binding of IgT-antigen complexes such as,

TABLE 7

INDUCTION OF HELPER CELLS FROM PURIFIED NONIMMUNE T-CELL POPULATIONS *

Helper Cells	% B	Challenge	Anti-DNP Response (AFC/Culture)
nil		nil	30
nil		TNP KLH	23
nil		DNP POL	1020
LN (10^5)	28.	TNP KLH	780
CRT (10^5)	0.2	↓	595
CRT, anti-Ig (10^5)	0.03	↓	610
CRT, anti-Ig, nylon wool (10^5)	0.002	↓	560

* Helper cells were induced by 4-day culture of LN (pooled mesenteric and peripheral) with 1 μg/KLH, or CRT (and derivatives) with 10^{-1} μg/ml KLH. Percentages of B-cells was established by staining with a fluoresceinated anti-Ig and a heterologous anti-B serum. Anti-DNP responses of normal spleen after 4 days culture in response to 10^{-1} μg/ml TNP KLH and 10^5 cultured "helper cells," or 1 μg/ml DNP POL. (Data from M. Feldmann, S. Kontiainen, and M .F. Greaves. 1974. Unpublished.)

the half-life of IgT, number of receptors, pattern of binding, and whether macrophages play an active role in cooperation. (2) Specific T-cell suppression is initiated by the direct binding of IgT-antigen complexes to the surface of lymphocytes. Basically this is envisaged as being analogous to antibody-mediated tolerance.[30] (3) Antigenic competition is envisaged as a blockage of the surface receptors for IgT, preventing the realization of an immunogenic concentration of IgT complexes, perhaps by inhibiting the formation of suitably sized matrices of antigenic determinants.[2] (4) Augmentation of IgG responses is the newest and least understood of the functions of IgT.[24] These 4 functions are represented in FIGURE 3.

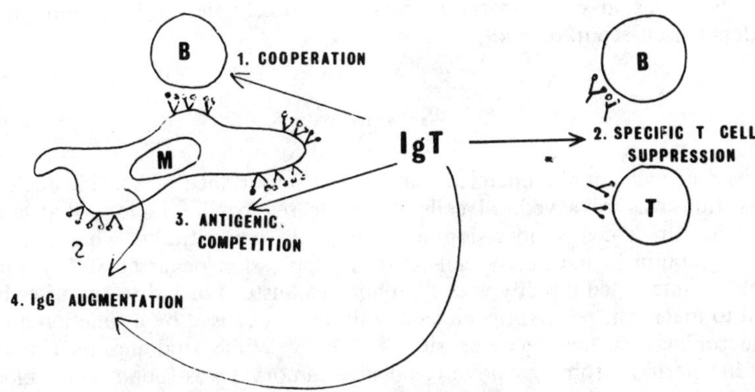

FIGURE 3. Scheme of actions of IgT.

It is possible to integrate these actions of IgT into a framework of cooperation that has a strong inbuilt component of self-regulation, based on the interaction of IgT with macrophages. Let us consider only the events *after* T-cells are activated and releasing IgT complexes, since those occurring before are even less understood.

Since IgT is highly cytophilic for macrophages but not T- or B-cells [11, 18] and macrophages are more common than antigen-specific T- or B-cells, IgT will be bound via the F_c segment to macrophages. Initially essentially all will be bound, leading to the formation of increasing numbers of IgT-antigen matrices, which can be envisaged as the "cooperative patches" upon which B-cells are triggered. Thus, with increasing numbers of T-cells (or of ATC supernatant) there is an incremental phase of the response. With the approaching saturation of IgT receptors, the number of cooperative patches is at a maximum, and cooperative capacity, and responses are at a maximum. With even more IgT released, sufficient will remain to bind to lymphocytes, inactivating them, and causing the descending shape of T-cell/antibody response curves. This is "T-cell suppression." Thus, this cooperative pathway has a fixed maximum set by the macrophages. Over immunization is prevented not only by this maximum, but also by the direct suppression of both T- and B-lymphocytes.[28, 29] Consequences of this pathway are the partial suppression of responses to other antigens, subsequently administered, manifest as "antigenic competition," and the increased IgG responses in the presence of large concentrations of IgT (TABLES 5 and 6). In support of this idea it has been reported that prior priming of T-cells alone can influence Ig class.[46]

There are, however, other influences in cooperative responses not yet fitted into this framework. The action of C3 in cooperation is such example.[47] Anti-C3 antibodies block cooperative but not thymus-independent responses *in vitro*.[48] Whether C3 acts at the macrophage or B-cell level is not yet known.

Genetic restrictions on responsiveness is another example. Recently it was thought that genetically nonresponder animals lacked functional T-cell receptors for that antigen, and that the lesion was due to the lack of a T-cell response (reviewed in ref. 44, challenged in 49). However this position can no longer be held, as there are many instances of "nonresponder" T-cells having receptors [49] and responding *in vivo* [e.g. 50–52] and *in vitro* [5, 53, 57] as assayed by immunologically specific proliferation,[50, 53, 54] or the release of specific helper factors.[51, 52] A lesion of cooperation seems the likely defect in genetic nonresponders (discussed in refs. 49, 55).

SUMMARY

The evidence for the chemical nature and importance of specific factors in cooperation was reviewed. T-cells also release specific factors that are of importance in T-cell suppression and antigenic competition, which are also immunoglobulin in nature. Specific T-cell suppression occurred if IgT-antigen complexes interacted directly with lymphocytes, instead of indirectly, after being bound to macrophages. Antigenic competition was caused by a functional block of macrophage surface-receptor sites for IgT. While studying Ig (immunoglobulin) purified from θ positive Ig positive tumors it was found that it blocked thymus-dependent (but not independent) antibody IgM responses, but at low concentrations augmented IgG responses. These four functions of IgT stress its importance as an effector of T-cell function in cell cooperation and its regulation, despite the fact that its biosynthesis by T-cells remains to be proven. Whether the 4 functions of IgT are all mediated by a single class of IgT, or by multiple classes is not yet known.

References

1. Miller, J. F. A. P. 1972. Lymphocyte interactions in antibody responses. Int. Rev. Cytol. **33:** 77–121.
2. Feldmann, M. 1974. Cell to cell interactions in the immune response. Series Haematol. In press.
3. Claman, H. N. & E. A. Chaperon. 1969. Immunologic complementation between thymus and marrow cells—a model of the two cell theory of immunocompetence. Transplant. Rev. **1:** 92–113.
4. Miller, J. F. A. P. & G. F. Mitchell. 1969. Thymus and antigen reactive cells. Transplant. Rev. **1:** 3–42.
5. Mitchison, N. A., K. Rajewsky & R. B. Taylor. 1970. Cooperation of antigenic determinants in the induction of antibodies. *In* Developmental Aspects of Antibody Formation and Structure. J. Sterzl, Ed. : 547–561. Czech. Acad. Sci. Prague.
6. Feldmann, M. & A. Basten. 1972. Cell interactions in the immune response *in vitro* III Specific cooperation across a cell impermeable membrane. J. Exp. Med. **136:** 49–67.
7. Feldmann, M. & A. Basten. 1972. Cell interactions in the immune response *in vitro* IV Comparism of the effects of antigen-specific and allogeneic thymus derived cell factors. J. Exp. Med. **136:** 722–736.
8. Feldmann, M. 1972. Cell interactions in the immune response *in vitro* V. Specific collaboration with complexes of antigen and thymus derived cell immunoglobulin. J. Exp. Med. **136:** 737–760.
9. Feldmann, M., R. E. Cone & J. J. Marchalonis. 1973. Cell interactions in the immune response *in vitro* VI. Mediated by T cell surface IgM. Cell Immunol. **9:** 1–11.
10. Gisler, R. H., F. Staber, E. Rude & P. Dukor. 1973. Soluble mediators of T-B interactions. Eur. J. Immunol. **3:** 650–653.
11. Rieber, E. P. & G. Riethmuller. 1974. Surface Immunoglobulin of thymus cells II. Release of heterologous anti-Ig antibodies from thymus cells as an immunogenic complex. Z. Immunitätsforsch. **147:** 262.
12. Lachmann, P. J. & H. E. Amos. 1971. Soluble factors in the mediation of the cooperative effect. Immunopathology **6:** 65–72.
13. Yu, K. & J. Gordon. 1973. Helper function in antibody synthesis mediated by soluble factors. Nature New Biol. **244:** 20–21.
14. Tada, T., K. Okumara & Masaru Taniguchi. 1974. Reagenic antibody formation in the rat: regulatory effects of soluble carrier specific T cell factors on hapter specific reagin production. Proc. VIII Int. Congress Allergology. Excerpta Medica. 473.
15. Nossal, G. J. V. & G. L. Ada. 1971. Antigens, Lymphoid Cells and the Immune Response. Academic Press. New York, N.Y.
16. Guttman, G. & I. L. Weissman. 1972. Lymphoid tissue architecture. Experimental analysis of the origin and distribution of T-cells and B-cells. Immunology **23:** 465–480.
17. Curtis, A. S. G. & M. S. B. de Sousa. 1973. Factors affecting adhesion of lymphoid cells. Nature New Biol. **244:** 45–46.
18. Cone, R. E., M. Feldmann, J. J. Marchalonis & G. J. V. Nossal. 1974. Adherence of T cell receptor Ig to the macrophage surface. Immunology **26:** 49–60.

19. FELDMANN, M. & J. W. SCHRADER. 1974. Mechanism of antigenic competition I. Induction by specific T cell products. Cell. Immunol. **14:** 255.
20. PLAYFAIR, J. H. L. & E. PURVES. 1971. Heterogeneity of B cells. Nature New Biol. **231:** 149–151.
21. GORCZYNSKI, R. M. & M. FELDMANN. 1974. B cell heterogeneity—difference in the size of B lymphocytes responding to T dependent and T independent antigens. Cell. Immunol. In press.
22. WALDMAN, H. & A. MUNRO. 1973. T cell dependent mediator in the immune response. Nature **243:** 256–7.
23. SCHRADER, J. W. 1973. Mechanism of activation of the bone marrow derived lymphocyte III. A distinction between a macrophage produced triggering signal and the amplifying effect on triggered B lymphocytes of allogeneic interactions. J. Exp. Med. **138:** 1466–1480.
24. FELDMANN, M., A. BOYLSTON & N. M. HOGG. 1974. Role of T cell immunoglobulin in the regulation of the immune response. Nature. In press.
25. KATZ, D. H. & B. BENACERRAF. 1972. The regulatory influence of activated T cells or B cell responses to antigen. Advan. Immunol. **15:** 1–92.
26. SCHIMPL, A. & E. WECKER. 1972. Replacement of a T cell function by a T cell product. Nature New Biol. **237:** 15–18.
27. DUTTON, R. W., R. FALKOFF, J. A. HURST, H. HOFFMAN, J. W. KAPPLER, J. R. KETTMAN, J. F. LESLEY & D. VANN. 1971. Is there evidence for a nonspecific diffusable chemical mediator in the initiation of the immune response? Progr. Immunol. **1:** 355–361.
28. FELDMANN, M. 1973. Induction of B cell tolerance by specific T cell products. Nature New Biol. **242:** 82–84.
29. FELDMANN, M. 1974. T cell suppression *in vitro* II. Nature of specific suppressive factor. Eur. J. Immunol. **4:** 664.
30. DIENER, E. & M. FELDMANN. 1972. Relationship between antigen and antibody mediated suppression of immunity. Transplant. Rev. **8:** 76–103.
31. SJOGREN, H. O., I. HELLSTROM, S. C. BANSAL & K. E. HELLSTROM. 1971. Suggestive evidence that the 'blocking antibodies' of tumor-bearing individuals may be antigen-antibody complexes. Proc. Nat. Acad. Sci. U.S. **68:** 1732–1738.
32. GERSHON, R. K. & K. KONDO. 1971. Infectious immunological tolerance. Immunology **21:** 903–914.
33. ADA, G. L. & M. COOPER. 1973. Personal communication.
34. BASTEN, A., J. F. A. P. MILLER, C. CHEERS & J. SPRENT. 1974. Submitted for publication.
35. HUCHET, R. & M. FELDMANN. 1974. Tolerance induction to a hepter-protein conjugate *in vivo:* are suppressor cells involved? Eur. J. Immunol. **4:** 768.
36. TAUSSIG, M. J. 1973. Antigenic competition. Curr. Top. Microbiol. Immunol. **60:** 125–162.
37. LIACOPOULOS, P. & S. BEN EFRAIN. 1974. Antigenic competition. Progr. Allergy. In press.
38. PROSS, H. & D. EIDINGER. 1974. Antigenic competition—a review of nonspecific antigen induced suppression. Advan. Immunol. In press.
39. SJOBERG, O. 1971. Antigenic competition *in vitro* of spleen cells subjected to a graft versus host reaction. Immunology **21:** 351–362.
40. BOYLSTON, A. 1973. Theta antigen and immunoglobulin on a tissue-cultured mouse lymphoma. Immunology **24:** 851–8.
41. HARRIS, A. W., A. D. BANKHURST, S. MASON & N. L. WARNER. 1973. Differentiated functions expressed by cultured mouse lymphona cells II. θ antigen, surface immunoglobulin and a receptor for antibody on cells of a thymoma cell line. J. Immunol. **110:** 431–8.
42. PERMS, B., J. F. A. P. MILLER, L. FORM & J. SPRENT. 1974. Immunoglobulin an activated T cells detected by indirect immunofluorescence. Cell. Immunol. In press.

43. WILLIAMS, A. F. & S. HUNT. 1973. Unpublished data.
44. McDEVITT, H. O. & M. LANDY, Eds. 1972. Genetics of Immune responsiveness. Academic Press. New York, N.Y.
45. RIEBER, E. P., G. RIETHMULLER & M. HADMAN. 1974. Demonstration of surface Ig in thymus cells. Protides Biol. Fluids **21:** 311–4.
46. CHEERS, C. & J. F. A. P. MILLER. 1972. Cell to cell interaction in immune response IX. Regulation of hapten specific antibody class by carrier priming. J. Exp. Med. **136:** 1661–1663.
47. PEPYS, M. B. Role of complement in induction of the allergic response. Nature New Biol. **237:** 157–159.
48. FELDMANN, M. & M. B. PEPYS. 1974. Role of C_3 in *in vitro* lymphocyte cooperation. Nature **249:** 159.
49. FELDMANN, M. 1973. H linked Ir genes—what do they do? Transplant. Proc. **5:** 1803–1807.
50. GERSHON, R. K., P. MAURER & C. MERRYMAN. 1973. A cellular basis for genetically controlled immunologic unresponsiveness in mice. Tolerance induction in T-cells. Proc. Nat. Acad. Sci. Su. U.S. **70:** 250–254.
51. MOZES, E. & M. J. TAUSSIG. 1974. Personal communication.
52. BEN EFRAIM, S. & P. LIACOPOULOS. 1969. The competitive effect of DNP-poly-L-lysine in responder and non-responder guinea pigs. Immunology **16:** 573–580.
53. PHILLIPS-QUAGLIATA, J. M. & J. McDONALD. 1973. Unpublished data.
54. FELDMANN, M. & D. B. KILBURN. 1974. Unpublished data.
55. ROELANTS, G. E., AINA RYDEN, LENA BRITT HAGG & FRANCIS LOOR. 1974. Active synthesis of immunoglobulin receptors for antigen by T lymphocytes. Nature. **247:** 106–108.

DISCUSSION OF THE PAPER

DR. J. F. A. P. MILLER: I believe we agree on the general principle that the immunoglobulin released from T-cells may not necessarily be synthesized by T-cells but may be perhaps passively absorbed from B-cells, as you mentioned. I would like to ask you if it is an immune complex that is on the macrophage which augments the responses of the B-cell; could the same complex produce tolerance of the B-cell?

DR. FELDMANN: Yes, that is the working hypothesis that we have at the moment. I think at the moment we can study effects, but we have really no idea as to biosynthetic origin of the factor. Direction of IgT complexes causes tolerance; indirect action, via macrophages, would cause an immune response.

DR. J. THORBECKE (*New York University, New York, N.Y.*): Will you please comment on whether you have any data regarding the histocompatibility requirements of the B- and T-cells or the macrophages?

DR. M. FELDMANN: We decided to investigate this problem. In fact, talking to Dr. Cudkowicz a few days ago he has done much more extensive studies and I do not think we will continue. The first system that was investigated was to see whether induction requires T-cells and macrophages. We have to have syngeneic T-cells and macrophages for inducing optimal "help." Dr. Cudkowicz has a lot of data that indicate a requirement for syngeneic T-cells and B-cells occurs in some circumstances, but not in others.

EFFECT OF THYMOSIN ON THYMOCYTE PROLIFERATION AND AUTOIMMUNITY IN NZB MICE

Norman Talal, Michael Dauphinee, Rao Pillarisetty, and Ronald Goldblum

Clinical Immunology and Arthritis Section
Veterans Administration Hospital, and Department of Medicine
University of California, San Francisco
San Francisco, California 94122

The New Zealand Black (NZB) and NZB/NZW F_1 hybrid mice are generally considered a model for human autoimmune disease, particularly systemic lupus erythematosus.[1-3] Genetic, immunologic and viral factors are all implicated in their disease.[4] These mice develop LE cells, antinuclear factor, antibodies to nucleic acids such as DNA and RNA, autoimmune hemolytic anemia and immune complex glomerulonephritis.[5-7] In addition, they have a generalized infiltration of many organs with lymphocytes and plasma cells. These findings appear after 16 weeks of age.

Over 30% of NZB/NZW F_1 mice greater than eleven months of age develop monoclonal macroglobulinemia.[8] A transplantable lymphoma producing monoclonal IgM was established from the spleen of one animal. Thus, NZB mice, in addition to their autoimmune disease, develop features of yet another human disorder, monoclonal (Waldenstrom's) macroglobulinemia. This disorder is considered to be a malignant proliferation of lymphocytes or lymphocytoid plasma cells, in many ways analogous to chronic lymphocytic leukemia.[9]

NZB mice show a progressive loss of T-cell functions during their lifespan.[4] Even prior to the onset of autoimmunity, their T-cells are resistant to the development of immunologic tolerance.[10-12] Later in life, they have marked deficiencies of various T-cell effector functions such as reactivity to mitogens[13] and ability to induce graft-vs-host (GvH) disease.[14] At this stage, they also have a deficiency of long-lived recirculating T-cells.[15, 16]

We have recently reported a thymocyte abnormality in NZB mice that was detected by measuring the DNA synthetic response to foreign transplantation antigens.[17] NZB thymocytes were injected into lethally irradiated C57Bl/6 mice and DNA synthesis measured as the incorporation of ^{125}iododeoxyuridine (^{125}IUDR) by spleen and lymph node seeking cells. Thymocytes from DBA/2 mice (who are the same H_2 type as NZB) were similarly injected into other C57Bl/6 mice as controls.

DBA/2 thymocytes from 2 and 8 week old donors and NZB thymocytes from 2 week old donors showed essentially the same proliferative response upon encountering the foreign histocompatibility antigens of the recipient animals. There was a rapid synthetic response that peaked on day 4 and was over by day 6. By contrast, thymocytes from 8 week old NZB mice showed a very different response. DNA synthesis was markedly delayed and did not begin until day 4.

These results suggested an alteration in the DNA synthetic response to histocompatibility antigens by NZB thymocytes occurring between 2 and 8 weeks of age. This may reflect an intrinsic abnormality of thymocyte differentiation, perhaps genetically determined or induced by a latent viral infection.

Bach *et al.* have recently demonstrated the presence of a thymosin-like material in normal mouse serum that is lacking in the serum of congenitally thymus-deficient ("nude") mice.[18] Such thymosin-like activity declines with age in normal mice and declines prematurely in the serum of NZB and NZB/NZW F_1 hybrid mice. By two months, a time when abnormal thymocyte proliferation and T-cell resistance to tolerance are already present, serum thymic activity is insignificant in NZB mice.[18] These findings raise the possibility that a deficiency of thymosin could contribute to the T-cell abnormalities characteristic of the NZB strain.

The present study was undertaken to determine the role of thymosin in the abnormal DNA synthetic response of NZB thymocytes. We have attempted to preserve a normal DNA synthetic response in 8 week old NZB thymocytes by treating the donor NZB mice with various regimens of thymosin. We find that treatment with thymosin can correct the abnormal DNA proliferation of NZB thymocytes. Preliminary experiments examining the effects of thymosin on antigen-induced depression and autoimmunity are also presented.

Materials and Methods

Mice

NZB mice were from our colony maintained at the Vivarium of the University of California, San Francisco. C57Bl/6 and DBA/2 mice were from Jackson Laboratory, Bar Harbor, Maine.

Irradiation Procedure

Recipient C57Bl/6 mice received 750 R total body x-irradiation from a Quadacondex Westinghouse x-ray machine with a 0.5 mm Cu and 1 mmAl. filter at 15 ma and 230 kVp. The dose rate was 122 R/min.

Preparation of Thymosin

Thymosin fraction 5 was kindly supplied by Dr. Allan L. Goldstein. The purification procedure through fraction 5 is as follows. Thymus tissue is homogenized in 3 volumes of 0.9% NaCl with 0.5% (vol/vol) octyl alcohol added to minimize foaming. The homogenate is centrifuged at $14{,}000 \times g$. Three liter portions of the supernatant are heated with stirring in a boiling water bath. When the temperature reaches 80° C, the sample is rapidly cooled in an ice-water bath. The heat-coagulated materials are removed by centrifugation and the supernatant is added to 5 volumes of acetone that has been cooled to −10° C. The precipitate that forms during this procedure is collected by filtration, washed several times with cold acetone, and then dried in a desiccator under reduced pressure. The white powder is suspended in 10 volumes of 10 mM $NaPO_4$ (pH 7) and is stirred at room temperature for one hour. After removing a small amount of insoluble residue by centrifugation, the sample is brought to 25% of saturation with a saturated $(NH_4)_2SO_4$ solution (pH 7).

The precipitate is discarded and the supernatant is adjusted to pH 4 with 10% acetic acid. Solid $(NH_4)_2SO_4$ is added to 50% of saturation. The resulting precipitate is collected by centrifugation, dissolved in 10 mM Tris HCl (pH 8) and subjected to ultrafiltration with the Amicon DC-2 hollow fiber system (concentration mode, HICP 10 membrane cartridge). The filtrate is concentrated by rotary evaporation under reduced pressure and desalted on a 50 × 80 cm column of Sephadex® G25 equilibrated with deionized water. The protein eluted prior to the salt and nucleotide peak is concentrated by rotary evaporation and dried by lyophilization. This thymosin preparation (fraction 5) is stored desiccated at −20° C and is readily soluble in phosphate-buffered saline.

Administration of Thymosin

Thymosin fraction 5 was injected intraperitoneally into 6 groups of NZB mice. Each group contained from 15–25 mice. The total amount of thymosin administered in 3–9 injections varied from 0.3–3.0 mg.

In 5 experiments age- and sex matched NZB mice received the same amount of bovine serum albumin (BSA) as a control for the thymosin protein. In a sixth experiment, untreated NZB mice served as controls.

Thymus Cell Suspensions

Thymus cells were prepared as previously described.[17] We injected 50×10^6 viable thymus cells intravenously (0.5 ml) into each recipient. Four to 8 recipient mice were used for each experimental determination. All recipient mice were put on 1 mg/ml Panamycin (Upjohn, Kalamazoo, Michigan) in their drinking water one week prior to lethal irradiation and during all subseqent testing.

DNA Synthesis

The procedure used followed Gershon and Hencin,[19] in which DNA synthesis is measured by uptake of ^{125}I-labeled 5-iodo-2-deoxyuridine (^{125}IUDR Amersham-Searle Corp., Des Plaines, Ill., specific activity 8.4 μCi/μg). The procedure has been described previously.[17] Each mouse received 2 μCi of ^{125}IUDR intraperitoneally in 0.2 ml of saline 24 hours before spleen and femoral lymph nodes were harvested. The % IUDR incorporated was determined according to the formula:

$$\frac{\text{organ (thymocyte injected recipient)} - \text{organ (noninjected recipient)}}{\text{total isotope injected} - \text{organ (noninjected recipient)}} \times 100 = \%\ ^{125}\text{IUDR Incorporation}$$

Cytotoxicity Assay

The *in vitro* cytotoxic activity of sensitized lymphocytes was determined according to the method of Brunner [20] with slight modifications. Cytotoxicity was measured against ^{51}Cr-labeled E1–4 lymphoma target cells. The procedure has been described previously.[17] Specific cytotoxicity was determined by measuring the release of ^{51}Cr into the medium compared to maximal release (water lysis) using the following formula:

$$\frac{\text{experimental } ^{51}\text{Cr release} - \text{spontaneous } ^{51}\text{Cr release}}{\text{maximal } ^{51}\text{Cr release} - \text{spontaneous } ^{51}\text{Cr release}} \times 100 = \% \text{ specific release}$$

Antigen-induced Depression of DNA Synthesis

Sheep erythrocytes (Mogul Diagnostics, Madison, Wisc.), 5×10^8, were injected intravenously in a volume of 0.2 ml. Control mice received 0.2 ml of phosphate-buffered saline. Six hours later, 2 μCi of ^{125}IUDR were injected intraperitoneally. Twenty hours later, mice were sacrificed. Spleens were weighed and assayed for isotope incorporation. Results are expressed as incorporation (cpm) per 100 mg spleen weight. Student's t test was applied to determine statistical significance.

Thymosin Effect on Autoantibodies

Twelve NZB/NZW F_1 female mice received 2 mg of thymosin fraction 5 in 20 intraperitoneal injections given twice weekly. Eight age- and sex-matched control mice received bovine serum albumin in the same protocol. Treatment was started at 4 months and maintained for 2½ months.

In a separate experiment, 9 female NZB/NZW F_1 mice were treated for 5 months starting at 1 month of age. Age- and sex-matched control mice were untreated. Mice received 200 μg weekly the first 3 months, 400 μg weekly for the next month, and then 800 μg weekly for the last month.

Mice were bled at intervals and sera assayed for antibodies to DNA and RNA by a filter radioimmunoassay method.[21]

Results

Thymocyte Proliferation

Following the transfer of NZB thymocytes into lethally irradiated C57Bl/6 recipients, DNA synthesis was studied separately in the spleen- and lymph-node-seeking populations. Two week spleen-seeking NZB thymocytes gave a normal response similar to that of control DBA/2 and other strains.[17] This response is characterized by a rapid incorporation of ^{125}IUDR with a peak between days 3 and 4, followed by decreased incorporation and return to baseline (Figure 1). By contrast, totally different kinetics were observed when 8-week NZB thymocytes were injected into C57Bl/6 recipients. Incorporation of ^{125}IUDR was delayed, the response starting between days 4 and 5. Maximum incorporation was achieved on day 6, the last day of assay. Thus there was no observed decrease in incorporation. This we call an abnormal response.

The results with lymph-node-seeking NZB thymocytes is similar (Figure 1). The DNA synthetic response of 2-week cells appeared earlier and was

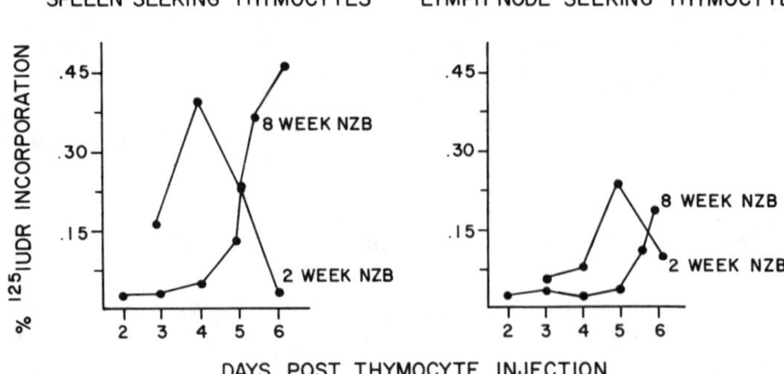

FIGURE 1 Incorporation of ^{125}IUDR by spleen-seeking (left) and lymph-node-seeking (right) thymocytes from 2 and 8 week old NZB donors injected into lethally irradiated C57B1/6 recipients.

over by day 6. The 8-week cells showed a delayed response which was maximal on day 6.

We attempted to maintain a normal DNA synthetic response in 8-week NZB thymocytes by treating donor NZB mice with thymosin starting at 14 days of age (TABLE 1, Group A). Nine injections of 0.9 mg of thymosin were injected over the 6-week period. Age- and sex-matched control NZB mice were untreated. At 8 weeks of age, both thymosin-treated and untreated mice were sacrificed, and thymocytes injected into irradiated C57Bl/6 recipients. As shown in FIGURE 2, the kinetics of DNA synthesis were markedly different in the two groups. Thymosin treated mice showed the response characteristic of 2 week NZB thymocytes whereas the untreated mice had the abnormal response expected at 8 weeks of age.

In groups B and C, treatment was started at 21 and 28 days for a total dose of 0.7 and 0.3 mg respectively. As a control, age- and sex-matched mice received the same quantity of bovine serum albumin (BSA) injected in an identical schedule. Mice receiving thymosin showed a DNA proliferative response characteristic of 2-week NZB thymocytes, whereas mice receiving BSA showed the customary delayed onset and abnormal response (FIGURE 3).

TABLE 1

PROLIFERATION OF 8-WEEK NZB THYMOCYTES AFTER THYMOSIN TREATMENT

Group	Age at Onset (Days)	Number of Mice	Number of i.v. Injections	Total Thymosin (mg)	Proliferative Response
A	14	9	9	0.9	normal
B	21	9	7	0.7	normal
C	28	12	3	0.3	normal
D	35	10	3	0.3	abnormal
E	35	8	3	3.0	normal
F	49	16	3	0.3	abnormal

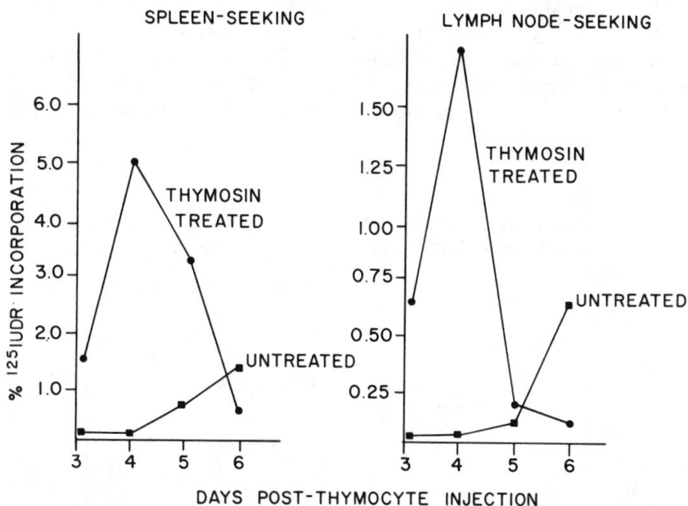

FIGURE 2 Incorporation of ^{125}IUDR by spleen-seeking and lymph-node-seeking thymocytes from thymosin-treated and untreated NZB donors. Treatment was started at 14 days.

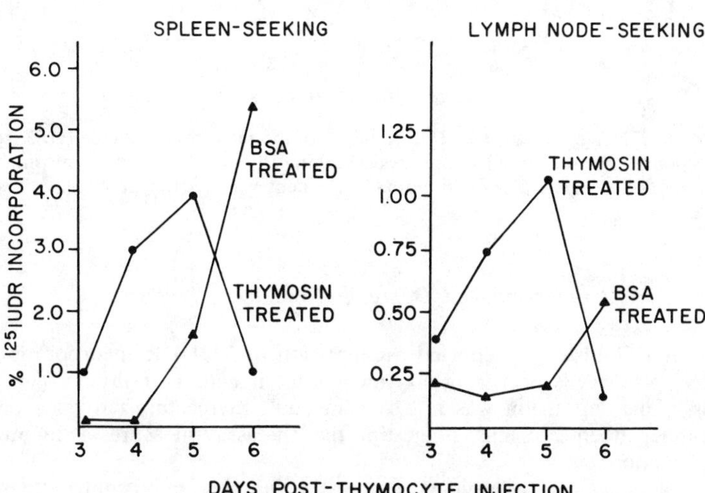

FIGURE 3 Incorporation of ^{125}IUDR by spleen-seeking and lymph-node-seeking thymocytes from thymosin-treated or albumin (BSA)-treated NZB donors. Treatment was started at 28 days.

Groups D and E started treatment at 35 days of age. Group D (receiving 0.3 mg of thymosin) behaved like untreated mice, showing an abnormal response. By contrast, group E (receiving 3.0 mg of thymosin) showed maintenance of the normal young response pattern. Group F, starting thymosin at 49 days and receiving only 0.3 mg of thymosin, showed no effect of treatment. Effector cell activity was assayed in this experiment and also showed no difference between thymosin-treated and BSA-treated mice (FIGURE 4). Thus, the ability of thymosin to maintain normal DNA synthetic response seems related to dose and duration of treatment.

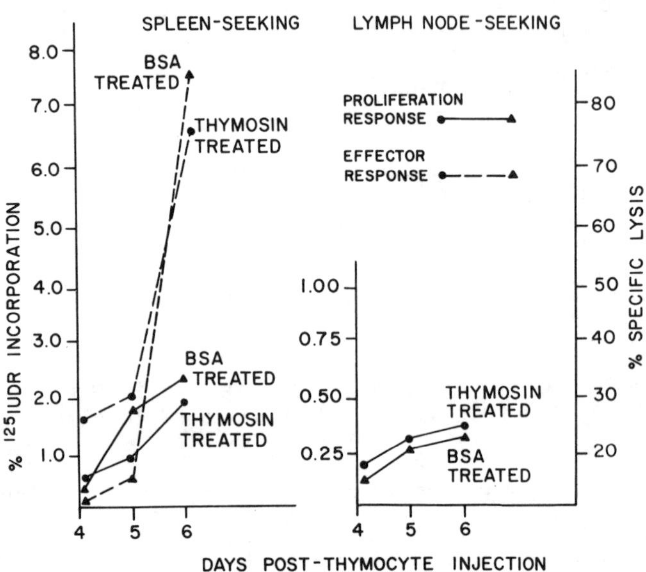

FIGURE 4 DNA synthetic (% IUDR incorporation) and effector cell (% specific lysis) responses of spleen and lymph node seeking thymocytes from thymosin-treated or albumin (BSA)-treated NZB donors. Treatment was started at 49 days and had no effect.

Antigen-induced Depression of DNA Synthesis

Zatz and Goldstein [22] reported a depression of ^{125}IUDR incorporation into DNA by spleen cells occurring six hours after injection of thymus-dependent antigens. This depression was not seen in adult thymectomized mice or with thymus-independent antigens, suggesting that the assay measures a thymus suppressor function.

Since a deficiency of thymus suppressor function may contribute to the emergence of autoimmunity, we decided to study antigen-induced depression of DNA synthesis in NZB and control CBA/J mice. The results in the normal

TABLE 2

ANTIGEN-INDUCED DEPRESSION OF DNA SYNTHESIS IN NORMAL MOUSE SPLEEN

Group	Number of Mice	Antigen	Mean CPM / 100 mg Spleen Wt ±SE	% Depression	Significance
CBA/J (5 week)	12	+	1330±240	49	p <0.01
	13	—	2630±520		
CBA/J (2 month)	14	+	1490±280	42	p <0.02
	14	—	2570±430		
CBA/J (4 month)	19	+	1746±166	29	p <0.02
	15	—	2465±250		
CBA/J (8 month)	15	+	1267±110	(0)	NS
	14	—	1128±108		

CBA/J mice are shown in TABLE 2. The antigen (sheep erythrocytes) resulted in significant depression in 5 week, 2 month and 4 month old animals. No depression was observed in 8 month old mice, suggesting that this activity may normally be lost as a consequence of aging.

The results in NZB mice are shown in TABLE 3. The only significant antigen-induced depression of DNA synthesis was seen in 5 week old mice. No depression was seen in NZB mice aged 2 months, 4 months or more than one year. These results suggest that antigen-induced depression is lost prematurely in NZB mice (between 5 and 8 weeks), at a time when the thymocyte proliferative response converts from normal to abnormal kinetics.

In a preliminary experiment, antigen-induced depression was studied in 3 month old NZB mice treated with 5 mg of thymosin or BSA given on 3 consecutive days. Sheep erythrocytes were injected one day later. Thymosin caused an increased incorporation in control NZB mice (given saline only) and a significant depression in animals receiving the antigen (TABLE 4). This result suggests that thymosin may be able to restore antigen-induced depression, just as it is capable of maintaining a normal DNA proliferative response.

TABLE 3

LOSS OF ANTIGEN-INDUCED DEPRESSION OF DNA SYNTHESIS IN NZB MOUSE SPLEEN

Group	Number of Mice	Antigen	Mean CPM / 100 mg Spleen Wt ±SE	% Depression	Significance
NZB (5 week)	12	+	1049±179	72	p <0.001
	13	—	3724±454		
NZB (2 month)	15	+	650±120	18	NS
	12	—	796±140		
NZB (4 month)	18	+	1566±209	9	NS
	17	—	1728±181		
NZB (<1 year)	15	+	1449±229	3	NS
	15	—	1502±79		

TABLE 4

RESTORATION OF ANTIGEN-INDUCED DEPRESSION OF SPLEEN DNA SYNTHESIS IN 3 MONTH OLD NZB MICE BY THYMOSIN TREATMENT

Treatment	Number of Mice	Antigen	Mean CPM / 100 mg Spleen Wt ±SE	% Depression	Significance
Thymosin	7	+	2225±127	30	$p < 0.05$
(15 mg)	7	—	3178±350		
BSA	7	+	2226±447	(0)	NS
	7	—	1945±185		

Autoimmunity

The experiments on thymocyte proliferation and antigen-induced depression suggest that an alteration of thymocyte differentiation is an important early event in NZB mice preceding the development of autoimmunity. The results with thymosin indicate the potential reversibility of this thymocyte abnormality.

The pathogenesis of autoimmunity in NZB mice is extremely complicated and dependent upon genetic, immunologic, and viral factors.[4] If maintenance of normal thymocyte function can suppress the emergence of autoantibody-producing B-cells, then thymosin has the theoretical potential of preventing or ameliorating autoimmune disease in NZB mice. This possibility is currently under investigation in our laboratory.

NZB and NZB/NZW F_1 mice spontaneously produce antibodies to DNA and RNA that can be measured using a filter radioimmunoassay method.[21] The formation of such antibodies is most pronounced in female NZB/NZW F_1 mice (FIGURE 5). We have treated female NZB/NZW F_1 mice with thymosin starting

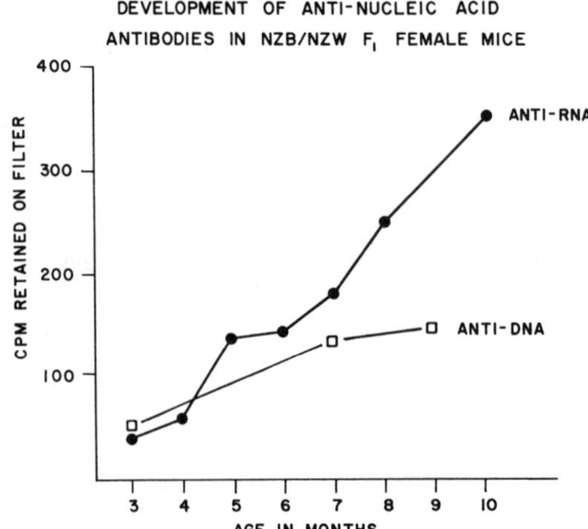

FIGURE 5 Antibodies to DNA and RNA develop progressively with age in NZB/NZW F_1 mice. Antibody activity was measured using a filter radioimmunoassay method.

TABLE 5

EFFECT OF THYMOSIN ON ANTINUCLEIC ACID ANTIBODIES

Thymosin Started at 1 Month Age (Months)	Total Thymosin (mg)	Ratio of Antibody-binding Activity $\frac{\text{Thymosin Treatment}}{\text{Controls}} \times 100$ RNA (p Value)	DNA (p Value)
4	2.4	32 (<0.001)	77 (<0.005)
5	4.0	69 (<0.001)	93 (NS)
6	7.2	100 (NS)	106 (NS)
Thymosin Started at 4 Months			
5	1.0	90 (NS)	
6½	2.0	95 (NS)	

at 1 month or 4 months of age. Thymosin was injected several times per week and antibodies measured at intervals during the treatment periods. Mice under treatment showed significantly less antibody to RNA and DNA at 4 months, and less antibody to RNA at 5 months (TABLE 5). By 6 months, there was no difference between thymosin-treated and untreated mice. When thymosin treatment was delayed until 4 months of age, no difference was observed at 5 or 6½ months. These results are preliminary, but suggest that early treatment with thymosin may delay the formation of antinucleic acid antibodies.

DISCUSSION

The immunologic abnormalities of NZB mice are now well documented (TABLE 6). Their status can generally be described as an immunologic imbalance in which B-cell activity is excessive and T-cell function is depressed.[4] Since T-cells play a major role in the regulation of immune responses, it seems likely that the B-cell abnormalities arise as a consequence of T-cell dysfunction. Moreover, certain T-cell defects are present within the first weeks of life, prior

TABLE 6

IMMUNOLOGIC ABNORMALITIES IN NEW ZEALAND BLACK MICE

(1) Premature development of competence in B- and T-cells.
(2) B-cells make excessive antibody responses and autoantibodies.
(3) T-cells are unable to develop and maintain tolerance.
(4) Abnormal DNA synthetic response of thymocytes.
(5) Loss of antigen-induced depression of DNA synthesis and suppressor function.
(6) Decreased serum "thymic activity."
(7) Spontaneous production of thymocytotoxic antibody.
(8) Deficient T-cell functions later in life (e.g., mitogen responses).
(9) Loss of recirculating T-lymphocytes.
(10) Loss of θ-positive cells late in life.

to the onset of autoantibody production by B-cells. The period between 3 and 6 weeks of life seems particularly critical, for it is at this time that the following abnormalities first appear: (1) inability to induce tolerance in T-cells, (2) alteration in kinetics of DNA synthesis by NZB thymocytes, (3) loss of antigen-induced depression of DNA synthesis, (4) loss of serum "thymic activity," and (5) appearance of thymocytotoxic antibody.

Evidence presented here and elsewhere by other investigators [23, 24] supports the hypothesis that suppressor T-cells may be deficient in New Zealand mice. It would follow, then, that B-cells would escape from this normal regulatory mechanism and go on to produce autoantibodies. Recent studies by Purves and Playfair indicate that B-cells of NZB mice have normal high-dose tolerance characteristics,[25] further evidence that the excessive B-cell antibody responses might arise not as a primary defect but rather secondary to a loss of T-cell regulation.

As the mice age and clinical disease becomes readily apparent, the more striking aspects of deficient T-cell function emerge with virtually complete loss of T-effector functions. It is noteworthy that autoreactive T-cells appear and remain present even while other T-cell activities are disappearing.[26]

The ultimate cause of the progressive loss of T-cell function is unknown, but almost certainly involves a deficiency of thymic humoral factors. Both an immunologic and an endocrine deficiency could result from an immunologic attack on the thymus, mediated either by antibody, by effector T-cells or, as seems likely, by more than one mechanism. Viral-induced alterations of thymocyte surface antigens could be an important initiating mechanism for such an attack. Profitt, Hirsch, and Black have recently shown that thymocytes infected with Moloney leukemia virus become cytotoxic for noninfected syngeneic fibroblasts.[27] They suggest that destruction of normal noninfected thymocytes could result from action of other autoaggressive infected thymocytes, leading to T-cell deficiency, autoimmunity and neoplasia. NZB thymocytes are infected with murine leukemia virus readily demonstrable by electron microscopy as C-type particles.[28, 29] If such viral infected thymocytes become cytotoxic for thymic epithelial cells and other thymocytes, a deficiency of thymosin and of thymic function might appear.

NZB mice produce, early in life, an autoantibody capable of destroying thymocytes from NZB and other mouse strains.[30] Such a thymocytotoxic antibody might also contribute to a state of thymic and T-cell deficiency.

Alternatively, a deficiency of thymosin could arise as a primary defect, perhaps as a direct expression of a genetic abnormality in NZB mice. The loss of serum thymic activity in NZB mice correlates in time with the abnormalities of thymic tolerance, proliferation and suppression. Thus, a logical case can be made for a primary thymic hormone deficiency leading to the abnormal state of thymocyte differentiation.

Our results support this hypothesis and suggest that abnormal thymocyte differentiation and loss of suppression can be prevented by administration of thymosin either prophylactically to young mice (under 28 days) or in larger doses to older mice (35 days). Our hope is that the abnormal thymocyte proliferation will correlate with the subsequent emergence of autoimmune disease and that treatment with thymosin may have therapeutic possibilities. Preliminary results presented here indicate that thymosin may delay the formation of antinucleic acid antibodies if treatment is started early in life. Much more work must be performed on mice already ill with disease, including examination of kidney function and survival, before the actual potential of thymosin treatment can be fully evaluated. These results suggest that thymosin might act either to induce the appearance of new T-cells with suppressor-like characteristics or to influence aberrant T-cells to revert to more normal modes of function. These results raise the interesting possibility that an endocrine disturbance may underlie many of the immunologic abnormalities associated with autoimmunity and lymphoid malignancy in New Zealand mice and, by analogy, in humans.

References

1. Howie, J. B. & B. J. Helyer. 1968. Advan. Immunol. **9:** 215–266.
2. Mellors, R. C. 1966. Int. Rev. Exp. Pathol. **5:** 217–252.
3. Talal, N. & A. D. Steinberg. 1974. Curr. Top. Microbiol. Immunol. **64:** 79–103.
4. Talal, N. 1970. Arthritis Rheum. **13:** 887–894.
5. Lambert, P. H. & F. J. Dixon. 1968. J. Exp. Med. **127:** 507–522.
6. Dixon, J. F., M. B. A. Oldstone & G. Tonietti. 1971. J. Exp. Med. **134:** 65s–71s.
7. Talal, N., A. D. Steinberg, M. E. Jacobs, T. M. Chused & A. F. Gazdar. 1971. J. Exp. Med. **134:** 52s–64s.
8. Sugai, S., R. J. Pillarisetty & N. Talal. 1973. J. Exp. Med. **138:** 989–1002.
9. Preud'homme, J. L. & M. Seligmann. 1972. Blood **49:** 777–794.
10. Staples, P. J., A. D. Steinberg & N. Talal. 1970. J. Exp. Med. **131:** 123–128.
11. Jacobs, M. E., J. K. Gordon & N. Talal. 1971. J. Immunol. **107:** 359–364.
12. Playfair, J. H. L. 1971. Immunol. **21:** 1037–1043.
13. Leventhal, B. G. & N. Talal. 1970. J. Immunol. **104:** 918–923.
14. Cantor, H., R. Asofsky & N. Talal. 1970. J. Exp. Med. **131:** 223–234.
15. Denman, A. M. & E. J. Denman. 1970. Clin. Exp. Immunol. **6:** 457–472.
16. Zatz, M. M., R. C. Mellors & E. M. Lance. 1971. Clin. Exp. Immunol. **8:** 491–500.
17. Dauphinee, M. J. & N. Talal. 1973. Proc. Nat. Acad. Sci. U.S. **70** (Part II): 3769–3772.
18. Bach, J. F., M. Dardenne & J. C. Salomon. 1973. Clin. Exp. Immunol. **14:** 247–256.
19. Gershon, R. K. & R. S. Hencin. 1971. J. Immunol. **107:** 359–364.
20. Brunner, K. T., J. Mauel, J. C. Cerottini & B. Chapuis. 1968. Immunol. **14:** 181–196.
21. Talal, N. & R. C. Gallo. 1972. Nature New Biol. **240:** 240.
22. Zatz, M. M. & A. L. Goldstein. 1973. J. Immunol. **110:** 1312–1317.
23. Allison, A. C., A. M. Denman & R. D. Barnes. 1971. Lancet **i:** 135–140.
24. Hardin, J. A., T. M. Chused & A. D. Steinberg. 1973. J. Immunol. **111:** 650–651.
25. Purves, E. C. & J. H. L. Playfair. 1973. Clin. Exp. Immunol. **15:** 113–122.
26. Liburd, E. M., A. S. Russell & J. B. Dassetor. 1973. J. Immunol. **111:** 1288–1291.
27. Profitt, M. R., M. S. Hirsch, P. H. Black. 1973. Science **182:** 821–823.
28. Mellors, R. C. & C. Y. Huang. 1966. J. Exp. Med. **124:** 1031–1038.
29. Prosser, P. R. 1968. Clin. Exp. Immunol. **3:** 213–226.
30. Shirai, T. & R. C. Mellors. 1971. Proc. Nat. Acad. Sci. U.S. **58:** 1412–1415.

Discussion of the Paper

Dr. B. Waksman: I do not wish in any way to call into question this really very beautiful study, but there was something in the theoretical formation that seems to me to neglect two questions. First of all, many of the autoantibodies that you see in many of these animals are the type of antibody that we normally think of as thymus-dependent. And you spoke of their formation in these animals as occurring because of an escape from tolerance. But what I feel you may have neglected in this is the question of whether you need T-cell cooperation in order to get the production of these autoantibodies. Now, the reverse of the same coin is the implication of the deficiency in the tolerance function that is seen in the very young NZB animals. One of the first implications would be that you ought to see autoimmunity of T-cell-mediated type. There has not been extensive investigations in the past on this question. I wonder if you'd comment on the possibility that somewhere in the earlier phases of the life of the NZB mouse one in fact finds T-cell mediated autoimmunity, something comparable to a graft-versus-host reaction in which the animal reacts against its own antigens.

Dr. N. Talal: I believe that to answer Dr. Waksman's question adequately, I would need as much time as I took to present the paper. Let me see what I can do quickly. Number one: these animals have helper T-cells early in life. In fact, they are born with full immunologic competence. They require no time at all to achieve adult levels of antibody-forming cells. And they probably have normal helper function even beyond the time that they lose suppressor function, although that is speculation at this point. They can make perfectly good T-dependent responses and probably do. Now, with regard to GvH, they develop a type of autoimmune reactivity, but it is late in life, not early. It is seen only as a consequence of age. They also develop antibodies to their own thymocytes, which again is an indication of an autoimmune reactivity. But this is not the cause of their autoimmune disease because we have recently found independent appearance of anti-RNA antibodies without prior development of antithymocyte antibodies.

THE ROLE OF CORTISONE-SENSITIVE THYMOCYTES IN DNA SYNTHETIC RESPONSES TO ANTIGEN *

P. Cohen and R. K. Gershon

Department of Pathology
Yale University School of Medicine
New Haven, Connecticut 06510

Introduction

It has long been established that corticosteroids cause a selective depopulation of the thymus.[1] More recently, several investigators have attributed distinctive characteristics to those cells that remain.

Warner, in 1964, showed that medullary cells of the chick thymus, selected by cortisone resistance, were a far more immunologically competent population than cortical cells, as judged by their ability to injure chick chorioallantoic membranes.[2] Weber, in 1966, showed that PHA-responding cells in the pig thymus were mostly cortisone-resistant and located in the thymus medulla;[3] in 1970 he demonstrated that those medullary thymocytes were able to participate in mixed lymphocyte reactions almost as well as spleen lymphocytes; in contrast, cortical thymocytes were said to show negligible participation.[4]

Blomgren and Andersson, in 1969, showed that cortisone resistant thymocytes were far more active in inducing graft-versus-host (GvH) splenomegaly in neonatal mice than were suspensions of untreated thymocytes.[5] The hypothesis that the cortisone-resistant thymocytes represented a population similar to peripheral lymph node lymphocytes was supported by the observation that the volume distribution of these two groups of cells was identical. Cortisone-resistant thymocytes were later shown to be more active than untreated thymocytes suspensions in cooperation with bone marrow in the humoral response to a number of antigens.[6]

Further experiments involving volume changes during blastoid transformation,[7] GvH reactivity,[8] cooperation with B-cells in the response to sheep red blood cells (SRBC),[9] generation of "killer cells,"[10–11] capacity to recirculate[12–13] rosette-forming ability[14] and PHA responsiveness[11–15] have established beyond reasonable doubt that cortisone-resistant thymocytes represent a highly active immunocompetent subpopulation within the thymus. However, the above findings have been interpreted to indicate that cortisone-resistant thymocytes are the only immunocompetent cells in the thymus.[5–11] We present evidence herein to the contrary, and propose that there may be several interacting populations within the thymus. Tigelaar and Asofsky have recently reached similar conclusions using a different assay system.[16]

Experimental Plan

Previous studies on the responsiveness of thymocyte populations, fractionated by sensitivity to cortisone, have been done by comparing the responses of

* This work was supported by Public Health Service Grants CA–08593 and AI 10,497 from the National Institute of Health.

† Richard K. Gershon is a recipient of a career development award CA 10,316 from the National Cancer Institute.

equivalent doses of cortisone-resistant cells with those of untreated thymocytes. Such comparisons have shown that the cortisone-resistant cells are more active on a cell-for-cell basis but do not rule out the possibility that the cortisone-sensitive cells are participating, at least somewhat, in the measured responses. To study this question we have tried to compare the response of equal numbers of cortisone-resistant cells in the presence and in the absence of cortisone-sensitive cells. To do this, we inoculated a given number of mice with cortisone. Two days later we harvested their thymuses and also the same number of thymuses from uninoculated controls. After making the cell suspensions and counting, we suspended the harvested cells from both groups of donors in an equal volume of diluent. Lethally irradiated recipient mice were inoculated with 0.2 ml of cells and thus all received the same percentage of the cell yield. If it is true that the treatment with cortisone did not affect the number of cortisone-resistant thymus cells this means that although recipients of normal cells got >15 times more total cells, they got approximately the same number of cortisone-resistant cells as those mice which got those cells only. There are no direct experimental data to validate the above assumption. However, the differences in response reported below cannot be explained by simply postulating that the cortisone treatment altered the number of recovered cortisone-resistant cells, as important qualitative as well as quantitative distinctions were observed.

The assay we used for the activity of the inoculated cells has been described in detail elsewhere.[17–20] It consists of inoculating the thymocytes into lethally irradiated recipients and using that amount of DNA they synthesize, after antigenic stimulation, as a measure of their response to that antigen. Normal thymocytes do not ordinarily synthesize measurable amounts of DNA in syngeneic recipients unless stimulated with antigen.[17–20] This assay yields results that are qualitatively indistinguishable from those which measure mitoses of chromosomally marked T-cells.[19]

Materials and Methods

Mice

Male C_3H, $CDF_1(C_3H \times DBA/2)$ and CBA mice were obtained from Jackson Laboratory, Bar Harbor, Maine. They were rested in our animal facility for one week before use. Thymocyte donors were 5 weeks old, recipients were 7–8 weeks old.

Irradiation

A Siemens 250 KV machine with a 2 mm aluminum filter was used for irradiation. Mice were placed in a plexiglass chamber on a rotating platform and received 900 R at a dose rate of 85 R per minute.

Sheep Erythrocytes

These were maintained in refrigerated Alsevers solution and washed three times before use. They were inoculated intraperitoneally (i.p.) into recipient mice in a volume of 0.2 ml.

Cell Suspensions

Donor mice were killed by cervical dislocation and thymuses carefully dissected out under sterile conditions. They were then gently squeezed between two sterile glass slides. The cell suspension thus obtained was filtered through three layers of gauze and washed twice in ice-cold sterile medium M-199 with 100 units/ml penicillin, streptomycin, kanamycin, and 10 units/ml heparin. Viable cell counts were made with a hemocytometer using the trypan-blue dye exclusion method.

Cortisone

Donor mice were given i.p. injections of 2.5 mg of cortisone acetate ("Cortone," Merck, Sharpe and Dome). These animals were sacrificed 48 hours later and cell suspensions made from their thymuses.

Cell Inoculations

These were given i.v. by tail vein, in a volume of 0.2 ml.

Technique for Assaying DNA Synthesis of Thymocytes

This technique has been described in detail elsewhere.[17] Lethally irradiated mice were inoculated with the appropriate experimental suspensions of thymocytes on the first day (Day 0) of the experiment. On the day of assay of DNA synthesis, they received an i.p. injection of two microcuries (μCi) of [^{125}I]UDR (5-iodo-2-deoxyuridine) in 0.2 ml (Amersham/Searle or New England Nuclear, specific activity 4–6 μCi/μg). The [^{125}I]UDR is incorporated into DNA in the place of thymidine.[21] Twenty-four hours later the animals were killed and their spleens and in some cases femoral lymph nodes were dissected out and placed in counting tubes containing formalin. At the termination of the experiment, the spleens and nodes were counted for six minutes in a Nuclear-Chicago gamma counter. Also counted at this time was a standard aliquot of 0.2 ml [^{125}I]UDR from the same lot used in inoculating test animals. The counts in the experimental tubes were divided by the counts of the standard, and the result expressed as percent uptake of isotope. All counts had been corrected for background.

Statistical Analysis

Results were analyzed using Students t-test.

Results

Response to SRBC in Syngeneic Recipients

Thirty CBA mice were inoculated with cortisone and thirty were left alone. Two days later thymus cell suspensions were made from both groups of mice. The normal thymuses yielded a total of 4.8×10^9 cells and the cortisone-treated thymuses 8.0×10^7 (a yield of approximately 1.8% of normal). Both cell suspensions were subdivided so that 1/40th of the total cell yield was present in 0.2 ml. Thirty-six lethally irradiated recipients were given 0.2 ml of cortisone-resistant cells (2.4×10^6 cells each) and 36 recipients were given 0.2 ml of normal thymocytes (2.4×10^6 cortisone-resistant cells each, in a total inoculum of 1.3×10^8 cells). Antigen (0.2 ml of 10% SRBC) was administered either on the day of irradition and thymocyte infusion, day 0 (12 mice in each group), on days 0 and 1 (12 mice each), on days 0, 1, and 2 (8 mice each) or on days 0, 1, 2, and 3 (4 mice each). DNA synthesis in the recipients' spleens was measured on days 2, 3, and 4 as described above. Data are expressed as the ratio of the total response of the cortisone-resistant thymocytes to the total response of the normal thymocytes; this ratio would be unity if the cortisone-resistant thymocytes were the only reactive cells in the thymus. A deviation from unity would imply participation by the cortisone-sensitive cells; in a positive fashion if less than one and in a negative fashion if greater. The responses of mice getting 1 or 2 doses of SRBC are the sums of the measurements made on days 2, 3, and 4 (4 mice each day). Mice getting 3 doses of SRBC were measured on days 3 and 4, and mice getting 4 doses only on day 4.

It can be seen (FIGURE 1) that the number of SRBC injections markedly influenced the ratio of the cortisone-resistant:normal thymocyte DNA synthetic response. The response of the cortisone-resistant fraction of thymocytes to one immunization with SRBC was significantly less than that of the whole population ($p < 0.05$); but became slightly better after a second immunization, ($p = \text{N.S.}$) became much better after 3 immunizations ($p < 0.01$) and became significantly less after the fourth immunization ($p < 0.05$). These results indicate that cortisone-sensitive thymocytes can partake in the DNA synthetic response elicited by SRBC. Their participation may be either positive or negative (or neutral) depending on the mode of immunization. It cannot be decided on the basis of these experiments if they respond directly to antigen or to signals they may receive from the cortisone-resistant cells. We have conconfirmed these findings in 2 other strains of mice ($C_3H \times DBA_2$ F_1 and $C_{57}Bl_6 \times A$ F_1 mice) with widely differing thymocyte doses as well as different doses of SRBC. It is clear that the cortisone-resistant fraction of a thymocyte inoculum cannot account for the entire activity of the whole inoculum.

Response to Histocompatibility Antigens and to SRBC in Allogeneic Recipients

It has been suggested that thymocytes may be particularly endowed with a capacity to react against the histocompatibility antigens possessed by other animals of the same species.[22] Therefore, we also compared cortisone-resistant thymocytes to unfractionated cell populations in response to the antigens coded for by the major histocompatibility locus of the mouse (H-2). In addition, we immunized some of the test animals with SRBC to see if multiple SRBC immunizations in an allogeneic system would produce similar alterations to those produced when the donor and host were syngeneic.

We divided the thymocyte field from 20 cortisone-treated and 20-untreated C_3H mice, so that approximately 1/25th of the total cell yield from each group of donors was in 0.2 ml of medium and inoculated this volume into 48 lethally irradiated CDF_1 ($C_3H \times DBA/2$) mice. The untreated thymuses yielded 1.1×10^9 total cells and the cortisone treated 7.7×10^7 (7%). (We have found that C_3H thymuses are consistently smaller than those of CBA mice and contain a higher proportion of cortisone-resistant cells resulting in a similar yield of cortisone-resistant cells from the thymuses of both strains.) Thus, in these experiments 24 F_1 mice were given approximately 3.2×10^6 cortisone-resistant thymocytes and 24 others were given the same number of cortisone-resistant cells in a total thymocyte inoculum of 4.5×10^7. Nine recipients of each thymocyte inoculum received no further treatment; 9 were given 0.2 ml of a 10% suspension of SRBC i.p. on the day of thymocyte inoculation (day 0) as well as on day 1; and 6 were given the SRBC inoculations on days 0, 1, and 2. DNA synthesis in the recipients spleens and lymph nodes was determined on days 2, 3, and 4 as described above. The data were computed and are presented (FIGURE 2) similarly to those in the previous experiment. It can be seen that the response of the thymocytes from cortisone-treated donors to the recipients histocompatibility antigens was clearly less than that of the thymocytes from untreated mice ($p < 0.02$ in spleens; < 0.05 in lymph nodes).

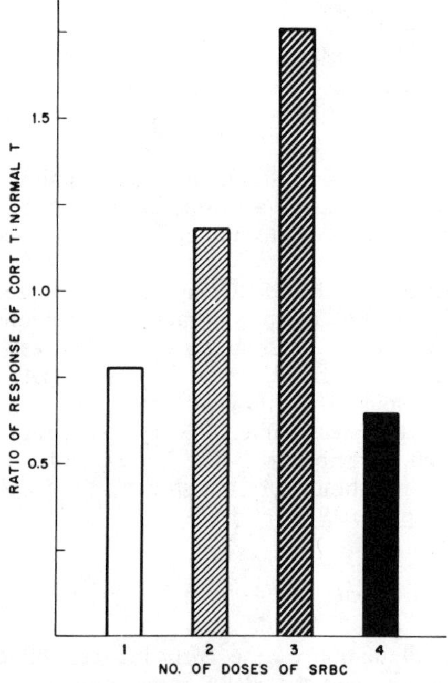

FIGURE 1. The total DNA synthetic response of the cortisone-resistant fraction of a thymus cell population divided by the response of the whole population, in response to different numbers of daily SRBC injections.

We have found cortisone-resistant:whole-thymocyte response ratios of approximately 1/2, in response to H-2 antigens in other strain combinations (AKR → AKR × DBA/2 and A → Balb/C × A) using differing cell doses.

In addition, the results show that inoculation of SRBC can alter the ratio of responsiveness between these cell populations. Similar to the results in syngeneic recipients, increasing amounts of antigen increase the response ratio of the cortisone-resistant:normal cells up to a point past which a decline occurs. These results are presented in greater detail in FIGURE 3 where the daily responses of the mice in each group are given. There it can be seen that the SRBC injections produced relatively small changes in the response of the normal thymocytes whereas they caused wide swings in the response of the cortisone-resistant cells. Thus, the differences in the ratio of responsiveness of

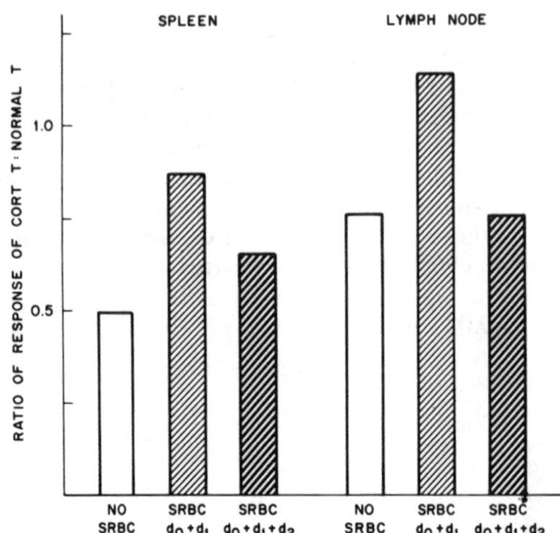

FIGURE 2. The total DNA synthetic response of the cortisone-resistant fraction of a thymus cell population divided by the response of the whole population in a GvH reaction with or without additional stimulation with SRBC.

cortisone-resistant thymocytes:unfractionated cells secondary to stimulation with different antigen dose schedules is mostly due to variations in the response of the cortisone-resistant cells. The presence of cortisone-sensitive cells appears to dampen these variations.

The nature of the changes produced by the SRBC injections in these experiments, particularly in the lymph nodes, is of special interest. Injections of SRBC on days 0 and 1 resulted in a marked synergistic reaction between the SRBC inoculations and the stimulation produced by the histocompatibility antigens of the host. (note: i.p. injections of the dose of SRBC used in these experiments do not ordinarily lead to any measurable DNA synthetic response in the femoral lymph nodes of syngeneic recipients). The injection of a third dose of SRBC on day 2 not only was nonstimulatory but shut off the response produced by the first two injections ($p < 0.05$).

Response in a Regulatory Role

The synergistic effects between stimulation of the cortisone-resistant cells with the hosts histocompatibility antigens and the SRBC inoculations, as well as the pronounced shut-off effect produced by the third SRBC injection indicate that significant cell interactions between the cortisone resistant cells occurred. The lack of such interaction effects between these cells when cortisone sensitive cells were present suggested that the latter cells might be acting in a regulatory fashion. We have previously reported that F_1 cells can regulate the response of parental thymocytes in lethally or sublethally irradiated F_1 mice.[18, 23–25] We therefore performed an experiment to see if the regulatory effects that F_1 thymocytes produce could be altered by separating the cortisone-resistant cells from the rest of the F_1 thymocyte population. To do this, we inoculated 36 lethally irradiated CDF_1 mice with 4×10^7 normal C_3H thymocytes; 12 of these mice got in addition ⅕ of a normal CDF_1 thymus (1×10^7 cells) and 12 got ⅕ of a thymus from a cortisone treated F_1 mouse (3×10^5 cells). Both F_1 thymocyte populations were irradiated with 900 R prior to injection, as this radiation dose has been shown to stop their DNA synthesis without stopping their regulatory effects.[25]

The cortisone-resistant cells significantly suppressed the response of the parental cells (FIGURE 4) in both the spleens and lymph nodes ($p < 0.005$ in both cases). However, their suppressive effect was abolished when cortisone-sensitive cells were present, as the untreated F_1 thymocytes did not significantly

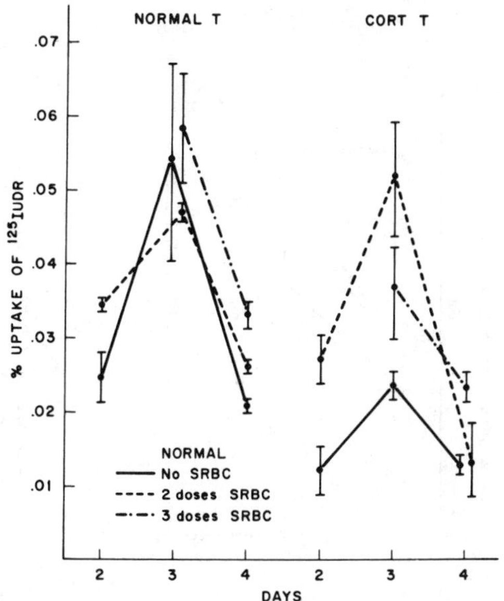

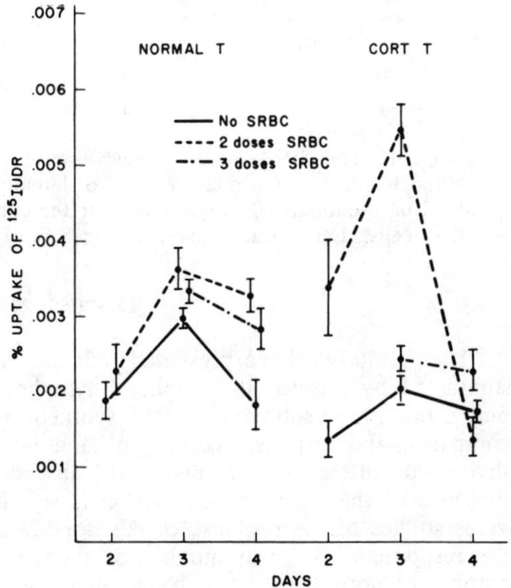

FIGURE 3. The daily DNA synthetic response of unfractionated thymocytes and the cortisone-resistant fraction of them in a GvH reaction, with or without additional daily stimulation with SRBC. *Upper:* response in the spleen; *Lower:* response in the femoral lymph nodes. Each point is the mean ± S.E. of 3 individual determinations.

alter the response of parental cells. These results support the notion that some cortisone-resistant thymocytes regulate the response of other cells and that cortisone-sensitive cells exert a modulating influence on this regulation. These results should not be interpreted to mean that unfractionated F_1 thymocytes cannot suppress the response of parental cells. Whether or not they will do so depends on a number of factors.[24, 25] The point is that one of these factors is the presence of cortisone-sensitive cells.

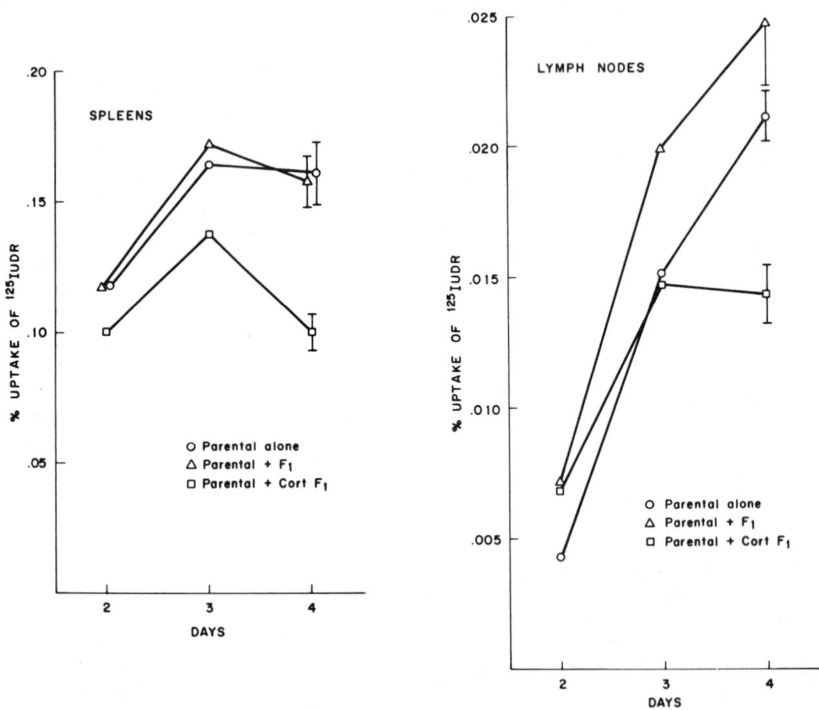

FIGURE 4. The DNA synthetic response of parental thymocytes in the spleens (*left*) and femoral lymph nodes (*right*) of lethally irradiated F_1 mice in the presence of added unfractionated F_1 thymocytes, or the cortisone fraction of them, or without added F_1 cells. Each point is the mean ± S.E. of 4 individual determinations.

DISCUSSION

The results we have presented indicate that when normal thymocytes are stimulated by antigen in peripheral lymphoid tissue, cortisone-sensitive cells play a role in the subsequent DNA synthetic response. We have shown this by comparing the response to antigen of a given number of cortisone-resistant thymocytes in the presence and in the absence of cortisone-sensitive cells. The presence of the cortisone-sensitive cells significantly alters the response. Previous studies of the response of cortisone-resistant thymocytes have compared the response of a given number of these cells to the response of an equal number of normal cells and have found the cortisone resistant fraction to be much more active on a cell-for-cell basis.[2–11] Our results also indicate that cortisone-resistant cells are a highly reactive subpopulation of thymocytes; indeed, with some antigen dose schedules they are *more* reactive when separated from the cortisone-sensitive cells than they are when cortisone-sensitive cells are present. This result suggests that cortisone-sensitive cells may suppress the response of resistant cell and point up a difficulty in interpretation of the data we have presented. Since we are unable to isolate populations of cortisone-sensitive cells, free of resistant ones and since cortisone-resistant cells respond quite well to antigen in the absence of cortisone-sensitive cells, we cannot determine whether the participation of the cortisone-sensitive cells is induced directly by the antigen or indirectly via signals from the respondng cortisone-resistant cells or both. Their ability to suppress the response of the cortisone-resistant cells suggests that regulatory interactions between these two cell populations do occur. Indeed, the marked dependence of the cortisone-resistant: normal thymocyte response ratio on antigen dose and timing is similar to previous reports of bidirectional regulatory interactions between thymocyte subpopulations.[23-25] In those studies it was shown that F_1 cells altered the GvH reaction produced by parental thymocytes. The regulatory F_1 thymocytes were shown to have a predilection for splenic localization[24] as do cortisone-sensitive cells.[12] In addition, their regulatory capacities were very sensitive to stress,[24] which is consistent with a sensitivity to cortisone. The F_1 cells could either increase or decrease the reaction. One of the factors that determined which of these effects the F_1 cells would produce was the dose of parental thymocytes used to produce the GvH reaction. The effects the cortisone-sensitive cells had in the present report was also dose-dependent; varying the immunizing SRBC dose could cause the influence of the cortisone-sensitive cells to change from helper to suppressor.

The experiments we did comparing the regulatory capacity of cortisone-resistant F_1 thymocytes to that of unfractionated cells also indicate that cortisone-sensitive cells may play an important regulatory role. We showed that cortisone-resistant F_1 cells were significantly better at suppressing the response of parental thymocytes to histocompatibility antigens when they were isolated from accompanying cortisone-sensitive cells. This observation suggests that the cortisone-resistant F_1 cells had a regulatory effect on the response of the parenteral cells and that the cortisone-sensitive cells regulated that regulation. Such an effect might be thought of as one of modulation.

The cortisone-sensitive cells also had a modulatory effect on the response to SRBC. Two injections of SRBC into F_1 mice that had received an inoculation of cortisone-resistant parental thymocytes produced a marked increase in thymocyte DNA synthesis. A third injection of the SRBC shut off the DNA synthesis the first 2 injections had produced. On the other hand, these SRBC injections had relatively little effect on the thymocyte DNA synthesis when cortisone-sensitive cells were present; another example of a modulating influence exerted by cortisone-sensitive cells.

As the story of the cellular events that lead to an immune response unfolds, it is becoming more apparent that quite complex interactions between cells occur.[16-18, 20, 23-27] These interactions are both of a specific and nonspecific nature.[28-33] Thus, teleologically, a "modulator cell" seems not to be a bad idea. That such a cell should be sensitive to cortisone also seems reasonable from a teleological point of view. Under conditions of stress when endogenous cortisone is released and extreme and rapid reactions are needed, modulation, such as might be required to prevent autoimmunity,[34] might not be biologically advantageous.

The relationship of the results we have presented to what transpires during an immune response under less experimentally contrived conditions is not absolutely clear. The possibility exists that cortisone-sensitive thymocytes are immature cells that would not leave the thymus unless they were forced to do so by the experimenter and thus, the results we have presented are artifacts of the experimental conditions. On the other hand, immature thymocytes (which have been referred to as T_1) may leave the thymus.[26] These cells are amongst the cortisone-sensitive fraction and the evidence that they ordinarily leave the thymus prior to the acquisition of cortisone resistance seems quite good (reviewed in Raff and Cantor [26]). Thus, it is possible that cortisone-sensitive cells subserve the same functions in peripheral tissues as their counterparts in the thymus. Their participation in GvH reactions seems to be consistently more positive than it does in the response to SRBC. Tigelaar and Asofsky have made similar observations.[16] This may explain why Wilson and Nowell find such high numbers of cells reacting in mixed lymphocyte reactions,[35] and also why so many of the reacting cells come from a population which has recently divided.[36] Cortisone-sensitive cells are much more mitotically active than are those cells that are resistant to the drug.[37]

In any case, our results clearly show that cortisone-sensitive thymocytes can partake in the DNA synthetic response to antigen, either directly or by influencing the response of those cells that are resistant to the drug. More recently we have been able to show similar modulating effects of cortisone-sensitive thymocytes in the generation of antitumor killer cells.[38] This work, in conjunction with the recent demonstration of interactions between cortisone-resistant and cortisone-sensitive thymocytes in the production of GvH splenomegaly and toxicity,[16] indicates a possible important function for cortisone-sensitive T-cells, not heretofore appreciated.

Summary

The role of cortisone-sensitive thymocytes in the *in vivo* DNA synthetic response to antigen was examined by comparing the response of a given number of cortisone-resistant thymocytes, which had been separated from cortisone-sensitive cells, to the response of the same number of cortisone-resistant cells in the presence of the cortisone-sensitive cells. The presence of cortisone-sensitive cells significantly altered the response. Inocula of unfractionated thymocytes synthesized more DNA in response to a single injection of SRBC or in a GvH reaction than could be accounted for by the response of their cortisone-resistant fractions, indicating that cortisone-sensitive thymocytes can contribute in a positive fashion in response to antigen. However, with certain schedules of hyperimmunization, the response of the unfractionated thymocytes was significantly less than that of the separated cortisone-resistant fraction, indicating that cortisone-sensitive cells may also act as "suppressor" cells. Multiple injections of SRBC led to marked alterations in the amount of DNA the separated cortisone-resistant cells synthesized without producing much change in the response of unfractionated cell populations. Thus, the presence of cortisone-sensitive cells had a modulating influence on the response of cortisone-resistant cells. Modulation by cortisone-sensitive cells was shown in another way. The separated cortisone-resistant fraction of an inoculum of F_1 thymocytes suppressed the response of parental thymocytes to F_1 antigens, but failed to do so when cortisone-sensitive F_1 cells were included in the inoculum. These results indicate that at least some cells within the cortisone-sensitive thymocyte population are not immunologically inert and may play a role in immunoregulation.

ACKNOWLEDGMENT

The expert technical assistance rendered by Ronald Hencin is greatly appreciated.

REFERENCES

1. DOUGHERTY, T. F. 1952. Physiol. Rev. **32:** 379–401.
2. WARNER, N. L. 1964. Aust. J. Exp. Biol. Med. Sci. **42:** 401–416.
3. WEBER, W. T. 1966. J. Cell Physiol. **68:** 117–126.
4. WEBER, W. T. 1970. Clin. Exp. Immunol. **6:** 919–940.
5. BLOMGREN, H. & B. ANDERSSON. 1969. Exp. Cell Res. **57:** 185–192.
6. ANDERSSON, B. & H. BLOMGREN. 1970. Cell Immunol. **1:** 362–371.
7. BLOMGREN, H. 1971. Clin. Exp. Immunol. **8:** 279–289.
8. COHEN, J. J., M. FISCHBACH & H. N. CLAMAN. 1970. J. Immunol. **105:** 1146–1150.
9. COHEN, J. J. & H. N. CLAMAN. 1971. J. Exp. Med. **133:** 1026–1054.
10. BLOMGREN, H., M. TAKASUGI & S. FRIBERG. 1970. Cell Immunol. **1:** 619–631.
11. BLOMGREN, H. & E. SVEDMYR. 1971. Cell Immunol. **2:** 285–299.
12. LANCE, E. M. & S. COOPER. 1970. Hormones and the Immune Response. Ciba Foundation Study Group **36:** 73–95.
13. BLOMGREN, H. & B. ANDERSSON. 1972. Clin. Exp. Immunol. **10:** 297–303.
14. BACH, J. F. & M. DARDENNE. 1971. C.R. Acad. Sci. **272:** 1318–1319.
15. ELLIOTT, E. V., V. WALLIS & A. J. S. DAVIES. 1971. Nature New Biol. **234:** 77–78.
16. TIGELAAR, R. E. & R. ASOFSKY. 1973. J. Immunol. **110:** 567–574.
17. GERSHON, R. K. & R. HENCIN. 1971. J. Immunol. **107:** 1723–1728.
18. BERSHON, R. K., P. COHEN, R. HENCIN & S. A. LIEBHABER. 1972. **108:** 586–590.
19. KRUGER, J. & R. K. GERSHON. 1972. J. Immunol. **108:** 581–585.
20. GERSHON, R. K. & S. A. LIEBHABER. 1972. J. Exp. Med. **136:** 112–127.
21. FOX, B. W. & W. H. PRUSOFF. 1965. Cancer Res. **25:** 234–240.
22. JERNE, N. K. 1971. Eur. J. Immunol. **1:** 1–9.
23. LIEBHABER, S. A., J. BARCHILON & R. K. GERSHON. 1972. J. Immunol. **109:** 238–243.
24. GERSHON, R. K., K. KONDO & E. M. LANCE. 1974. J. Immunol. **112:** 546–554.
25. GERSHON, R. K., S. A. LIEBHABER & S. RYU. Immunology. In press.
26. RAFF, M. C. & H. CANTOR. 1971. *In* Progress in Immunology. : 83–93. Academic Press. New York, N.Y.
27. ASOFSKY, R., H. CANTOR & R. E. TIGELAAR. 1971. *In* Progress in Immunology. : 369–381. Academic Press. New York, N.Y.
28. GERSHON, R. K. & K. KONDO. 1970. Immunology. **18:** 723–737.
29. GERSHON, R. K. & K. KONDO. 1971. Immunology. **21:** 903–914.
30. GERSHON, R. K. & K. KONDO. 1971. J. Immunol. **106:** 1524–1531.
31. KATZ, D. H., W. E. PAUL, E. A. GOIDL & B. BENACERRAF. 1971. J. Exp. Med. **133:** 169–186.
32. WU, C. Y. & B. CINADER. 1971. J. Exp. Med. **134:** 693–712.
33. FELDMAN, M. & A. BASTEN. 1972. J. Exp. Med. **136:** 49–67.
34. ALLISON, A. C., A. M. DENNAM & R. D. BARNES. 1971. Lancet **ii:** 135–140.
35. WILSON, D. B. & P. C. NOWELL. 1971. J. Exp. Med. **133:** 442–453.
36. NOWELL, P. C. & D. B. WILSON. 1971. J. Exp. Med. **133:** 1131–1148.
37. ESTEBAN, J. N. 1968. Anat. Rec. **162:** 349–356.
38. FRANK, G., L. FREEDMAN & R. K. GERSHON. J. Immunol. Submitted

TRANSFER OF DELAYED HYPERSENSITIVITY BY THYMIC EXTRACT

Elias G. Elias and Robert M. Cohen

Department of General Surgery
Roswell Park Memorial Institute
New York State Department of Health
Buffalo, New York 14203

Introduction

It has been reported that thymic extracts administered to animals with intact thymuses would result in lymphocytosis [1, 2] and lymphopoiesis.[3, 4] On the other hand, the administration of thymic extracts to neonatally thymectomized mice resulted in a rise in the lymphocyte count, prevention of the wasting disease,[5, 6] improvement of the ability to develop cutaneous delayed hypersensitivity (DHS) response,[7] and the capacity of the spleen cells to mount a graft-versus-host (GvH) reaction.[8, 9] All these experiments measured the T-cell function and suggested that the T-cell differentiation was stimulated by some component of the thymic extracts. It had also been reported that the extracts of human peripheral blood leukocytes were effective in transferring cutaneous delayed hypersensitivity in man.[10, 11]

The purpose of this report is to present data indicating successful transfer of delayed skin hypersensitivity to 2,4-dinitrochlorobenzene (DNCB) and to purified protein derivative of tuberculin (PPD) with thymic extracts in guinea pigs.

Materials and Methods

Animals: The guinea pigs used in these experiments were Hartley strain (Camm/Hartley strain from Camm Research Institute, Wayne, New Jersey) females. Young guinea pigs (GP) that weighed between 175–200 g were the donors of the thymic extract, while adult GP weighed between 600–700 g were the recipients.

The young donors were divided into three groups. One group was sensitized by DNCB, another by BCG, and the third group was left unsensitized (controls).

DNCB Sensitization

The guinea pigs were sensitized to DNCB by applying 0.005 ml of a 50% DNCB solution in acetone to the dorsal surface of the right ear as described by Turk.[12] These animals were skin tested to confirm DNCB sensitivity, 6 days later, by applying 0.1% DNCB cream (acid mantle vehicle) to skin that had been clipped. Those who showed delayed hypersensitivity were used as donors and were sacrificed on the 8th day.

PPD Sensitization

The animals were sensitized to PPD by injecting 1 mg of Connaught BCG intradermally in the back of the neck. Seven days later, the dorsal hair was clipped and each animal was tested with 0.1 ml (250 TU) of Connaught PPD by intradermal injection. Those who showed delayed hypersensitivity were used as donors on the 9th day.

Preparation of Thymus Extract

Three groups of animals were used. All of them were young females and each weighed between 175–200 g. One group was used as a control, i.e. they were not previously sensitized. The other 2 groups were previously sensitized, one with DNCB, and the other received BCG and became PPD positive. All the animals were sacrificed with ether, and the thymus glands were dissected out; the animals in each group were pooled together and treated similarly.

The harvested thymus glands in each group were hand ground in Hank's buffered saline, and centrifuged at $250 \times g$ for ½ hour. The supernatant (TE) was used for the transfer. The controls donated TE^0, the DNCB sensitized animals donated TE^{DNCB}, and the last group that was sensitized to BCG donated TE^{PPD}. The extracts were measured and calculated per gland.

Administration of Thymic Extracts

DNCB Transfer

In this part of the experiment, 30 adult animals were used as recipients. All the animals received thymus extract equivalent to 0.25 of a thymus. Two experiments were then carried out:

Experiment 1. Twelve recipients were used. All thymic extract in this experiment was freshly prepared. Eight animals received TE^{DNCB} by intradermal or intramuscular injections, while the other 4 recipients received TE^0 by the same methods. Some of the animals were then tested for delayed hypersensitivity to DNCB 12 hours after the thymic injections, while the rest of them were tested at 6 days. The delayed hypersensitivity to DNCB was tested as described below.

Experiment 2. Eighteen recipients were used in this part of the experiment. Eight animals received freshly prepared thymic extract while the other 8 received thymic extract that had been stored in deep freeze (−80° C) for 6 days and thawed just before being used. All the animals received the thymic extracts by the intradermal route. Furthermore, 2 animals received stored thymic extract that was ultracentrifuged at $60{,}000 \times g$ for 1 hour and then passed through 0.22 μ Millipore® filter. All the animals were tested 24 hours later for DNCB delayed hypersensitivity.

PPD Transfer

Twenty-four recipients were used for this part of the experiment. All the animals were initially tested for PPD delayed hypersensitivity and were negative.

Experiment 3. Eight animals were utilized in this experiment; 6 of them received TE^{PPD} at different dose levels that ranged from 0.125 to 0.50 of a thymus. The other two received TE^{0} at the 0.50 dose level. Half of the number received the thymic extract intradermally while the others received similar dosage subcutaneously. All the thymic extracts used in this experiment had been stored at —80° C for 24 hours after extraction and thawed just before use. The animals were then tested for DHS to PPD.

Experiment 4. Sixteen animals were used as recipients. All of them received TE^{PPD} that had been stored at —80° C for 3 months before being thawed and utilized in this experiment. These animals received the TE^{PPD} intradermally at different dose levels that ranged from 0.10 to 0.50 of a thymus. The animals were then repeatedly tested by PPD at different intervals to determine the duration of the transfer.

TABLE 1

DNCB TRANSFER: METHODS OF ADMINISTERING THYMIC EXTRACT *

Number of GP	TE Dosage and Type	Route of TE Administration	Positive Skin Tests (DHS) to DNCB at: † 12 hours	6 days
4	0.25 TE^{DNCB}	i.d.‡	2/2	2/2
4	0.25 TE^{DNCB}	i.m.	2/2	2/2
2	0.25 TE°	i.d.	0/2	—
2	0.25 TE°	i.m.	0/2	—

* All thymus extracts were freshly prepared.

† DHS to DNCB was tested by applying 0.01% DNCB cream (acid mantle base) to skin.

‡ Abbreviations: i.d.=intradermally; i.m.=intramuscularly; s.c.=subcutaneously.

Skin Testing

The dorsal surface was clipped with an electric clipper (Oster, blade 0000). For DNCB testing; 0.01% DNCB cream (acid mantle vehicle) was applied to the skin surface to an area of 4 × 3 inches. For PPD testing; 0.1 ml (250 TU) Connaught was injected intradermally. Skin reactions were observed at 24 and 48 hours. Although there were some variations in the intensity of the reactions, all the animals could unequivocally be graded as either positive or negative.

RESULTS

It was clear that transfer of delayed hypersensitivity to DNCB and PPD was established in the guinea pigs by using unpurified thymic extracts. TABLE 1 shows the results of Experiment 1, and it clearly indicates that the thymic

TABLE 2

DNCB TRANSFER: THE EFFECT OF DEEP FREEZE ON THYMIC EXTRACT

Number of GP	TE Type and Dose	Route of TE Administration	Positive Skin Tests (DHS) to DNCB at 24 hours *
4	TE^{DNCB} 0.25 (fresh)	i.d.	4/4
4	TE^{DNCB} 0.25 (stored) †	i.d.	4/4
4	TE° 0.25 (fresh)	i.d.	0/4
4	TE° 0.25 (stored) †	i.d.	0/4
2	TE^{DNCB} 0.25 (stored filtrate) ‡	i.d.	2/2

* DHS to DNCB was tested by applying 0.01% DNCB cream to skin.
† Stored at −80° C for 6 days then thawed just before use.
‡ Filtrate—TE was ultracentrifuged (60,000 × *g* for 1 hour) then passed through 0.22μ millipore filter.

extract from animals previously sensitized to DNCB established a transfer of delayed hypersensitivity, to DNCB, whether administered intradermally or intramuscularly. The delayed hypersensitivity to DNCB could be detected when the animals were tested 12 hours and 6 days after receiving the specific thymic extract.

TABLE 2 shows that stored or fresh thymus extracts can transfer delayed hypersensitivity to DNCB and it also indicates that the thymic filtrate may have the same activity as the unpurified extracts.

The results of Experiment 3 as shown in TABLE 3, demonstrate that PPD delayed hypersensitivity can be transferred by the intradermal as well as by the

TABLE 3

PPD TRANSFER: DOSE LEVEL AND DIFFERENT ROUTE OF ADMINISTRATION OF THYMIC EXTRACT

Number of GP *	TE Type and Dosage †	Route of TE Administration	Skin Tests (DHS) 2 days	3 days	5 days	3 months
2	TE^{PPD} 0.125	1 i.d.	+ ‡	+	+	—
		1 s.c.	+	—	+	—
2	TE^{PPD} 0.25	1 i.d.	+	+	+	—
		1 s.c.	+	+	+	—
2	TE^{PPD} 0.50	1 i.d.	+	+	—	—
		1 s.c.	+	+	—	—
2	TE° 0.50	1 i.d.	—	—	—	—
		1 s.c.	—	—	—	—

* All were PPD (250 TU) negative before receiving TE.
† All TE was stored at −80° C for 24 hours.
‡ +=positive for DHS; —=negative for DHS.

subcutaneous route, and it seemed that as little as 0.125 of a thymic extract was sufficient to establish a transfer.

Finally, the results of Experiment 4 as expressed in TABLE 4, show the effect of a single injection of stored thymic extracts at different dose levels, and again it seemed that 0.10 of a thymus was sufficient to establish transfer of delayed hypersensitivity, which seemed to reach a maximum at the second week, but some activity was also noted at 6 weeks.

DISCUSSION

It is clear from the above results that a small dosage of thymic extracts can transfer delayed hypersensitivity to DNCB and PPD in the guinea pigs, known to be very resistant to the Lawrence transfer factor (that is obtained from the peripheral leukocytes).[13] Indeed, as little as 0.10 of a thymus was required to establish this transfer. The deep freeze storage of the thymic extracts did not

TABLE 4

PPD TRANSFER: THE EFFECT OF SINGLE INJECTION OF STORED THYMIC EXTRACT *

Number of GP	TE^{PPD} Dosage †	Positive Skin Tests for DHS, to 250 TU PPD					
		2 D ‡	1 W	2 W	3 W	4½ W	6 W
5	0.10	2/5	4/5	5/5	5/5	5/5	3/5
6	0.30	3/6	3/6	4/6	2/6	4/6	0/6
5	0.50	2/5	3/5	4/5	2/5	2/5	1/5

* TE^{PPD} was stored at —80° C for 3 months.
† TE^{PPD} was given intradermally to all recipients.
‡ D=days; W—weeks.

abolish their ability to transfer delayed hypersensitivity. The duration of the transfer seemed to reach a maximum in 2 weeks, and there was some activity even at 6 weeks after a single dose of thymic extract. This was demonstrated in the PPD system but not in the DNCB simply because we do not retest any animal that had been exposed to DNCB.

These results would suggest that some component of the thymic extract could stimulate T-cell differentiation *in vivo*.

SUMMARY

Successful transfer of cutaneous delayed hypersensitivity to DNCB and PPD was established in the guinea pigs utilizing thymic extracts. As little as 0.10 of a thymus (extract) was sufficient to establish this transfer. The storage of these thymic extracts in deep freeze for 3 months did not abolish its activity or ability to transfer DHS.

References

1. Rehn, E. 1940. Deut. Med. Wochenschr. **66:** 594.
2. Bomskow, C. H. & L. Slavodic. 1940. Deut. Med. Wochenschr. **66:** 589.
3. Klein, J. J., A. L. Goldstein & A. White. 1965. Proc. Nat. Acad. Sci. U.S. **53:** 812.
4. Trainin, N., M. Burger & A. M. Kaye. 1967. Biochem. Pharmacol. **16:** 711.
5. DeSomer, P., P. Denyo, Jr. & R. Layten. 1963. Life Sci. **11:** 810.
6. Trainin, N., A. Bejerano, M. Stahilevitch, D. Goldring, & M. Small. 1966. Israel J. Med. **2:** 549.
7. Jankovic, B. D., K. Isakovic & J. Horvat. 1965. Nature **208:** 356.
8. Bach, J., M. Dardennc, A. L. Goldstein, A. Guha & A. White. 1971. Proc. Nat. Acad. Sci. U.S. **68:** 2734.
9. Goldstein, A. L., Y. Asanuma, J. R. Battisto, M. A. Hardy, J. Quint & A. White. 1970. J. Immunol. **104:** 359.
10. Lawrence, H. S. 1954. J. Clin. Invest. **33:** 951.
11. Lawrence, H. S. 1969. Advan. Immunol. **2:** 195.
12. Turk, J. L. 1967. Delayed Hypersensitivity. North Holland Pub. Co. Amsterdam, The Netherlands; and J. Wiley & Sons, Inc. New York, N.Y.
13. Jeter, W. S., M. M. Tremaine & P. M. Seebohm. 1954. Proc. Soc. Exp. Biol. Med. **86:** 251.

THE RELATIONSHIP BETWEEN CFU KINETICS AND THE THYMUS

E. Frindel and H. Croizat

Institut de Radiobiologie Clinique INSERM
Institut Gustave-Roussy
Villejuif, France

Introduction

Colony forming units (CFU) in the marrow of rodents have been extensively studied since the pioneering work of Till and McCulloch.[1] In the mouse, these cells seem to be able to differentiate along any one of several hematological lines although the mechanism of the "choice" of the CFU towards one or the other series is not known. Some work has been done which suggests a "microenvironmental" influence,[2] but little is known of the nature of this influence. It seems that once development of a colony has proceeded to a certain point the cell population will only differentiate to one type of hematological cell. It is believed that beyond a certain stage of differentiation in any developing colony that the completion of the process is affected by promoting factors such as erythropoietin on erythropoiesis and possibly colony-stimulating factor on granulocytopoiesis. As far as the lymphoid system is concerned, it is not known whether there are any promotory influences.

Becker and McCulloch[3] have shown that a large proportion of CFU are quiescent and only a small fraction of these cells are suicidable by lethal doses of [^{3}H]TdR. However, this proportion can increase under a great variety of circumstances such as stimulation by erythropoietin,[4] endotoxin and bleeding.[5]

In our animal colony, we found a relatively high proportion of CFU in DNA synthesis (S), and this proportion increased during an outbreak of infectious disease. It thus seemed interesting to try and find out if the presence of microorganisms could influence CFU proliferation and if so, by what mechanism.

In the present paper we wish to report the experiments that were undertaken to try and elucidate the problem of the proliferative status of CFU under these circumstances and explore the possibility that immunological processes might be involved in the triggering of CFU.

It is known that the thymus plays a very important role in immunological responses[6] and we wished to see if it also played a role in CFU proliferation and differentiation. Some authors have shown[7] that the number of CFU may vary after neonatal thymectomy.

Materials and Methods

Animals

All experiments were performed on C3H female mice unless otherwise stated. They were aged from 2 to 3 months and were either axenic, holoxenic or neoholoxenic. The neoholoxenic mice were germ-free mice placed in a nonsterile environment for 21 days after 5 days of monocontamination by a clostridium.

Antigen

The antigen used was either Salmonella typhosa (Institut Pasteur) injected intraperitoneally at a dose of 5×10^7 bacteria in 0.10 ml or peroxidase type VII-L at a dose of 250 μg per mouse injected subcutaneously.

Diffusion Chambers

Cell impermeable Millipore® chambers (0.22 μm) were inserted in the peritoneal cavity of the mice. They were either empty or contained one adult thymus lobe per chamber.

Thymectomy

Neonatal thymectomy was performed in the first 18 hours after birth following the technique of Bealmear and Wilson.[8] Adult thymectomy was performed at 8 weeks of age.

CFU Quantitation

The number of CFU was determined by the method of Till and McCulloch and the proportion of CFU in DNA synthesis was assessed by the method of Becker and McCulloch. Recipient mice aged from 2 to 3 months were irradiated with a dose of 900 rads (200 Kv, 12 mA, HVL 0.87 Cu) 24 hours before injection of the marrow. The mice were killed nine days later and spleens fixed in Bouin's for 24 hours before the nodules were counted. The donor bone marrow was divided into two groups: (a) cells were incubated for 20 minutes at 37° C in 2 ml of Eagle's or Hank's medium with 500 μCi of [^{3}H]TdR; (b) cells were incubated in the same conditions but without [^{3}H]TdR. The percentage of CFU in S was calculated by the following formula: $S = \frac{(b) - (a)}{(b)}$; 10^5 donor cells were injected per mouse.

Results

Response of CFU's to Antigenic Stimulation in Axenic, Holoxenic, and Neoholoxenic Mice

Table 1 summarizes the results. A pool of bone marrow from three mice was injected into 24 mice for each group of experiments. Table 2 shows the results of 5 replicate experiments.

There is a significant difference between the proportion of suicidable CFU

TABLE 1

NUMBER OF CFU/10^5 CELLS AND THE PROPORTION OF CFU UNDERGOING DNA SYNTHESIS IN AXENIC, HOLOXENIC, AND NEOHOLOXENIC MICE

Donors		Holoxenic Mice	Axenic Mice	Neoholoxenic Mice	Days after Stimulation with Antigens of Axenic Mice: 2 days	11 days
Average number of nodules	Incubation with [^{3}H]thymidine	8.5 ± 3.5	16.68 ± 4.2	8.8 ± 4.2	17.2 ± 4.8	17.1 ± 3.8
	Incubation without [^{3}H]thymidine	11.3 ± 2.9	16.78 ± 4.3	11.5 ± 2.5	20.2 ± 3.3 *	25.4 ± 4.8 *
% of CFU in DNA synthesis		25	0	24	13	33

* Significantly different from nonstimulated axenic mice ($p < 0.05$).

TABLE 2

PROPORTION OF CFU IN S IN AXENIC MICE

Experiment	Axenic Mice Without ^{3}H	With ^{3}H	% in S
I	18.5 ± 3.58	18.5 ± 2.44	0
II	12 ± 3.48	12 ± 3.68	0
III	13.1 ± 2.44	13.1 ± 2.56	0
IV	16 ± 4.25	15 ± 7.09	8
V	18.1 ± 2.64	18.4 ± 2.5	0

in holoxenic and axenic mice, whereas the neoholoxenic mice are similar to the holoxenic ones. In the axenic mice we could not demonstrate any CFU in S, whereas in holoxenic and neoholoxenic mice about 25% of the CFU were in DNA synthesis. Two and 11 days after the injection of Salmonella O antigen, the percent of suicidable CFU increased in axenic mice.

The Effect of Neonatal Thymectomy on the Proliferative Status of CFU in Axenic Mice

These experiments were conducted using 52 donors and 340 recipients. TABLE 3 shows that peroxidase has an effect on the proportion of CFU in S, which increases from 0 to 33% at 8 days after injection and gradually returns to normal by 36 days. Peroxidase had practically no effect on neonatally thymectomized mice whether the CFU were investigated at 8 days or 26 days after immunization. TABLE 4 shows that in axenic mice the thymus graft does not modify the proportion of CFU in S (it is 0 in control axenic mice). However, this percentage increased to 35% 16 days after antigen stimulation. In thymectomized axenic mice, the thymus graft does not increase the proportion of CFU in S since in mice with an intact thymus this proportion is 0. However, the thymus graft restores the capacity of CFU to respond to antigen and the proportion of CFU in S increases to 39% after injection of peroxidase.

TABLE 3

EFFECT OF THYMECTOMY ON CFU RESPONSE TO ANTIGEN

Time after injection (days)	Axenic Mice			Thymectomized Axenic Mice		
	Without ^{3}H	With ^{3}H	% in S	Without ^{3}H	With ^{3}H	% in S
8	21.7±5.3	14.8±2.5	33	24.3±4.8	22.7±3.7	7
11	18.3±3.0	13.8±2.8	25	—	—	—
16	19.5±1.2	14.2±2.9	29	—	—	—
26	—	—	—	15.8±5.5	13.6±6.6	13
29	18.2±5	16±4.3	12	—	—	—
36	18.8±3.9	19.6±5.3	0	—	—	—

TABLE 4

EFFECT OF THYMUS GRAFT IN THYMECTOMISED MICE

	Without ^{3}H	With ^{3}H	% in S	Without ^{3}H	With ^{3}H	% in S
40 days after thymus graft	19.1±4.3	19±3.8	0	19.1±2.1	18.5±2.1	3
40 days after thymus graft & 15 days after antigen injection				18±5.1	11±2.4	39
16 days after simultaneous thymus graft & antigen injection	19.8±1.7	13±7.2	35	20.5±4.5	14.6±5.3	29

The Effect of Adult Thymectomy on CFU Response in Holoxenic Mice

A pool of 3 to 5 donors and 24 recipients was used for each experimental point. On an average 2 to 3 replicate experiments were done for each group. The results were obtained from 493 surviving recipients. The antigen used was Salmonella O and the proliferative status of CFU was tested 14 days after thymectomy and 2 and 10 days after antigen challenge.

TABLE 5 demonstrates the fact that as early as 7 days after adult thymectomy and during the 8 months of observation the proportion of CFU in S was consistently nil, whereas in sham thymectomized mice this proportion varied from 17 to 26%. The number of CFU per leg was very slightly lower in the thymectomized animals and the bone marrow cellularity did not show any significant difference in the two groups of mice.

TABLE 6 shows that 2 days and 10 days after injection of Salmonella O antigen, the percentage of CFU in S increases to about 30% in sham thymec-

TABLE 6

ANTIGEN STIMULATION (SALMONELLA O)

Time after Stimulation		2 days: Sham Thymectomy	2 days: Thymectomy	10 days: Sham Thymectomy	10 days: Thymectomy
Cells per leg × 10^6		14.3	14.1	20	20
Number of CFU per leg		2,290	1,840	2,360	2,000
CFU per 10^5 nucleated cells±σ	Incubated without [^{3}H]TdR	16±1.8	13±3	11.8±2.2	10±1.7
	Incubated with [^{3}H]TdR	11±1.4	13±3	8±2.5	10.6±1.8
% CFU in S phase		31	0	32	0

TABLE 5

THYMECTOMY AT 8 WEEKS OF AGE

Time after thymectomy		7 days		14 days		30 days		11 weeks		8 months	
		Sham Tx	Tx	Sham Tx	Tx	Sham Tx	Tx	Sham Tx	Tx	Sham Tx	Tx
Cells per leg $\times 10^6$		19.8	23.6	27.6	17.0	—	21.0	26.0	33.0	24.6	21.5
CFU per 10^5 nucl. cells±σ	Incubated without [³H]TdR	15.8±2.5	10.9±3	12.5±2.5	15.8	—	11.6±2.9	10.6±3	7±1.8	13.3±3.6	10±2
	Incubated with [³H]TdR	13±8	10.9±3	9.2±1.8	16	—	11.5±2.2	8.3±2.4	7.1±1	11±2	10.5±4
% CFU in S phase		18	0	26.4	0	—	0	20	0	17	0
Number of CFU per leg		3,130	2,580	3,440	2,680	—	2,440	2,760	2,310	3,270	2,150

TABLE 7

BLEEDING

		Sham Thymectomy	Thymectomy
Number of nucleated cells per leg $\times 10^6$		16.5	16.5
Number of CFU per 10^5 nucleated cells$\pm\sigma$	Incubated without [^{3}H]TdR	16.2±2.6	17.5±1.9
	Incubated with [^{3}H]TdR	10±2	13.2±1.8
% CFU in S phase		38	25
Number of CFU per leg		2,670	2,880

tomized mice, whereas it remains at 0 in thymectomized mice. When these mice were bled (TABLE 7) or challenged with colony-stimulating factor, the CFU were triggered into synthesizing DNA in the absence of the thymus as well as in the presence of the thymus.

CFU Response to a "Thymic Factor"

C3H female mice were thymectomized at 8 weeks of age and another group of mice was sham thymectomized at the same age. Millipore chambers, each either empty or with a thymus lobe from an 8-week old mouse, were inserted into the peritoneal cavity on the same day as thymectomy or sham thymectomy. In one group of mice Salmonella antigen was injected 10 days after thymectomy and diffusion chamber insertions.

One-hundred and sixty recipient mice were used in 3 replicate experiments using 2 groups of mice: thymectomized mice having either empty or "full" chambers. The results are summarized in TABLE 8.

TABLE 8

EFFECT OF EMPTY OR THYMUS-CONTAINING DIFFUSION CHAMBERS ON CFU PROLIFERATION

		Number of CFU/10^5 Cells			
Experiment	Diffusion Chamber	Without [^{3}H]TdR	[^{3}H]TdR	% in S	Number of Mice
I	empty	14.5±3.6	14.8±4.5	0	30
	containing thymus	14.4±3.6	12.5±2.6	13	27
II	empty	16.5±3.4	16.3±2.3	0	27
	containing thymus	13.4±4.8	10.3±2.4	20.5	27
III	empty	13.6±3	13.6±5.9	0	26
	containing thymus	14.8±5.7	12±5.6	19	19

As can be seen, in all three experiments, the percentage of CFU in S was nil in those thymectomized mice which had empty diffusion chambers whereas it was almost normal in mice which had diffusion chambers containing a thymus lobe. In sham thymectomized mice, diffusion chambers did not have a constant effect.

In the next series of experiments using 110 recipients (TABLE 9) thymectomized mice were challenged with Salmonella antigen and CFU tested 10 and 14 days later. It can be seen that antigen had very little effect when the diffusion chambers were empty, but the effect was restored when diffusion chambers contained thymus. In sham thymectomized mice, the effect of diffusion chambers was variable. In one experiment, a single neonatal thymus was included in the Millipore chamber but it showed no effect.

TABLE 9

EFFECT OF EMPTY OR THYMUS-CONTAINING DIFFUSION CHAMBERS ON CFU PROLIFERATION AFTER ANTIGEN STIMULATION

Time after Ag Stimulation (days)	Diffusion Chamber	Number of CFU/10^5 Cells		% in S	Number of Mice
		Without [^{3}H]TdR	[^{3}H]TdR		
10	empty	14.3±3.7	12.7±3	11.4	27
	containing thymus	16±2.8	12.5±2.6	22	27
14	empty	11.8±2.3	10±2.6	14.4	27
	containing thymus	13.9±2.6	11.2±2	20	29

DISCUSSION

It has been shown that bone marrow stem cells are mostly quiescent. The fact that sometimes, in apparently normal mice, the quiescent state can be disrupted, was intriguing. The same strain of mice kept in either holoxenic or axenic conditions had very different percentages of suicidable CFU. It could be suggested that the bacterial flora provoked some gastrointestinal modifications, such as inflammation or microscopic bleeding, that could explain the high proportions of CFU in S in holoxenic mice.

Therefore, axenic mice were used as a model for determining whether there was some specific effect of antigens on CFU either directly or by some indirect mechanism. It was found that CFU were indeed quiescent in axenic mice but that they could be stimulated into DNA synthesis by the injection of two different types of antigen or by taking the mice out of sterile conditions. It has been shown that when axenic mice are removed from the germ-free environment there is a significant increase in the immunoglobulin level.[9]

To determine whether the effect observed was a direct one on CFU or was in some way connected to an immunological process, thymectomies were performed on neonatal and adult mice. Thymectomy reduced the proportion of suicidable CFU in all cases and seemed to render CFU unresponsive to antigen stimulation. However, one cannot affirm that the unresponsiveness is complete. It may be delayed or a greater quantity of antigen may be necessary in the absence of the thymus to trigger the CFU.

One should note that thymectomy did not modify the response of CFU to bleeding nor to CSF stimulation.

Our results suggest that antigen has no direct effect on CFU and that the CFU response to antigen is thymus-dependent. The exact mechanism of this dependency has not yet been elucidated. In response to antigen stimulation, either exogenous or endogenous, some modification may occur in the process of T- and/or B-cell differentiation and proliferation. This may in turn have an effect on CFU if one believes that the latter cell is pluripotential and a precursor of the lymphocyte series. In the absence of the thymus, these modifications cannot occur for some, as yet unknown, reason.

It is a suggestion that thymus may secrete some "factor" comparable to erythropoietin and that this factor is necessary for the processes triggered by antigen stimulation. This does not exclude the possibility of other tissues secreting this "factor" as well and we are now testing various organs in diffusion chambers and under the kidney capsule.

An alternative possibility is that the thymus secretes a factor that could be quite independent of any immunological processes and that might trigger off a whole cascade of events resulting in CFU proliferation.

The preliminary results imply that there is a definite relationship between the thymus and the proportion of suicidable CFU. The experiments using the diffusion chambers, although they give some indication that a factor may be operating, do not entirely satisfy us. Therefore, injection of purified thymic factor is now envisaged.

In conclusion one may say that there is a relationship between the thymus and the proportion of suicidable CFU. Antigen seems to stimulate CFU into DNA synthesis and this stimulation is thymus-dependent. Preliminary experiments seem to suggest that some "thymic factor" is involved in the process, but there are not enough data as yet to testify definitely that it is via this "factor" that the thymus plays a role in CFU kinetics.

References

1. McCulloch, E. A. & J. E. Till. 1961. Radiat. Res. **14:** 213.
2. Wolf, N. S. & J. J. Trentin. 1968. J. Exp. Med. **127:** 205.
3. Becker, A. J., E. A. McCulloch & J. E. Till. 1965. Blood **26:** 296.
4. Feldman, M. 1969. *In* Effects of Radiation on Cellular Proliferation and Differentiation. : 223. International Atomic Energy Agency. Vienna, Austria.
5. Boggs, D. R., J. C. Marsh, P. A. Chevernick, G. E. Cartwright & M. M. Wintrobe. 1968. Radiat. Res. **35:** 68.
6. Miller, J. F. A. P. 1961. Lancet **2:** 748.
7. Resnitsky, P., D. Zipori & N. Trainin. 1971. Blood **37:** 634.
8. Bealmear, P. M. & R. Wilson. 1967. Cancer Res. **27:** 358.
9. Sell, S. & J. L. Fahey. 1964. J. Immunol. **93:** 81.

THE ABSOLUTE REQUIREMENT FOR T-CELLS IN THE INDUCTION OF IgM-SECRETING CELLS, *IN VITRO*

Ko Okumura and Milton Kern

National Institute of Arthritis, Metabolism,
and Digestive Diseases
National Institutes of Health
Bethesda, Maryland 20014

The helper cell function of thymus-derived (T) cells in mouse has been well documented by the demonstration that the production of immunoglobulins by bone marrow derived (B) cells is stimulated by T-cells.[1, 2] As a consequence of this operational definition, the term helper cell carries with it the connotation that such T-cells aid but are not necessarily requisite for immunoglobulin production by B-cells. Moreover, in a number of reports based on *in vivo*[3, 4] as well as *in vitro*[5, 6] studies the effect of bacterial lipopolysaccharide has been described as T-cell independent. Indeed, it has been reported that lipopolysaccharide can induce immunoglobulin production in the absence of T-cells.

In order to study the role of T-cells in the induction process, rabbit lymph node cells cultured in the absence of antigen provide a simple means of assessing the induction of IgM secreting cells.[7, 8] Under these circumstances, the induction of IgM production reflects the activities of a much larger population than that measured by focusing on antigen-stimulated cells of a single specificity, but it suffers the limitation that antigen involvement cannot be assessed. Nevertheless, using cells cultured in the absence of antigen, evidence for an absolute requirement for T-cell involvement in the induction of IgM secreting cells will be demonstrated herein, along with our evidence indicating that lipopolysaccharide stimulation of immunoglobulin production is T-cell dependent.

Materials and Methods

The materials used and the procedures followed for the immunization of rabbits have been described.[9, 10] Conditions for the isolation of popliteal lymph nodes[11, 12] were as before except that sterile techniques were used. The cell culture technique as well as the conditions for the labeling of immunoglobulins after cell culture incubation have also been previously described.[7, 8] ^{3}H-labeled immunoglobulin secreted into the extracellular fluids was assayed by specific immune coprecipitation.[13]

Anti-rabbit thymocyte serum was prepared in a goat injected with 2×10^{10} rabbit thymocytes in Freund's complete adjuvant and boosted with the same material on two occasions at 14 day intervals. The serum obtained two weeks after the third injection was heated at 56° C for 30 minutes and then absorbed with rabbit erythrocytes until no hemagglutination was detected. The serum was further absorbed with 1/20 volume of normal rabbit bone marrow cells and then absorbed with the IgM-rich euglobulin fraction of serum covalently linked to Sepharose®-4B. Finally, the serum was tested for its cytotoxic activity against various lymphoid cells by the dye exclusion test. The serum used in these studies maximally killed virtually 100% of thymus cells, 20% of spleen cells, 30% of lymph node cells and <2% of bone marrow cells. The highest dilution of antithymocyte serum yielding 50% cytototoxicity for thymocytes was 1:2048.

In tests to assess the specificity of antithymocyte serum, 1.0 ml of serum was absorbed with 2×10^{10} thymocytes at 3° C for 1 hour and after centrifugation to remove cells the process was repeated. As a control, bone marrow cells were similarly used for absorption.

Antisera preparations digested with pepsin [14] were reduced with dithiothreitol at a final concentration of 0.01 M and alkylated with excess iodoacetamide to produce univalent antibody.[15]

TABLE 1

EFFECT OF ANTITHYMOCYTE SERUM ON THE INDUCTION OF IGM SYNTHESIS *in Vitro* *

Antiserum used	Treatment	Volume (ml)	Inhibition (%)
ATS	DEAE	0.5	100
		0.1	95
		0.001	34
ATS	pepsin	0.5	99
		0.1	91
		0.001	26
ATS	pepsin R/A	0.5	96
AOv (control)	pepsin R/A	0.5	0

* Rabbit lymph node cells, goat anti-rabbit thymocyte serum (ATS) and goat anti-ovalbumin serum (AOv) were used in these experiments. DEAE treatment refers to purification of antiserum by diethylaminoethyl-cellulose chromatography. Pepsin digestion and reduction and alkylation (R/A) of the pepsin product were performed by standard techniques. Immunoglobulin production was assessed after 72 hours of cell culture.

Results

We have previously demonstrated [7, 8] that freshly isolated popliteal lymph node cells synthesize and secrete principally IgG together with a relatively small amount of IgM. After incubation in cell culture for 48 hours in the absence of added antigen, such IgG production approached zero while IgM production was enhanced about 10-fold. Therefore, the capacity of cells to secrete immunoglobulins after incubation in culture for 72 hours can be used as a convenient measure of the induction of IgM producing cells.

The data of TABLE 1 show that the presence of antithymocyte serum during cell culture results in virtually complete inhibition of the induction of immunoglobulin production. Pepsin-digested antithymocyte serum as well as univalent antithymocyte antibody derived by reduction and alkylation of the pepsin digestion product were similarly inhibitory, whereas a control antiserum specific for ovalbumin was without effect.

TABLE 2

LOSS OF INHIBITORY ACTIVITY OF ANTITHYMOCYTE ANTIBODY AFTER ABSORPTION WITH THYMOCYTES *

	Inhibition by Antithymocyte Serum		
Volume of serum	Unabsorbed (%)	Absorbed with Thymocytes (%)	Absorbed with Bone Marrow Cells (%)
0.5	88	28	88
0.1	87	17	87
0.03	24	0	38

* ATS preparations were digested with pepsin after absorption with cells. Immunoglobulin production was assessed after 72 hours of cell culture.

Since antithymocyte serum was prepared from thymus cells it was necessary to establish that the antiserum was directed toward thymocyte surface antigens that are specific for T-cells. Clearly, absorption of antithymocyte serum with thymocytes reduced the inhibitory capacity of the antiserum, whereas absorption of antiserum with bone marrow cells had no effect on the extent of inhibition due to antiserum (TABLE 2).

The fact that antithymocyte serum affected the induction of immunoglobulin production rather than immunoglobulin synthesis and secretion per se, was indicated by the finding that addition of antiserum at 48 hours did not inhibit the amount of immunoglobulin that cells could ultimately produce after 72 hours in culture (TABLE 3). Under these same circumstances, antithymocyte serum was inhibitory when added to cells at 24 hours, i.e., at a time prior to completion of the induction process. Furthermore, a brief treatment of cells with antithymocyte serum was sufficient to inhibit the induction of immunoglobulin production. Thus, lymph node as well as spleen cell populations briefly incubated with antithymocyte serum and washed before being cultured for 72 hours produced very small amounts of immunoglobulin (TABLE 4).

TABLE 3

EFFECT OF DELAYED ADDITION OF ANTITHYMOCYTE ANTIBODY ON THE INDUCTION OF IMMUNOGLOBULIN PRODUCTION *

Time of Addition of ATS †	Inhibition (%)
0 hr	94
24 hr	87
48 hr	0

* Cells were incubated in culture for a total of 72 hours and antithymocyte serum (ATS) was added at the time indicated. Immunoglobulin production was assessed after incubating the cells in tissue culture for 72 hours.

† 0.5 ml of pepsin digested antithymocyte serum was added to each culture bottle.

TABLE 4

EFFECT OF THE ADDITION OF THYMOCYTES ON CELLS TREATED WITH ANTITHYMOCYTE SERUM *

Cell Mixtures	^{3}H-Labeled Immunoglobulin Production (cpm)
Lymph node (2)	12,110
ATS-lymph node (2)	770
ATS-lymph node (2) + thymus (2)	1,100
Thymus (2)	0
Spleen (2)	1,190
ATS-spleen (2)	90
Thymus (4)	0
ATS-spleen (2) + thymus (2)	1,110
↓ (4)	2,250
↓ (6)	3,330
Spleen (2)	1,190
Spleen (2) + thymus (4)	2,640
↓ + (4)	4,110
↓ + (6)	5,700
Lymph node (2)	6,280
Lymph node (2) + thymus (2)	6,360
Thymus (2)	80

* Cells treated with antithymocyte serum (ATS) were incubated with ATS in tissue culture incubation medium at 3° C for 1 hour. The cells were washed and resuspended in fresh medium prior to tissue culture incubation. Immunoglobulin production was assessed after 72 hours in tissue culture. The values in parentheses refer to number of cells × 10^8 that were added per 10 ml of culture medium. ATS-spleen and ATS-lymph node refer to ATS-treated spleen and lymph node cells, respectively. ATS was digested with pepsin prior to use.

Subsequent to their treatment with antithymocyte serum, lymph node and spleen cells differed in their behavior upon culture in the presence of untreated thymocytes. In many experiments, such treated lymph node cells cultured with thymocytes from the same animal produced, at best, only a marginally greater quantity of immunoglobulin. On the other hand, spleen cells treated with antithymocyte serum routinely responded substantially to the presence of thymocytes. Untreated spleen and untreated lymph node cells also differed in regard to their behavior when cultured with thymocytes. Although spleen cells exhibited an enhanced immunoglobulin production, untreated lymph node cells were essentially unaffected by the presence of thymocytes during cell culture.

In view of the reports that immunoglobulin production in response to bacterial lipopolysaccharide is T-cell independent,[3-6] it was of interest to test the effect of lipopolysaccharide on untreated as well as antithymocyte-treated cells. To begin with, both untreated spleen and lymph node cells showed a 2- to 4-fold lipopolysaccharide-mediated enhancement of immunoglobulin production.[8] However, lipopolysaccharide did not replace the requirement for T-cells as judged from the relatively small increase in immunoglobulin production resulting from the incubation of cells treated with antithymocyte serum in culture with lipopolysaccharide (TABLE 5). For example, untreated spleen cells yielded a lipopolysaccharide-mediated stimulation of immunoglobulin production of about 6000 cpm (see TABLE 5), whereas after antithymocyte serum treatment of spleen cells the lipopolysaccharide-mediated stimulation of immunoglobulin production was only 600 cpm.

Discussion

These experiments show that the presence of antiserum specific for T-cells totally inhibited the induction of immunoglobulin production by lymph node cells, *in vitro*. Whether or not the antithymocyte antibody reacts with T-cell sites that are necessary for interaction with B-cells or if such T-cell sites are sterically hindered by the presence of antibody cannot be decided from these data. However, the finding that univalent antithymocyte antibody also inhibited the induction process provides evidence that complement-mediated reactions that are dependent on bivalent antibody, such as cytotoxic reactions, are not involved in the mechanism of inhibition.

Before considering the effect of thymocytes on spleen and lymph node cells treated with antithymocyte antibody, it is convenient to first discuss the effect of thymocytes on untreated lymph node and spleen cells. First of all, no simple explanation can be offered to account for the difference in the behavior of lymph node and spleen cell populations incubated with thymocytes. Despite the fact that lymph node and spleen cells were derived from the same animal, only spleen cells showed an enhanced immunoglobulin production when cultured in the presence of thymocytes. Such results may indicate that spleen cell populations are deficient in the pertinent T-cells and therefore respond to thymocytes.

TABLE 5

EFFECT OF LIPOPOLYSACCHARIDE ON ANTITHYMOCYTE-TREATED CELLS

Cell Source	Cells Initially Incubated with	Lipopolysaccharide Added (μg/ml)	Immunoglobulin ^{3}H-Labeled Production (cpm)
Lymph node	culture medium	0	11,970
	culture medium	5	20,630
	ATS	0	900
	ATS	5	2,040
Spleen	culture medium	0	5,210
	culture medium	5	11,330
	ATS	0	500
	ATS	5	1,110

* Cells were initially incubated with culture medium or pepsin-digested antithymocyte serum (ATS) in culture medium at 4° C for 1 hour. The cells were washed, suspended in culture medium, and lipopolysaccharide was added as indicated. Immunoglobulin production was assessed after 72 hours of culture.

On the other hand, the difference in the behavior of lymph node and spleen cell populations may be a consequence of differences in the B-cell population. This possibility is suggested by the fact that spleen cell populations treated with antithymocyte antibody responded to thymocytes whereas similarly treated lymph node cell populations did not. Implicit in this view is the notion that certain cells, possessed in common by both lymph node and spleen, are irreversibly inactivated with regard to the induction of immunoglobulin production as a consequence of treatment with antithymocyte antibody and that spleen cell populations in addition possess cells capable of reacting with thymocytes under the conditions used. Regardless of which interpretation ultimately proves to be correct it is clear that thymocytes, as a T-cell source, substantially enhanced the induction of immunoglobulin production by spleen cells treated with antithymocyte antibody.

There is presently considerable controversy over whether or not lipopolysaccharides can stimulate the induction of immunoglobulin production in the absence of T-cells.[16, 17] Clearly, in the present study, a T-cell dependence for lipopolysaccharide was indicated by the inhibitory effects of antithymocyte antibody. In the absence of evidence herein for T-cell independence of lipopolysaccharide, the mechanism of stimulation of induction of immunoglobulin production by lipopolysaccharide remains unexplained. Two attractive possibilities are that lipopolysaccharide may exert its influence by providing for a firmer link between B- and T-cells or that lipopolysaccharide may function as a general mitogenic stimulus perhaps augmenting the specific mitogenic stimulus provided by T-cells.

Summary

Anti-rabbit thymocyte antibody can totally inhibit the induction of IgM production that ordinarily is observed when lymphoid cells are incubated, *in vitro,* in the absence of added antigen. Univalent as well as bivalent antithymocyte antibody preparations were inhibitory when added to cells before the induction of immunoglobulin production had occurred but not afterwards.

Spleen cells that had been treated with antithymocyte antibody and then cultured with thymocytes for 72 hours exhibited an enhanced induction of immunoglobulin production. Untreated spleen cells also showed this property, although both untreated lymph node cells and lymph node cells treated with antithymocyte antibody did not respond to thymocytes.

The enhancement of the induction of immunoglobulin production by lipopolysaccharide was found to be T-cell dependent as judged from studies using antithymocyte antibody.

Acknowledgment

We wish to thank Mr. Charles Rabkin for technical assistance during the course of this study.

References

1. Miller, J. F. A. P. & G. F. Mitchel. 1969. Transplant. Rev. **1:** 3.
2. Claman, H. N. & E. A. Chaperon. 1969. Transplant. Rev. **1:** 92.
3. Schmidtke, J. & F. J. Dixon. 1972. J. Exp. Med. **136:** 392.
4. Jones, J. M. & P. D. Kind. 1972. J. Immunol. **108:** 1453.
5. Sjöberg, O., J. Andersson & G. Möller. 1972. Eur. J. Immunol. **2:** 326.
6. Watson, J. R., R. Epstein, I. Nakoinz & P. Ralph. 1973. J. Immunol. **110:** 43.
7. Zimmerman, D. H. & M. Kern. 1973. J. Immunol. **111:** 761.
8. Zimmerman, D. H. & M. Kern. 1973. J. Immunol. **111:** 1326.
9. Kern, M., E. Helmreich & H. N. Eisen. 1959. Proc. Nat. Acad. Sci. U.S. **45:** 862.
10. Helmreich, E., M. Kern & H. N. Eisen. 1961. J. Biol. Chem. **236:** 464.
11. Swenson, R. M. & M. Kern. 1967. Proc. Nat. Acad. Sci. U.S. **57:** 417.
12. Sutherland, E. W., III, D. H. Zimmerman & M. Kern. 1970. Proc. Nat. Acad. Sci. U.S. **66:** 987.
13. Swenson, R. M. & M. Kern. 1968. Proc. Nat. Acad. Sci. U.S. **59:** 546.
14. Utsumi, S. & F. Karush. 1965. Biochemistry **4:** 1766.
15. Nisonoff, A., F. C. Wissler, L. M. Lipman & D. L. Woernley. 1960. Arch. Biochem. Biophys. **89:** 230.
16. Coutinho, A. & G. Möller. 1973. Nature New Biol. **245:** 12.
17. Kagnoff, M. F., P. Billings & M. Cohn. 1974. J. Exp. Med. **139:** 407.

IN VIVO STUDIES OF DIFFERENTIATION OF THYMUS-DERIVED LEUKEMIC CELLS *

Anna D. Barker and Samuel D. Waksal †

Biomedical Sciences Section
Battelle's Columbus Laboratories
Columbus, Ohio 43201

Introduction

That thymus-derived lymphocytes (T-cells) are a heterogeneous population of cells is suggested by differences in surface antigens,[1, 2] recirculation properties,[3] and sensitivity to corticosteroids,[4] x-irradiation,[5] and antilymphocyte serum.[6] This heterogeneity is thought to be a result of changes occurring in these cells during maturation. These differences have been more clearly delineated in experiments designed to determine the capacity of thymus cells and T-cells to effect or participate in humoral and/or cell-mediated immune responses.[7, 8]

If, as has been suggested by Pilgrim,[9] neoplastic cells maintain many of the functions of their normal counterparts, subpopulations of T-cells would be expected to occur in animals with a thymus-derived lymphoid leukemia. Indeed, we recently have demonstrated such functional heterogeneity in T-cells derived from AKR mice with a spontaneous viral-induced lymphoma.[10] The administration of lymphoid cells derived from the thymuses (LTC_1), spleens (LSC_1), or lymph nodes ($LLNC_1$) produced three different and distinct disease pathologies in preleukemic recipients. The resultant disease patterns correlated with the homing patterns of these T-cell subpopulations. These differences were further reflected in the differential reactivity of these leukemic T-cells to mitogens and the T-dependent antigen, sheep erythrocytes.[11]

The present report describes the changes in differentiation patterns noted in these neoplastic T-cell subpopulations following second and third *in vivo* passage of these cells. Further, the behavior of certain of these leukemic T-cell subpopulations in splenectomized and thymectomized preleukemic mice is presented.

Materials and Methods

Six 8-week-old and 8 10-month-old AKR mice were obtained from Jackson Laboratories, Bar Harbor, Maine and allowed food and water *ad libitum*.

The thymuses, spleens, and lymph nodes were removed from aged animals with advanced spontaneous lymphoma, the organs weighed, separately pooled in Hank's balanced salts solution (HBSS), and the lymphoid cells were teased

* This study was supported in part by National Institutes of Health Grant 5 SO1–RR05723–03.

† Present Address: Department of Anatomy, College of Medicine, The Ohio State University, Columbus, Ohio, 43210.

free of the tissue. The cells were washed twice in HBSS and the viability was determined by trypan blue exclusion. The cell suspensions were preserved in liquid nitrogen or used immediately for transplant into 8-week-old syngeneic recipients (first transplant). Cells used in second and third transplant experiments were also prepared in this manner.

Eighteen days following intraperitoneal injection of 10^5 LTC_1, LSC_1, or $LLNC_1$ (this cell concentration was used in all experiments), the recipients were sacrificed and their lymphoid tissues removed and weighed. As shown in FIGURE 1, selected lymphoid cell populations from first passage mice were reinoculated into 8-week-old AKR mice (second passage). Cells chosen for

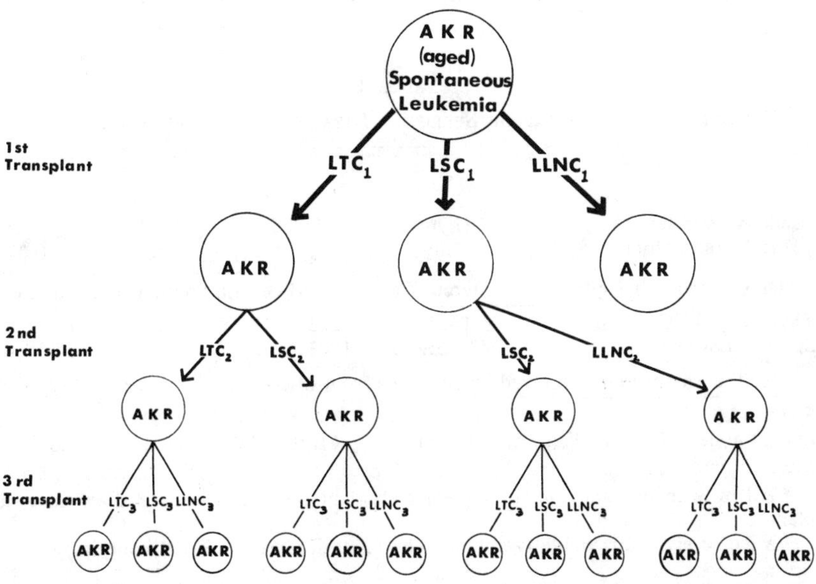

FIGURE 1. Experimental design employed in studies of the *in vivo* differentiation patterns of thymus-derived leukemic cells.

second passage were LTC_2 and LSC_2, and LSC_2 and $LLNC_2$ from first transplant mice originally administered LTC_1 and LSC_1, respectively. The second transplant mice were sacrificed 18 days postimplant, their lymphoid organs removed and weighed, and LTC_3, LSC_3, and $LLNC_3$ were again implanted into 8-week-old recipients (third transplant). These mice were sacrificed 18 days later, and all animals were autopsied and lymphoid tissues were weighed.

In experiments requiring splenectomized or thymectomized mice, 6-week-old mice were used and tested 2 weeks later. At the conclusion of these studies, all mice were routinely examined for thymic or splenic remnants. If residual thymic or splenic tissues were present, these animals were excluded from the studies.

Results

In the original experiments, it was established that transplantation of 10^5 LTC_1, LSC_1, or $LLNC_1$ from AKR mice with spontaneous leukemia into preleukemic AKR mice resulted in three different disease pathologies. Animals given LTC_1 exhibited thymomas, moderate splenomegaly, and lymph node enlargement, whereas complete thymic atrophy and marked splenic and lymph node enlargement were noted in mice given LSC_1. The thymuses of mice given $LLNC_1$ appeared normal and were associated with gross splenic and lymph node enlargement. The mean survival time of mice receiving LTC_1 or LSC_1 was similar, but it was significantly reduced in animals given $LLNC_1$.

It was assumed that first transplant mice receiving LTC_1 or LSC_1 received a greater proportion of undifferentiated T-cells than those given $LLNC_1$. As

TABLE 1

SECOND *in Vivo* PASSAGE OF SELECTED THYMUS-DERIVED LEUKEMIA CELLS

Cells Administered * (2nd Transpalnt)	Weights Thymus (mg)	Spleen (mg)	Lymph Node (mg)	Liver (g)
1st Transplant Mice Received Thymus Cells from Mice with Spontaneous Disease				
Thymus † (LTC_2)	16± 6.7	263± 18.4	25±12.0	1.48±0.3
Spleen (LSC_2)	43.3±20.3	1043± 72.0	30± 5.0	2.78±0.6
1st Transplant Mice Received Spleen Cells from Mice with Spontaneous Disease				
Spleen (LSC_2)	165± 9.9	798± 95.4	79±19.9	3.4 ±0.4
Lymph node ($LLNC_2$)	95±15.0	610±109.0	37±11.0	1.8 ±0.4

* All mice in this and the subsequent transplant were sacrificed 18 days after implant.

† Mice received 10^5 viable lymphoid cells (20 mice/group) in all experiments.

shown in TABLE 1, second transplant experiments were performed on selected populations of thymus-derived leukemic cells from these two groups. Groups of mice implanted with either LTC_2 or LSC_2 (from first transplant mice given LTC_1) exhibited the pathology associated with animals receiving LSC_1 (i.e., thymic atrophy, splenomegaly, and moderate lymph node enlargement). However, thymic atrophy was less pronounced in mice given LSC_2. Mice administered LSC_2 or $LLNC_2$ (derived from first transplant mice given $LLNC_1$) demonstrated the disease pathology characteristic of first transplant mice receiving $LLNC_1$ (TABLE 1).

The lymphoid cells from these four groups of mice were repassaged into preleukemic recipients. In this series of experiments, the effects of LTC_3, LSC_3, and $LLNC_3$ were assessed. The results of these third passage studies are summarized in TABLES 2 and 3. As shown in TABLE 2, all groups of mice exhibited the distinct disease pattern seen in animals originally implanted with $LLNC_1$. Slight thymic atrophy was noted in mice receiving LSC_3 (from LTC_2 mice).

TABLE 2

THIRD *in Vivo* PASSAGE OF THYMUS-DERIVED LEUKEMIC THYMUS, SPLEEN, AND LYMPH NODE CELLS

Group Number	Cells Administered (3rd Transplant)	Weights: Thymus (mg)	Spleen (mg)	Lymph Node (mg)	Liver (g)
	2nd Transplant Mice Received Thymus Cells *				
1.	Thymus † (LTC_3)	124±10.3	780±71	41±4	2.3±0.2
2.	Spleen (LSC_3)	48±16.0	780±30	47±9	2.8±0.2
3.	Lymph node ($LLNC_3$)	71± 8.7	826±36	58±8	2.8±0.4
	2nd Transplant Mice Received Spleen Cells				
4.	Thymus (LTC_3)	65± 2.9	714±18	64±21	2.1±0.1
5.	Spleen (LSC_3)	117±17.6	845±177	40±15	2.7±0.5
6.	Lymph node ($LLNC_3$)	90± 4.0	870±63	58±3	2.5±0.2

* Some mice in groups 4, 5, and 6 died before 18 days postimplant (maximum 2/group). The mean represents the mean obtained from those mice dying from disease and survivors.

† 10 mice/group.

TABLE 3

THIRD *in Vivo* PASSAGE OF THYMUS-DERIVED LEUKEMIC THYMUS, SPLEEN, AND LYMPH NODE CELLS

Group Number	Cells Administered (3rd Transplant)	Weights: Thymus (mg)	Spleen (mg)	Lymph Node (mg)	Liver (g)
	2nd Transplant Mice Received Spleen Cells *				
1.	Thymus † (LTC_3)	90±12	750±90	45±15	2.9±0.4
2.	Spleen (LSC_3)	80±15	760±65	32±5	2.4±0.3
3.	Lymph node ($LLNC_3$)	50±9	756±49	23±5	2.4±0.1
	2nd Transplant Mice Received Lymph Node Cells				
4.	Thymus (LTC_3)	31±5	700±58	24±3	2.3±0.2
5.	Spleen (LSC_3)	15±4	560±92	15±2	1.6±0.2
6.	Lymph node ($LLNC_3$)	24±1.2	672±38	24±7	2.0±0.1

* Several mice in groups 2, 3, 5, and 6 died before 18 days postimplant. The values represent the means obtained from those mice dying of disease (maximum 5/group) and survivors.

† 10 mice/group.

Additionally, one or two animals died in groups receiving LTC_3, LSC_3, and $LLNC_3$ before 18 days postimplant (from LSC_2 mice). The disease pathology noted in mice dying of leukemia and the survivors in these groups at day 18 was similar.

It can be seen in TABLE 3 that preleukemic mice implanted with LTC_3, LSC_3, or $LLNC_3$ (from LSC_2 mice) also displayed enlargement of lymphoid tissues reminiscent of mice given $LLNC_1$. Although several mice in these groups died prior to 18 days postimplant, the pattern of disease development was similar in all of these animals.

The three groups of mice receiving LTC_3, LSC_3, or $LLNC_3$ (from $LLNC_2$ mice) showed the largest percentage of animals dying before the 18-day termination date (4–5 mice/group). All mice demonstrated thymic atrophy, gross splenomegaly, and moderate lymph node enlargement.

The three different types of disease pathology observed in the original studies indicated that the *in vivo* metastatic behavior of the leukemic T-cell subpopulations resulted from a sequential differentiation process. To examine the possible lymphoid organ dependence of this process, selected populations of leukemic T-cells (LTC_1 and LSC_1) were passaged into 8-week-old thymectomized or splenectomized AKR mice. The results of these studies are shown in TABLES 4 and 5. Marked splenomegaly and lymph node enlargement were observed in thymectomized animals receiving LTC_1 or LSC_1 with 20 percent of the mice given LSC_1 surviving through 30 days.

Thymic atrophy was seen in splenectomized animals administered LTC_1 or LSC_1, but was most pronounced in the latter group. It appears that in the absence of a spleen depletion of thymocytes occurs in mice receiving LTC_1, but at a much slower rate than in the group given LSC_1. Mean survival in the thymectomized and splenectomized groups was not significantly increased over that observed in normal preleukemic recipients.

Discussion

The present studies further support our earlier findings that subpopulations of leukemic T-cells exist in mice with a thymus-derived leukemia.[10] The stage of differentiation of these subpopulations is apparently related to the lymphoid

TABLE 4

SURVIVAL AND ORGANOMEGALY IN THYMECTOMIZED PRELEUKEMIC AKR MICE ADMINISTERED THYMUS OR SPLEEN CELLS FROM LEUKEMIC AKR MICE

Cells Administered *	Survival (Days)	Survivors (%)	Weights: Spleen (mg)	Weights: Node (mg)	Weights: Liver (g)
Leukemic thymus cells (10^5) (LTC_1)	27±1.8	10	777.5± 83.7	40± 3.6	2.3±0.4
Leukemic spleen cells (10^5) (LTC_1)	31±2.5	20	923 ±133	50±13.3	2.3±0.2

* Cells derived from AKR mice with spontaneous leukemia (20 mice/group).

TABLE 5

SURVIVAL AND ORGANOMEGALY IN SPLENECTOMIZED PRELEUKEMIC AKR MICE ADMINISTERED THYMUS OR SPLEEN CELLS FROM LEUKEMIC AKR MICE

Cells Administered *	Survival (Days)	Survivors (%)	Thymus (mg)	Weights Node (mg)	Liver (g)
Leukemic thymus cells (10^5) (LTC_1)	26 ± 1.3	0	56 ± 12.7	36 ± 4.2	1.9 ± 0.2
Leukemic spleen cells (10^5)	26 ± 1.4	25	< 10	29 ± 4.2	1.6 ± 0.1

* Cells derived from AKR mice with spontaneous leukemia (20 mice/group).

compartment from which they are derived, with thymus containing primarily undifferentiated cells, spleen being comprised of cells in various stages of differentiation, and lymph nodes containing the greatest proportion of highly differentiated leukemic T-cells. The distinct disease pathologies that result following transplantation of subpopulations from animals with spontaneous leukemia correlated with the expected recirculation properties of these leukemic T-cells.

In studies of normal T-cell differentiation, cells have been shown to be heterogeneous, but the question of whether or not these subpopulations arise from a single line of sequential differentiation or are derived from several precursors has not been resolved. The functional heterogeneity of normal T-cells has been convincingly demonstrated in graft vs. host reactions,[12, 13] the anti-sheep erythrocyte rosette response,[14] and reactivity to mitogens.[15] In addition, the tissue distribution of mature T-cells correlates with that expected for long-lived recirculating T-cells, whereas less mature T-cells are found primarily in thymus and spleen.[8]

Normal T-cell differentiation in the peripheral lymphoid tissues is thought to be influenced by at least two mechanisms. The first results from the action of normal humoral control mechanisms (i.e., thymosin) whereas the second is thought to result from continued antigenic stimulation. Recent work in our laboratory has shown that thymocytes and splenic lymphocytes, cultured *in vitro* with alloantigens, change their migration patterns and behave like lymphocytes derived from lymph nodes.‡ This may represent the normal correlate of the experiments in the present studies which show that continued *in vivo* passage of leukemic T-cells results in uniform disease pathology by the third passage. The disease pathology noted in the third passage studies correlates with the pathology noted in the first transplant following administration of $LLNC_1$. The exception to this is the pathology effected by LTC_3, LSC_3, or $LLNC_3$ derived from animals that had received $LLNC_2$ in the second transplant. The variation seen here is similar to the disease pathology noted in the first transplant in animals receiving LSC_1. This may be due to the existence of a highly differentiated population of $LLNC_3$ with properties that enable them to shut off feedback mechanisms similar to the effect produced by LSC_1. The reduced thymus weights may be due to continued antigenic stimulation of the leukemic cells, or simply reflect the clonal expansion of a single T-cell subpopulation. An

‡ S. D. Waksal, A. D. Barker, and R. L. St. Pierre. Submitted for publication.

alternative explanation for this observation is that subpopulations of leukemic cells have varied effects on normal cells by initiating virus replication.

Although the differentiation of neoplastic T-cells appears to occur sequentially, the removal of key lymphoid tissue apparently does not block this process. Removal of the thymus resulted in increased splenomegaly and lymph node enlargement following administration of LTC_1 or LSC_1. The LTC_1 population may contain a population of differentiated cells which can further proliferate in the spleen and/or a population of undifferentiated thymus cells which are induced to differentiate in the spleen in the absence of a thymus. When recipients were splenectomized and given LTC_1 or LSC_1, thymic atrophy occurred. Although it appears that the spleen may exert a significant influence on the differentiation and release of thymocytes, similar control can be exerted in the absence of a spleen. It is not currently known whether the complete release of thymus cells seen in normal and splenectomized preleukemic animals receiving LSC_1 is due to the same mechanism, but both could result from proliferation of a subpopulation of T-cells that would ultimately effect feedback control processes.

The functional heterogeneity of leukemic T-cells is readily demonstrable in the *in vivo* differentiation studies presented. The capacity of these cells to induce a specific disease pattern in syngeneic recipients provides an objective indicator of the stage of differentiation in leukemic T-cells that is not available in studies of normal T-cell differentiation.

Studies are in progress to determine the possible host factors responsible for the differentiation of thymus-derived leukemic cells following sequential transplantation into syngeneic recipients.

These data continue to suggest that, like their normal T-cell counterparts, leukemic thymus-derived cells exist as subpopulations in various stages of differentiation. The evidence also shows that these leukemic cells retain many characteristics of normal T-cells. Thus, the study of the *in vivo* and *in vitro* characteristics and differentiation patterns of subpopulations of leukemic T-cells from this thymus-derived neoplastic disorder may provide a basis for understanding the differentiation sequence and ultimately the functional heterogeneity of normal T-cells.

Finally, since these cells do maintain many of the characteristics of their normal T-cell counterparts, it may be possible to determine metastatic patterns in this disease which will allow for a greater understanding of leukemogenesis and possible approaches to treatment.

References

1. RAFF, M. C. & H. H. WORTIS. 1970. Thymus dependence of θ bearing cells in peripheral lymphoid tissues of mice. Immunology **18:** 931–942.
2. RAFF, M. C. & J. J. T. OWEN. 1971. Thymus-derived lymphoctyes: Their distribution and role in the development of peripheral lymphoid tissues of the mouse. Eur. J. Immunol. **1:** 27–30.
3. ZATZ, M. M. & E. M. LANCE. 1970. The distribution of chromium 51-labeled lymphoid cells in the mouse. Cell Immunol. **1:** 3–17.
4. SEGAL, S., I. R. COHEN & M. FELDMAN. 1972. Thymus-derived lymphocytes: Humoral and cellular reactions distinguished by hydrocortisone. Science **175:** 1126–1128.
5. DAVIES, A. J. S. & R. L. CARTER. 1972. Systems of lymphocytes in mouse and

man: An interim appraisal. *In* Contemporary Problems in Immunology. **1:** 1–26.

6. CANTOR, H. & R. ASOFSKY. 1972. Synergy among lymphoid cells mediating the graft versus host response. III. Evidence for interaction between two types of thymus-derived cells. J. Exp. Med. **135:** 764–779.
7. RAFF, M. C. & H. CANTOR. 1971. Subpopulations of thymus cells and thymus-derived lymphocytes. *In* Progress in Immunology. **1:** 83–93.
8. CANTOR, H. 1972. T-cells and the immune response. *In* Progress in Biophysics. **25:** 73–82.
9. PILGRIM, H. I. 1972. Relationship of the selective metastatic behavior of tumors of reticular tissues to the migration patterns of their normal cells of origin. J. Nat. Cancer Inst. **49:** 3–6.
10. BARKER, A. D. & S. D. WAKSAL. 1974. Thymus-derived lymphocyte differentiation and lymphocytic leukemias. I. Evidence for the existence of functionally different subpopulations of thymus-derived cells in leukemic AKR mice. Cell Immunol. In press.
11. BARKER, A. D. & S. D. WAKSAL. 1974. Immunologic profiles of AKR leukemic mice. J. Reticuloendothelial Soc. In press.
12. BLOMGREN, H. 1973. Synergism between thymocytes and lymph node cells in the graft versus host response. Effect of cortisone treatment of the thymus cell donor. J. Immunol. **110:** 144–147.
13. CANTOR, H. & R. ASOFSKY. 1970. Synergy among lymphocytic cells mediating the graft versus host response. II. Synergy in graft versus host reactions produced by BALB/c lymphoid cells of differing anatomic origin. J. Exp. Med. **131:** 235–251.
14. BACH, J. F., M. DARDENNE & A. S. S. DAVIS. 1971. Early effects of adult thymectomy. Nature New Biol. **231:** 110–113.
15. STOBO, J. D. 1972. Phytohemagglutin and concanavalin A: Probes for maurine "T" cell activation and differentiation. Transplant. Rev. **11:** 60–86.

INDUCTION OF T-CELL DIFFERENTIATION *IN VITRO* BY THYMUS EPITHELIAL CELLS *

Samuel D. Waksal,† Irun R. Cohen,‡ Harlan W. Waksal,† Hartmut Wekerle,‡ Ronald L. St. Pierre,† and Michael Feldman‡

† Department of Anatomy
Ohio State University College of Medicine
Columbus, Ohio 43210

‡ Department of Cell Biology
The Weizmann Institute of Science
Rehovot, Israel

Introduction

The thymus is responsible for the induction of differentiation and subsequent maturation of thymus-derived lymphocytes (T-cells).[1] T-cells are responsible for such cell-mediated reactions as homograft rejections, graft-versus-host reactivity (GvH) and helper activity in the antibody response to thymic-dependent antigens.[2-4] The thymus effects T-cell differentiation by a mechanism that is not fully understood. The thymic parenchyma consists of an epithelium of cells infiltrated by developing thymocytes.[5] These reticular epithelial cells (TE cells) of the thymus putatively secrete glycoproteins, which have the ability to induce T-cell development.[6,7] Precursor cells arise from the yolk sac and the fetal liver during embryogenesis and from the bone marrow in adult life.[8,9] These cells migrate to the thymus where the differentiation process takes place. The present report describes a system by which thymus epithelium can be grown in cell culture, devoid of any contaminating thymocytes, and used to induce T-cell differentiation *in vitro.* This system allows for an analysis of the development of T-cells *in vitro,* closely imitating *in vivo* conditions.

Materials and Methods

Animals

Four to 6-week-old female C57Bl/6 and BDF_1 mice, and female Lewis (Le) rats obtained from Jackson Laboratories, Bar Harbor, Maine, were maintained on Purina Laboratory Chow and water *ad libitum.*

T-deficient mice

Six to 8-week-old mice were thymectomized and 2 weeks later were irradiated with 900 R, using a 60 cobalt source. After irradiation, the mice were injected with 5×10^6 syngeneic bone marrow cells. All T-deficient mice were used as cell donors after 2 months.

* Supported in part by a grant from the American Cancer Society, Inc.

Supporting Cell Monolayers

Thymus-epithelial monolayers were prepared by asceptically removing thymuses from animals and mincing them until all solid pieces were removed. The minced thymus was put into a flask containing .05% collagenase solution (Type III, Sigma Chemical Company) and allowed to digest overnight at 4° C. Collagenase was then poured off and the minced thymus trypsinized for 10 and 20 minutes. The cells were centrifuged at 800 × *g* and washed in cold Hank's balanced salt solution (HBSS). The cells were then suspended in minimum essential Eagle's medium (MEM) without serum and plated on 60 mm falcon dishes. One 60 mm dish was used per mouse thymus. After two days of culture, the falcon dishes were washed with cold HBSS, MEM +15% fetal calf serum (FCS) was added and the cells maintained as a continuous line. Secondary cell cultures were prepared by trypsinizing the primary cell cultures with 0.1% trypsin. Fibroblast monolayers were prepared from 14- to 16-day-old mouse embryos and maintained on MEM +15% FCS.

Electron Microscopy

Cell monolayers were fixed in 2.5% gluteraldehyde solution in phosphate buffer containing 4% polyvinylpyrrolidone and 1% sucrose pH 7.4 for 18 minutes at room temperature. The cells were rinsed in buffer, dehydrated through graded ethanols and embedded in Araldite 502.

Cell Cultures

Spleens were removed asceptically from mice and teased in cold, sterile HBSS to obtain a single cell suspension. The cells were collected by centrifugation at 180 × *g* for 10 minutes at 4° C and resuspended in RPMI 1640 +10% FCS at a concentration of 1×10^6 per ml. Responses to concanavalin A (con-A, Miles-Yeda Laboratories) were assessed using 13 × 75 mm plastic tubes (Falcon Plastics, Division of Bioquest) at 37° C in a humidified 10% CO_2 atmosphere.

Mitogen Stimulation

One μg per ml final concentration of con-A was used for stimulation. Cells were cultured at a density of 1×10^6 per ml in 1 ml volumes. DNA synthesis was assayed at 72 hours. Twenty-four hours prior to harvest, 0.5 μci tritiated thymidine was added to each culture tube. Cultures were washed twice with cold HBSS, twice with cold 5% trichloracetic acid, and once with cold 95% ethanol. The precipitates were dissolved in 15 ml of Aquasol® liquid and placed in plastic screw-cap tubes and counted in a Beckman scintillation spectrometer. Triplicate cultures were performed for each experimental group.

Graft-versus-Host Response

We removed 10^7 nucleated cells from the thymus-epithelial cultures or from the control fibroblast cultures and suspended them in a volume of 0.05 ml of

HBSS and injected them into the right footpads of BDF_1 recipient mice, using a syringe with a 27 gauge needle. Each group contained 6 mice. The right and left popliteal lymph nodes were removed after 6 days and weighed. The lymph node index was computed as a mean ratio of the right to left lymph node weight ± the standard deviation. Statistical significance of the difference between experimental groups and control groups was measured using the student t-test.

Results

Thymus Reticular Epithelial Cell Cultures

The TE cells were shown to adhere after the first day of culture. The cells formed confluent monolayers between days 7 and 10 of culture. The TE cells appeared as large irregular cells with numerous refractile granules in their cytoplasm. The nuclei usually contained 2 or more dense nucleoli. Electron micrographs (Figure 1) showed a highly active metabolic cell with numerous cytoplasmic granules. The nucleus was euchromatic with two dense nucleoli. There were some formed vesicles in the cytoplasm along with free ribosomes. Ribosomes were also associated with endoplasmic reticulum containing large cisternae.

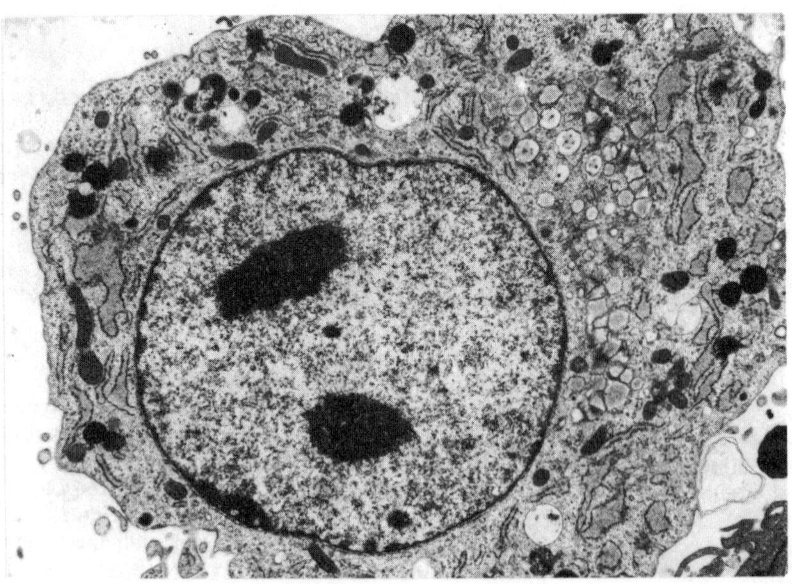

Figure 1. An electron micrograph of a thymus epithelial cell from cultures used in the study of T-cell differentiation. The nuclear pattern is euchromatic with two dense nucleoli. The cytoplasm is characteristic of highly metabolic cells, containing numerous granules and ribosomes associated with endoplasmic reticulum containing dilated cisternae (× 4250).

TABLE 1

EFFECT OF THYMUS EPITHELIUM ON CON-A RESPONSES OF SPLEEN CELLS *

Mouse Spleen Cells	Supporting Syngeneic Cell Monolayers	[^{3}H]Thymidine Uptake Con-A Treated	Control	Ratio—Exp/Control †
normal C57 BL/6	fibroblasts	8127±836	3147±421	2.58
AT×BM C57 BL/6	fibroblasts	1427±123	1623±89	.87
AT×BM C57 BL/6	TE cells	3142±192	1561±213	2.0

* Spleens from normal C57 BL/6 mice and C57 BL/6 mice that were thymectonized, lethally irradiated, and bone marrow protected (AT×BM) were cultured on syngeneic thymic epithelial (TE) cells or control fibroblast monolayers. TE cells were able to reconstitute the con-A response of T-deficient mice.

† Con-A ratios were computed by dividing the con-A treated CPM by the control CPM.

Induction of Mitogen Responsiveness

Single cell suspensions of splenic cells derived from normal or T-deficient C57Bl/6 mice were cultured on syngeneic TE monolayers or control fibroblasts for a period of 48 hours. The cells were collected and assessed for their ability to respond to con-A (a T-cell mitogen).

TABLE 1 shows the con-A responses of these cell populations as measured by uptake of [^{3}H]thymidine. The results are expressed as the ratio of the con-A treated group divided by the control group. The normal spleen cells show con-A ratios of 2.58, whereas cells from T-deficient mice show a greatly diminished con-A response (ratio .87). After 48 hours of culture on TE monolayers, the con-A response of the cells from T-deficient mice was reconstituted.

Comparative Effects of Syngeneic and Xenogeneic TE Monolayers

Since thymic extracts have been shown to cross species barriers in the induction of T-cell differentiation, it was decided to compare the effects of xenogeneic Le rat TE-cell monolayers to those produced by syngeneic mouse TE cells. Spleens from T-deficient C57Bl/6 mice were cultured for 48 hours on either xenogeneic Le TE-cell monolayers or syngeneic TE-cell monolayers. The cells were collected and examined for their ability to respond to con-A. TABLE 2 shows that xenogeneic TE cells are as effective in the induction of con-A responsiveness as syngeneic TE cells.

Induction of GvH Reactivity

Spleen cells from normal and T-deficient mice were cultured on TE-cell or fibroblast monolayers for 48 hours. The cells were collected and 10^7 nucleated cells suspended in 0.05 ml of HBSS and injected into the footpads of C57Bl/6 × DBA/2, F_1 hybrids (BDF_1), as described earlier.

TABLE 2

COMPARATIVE EFFECT OF SYNGENEIC AND XENGENEIC THYMUS EPITHELIAL CELLS ON CON-A RESPONSE OF SPLEEN CELLS FROM T-CELL DEFICIENT MICE *

Spleen Cell Reactivity	Supporting Cell Monolayers Rat Fibroblasts (Le)	Rat TE Cells (Le)	C57 BL/6 Fibroblasts	C57 BL/6 TE Cells
[^{3}H]thymidine uptake in CPM	1278±291	2877±628	1561±213	3142±192

* TABLE 2 shows the effect of culturing spleen cells from T-deficient C57 BL/6 mice (AT×BM) on either xenogeneic Lewis (Le) rat thymic epithelial (TE) monolayers or syngeneic thymic epithelial monolayers. Results are expressed in the uptake of [^{3}H]thymidine in counts per minute.

TABLE 3 shows that normal spleen cells cultured on either syngeneic TE or control monolayers give an equally strong GvH response (5.4–5.9 lymph node index). Cells from T-deficient mice cultured on fibroblast monolayers show poor GvH reactivity (2.1) index, whereas cells cultured on TE monolayers give a GvH response of the same magnitude as normal splenic lymphocytes.

DISCUSSION

This study has demonstrated that thymus reticular epithelial cells, grown *in vitro,* devoid of any lymphocytic elements have the capacity to restore con-A responsiveness and GvH reactivity to spleen cells from immunologically deficient mice. This suggests that the thymus epithelium interacts with T-cell precursors in the induction of functional T-cells. Studies in our laboratory have also shown thymus epithelial cell cultures to affect the differentiation of T-cells from their precursors in nude (nu/nu) mice *in vitro.*[10] In culture, thymic epithelial cells were found to be morphologically similar to those cells described

TABLE 3

EFFECT OF THYMUS EPITHELIUM ON GvH RESPONSES *

Cell Source Mouse Spleen Cells	Supporting Syngeneic Cell Monolayers	Lymph Node Index-Popliteal Node Assay in BDF 1 Mice †
normal C57 BL/6	fibroblasts	5.4±1.2
normal C57 BL/6	TE cells	5.9±1.4
AT×BM C57 BL/6	fibroblasts	2.1±.8
AT×BM C57 BL/6	TE cells	5.9±1.8

* Spleen cells from normal and T-deficient mice were cultured on thymus epithelial cells for 48 hours and injected (10^{7} cells/.05 ml HBSS) into the right foot pad of BDF1 (C57 BL/6×DBA/2 F1 hybrids) mice to examine GvH response.

† Lymph node index was computed by comparing the lymph node weight of the right foot pad to the left foot pad.

earlier by Clark in whole thymus sections.[6] It has been suggested that these cells are the secretory component of the thymus by audioradiographic studies.[7] Thymic extracts or thymosin also affect T-cell development and may be the mechanism of action by which the thymus epithelium functions.[11, 12]

It is well known that the thymus is essential for T-cell development.[1] Precursor cells migrate from the yolk sac during embryogenesis and from bone marrow in adult life to the thymus where development and maturation takes place.[8, 9] During the maturation process, thymocytes migrate from cortical areas, where immature cells reside, to medullary regions where more highly differentiated cells are located.[13] This maturation process is characterized by changes in surface antigens and functional properties.[14, 15] The mechanism by which this maturation takes place is not yet understood.

The present study adds further substance to the understanding of the important role the thymus epithelium plays in the differentiation of T-cells. It is proposed that the thymic microenvironment is the key to cell-mediated immunologic competence. The thymus epithelium may affect not only T-cell differentiation, but may also influence thymocytes during their various maturational changes.

The system described in this study provides an easy method of examining the events that take place during T-cell differentiation from their precursors.

Summary

Thymus-reticular epithelial cells (TE-cells) were grown in a cell culture devoid of any lymphocytic elements. These cells were able to induce T-cell differentiation in spleen cells from T-deficient mice as expressed by con-A responsiveness and GvH reactivity. It was also shown that xenogeneic rat TE cells were as effective in the induction of T-cell differentiation *in vitro* as syngeneic TE cells. This system is therefore ideal for the study of T-cell development.

Acknowledgment

The authors wish to thank Dr. Jeptha R. Hostetler, Department of Anatomy, Ohio State University, for his assistance with the electron microscopy.

References

1. Good, R. A. 1972. *In* Clinical Immunobiology. F. H. Bach & R. A. Good, Eds. Vol. 1: 1–26. Academic Press, New York, N.Y.
2. Burnet, F. M. 1970. Cellular Immunology. Melbourne Univ. Press. Melbourne, Australia.
3. Cantor, H. & R. Assofsky. 1972. J. Exp. Med. **135:** 764.
4. Miller, J. F. A. P. & G. F. Mitchell. 1969. Transplant. Rev. **1:** 3.
5. Clark, S. L. 1973. Contemporary Topics in Immunobiology. M. G. Hanna, Ed. Plenum Press, New York, N.Y.
6. Clark, S. L. 1963. Am. J. Anat. **112:** 1.
7. Clark, S. L. 1968. J. Exp. Med. **128:** 927.
8. Owen, J. J. T. & M. A. Ritter. 1969. J. Exp. Med. **129:** 431.

9. Ford, C. E., H. S. Micklem, E. P. Evans, J. G. Cray & D. A. Ogden. 1966. Ann. N.Y. Acad. Sci. **129:** 283.
10. Waksal, S. D., I. R. Cohen, H. W. Waksal & R. L. St. Pierre. 1974. Fed. Proc. **33:** 736.
11 Small, M. & N. Trainin. 1971. J. Exp. Med. **134:** 786.
12. White, A. & A. L. Goldstein. 1970. Control Processes in Multicellular Organisms. Ciba Fund. Symposium. **:** 210.
13. Weissman, I. L. 1973. J. Exp. Med. **137:** 504.
14. Waksal, S. D., R. L. St. Pierre, J. R. Hostetler & R. M. Folk. 1974. Cell. Immunol. **12:** 66.
15. St. Pierre, R. L. & S. D. Waksal. 1974. J. Reticuloendothel. Soc. **15:** 22.

THE EFFECT OF ANTITHYMOSIN GLOBULIN ON THE RECOVERY OF T-CELLS IN ATS-TREATED MICE *

Marion M. Zatz,†‡ Abraham White,§ Richard S. Schulof,¶ and Allan L. Goldstein **

Introduction

There is now extensive evidence (this volume) that the thymus produces a hormone(s) that influences T-cell differentiation and function.[1] One of the partially purified thymus products with such biological activity is thymosin.[2, 3] The present report deals with the *in vivo* effects of a rabbit antibovine thymosin antibody.

The gamma globulin fraction of this antiserum was administered daily for 1 to 4 weeks to mice previously treated with antithymocyte serum. The influence of the antithymosin globulin, or a control normal rabbit globulin, on the recovery of circulating lymphocytes and PHA responsive cells was then measured.

Methods

Animals

CBA/J mice of either sex, 6 to 8 weeks of age, were obtained from the Jackson Memorial Laboratories, Bar Harbor, Maine.

Antiserum Production (Anti-ECTEOLA)

The antiserum was prepared in adult female New Zealand White rabbits. One group of rabbits was immunized with 2 mg of bovine thymosin (ECTEOLA fraction 6) [2] in 1 ml of 0.15 M NaCl, homogenized with an equal volume of Freund's complete adjuvant. Booster injections contained 1 mg of fraction 6 in 1 ml of 0.15 M NaCl homogenized with an equal volume of freund's incomplete adjuvant, and they were administered in two subcutaneous and two intramuscular sites. Animals were boosted three times at 3 week intervals, and bled 10 days after the last injection.

* This work was supported in part by grants from the United States Public Health Service (RO1 CA 14108 and RO1 CA 14216).

† Address reprint requests to: Marion M. Zatz, Immunology Branch, National Cancer Institute, Bethesda, Maryland 20014.

‡ Departments of Microbiology and Surgery, Yale University School of Medicine, New Haven, Connecticut 06510.

§ Syntex Research, Palo Alto, California 94304.

¶ Department of Biochemistry, Albert Einstein College of Medicine, Bronx, New York 10461.

** Division of Biochemistry, University of Texas Medical Branch, Galveston, Texas 77550.

The sera from immunized or normal control rabbits were heat-inactivated and then subjected to $(NH_4)_2SO_4$ precipitation at 40% saturation. The resulting precipitate was redissolved in 0.1 M phosphate buffer, pH 7.2 and dialyzed overnight against several liters of 0.01 M PO_4, pH 7.2 with 2 changes. The dialyzed material was percolated through a column of DEAE-cellulose. The gamma globulin fraction that eluted in the void volume was pooled and concentrated using Amicon ultrafiltration, brought to a concentration of 15 mg protein per ml in 0.15 M NaCl, passed through a 0.45 μ Millipore® filter, and stored frozen at —20° until used.

The resulting anti-ECTEOLA globulin (AEG) was not cytotoxic for lymph node, spleen, thymus, or bone marrow cells, and formed specific lines of precipitation against thymosin (fraction 6) upon immunodiffusion in Ouchterlony plates (R. S. Schulof, unpublished results).

Lymph Node-Seeking Cell Assay

The percentage of recirculating lymphocytes in lymph node, spleen, and thymus cells was determined using the ^{51}Cr migration assay, which has been described in detail elsewhere.[4] Briefly, cell suspensions were labeled *in vitro* with [^{51}Cr]sodium chromate, and injected intravenously into normal syngeneic recipients. Twenty-four hours later, the recipients were killed, and the inguinal, axillary, brachial, and mesenteric nodes were removed, pooled, and counted in a gamma well spectrometer. Results were expressed as the percentage of injected radioactivity localizing in recipient lymph nodes. These lymph node-seeking cells (LNSC) have been shown to correspond to a recirculating, anti-thymocyte serum-sensitive, T-cell subpopulation.[4, 5]

Response to Phytohemagglutinin (PHA)

Spleen cell suspensions were prepared in an RPMI 1640 containing 5% FCS (GIBCO, Grand Island, N.Y.), and penicillin and streptomycin. Two ml of cells, at a concentration of 10^6 cells per ml, were incubated with and without 2.5 μl PHA (Burroughs-Wellcome, England) for 48 hours at 37° C in a humidified 5% CO_2 atmosphere. During the last 24 hours of culture, 2.5 μCi of [^{3}H]thymidine were added to the cells, which were harvested by Millipore filtration.

Experimental Protocol

Groups of CBA/J mice were injected subcutaneously (s.c.) on day 0 with 0.4 ml normal rabbit serum (NRS) or rabbit-anti-mouse thymocyte serum (ATS) (Microbiological Associates, Bethesda, Md.). The NRS and ATS animals were then injected daily with 1.5 mg AEG or NRG s.c. for 1 or 4 weeks. On the day following the last AEG or NRG injection, the 4 groups of mice, i.e. NRS-NRG, NRS-AEG, ATS-NRG, ATS-AEG, were sacrificed, and the lymph nodes, spleen, and thymuses from 2–5 donors were pooled and assayed for LNSC and responsiveness to PHA.

Statistics

Significance between groups was determined by Student's t-test.

RESULTS

Recovery of LNSC

The percentage of LNSC was measured in cell suspensions obtained from NRS-NRG, NRS-AEG, ATS-NRG, and ATS-AEG treated donors, sacrificed 1 or 4 weeks following NRS or ATS treatment, and daily injections of NRG or AEG. The results are shown in TABLE 1. ATS treatment results in a marked

TABLE 1

LYMPH NODE-SEEKING CELLS

Treatment	Percent Lymph Node-Seeking Cells: Lymph Node *		Spleen †		Thymus †	
+1 week	X SD	p<	X SD	p<	X SD	p<
NRS-NRG	13.2±2.7		— —	—	— —	—
NRS-AEG	14.0±3.0	NS	— —	—	— —	—
ATS-NRG	3.0±1.6		— —	—	— —	—
ATS-AEG	2.9±0.9	NS	— —	—	— —	—
+4 weeks						
NRS-NRG	14.7±3.4		7.8±0.5		1.0±0.1	
NRS-AEG	12.5±1.1	NS	7.6±0.9	NS	1.1±0.1	NS
ATS-NRG	8.3±1.8		6.4±0.4		1.1±0.2	
ATS-AEG	5.6±0.7	.01	3.9±0.3	.001	1.2±0.1	NS

* The mean % LNSC values for ^{51}Cr-labeled lymph node cells are based on 4 experiments, in which cells were obtained from 2–3 donors and injected into 3–4 recipients.

† The mean % LNSC values for ^{51}Cr-labeled spleen and thymus cells are based on a single experiment using cells obtained from 5 donors and injected into 4 recipients.

depletion of LNSC in lymph nodes at +1 week. These results confirm earlier studies,[5] showing that LNSC are an ATS-sensitive, recirculating T-cell population. No effect of AEG or NRG on the percentage of LNSC in either group is seen at 1 week after treatment.

At 4 weeks after NRS or ATS injection, there is a substantial recovery of LNSC in ATS-NRG lymph nodes and spleen, as compared to the NRS-treated groups. However, AEG treatment results in a diminished recovery of LNSC in lymph nodes and spleen. The differences between % LNSC in ATS-AEG vs. ATS-NRG lymph node cells (8.3 vs. 5.6%) and spleen cells (6.4 vs. 3.9%) are highly significant, ($p < .01$ and $< .001$ respectively). No influence of AEG upon LNSC is seen in the control NRS-treated group, and no effect of ATS or AEG on thymocyte LNSC is observed at +4 weeks.

Cell Yields

The average cell yields per donor mouse, 4 weeks after treatment, are recorded in TABLE 2. No significant effect of AEG upon recovery of cell numbers following ATS treatment is observed. Thus the differences in the percentage LNSC between the ATS-NRG and ATS-AEG groups represent actual differences in the numbers of LNSC in these two groups.

Response to PHA

The responsiveness of spleen cells to PHA was measured 1 and 4 weeks after NRS or ATS treatment and daily injections of NRG or AEG (TABLE 3). A marked recovery of the splenic response to PHA is seen by 4 weeks after treatment in the ATS-NRG group (15,000 cpm vs. 32,414 cpm), however the degree of recovery is diminished in the ATS-AEG group; the difference between the ATS-NRG and ATS-AEG group is significant ($p < .02$). No effect of AEG treatment is observed at 1 or 4 weeks on the response to PHA in the NRS-treated group.

TABLE 2

AVERAGE CELL YIELDS $\times 10^6$ PER DONOR MOUSE, AT + 4 WEEKS

Treatment	Lymph Node	Spleen	Thymus
NRS-NRG	62.5 (12) *	112 (5)	143 (5)
NRS-AEG	67.0 (12)	110 (5)	95.5 (5)
ATS-NRG	37.5 (12)	127 (5)	101 (5)
ATS-AEG	39.2 (12)	138 (5)	95.2 (5)

* The values in parentheses represent the number of donor mice on which the average is based.

DISCUSSION AND CONCLUSIONS

These results demonstrate that *in vivo* administration of antithymosin globulin modifies the recovery of PHA-responsive, circulating T-cells in ATS-treated mice.

From the data presented, it is possible to speculate on the mechanism whereby AEG exerts its effect on the peripheral T-cell population. It seems likely that AEG treatment diminishes regeneration of the thymus-dependent, ATS-sensitive population, rather than destroying or inactivating newly formed PHA-responsive, LNSC cells. The latter explanation is rendered unlikely by the observation that AEG has little or no effect upon the lymph node and spleen lymphocytes of the NRS-treated mice. The absence of cytotoxicity of AEG for lymph node and spleen cells (R. S. Schulof, unpublished observations) provides further evidence against a direct action of AEG on the circulating T-cell pool. Although AEG reduces recovery of circulating T-cells, we cannot at present distinguish between the possibilities that AEG functions at the level of the thymus to block thymosin production, or acts in the periphery by

TABLE 3

RESPONSE OF SPLEEN CELLS TO PHA *

Treatment	+1 week			+4 weeks		
	−PHA	+PHA	+PHA / −PHA	−PHA	+PHA	−PHA / +PHA
NRS-NRG	3432 (3041–3696)	16131 (15523–16740)	4.70	4990 (4591–5390)	32414 (28681–36148)	6.49
NRS-AEG	3191 (2801–3582)	13295 (10108–16482)	4.16	5007 (4313–5702)	30330 (23850–36810)	6.05
ATS-NRG	1453 (1260–1647)	1830 (893–2767)	1.25	3359 (3009–3710)	15181 (13819–16544)	4.51
ATS-AEG	2138 (1961–2316)	2018 (1759–2278)	0.94	4891 (4102–5680)	9029 (8664–9394)	1.84

* Results in counts per minute of two experiments performed in triplicate. The numbers in parentheses represent the range of cpm. The difference between the ATS-NRG and ATS-AEG groups at +4 weeks was significant ($p < .02$).

reducing circulating thymosin levels. It is known that thymosin activity is found in serum,[6] and that the serum levels correlate with immunocompetence (A. L. Goldstein, unpublished observations). In fact these two mechanisms are not mutually exclusive, and may both operate.

The present findings are in contrast to an earlier report by Lance *et al.*[7] suggesting that thymosin does not influence regeneration of the recirculating LNSC population. In those studies, thymosin fraction 3 was administered for 1 week following thymectomy, and irradiation or ALS treatment; the effect upon the LNSC population was then measured. The negative results obtained may have been due to an inactive fraction or inappropriate dose schedule of the thymosin used in those experiments. These studies should now be repeated with more purified thymosin preparations (e.g. fraction 6), which have been shown to be active in other assays.[2, 3]

The effect of AEG on the peripheral T-cell population, which we report here, is consistent with earlier work showing prolongation of skin-graft survival in mice treated with an antithymosin serum prepared against a crude thymus extract.[8]

The question of precisely how thymosin and antithymosin operate at the cellular level to influence regeneration of a peripheral T-cell population remains to be answered. It is unclear from the results of the present studies whether antithymosin diminishes the recovery of a single subpopulation with both LNSC-and PHA-responsive properties, or acts upon two separate subpopulations. Experiments now in progress should help to answer these important, but unresolved questions.

To summarize, the recovery of circulating, PHA-responsive cells normally occurs following ATS-treatment, provided the animal has an intact thymus. The degree of this recovery can be diminished by injecting ATS-treated mice with an antibody prepared to thymosin, fraction 6. These findings suggest that such thymus-mediated, circulating T-cell recovery, is at least partially dependent upon elaboration of a thymus product with the properties of thymosin.

Acknowledgments

We wish to thank Norma Roberts, Margaret Freund, Susan M. Baker, and James Oliver for their expert technical assistance.

References

1. Goldstein, A. L. & A. White. 1973. Contemporary Topics in Immunobiology, Vol. 2. A. J. S. Davies & R. L. Carter, Eds. : 339–350. Plenum Publishing Corp. New York, N.Y.
2. Goldstein, A. L., A. Guha, M. M. Zatz, M. A. Hardy & A. White. 1972. Proc. Nat. Acad. Sci. U.S. **69:** 1800.
3. Goldstein, A. L., J. A. Hooper, R. S. Schulof, G. H. Cohen, G. B. Thurman & M. C. McDaniel. 1974. Fed. Proc. In press.
4. Zatz, M. M. & E. M. Lance. 1970. Cell Immunol. **1:** 3.
5. Taub, R. N. & E. M. Lance. 1971. Transplantation **11:** 536.
6. Dardenne, M. & J. F. Bach. 1973. Immunology **25:** 343.
7. Lance, E. M., S. C. Gillette, A. L. Goldstein, A. White & M. M. Zatz. 1973. Cell. Immunol. **6:** 123.
8. Hardy, M. A., J. Quint, A. L. Goldstein, D. State & A. White. 1968. Proc. Nat. Acad. Sci. U.S. **61:** 875.

PART VI. ROLE OF THYMUS FACTORS IN IMMUNITY: PERSPECTIVES

THE NATURE AND FUNCTION OF T-CELL ANTIGENS

M. Schlesinger, E. Israel, M. Chaouat, and I. Gery

The Hebrew University-Hadassah Medical School
Jerusalem, Israel

Subpopulations of lymphocytes are endowed with different cell-surface antigenic properties.[1-3] In mice, T-lymphocytes are characterized by their possession of the θ- and Ly-alloantigens[4,5] whereas B-lymphocytes are characterized by their readily demonstrable cell-surface immunoglobulin coat[5] and by their distinctive antigens.[6,7] Subsets of both T- and B-lymphocytes have been shown to differ antigenically. Plasma cells are characterized by specific antigens.[7,8] Subpopulations of thymus cells[9,10] and of peripheral T-lymphocytes[11] have been shown to differ not only in their functional capacities but also in their cell-surface antigenicity.

Little is known about the possible functions of the cell-surface structures detectable as cell-surface antigens (see Reference 3). Immunoglobulin molecules, on the surface of B-lymphocytes, have been shown to play a major role as receptors involved in the recognition of antigens.[12,13] Similar cell-surface immunoglobulins probably also exist on the surface of T-lymphocytes, and they too seem to function as receptors for antigens.[14] The possible functions of cell-surface antigens such as the H-2, Ly, and θ-antigens is obscure.

The identification of functions of cell-surface antigens is fraught with many difficulties. It is relatively easy to demonstrate that cells endowed with a distinctive antigenic marker have a certain functional capacity. It is a much more complicated problem to show that an antigen is directly involved in the specific function carried out by the cell possessing the antigen. A correlation between cell-surface antigens and cell function may, however, be meaningful if in a large number of cell populations the same correlation between a given biological function and a distinct antigen can be found. By the same token, if cells of similar antigenicity differ in their function, or if functionally similar cells vary in their antigenic properties, it would seem reasonable to conclude that the function studied is not mediated through the cellular antigen analyzed. Another approach to the analysis of the function of T-cell antigens is to test the effect of antibodies, in the absence of complement, on the various functions carried out by T-lymphocytes. This approach is, of course, complicated by the possibility that the attachment of antibodies to the cell surface may interfere with cell functions in a nonspecific way, rather than by blocking of specific sites.

The present report summarizes some of our findings regarding the antigenic properties of subpopulations of T-lymphocytes, which differ in their capacity to localize in either the spleen or the lymph nodes, and which vary in their capacity to respond to mitogens. Attempts were made to determine whether any known antigenic cell-surface structure is directly involved either in the "homing" pattern of lymphocytes or in their response to mitogens.

Materials and Methods

Mice

Mice of the A/J and C3H inbred strains were used both as donors of lymphoid cells used for labeling with ^{51}Cr and as syngeneic cell recipients. Mice of the A/J and C3H strains also served as donors of the thymus and spleen cell suspension used in experiments on stimulation with various mitogens.

Additional strains of mice, used for the production of antisera were the AKR/J, BALB/c, and C57BL/6 strains.

Antisera

Alloantisera were prepared as described previously.[15] The H-2 antiserum used was elicited in C57BL mice by immunization with spleen cells from A/J mice. Antisera against the θ-C3H antigen[16] were prepared by immunizing AKR/J mice with C3H spleen cells. Antisera against the Ly-A.1 antigen[17] were elicited by immunization of (AKR/JX C57BL) F_1 hybrid mice with C3H thymus cells. Antisera against the TL-1 and TL-3 antigens[18] were raised in (BALB/c $\times$ C3H)F_1 hybrid mice by immunization with strain-A thymus cells. Guinea-pig serum (GPS) was obtained from normal guinea-pigs bred at the animal colony of the Department of Experimental Medicine and Cancer Research. Agar-absorbed guinea-pig serum was used as complement source.[19]

Preparation of Fab Fragments

The technique used was adopted from that described by Porter.[20] The IgG fraction of C57BL anti-A spleen serum was obtained by elution from a DEAE-cellulose column (Whatman, Balston Ltd, England) with a 0.01 M phosphate buffer, pH 8.0. To 50 mg protein eluted was added 0.5 mg papain (Sigma 2$\times$ crystalized) dissolved in 0.1 M phosphate buffer, pH 6.6, containing 0.01 M cysteine and 0.002 M EDTA. The immunoglobulin fraction was incubated with papain at 37° C for 16 hours, and was then dialysed against phosphate-buffered saline (PBS) (pH 7.2) for 40 hours at 4° C with repeated changes. The protein digest was filtered through a Sephadex® G-100 column, (Pharmacia, Uppsala) and the third elution peak, containing the Fab and Fc fragments was collected, concentrated by pervaporation, and dialyzed against PBS. In some experiments the Fab fraction was further purified by filtration through a Sephadex G-75 column, and collection of the second protein peak eluted.

Radioactive Labeling of Cells

Lymphoid cells were labeled with ^{51}Cr by incubation with isotonic sodium chromate solution (Radio-chemical Center, Amersham, Bucks.) according to the method of Wigzell.[21] Details of the technique were described previously.[9] Red blood cells present in the spleen cell suspensions were lysed by exposure to 0.83% NH_4Cl, according to the method of Boyle,[22] prior to labeling with ^{51}Cr.

Exposure of Labeled Cells to Antisera

^{51}Cr-labeled cells were exposed to various antisera as described previously.[23, 24] A similar procedure was used for the exposure of labeled cells to Fab fragments.

Exposure of Labeled Cells to Lectins

^{51}Cr-labeled lymphocytes were washed 4 times in normal saline, resuspended at a concentration of 80×10^6 cells per ml, and 0.5 ml of cell suspension was

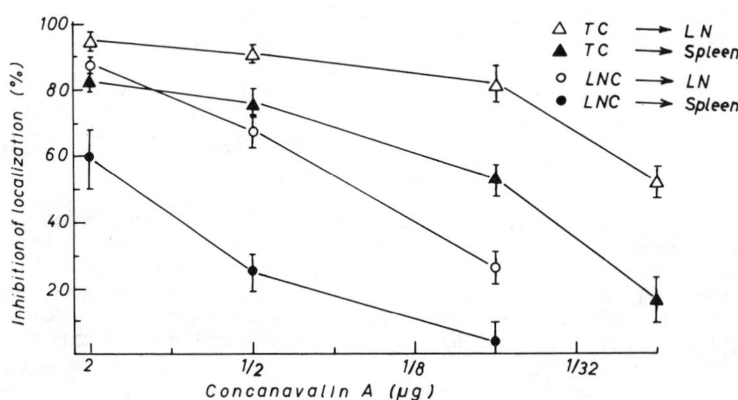

FIGURE 1. The effect of various concentrations of concanavalin-A on the localization of ^{51}Cr-labeled lymphoid cells of strain-A mice in the spleen and lymph nodes of syngeneic recipients. *Triangles:* labeled thymus cells. *Circles:* labeled lymph node cells. *Open symbols:* cells localizing in lymph nodes. *Filled symbols:* cells localizing in the spleen. The inhibition of the localization of Con-A-treated cells is calculated from the radioactivity recovered in organs of the recipients according to the formula:

$$100 - \frac{\%\text{ radioactivity injected, Con-A-treated cells}}{\%\text{ radioactivity injected, untreated cells}} \times 100$$

Each point represents the mean of results obtained in 6 mice ($\pm$SE).

delivered into plastic test tubes. In experiments with concanavalin A (Con-A) (Miles Yeda, Rehovot), 0.05 ml of serial fourfold dilutions of the lectin in normal saline was added to each test tube. The concentration of Con-A given in FIGURE 1 refers to the amount of lectin (in μg) added to 0.5 ml. of the labeled cell suspension. In experiments with PHA (Wellcome Research Laboratory, Beckenham) tenfold dilutions of the lectin in saline were set up, and 0.1 ml of the PHA dilution was added to each test tube. The dilutions shown in FIGURE 2 refer to the dilution of PHA prior to its addition to the cell suspension. Following the addition of the lectins, the suspensions were incubated at room temperature for 30 minutes. Just prior to the injection of the labeled cells, 0.05 ml of fresh normal, syngeneic mouse serum and 1.0 ml normal saline

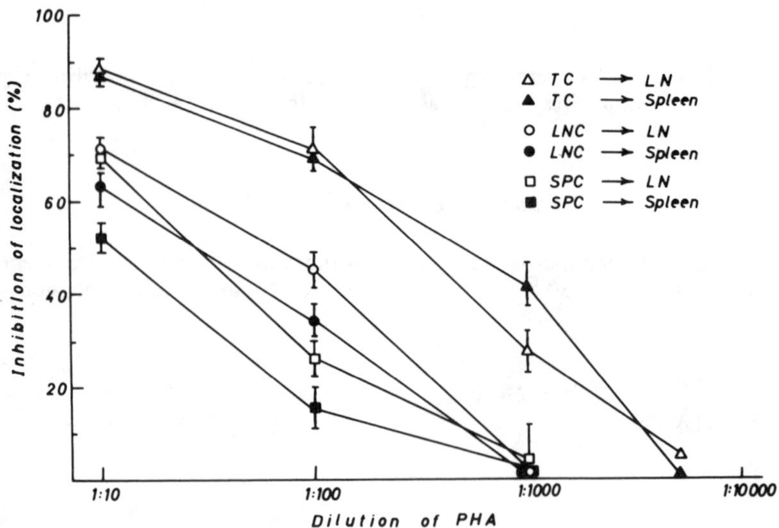

FIGURE 2. The effect of various concentrations of PHA on the localization of ^{51}Cr-labeled lymphoid cells of strain-A mice, in the spleen and lymph nodes of syngeneic recipients. *Triangles:* labeled thymus cells. *Circles:* labeled lymph-node cells. *Quadrangles:* spleen cells. *Open symbols:* cells localizing in lymph nodes. *Filled symbols:* cells localizing in the spleen. Inhibition of localization calculated as for FIGURE 1. Each point represents the mean of results obtained in 4 to 8 mice (±SE).

were added to each test tube. A volume of 0.6 to 0.7 ml of the suspensions was injected into syngeneic mice.

The Distribution of Labeled Cells

The localization of labeled cells in the lymph nodes (axillary, brachial, inguinal and mesenteric), spleens, and livers of the recipients was determined as described previously.[9, 24]

Exposure of Cells to Antisera Prior to Their in Vitro *Culture*

Suspensions of either thymus or spleen cells were prepared at a concentration of 25×10^6/ml in minimal essential medium-Spinner (MEM-S). Various amounts of either NMS, alloantisera, or GPS were added to 1–2 ml of the cell suspensions, and the cells were incubated for 45 minutes at 37° C. Thereafter, the suspensions were spun at $300 \times g$ for 10 minutes, and either washed once in MEM-S or incubated with C′ for 45 minutes at 37° C. The final concentration of C′ used for the lysis of thymus cells was 1:10, whereas for the lysis of spleen cells a final C′-concentration of 1:6 was used.

Culture Conditions

Following incubation in various antisera, in the presence or absence of guinea-pig C′, the cells were washed in MEM-S, and suspended in MEM-S supplemented with 5% human serum, at volumes that contained either 2.5×10^6 or 5.0×10^6 cells of the original suspensions per ml. No adjustment was made for the reduced number of cells remaining following exposure to antiserum and C′. Aliquots of 1.0 ml. of cell suspensions were delivered into plastic culture tubes (Falcon 2001). Cultures were stimulated by Con-A (Nutritional Biochemical Co.), by phytohemagglutinin (PHA; Difco), by pokeweed mitogen (PWM; Grand Island Biological Co.) or by bacterial lipopolysaccharide (LPS, Difco, *E. coli* 055: B5) The concentration of Con-A used was usually 5 μg/ml for the stimulation of thymus cells cultures, and 2 μg/ml for the stimulation of spleen cell cultures, whereas the concentration of PHA used for cultures of both cell types was 1 μl/ml. In some experiments, other concentrations of Con-A and PHA were employed.

The concentration of either PWM or LPS used was 50 μl/ml. The level of mitotic response of the cultures was determined according to the incorporation of tritiated thymidine ([^{3}H]T) as described elsewhere.[25]

Results

The Effect of Various Sera on the in Vivo *Migration of Lymphocytes*

Lymphoid cells from various sources were labeled with ^{51}Cr, exposed *in vitro* to antisera, and their localization in organs of syngeneic recipients was determined 18 to 20 hours later.[23, 24] Exposure of lymphocytes to various antisera impaired to a different extent their localization in either the spleen or the lymph nodes. The difference between spleen-seeking and lymph node-seeking thymocytes was particularly pronounced, and it was possible to delineate the antigenic profiles of these two subpopulations (Table 1). Particularly striking was the differential effect of H-2 antisera and of normal GPS on these two migration streams. H-2 antisera had a much stronger inhibitory effect on the localization of thymus cells in the lymph nodes than on their localization

Table 1

Comparative Concentration of Antigens on Spleen-seeking and Lymph Node-seeking Thymus Cell Subpopulations

Antigen	Spleen-seeking Subpopulation	Lymph Node-seeking Subpopulation
H–2	+	+++
θ	+++	++
Ly–A	+++	++++
TL	+++	+
Antigen reactive with GPS	+++	±

in the spleen, whereas GPS had the converse effect, and eliminated the migration of thymocytes to the spleen without affecting the migration to the lymph nodes. H-2 antisera were also found to exert a greater inhibitory effect on the migration of lymph node and spleen cells to the lymph nodes as compared to their localization in the spleen.[23]

The Effect of Fab Fragments of H-2 Antibodies on Lymphocyte Migration

The inhibitory effect of H-2 antisera on the localization of lymphocytes in lymphoid organs, results from opsonization of the cells and their elimination by the reticulo-endothelial system. This is supported by the fact that the livers of animals injected with antibody-coated ^{51}Cr-labeled lymphocytes showed an increased amount of radioactivity. The differing effect of antibodies, on the spleen- and lymph node-seeking streams largely reflects antigenic differences between the cells localizing in each of these organs. There is, however, the

TABLE 2

THE EFFECT OF MONOVALENT FAB FRAGMENTS OF C57BL ANTI-A SERUM ON THE MIGRATION OF STRAIN-A THYMUS AND LYMPH NODE CELLS

Cells Inoculated	Time After Injection (hrs)	Localization in: Lymph Nodes	Spleen	Liver
Lymph node cells	8	71 *	82	93
Lymph node cells	18	78	87	117
Thymus cells	8	61	101	103
Thymus cells	18	73	86	97

* The localization of Fab-treated cells is expressed as a percentage of the localization of cells exposed to NMS.

possibility that cell-surface antigenic determinants are directly involved in the process of selective localization of lymphocytes in either the lymph nodes or the spleen. To test the possibility that H-2 antigenic determinants are involved in the localization of lymphocytes, the effect of monovalent Fab-fragments of H-2 antibodies on the distribution of ^{51}Cr-labeled lymphocytes was tested. As shown in TABLE 2, exposure of either lymph node cells or thymus cells to Fab fragments of C57BL anti-A spleen serum reduced the proportion of cells localizing in lymph nodes, and, to a lesser degree, also reduced the proportion of cells localizing in the spleen. Unlike the effect of complete H-2 antibodies, coating of cells with their Fab fragments did not seem to result in elimination of the cells by the reticulo-endothelial system, as judged by the absence of significant changes in the radioactivity detected in the liver. At present it is not clear, however, whether the effect of a Fab fragment is due to its interaction with a distinctive receptor on the surface of lymphocytes, which is involved in the migration of lymphocytes, or whether the mere attachment of a Fab fragment to the surface of lymphocytes impairs their capacity for migration. Studies with Fab fragments of other antisera should clarify the problem.

The Effect of Con-A on the Migration of Lymphocytes

A number of previous studies have indicated that glycoproteins on the cell surface of lymphocytes are involved in the distinctive localization of lymphocytes in lymph nodes. Thus, exposure of lymphocytes to glycosidase,[27] trypsin,[28] neuraminidase,[29] or to potassium periodate [30] inhibited the localization of lymphocytes in lymph nodes. In the present study, exposure of lymphocytes to Con-A inhibited their migration to lymph nodes, to a greater extent than their migration to the spleen. For all the concentrations of Con-A tested (1⁄16 μg to 2 μg) the migration of lymph node and spleen cells to the lymph nodes was inhibited to a significantly greater extent than their migration to the spleen (FIGURE 1). The effect of Con-A on thymus cells was different among the strains tested. Con-A affected the lymph node-seeking migration stream of strain A thymocytes to a significantly greater extent than the spleen-seeking stream. In contrast, both migration streams of thymus cells of C3H mice were inhibited to a similar degree.

The Effect of PHA on the Migration of Lymphocytes

The *in vitro* exposure of lymphocytes to PHA inhibits their migration to either the lymph nodes or the spleen (FIGURE 2). In contrast to the activity of Con-A, the inhibitory effect of PHA on the lymph node-seeking and spleen-seeking migration streams were not significantly different. The migration of thymus cells proved to be very sensitive to the effect of PHA. A 1:1000 dilution of PHA still inhibited the migration of thymus cells, but failed to affect the migration of the other types of lymphocytes tested. Tests on the effects of PHA on the migration of lymphocytes from A/J and C3H mice yielded concordant results.

The Mechanism of the Inhibition of Cell Migration by Con-A

The inhibitory activity of Con-A on the migration of lymphocytes was not a result of its cytotoxic activity on the cells during their *in vitro* exposure. Incubation of lymphocytes *in vitro* with Con-A (1:8 μg/ml) in the presence of α-methyl-mannopyranoside (15 mg/0.5 ml) prevented the inhibitory activity of Con-A. Moreover, when α-methyl-mannopyranoside was added to lymphoid cells following their coating with Con-A, the cells were found to regain their capacity for migration to the lymph nodes. While these experiments indicate that Con-A does not kill lymph node-seeking lymphocytes *in vitro,* it was possible that prolonged contact with Con-A may specifically eliminate this subpopulation *in vivo.* To analyse this problem, the effect of Con-A was studied on lymphocytes that had localized in the lymph nodes of primary hosts, and which are known to constitute a relatively homogenous population of recirculating cells.[31] ^{51}Cr-labeled lymph node or spleen cells were injected into primary hosts; 20 hours later the primary hosts were killed and suspensions were prepared from their lymph nodes or their spleen. Part of the suspension was exposed to Con-A (0.5 μg per 20^6 cells) prior to injection into secondary hosts, while another part of the suspension was injected without further treatment. If Con-A acted by eliminating the lymph node-seeking population, one would expect that exposure to Con-A of the cells that had localized in the lymph nodes of primary hosts would eliminate their migration to the lymph nodes and the spleen of the secondary hosts to the same extent. The results showed, however, that Con-A affected only the migration of cells to the lymph nodes of the secondary hosts, but failed to affect their migration to the spleen of secondary hosts. (TABLE 3)

The Effect of Antisera and Complement on the Response of Thymus Cells to Mitogens

The mitotic response of thymus cells to PHA is much weaker than to Con-A.[11] The addition of a supernatant from cultures of peritoneal macrophages (SUP) causes a marked increase in the response of thymocytes to PHA.[26] It is now clear that only a small subpopulation of thymus cells, of relatively low bouyant density, responds to PHA, whereas an additional subpopulation of thymocytes, of higher bouyant density, responds to PHA in the presence of SUP.[26, 32] A still higher proportion of cells responds to Con-A.

TABLE 3

THE EFFECT OF CON-A ON THE LOCALIZATION OF ^{51}CR-LABELED LYMPHOCYTES IN SECONDARY SYNGENEIC HOSTS

Original Inoculum	Localization in Primary Host: Lymph Nodes	Localization in Primary Host: Spleen	Source of Cells in Primary Host	Localization in Secondary Host, Without Con-A: Lymph Nodes	Without Con-A: Spleen	Con-A Added: Lymph Nodes	Con-A Added: Spleen
Lymph node cells	12.65 *	15.89	lymph nodes	20.28	18.99	7.85	21.82
Spleen cells	2.89	12.51	spleen	2.81	11.29	0.80	10.03
Spleen cells	3.35	16.26	lymph nodes	12.78	16.80	3.97	13.08

* Percentage of total radioactivity injected (mean of results obtained in 2 to 4 mice).

The response of thymus cells to PHA alone was practically unaffected by exposure to anti-θ serum or anti-Ly serum and complement (C′).[31] Exposure of thymus cells to GPS, a procedure that killed over half of the cells, strikingly increased the response to PHA (FIGURE 3). TL-antiserum and C′ caused a moderate inhibition of the response to PHA (FIGURE 4) and H-2 antiserum and C′ had a pronounced inhibitory effect on the stimulation by PHA alone (FIGURE 5). The cells responding to PHA in the presence of SUP showed a different antigenic profile. They were inhibited by exposure to either anti-TL (FIGURE 4), anti-θ or anti-Ly sera and C′. Again, H-2 antiserum had a strong

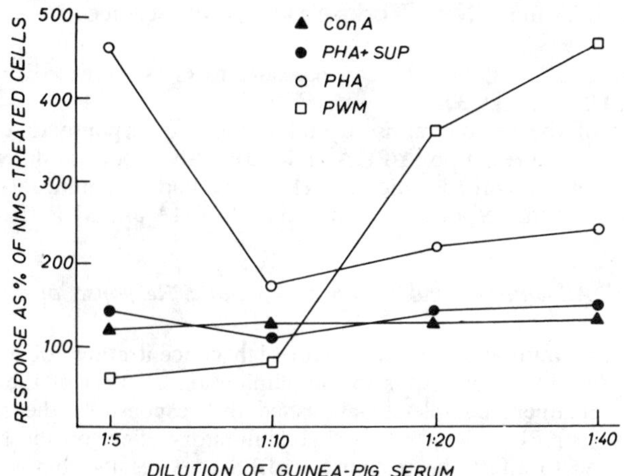

FIGURE 3. The response of C_3H thymus cells treated with dilutions of guinea-pig serum to various mitogens. The response of the cells is expressed as a percentage of the mitotic response of thymus cells exposed to normal mouse serum. The cells were exposed to Con-A (▲), to PHA (○), to PHA and a supernatant from cultures of peritoneal cells (●), or to pokeweed mitogen (□).

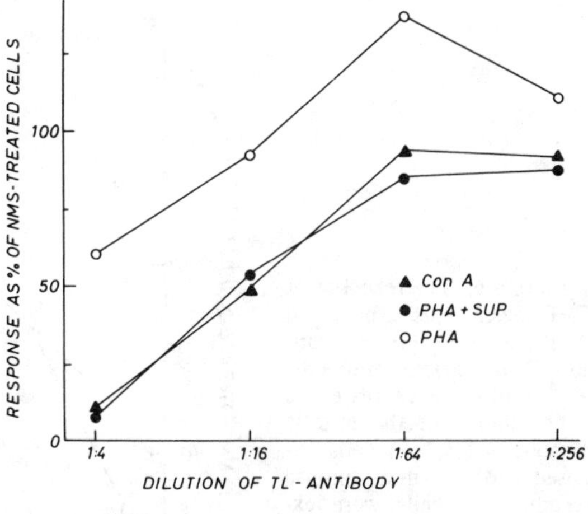

FIGURE 4. The response of strain-A thymus cells exposed to dilutions of anti-TL serum and C′ to various mitogens. Symbols as in FIGURE 3.

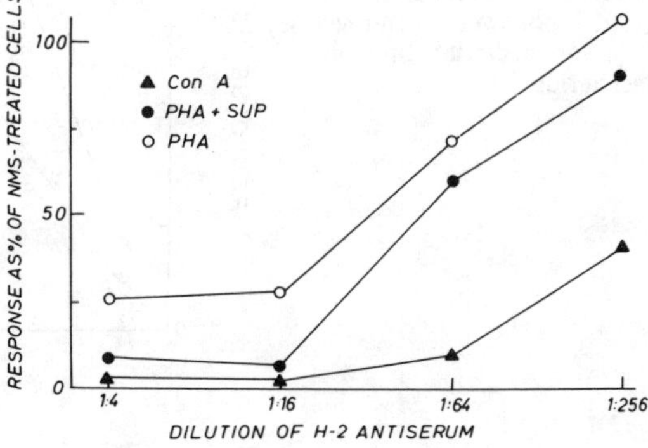

FIGURE 5. The response of C_3H thymus cells exposed to dilutions of anti-H-2 serum (C57BL anti-A spleen) and C′, to various mitogens. Symbols as in FIGURE 3.

inhibitory effect (FIGURE 5), whereas exposure to GPS increased the response to PHA and SUP (FIGURE 3).

The effect of the various antisera and C′ on the response to Con-A was similar to that on the response to PHA and SUP. An important difference was, however, that anti-θ, anti-Ly, and anti-H-2 sera had a significantly stronger inhibitory effect on the response to Con-A than to PHA and SUP (FIGURE 5).[32]

The Effect of Alloantisera and C′ on the Mitotic Response of Spleen Cells

Incubation of murine spleen cells with high concentrations of anti-θ-serum and C′, is a procedure that results in the elimination of most of the peripheral T-cells. This treatment completely abolished the response of the spleen cells to either Con-A or PHA, had only a slight inhibitory effect on the response to PWM, but failed to affect the response to LPS (see results obtained with the 1:4 serum dilution in FIGURE 6). Low concentrations of θ-antiserum still showed an inhibitory effect on the response to PHA, whereas the response to Con-A was either unaffected or even accelerated. This finding is in accordance with the observations of Stobo and Paul.[11, 33] The results obtained with anti-Ly serum and C′ resembled those obtained with anti-θ serum and C′. Again, the response to PHA was inhibited by serum dilutions that failed to affect the mitotic response to Con-A.

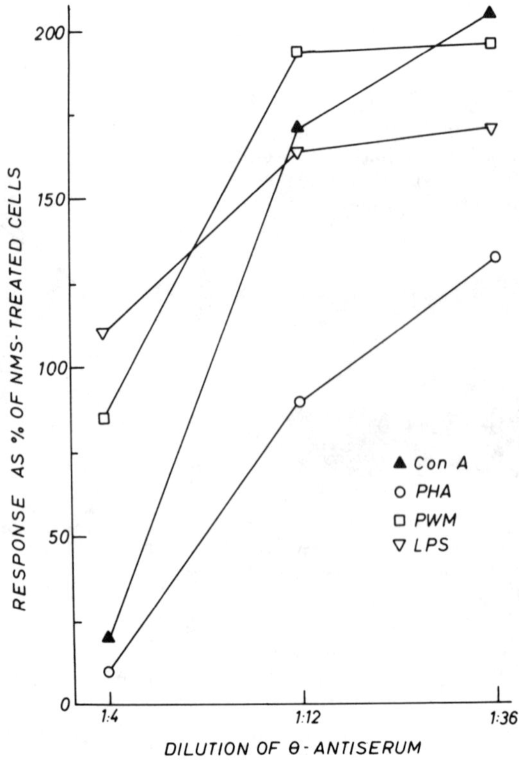

FIGURE 6. The response of C_3H spleen cells exposed to dilutions of anti-θ serum and C′ to various mitogens. The results are expressed as a percentage of the mitotic response of spleen cells exposed to normal mouse serum. The cells were exposed to Con-A (▲), PHA (○), pokeweed mitogen (□) or bacterial lipopolysaccharide (▽).

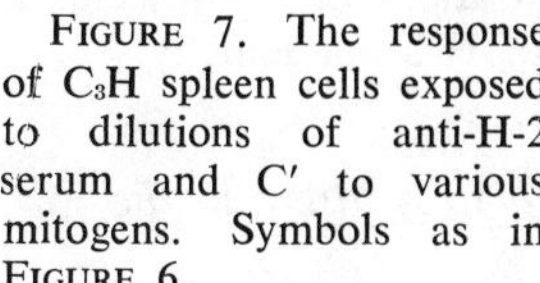

FIGURE 7. The response of C_3H spleen cells exposed to dilutions of anti-H-2 serum and C′ to various mitogens. Symbols as in FIGURE 6.

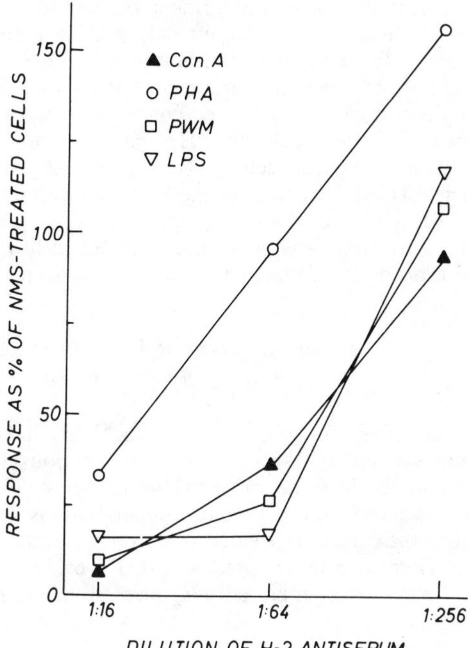

Exposure of spleen cells to H-2 antiserum and C′ had a strong inhibitory effect on their response to Con-A, PWM, and LPS. The response to PHA was affected to a lesser extent (FIGURE 7). In the experiment illustrated in FIGURE 7, a 1:64 dilution of H-2 antiserum and C′ inhibited the response to Con-A, PWM, and LPS by about 60 to 70%, while not inhibiting their response to PHA at all. It is clear, therefore, that the cells involved in the response to PHA have a significantly lower H-2 antigenicity than those cells which respond to other mitogens.

The Response of Cells Incubated with H-2 Antiserum and C′ to Various Concentrations of Lectins

Lymphoid cells show a maximal mitotic response to well-defined optimal concentrations of lectins.[11] In our experience the maximal mitotic response of spleen cells is elicited by a concentration of about 2 μg Con-A/ml or by 1 μl PHA/ml. Exposure of spleen cells to either higher or lower concentrations of the lectins results in a suboptimal stimulation of the cells. It was of interest to determine the effect of various concentrations of PHA and Con-A on the spleen cells that resisted exposure to H-2 antiserum and C′, *i.e.* the spleen cells that possess the lowest H-2 antigen concentration. As expected, concentrations of PHA or Con-A that were either higher or lower than the optimal concentration gave relatively weaker mitotic stimulation. Exposure of spleen cells to H-2 antiserum and C′ did not alter the pattern of response of spleen cells to various concentrations of Con-A. Spleen cells low in H-2 antigenicity showed a similar degree of impairment of their response to all Con-A concentrations tested (FIGURE 8). Completely different results were obtained with PHA. Here, cells exposed to H-2 antiserum and C′ had a marked reduction in their response to low concentrations of PHA, but did not differ from untreated cells in their response to higher concentrations of PHA (FIGURE 8). Indeed, exposure of these cells to PHA concentration of 16 μl/ml elicited a stronger response in spleen cells treated with H-2 antiserum and C′ than in untreated cells. These experiments indicate that response of cells to low concentrations of PHA is a distinctive property of cells possessing a high concentration of H-2 antigenicity, whereas the response to low concentrations of PHA seems to be a property of cells possessing low concentrations of H-2 antigenicity.

The Mitotic Response of Lymphocytes Exposed to Antisera in the Absence of Complement

In order to gain some insight into the relationship between cell-surface antigens and the receptor sites for various lectins, lymphocytes were coated with antibody alone, prior to stimulation with mitogens. This procedure avoided the selective elimination of subpopulations of lymphocytes that was observed when the cells were treated with antisera and C′.

Thymus cells exposed to either θ-or Ly-antisera, in the absence of C′, did not show any impaired response. Indeed, some degree of stimulation was

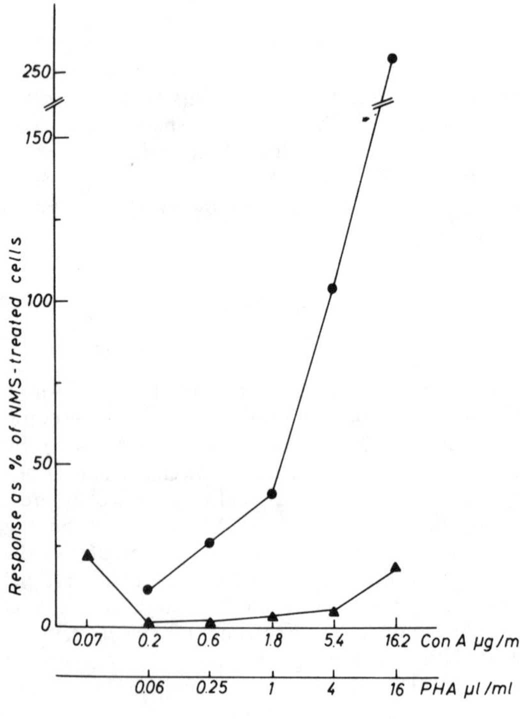

FIGURE 8. The response of C_3H spleen cells incubated with a 1:16 dilution of H-2 antiserum (C57BL anti-A spleen) and C′ to various concentrations of either PHA or Con-A. For each concentration of lectin the results are expressed as a percentage of the response of spleen cells incubated in normal mouse serum. *Circles:* inhibition of response to PHA. *Triangles:* inhibition of response to Con-A.

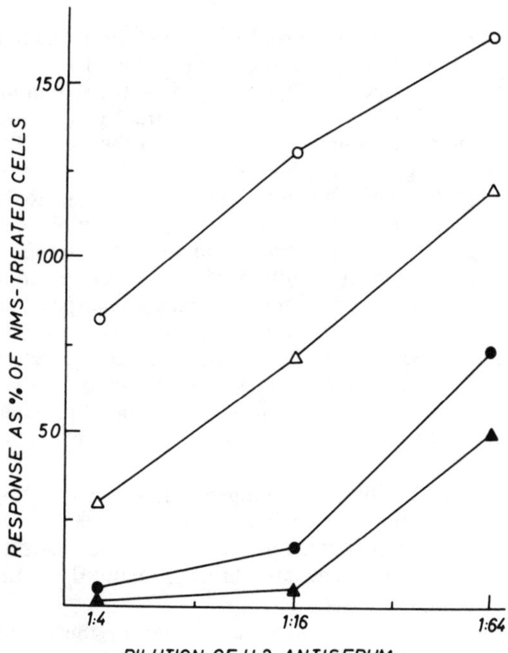

FIGURE 9. The response of C_3H thymus cells exposed to dilutions of anti-H-2 serum, in the presence or absence of guinea-pig complement. *Triangles:* response to Con-A. *Circles:* response to PHA and SUP. *Open symbols:* cells exposed to antibody in the absence of C′. *Filled symbols:* cells exposed to antibody in the presence of C′. The results are expressed as a percentage of the mitotic response of cells exposed to normal mouse serum.

frequently noted.[32] In contrast, exposure to H-2 antiserum alone caused a striking inhibition of the response to Con-A and a minor inhibition of the response to PHA and SUP (FIGURE 9). In repeated experiments with spleen cells, H-2 antiserum, in the absence of C′, caused only a moderate inhibition of the response to Con-A. Usually the response of antibody-treated spleen cells was about 30% lower than that of cells exposed to NMS. Variation in the concentration of Con-A did not change the degree of inhibition by antibody alone.

DISCUSSION

The two major antigen systems that differentiate murine T-lymphocytes from B-lymphocytes are the θ- and Ly-alloantigens.[2, 3] It is now becoming clear that rabbit antibodies specific for murine T-lymphocytes are directed against these same cell-surface antigens.[34] Rabbit antibodies specific for murine T-cells (MSLA) [35] seem to constitute antibodies that cross-react with various Ly-alloantigens.[34] The cell surface of T-cells probably is also endowed with immunoglobulins, although this is difficult to demonstrate.[14] Like all other tissues of the mouse, murine T-cells possess H-2 antigens. In addition to antigenic markers found on peripheral T-cells, murine thymus cells may possess thymus-distinctive TL-antigens [18] and are highly sensitive to the cytotoxic effect of guinea-pig serum.[19]

A number of studies have correlated the quantitative variations of the antigens present on the cell-surface of thymocytes and of peripheral T-lymphocytes with their capacity to carry out their specialized functions. Fractionation of thymus cell suspensions on BSA gradients have shown that cells of different bouyant densities vary both in their antigenic properties and in their immune reactivity. The higher the bouyant density of the cells, the greater was their TL-, θ-, and Ly-antigenicity, the more pronounced was their sensitivity to GPS, and the lower was their H-2 alloantigenicity.[9, 10, 36] As far as their function was concerned, only cells of relatively low bouyant density were found to be capable of carrying out functions characteristic for T-cells. Cells of low bouyant density had a high capacity for localization in lymph nodes,[9, 37] for response to PHA,[10, 26] for reaction in mixed lymphocyte cultures,[10] and for cooperation with B-lymphocytes in immune reactions.[10] Exposure of thymus cell suspensions to anti-θ serum and C′ under conditions that would kill a large proportion of the thymus cell suspension, was found to selectively spare the subpopulation of cells responding to PHA.[38] Peripheral T-lymphocytes that varied in their θ-antigenicity were shown to differ in their relative capacity to respond to either PHA or Con-A [28] and in their tendency to localize either in the lymph nodes or in the spleen.[11, 28]

The present paper summarizes our findings on antigenic differences among subpopulations of T-lymphocytes that differ in their migration pattern *in vivo* and that vary in their *in vitro* response to mitogens. Attempts were made to determine to what extent cell-surface antigens are directly involved in the specialized functions of T-lymphocytes.

Subpopulations of thymocytes migrating to either the spleen or the lymph nodes were found to differ antigenically.[24] Particularly striking was the high H-2 antigenicity of the lymph node-seeking subpopulation and the sensitivity to GPS of the spleen-seeking subpopulation. Since H-2 antiserum also inhibited to a greater extent the lymph node-seeking migration stream of spleen or lymph node cells [23] it was of interest to determine whether cell-surface H-2 antigenic determinants were directly involved in the localization of lymphocytes in the lymph nodes. Exposure of either lymph node cells or thymus cells to monovalent Fab fragments of an H-2 antiserum had only a weak inhibitory effect on lymphocyte migration. The lymph node-seeking stream was inhibited to a slightly greater extent than the spleen-seeking stream. Whatever inhibitory effect was exerted by the Fab fragments, it is not clear whether they block specific sites involved in the migration of lymphocytes or whether the attachment of the fragments impedes the migration of the cells in a nonspecific way. On the other hand, it should be pointed out that the relative weakness of the inhibitory effect of monovalent H-2 antibody fragments could be caused by shedding or pinocytosis of antibody-antigen complexes on the cell surface accompanied by resynthesis of new H-2 antigenic determinants.

Several lines of evidence indicate that the localization of lymphocytes in lymph nodes depends on glycoprotein receptors on the membrane of the lymphocytes.[27–30] In the present study ^{51}Cr-labeled lymphocytes were exposed *in vitro* to PHA or Con-A and their localization *in vivo* was analysed. Exposure of lymphocytes to PHA was found to inhibit the migration of lymphocytes to the lymph nodes and to the spleen to a similar extent. In contrast, Con-A inhibited the migration of lymphocytes to the lymph nodes to a significantly greater extent than to the spleen. Exposure of lymphocytes to other lectins, such as wheat-germ agglutinin and fucose-binding protein, had no effect on their migration (unpublished data). The inhibitory activity of Con-A on lymphocyte migration did not result from elimination of the subpopulation of lymph node-seeking cells. It resulted from a specific interaction with carbohydrates on the cell-surface of lymphocytes, which could be reversed by the addition of α-methyl-mannopyranoside. The concentration of Con-A that inhibited the migration of lymphocytes to the lymph nodes was much lower than that required for impairment of the free fluidity of the cell membrane.[39] While it remains possible that Con-A affects the migration of lymphocytes to lymph nodes in a nonspecific way, it is tempting to suggest that Con-A binds to the carbohydrate-containing receptors on the cell membrane, which are believed to determine the "homing" of lymphocytes to lymph nodes. Similar conclusions were reached recently by Gilette *et al.*[40] Subpopulations of T-lymphocytes that differed antigenically were found to differ in their responsiveness to various mitogens. Exposure of spleen cells to dilutions of θ-antiserum, in the presence of complement, inhibited the mitotic response to PHA to a greater extent than that to Con-A, in agreement with the observations of Stobo and Paul.[33] Exposure to Ly-antiserum and C′ was found to have the same effect. In contrast, exposure of spleen cells to H-2 antiserum and complement had a stronger inhibitory effect on their response to Con-A than on their response to PHA. Thus, the subset of spleen cells that has a relatively strong capacity to respond to PHA has a high concentration of the θ-and Ly-antigens. There was a correlation between H-2 antigenicity and capacity to respond to various concentrations of PHA. The subpopulation of T-lymphocytes that responded to low doses of PHA seemed to possess a high H-2 antigenicity. In contrast, the cells that responded to high concentrations of PHA seemed to have a very low H-2 antigenicity.

It is commonly believed that in the thymus only the subpopulation that resembles peripheral T-lymphocytes is capable of responding to lectins. It was found that only the thymus subpopulation responding to PHA had these attributes, since it had little TL-antigenicity, was resistant to GPS, had low θ- and Ly-antigenicities, and a relatively high H-2 antigenicity. In contrast, cells responding to Con-A had not only higher levels of θ- and Ly-antigenicity but also possessed the TL-antigen. Cells responding to PHA in the presence of a supernatant obtained from peritoneal macrophages had antigenic properties similar, although not identical to the cells responding to Con-A. Like peripheral T-lymphocytes, the subset of thymus cells responding to PHA and SUP had a slightly higher θ-antigenicity than those responding to Con-A. Also, H-2 antiserum and C′ inhibited the response to Con-A to a greater extent than that to PHA and SUP.

In the search for any correlation between cell-surface antigens and the receptors for mitogens, lymphocytes were exposed to antibodies, in the absence of C′, and their mitotic response was assayed. The response of thymus cells to Con-A was markedly inhibited by exposure to H-2 antibodies, while θ-or Ly-antisera failed to inhibit the response, or even augmented it.[32] H-2 antisera had only a weak (though reproducible) inhibitory effect on the response of spleen cells to Con-A. The results obtained with thymus cells indicate that cell surface H-2 antigenic determinants are closely related to Con-A binding sites, or at least to "productive" Con-A binding sites.[41] The fact that H-2 antibodies show only a weak inhibitory effect on the response of spleen cells to Con-A may indicate that productive Con-A binding sites and H-2 determinants on the surface of peripheral T-cells are not as closely related as on the surface of thymocytes. The possible importance of H-2 antigenicity for the Con-A response of spleen cells is shown by the fact that splenic lymphocytes selected for low H-2 antigen content may respond to high concentrations of PHA as well as control cells, but fail to respond to any concentration of Con-A.

It is of interest that of the various alloantigens tested, evidence for direct implication in T-cell function was so far obtained only for H-2 antigenicity. Recent studies on the modulation of the H-2 antigenicity of peritoneal macrophages [42] have indicated that K-end H-2 determinants on the cell surface of macrophages are closely associated with EAC′-receptors.[43]

It was suggested, that the close association of H-2 antigenicity and EAC′-receptors on the surface of macrophages may play a role in the regulation of the immune response by H-2 antigens (FIGURE 10). Possibly the close genetic linkage of many Ir genes to H-2 genes [44] may reflect a close association between H-2 antigens and various receptors on the surface of lymphocytes and of macrophages.

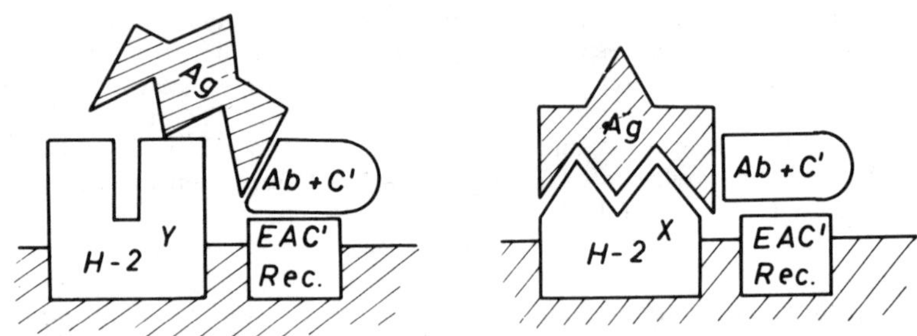

FIGURE 10. A model for the effect of the close association of H-2 determinants on the surface of macrophages and EAC′-receptors on immune responsiveness. On the right: The presence of H-2 determinants of the $H\text{-}2^x$ allele enables a firm attachment of complexes of antigen (Ag), antibody (Ab), and C′ through EAC′-receptors to the cell surface of macrophages. It is suggested that in this form the antigens are highly immunogenic. On the left: The presence of H-2 determinants of the $H\text{-}2^y$ allele do not allow a firm attachment of antigen-antibody-C′ complexes to the surface of macrophages, thus reducing the immunogenicity of the complex.

SUMMARY

T-lymphocytes differ antigenically from B-lymphocytes. In the present study attempts were made to determine the role of surface antigens of T-cells, in their migration *in vivo* and in their response to mitogens. Exposure of thymus cells to anti-H-2 sera inhibits migration to the lymph nodes (LN) to a greater extent than to the spleen. Fab fragments of H-2 antisera had only a slight effect on lymphocyte migration, inhibiting the LN-seeking stream only slightly more than the spleen-seeking stream. The interaction of Con-A with carbohydrates on the cell-surface of lymphocytes inhibits preferentially their localization in LN. Studies on the migration of lymphocytes that had localized either in the LN or spleens of primary hosts indicate that Con-A does not eliminate LN-seeking cells, but rather inhibits their active localization in LN. The subpopulation of lymphocytes, in both thymus and spleen, that responds to Con-A was found to possess a higher H-2 antigenicity and a lower Ly and θ-antigenicity than the cells responding to PHA. Spleen cells responding to low concentrations of PHA had a relatively high H-2 antigenicity, whereas those responding to high concentrations of PHA had a low H-2 antigenicity. Exposure of thymus cells to H-2 antiserum alone markedly inhibited their response to Con-A. Similar treatment of spleen cells had only a weak inhibitory effect.

References

1. Boyse, E. A. & L. J. Old. 1969. Ann. Rev. Genet. **3:** 269.
2. Raff, M. C. 1971. Transplant. Rev. **6:** 52.
3. Schlesinger, M. 1972. Progr. Allergy **16:** 214.
4. Schlesinger, M. & I. Yron. 1970. J. Immunol. **104:** 798.
5. Raff, M. C. & H. H. Wortis. 1970. Immunology **18:** 931.
6. Raff, M. C., S. Nase & N. A. Mitchison. 1971. Nature New Biol. **230:** 50.
7. Laskov, R., R. Rabinowitz & M. Schlesinger. 1973. Immunology **24:** 939.
8. Takahashi, T., L. J. Old & E. A. Boyse. 1970. J. Exp. Med. **131:** 1325.
9. Schlesinger, M., S. Gottesfeld & Z. Korzash. 1973. Cell Immunol. **6:** 49.
10. Smith, R. T. 1972. Transplant. Rev. **11:** 178.
11. Stobo, J. W. 1972. Transplant. Rev. **11:** 60.
12. Ada, G. L. 1970. Transplant. Rev. **5:** 105.
13. Sulitzeanu, D. 1971. Current Topics Microbiol. Immunol. **54:** 1.
14. Roelants, G. E. & A. Ryden. 1974. Nature **247:** 104.
15. Schlesinger, M. & D. Hurvitz. 1969. Transplantation **7:** 132.
16. Reif, A. E. & J. M. V. Allen. 1964. J. Exp. Med. **120:** 413.
17. Boyse, E. A., M. Miyazawa, T. Aoki & L. J. Old. 1968. Proc. Roy. Soc. Lond. B. **170:** 175.
18. Boyse, E. A., L. J. Old & S. Luell. 1963. J. Nat. Cancer Inst. **31:** 987.
19. Schlesinger, M. & A. Cohen. 1970. Transplantation **10:** 130.
20. Porter, R. R. 1959. Biochem. J. **73:** 119.
21. Wigzell, H. 1965. Transplantation **3:** 423.
22. Boyle, W. 1968. Transplantation **6:** 761.
23. Schlesinger, M. & Z. Korzash. 1973. *In* Advances in Experimental Medicine and Biology Vol. 29 (Microenvironmental Aspects of Immunity). B. D. Janković & K. Isaković, Eds. : 71–77. Plenum Press. New York, New York.
24. Schlesinger, M., Z. Shlomai-Korzash & E. Israel. 1973. Eur. J. Immunol. **3:** 335.
25. Ron, N., A. Laufer & I. Gery. 1973. Immunology **25:** 433.
26. Gery, I., R. K. Gershon & B. H. Waksman. 1972. J. Exp. Med. **136:** 128.
27. Gesner, B. M. & R. Ginsburg. 1964. Proc. Nat. Acad. Sci. U.S. **52:** 750.
28. Woodruff, J. & B. M. Gesner. 1968. Science **161:** 176.
29. Woodruff, J. & B. M. Gesner. 1969. J. Exp. Med. **129:** 551.
30. Zatz, M. M., A. L. Goldstein, O. O. Blumfeld & A. White. 1972. Nature New Biol. **240:** 253.
31. Lance, E. M. & R. N. Taub. 1969. Nature **221:** 841.
32. Schlesinger, M., M. Chaouat & I. Gery. 1974. *In* Lymphocyte Recognition and Effector Mechanisms. K. Lindahl-Kiessling & D. Osoba, Eds. : 645–650. Academic Press. New York, New York.
33. Stobo, J. W. & W. E. Paul. 1973. J. Immunol. **110:** 363.
34. Rabinowitz, R., A. Cohen, R. Laskov & M. Schlesinger. 1974. J. Immunol. **112:** 683.
35. Shigeno, N., U. Hämmerling, C. Arpels, E. A. Boyse & L. J. Old. 1968. Lancet **2:** 320.
36. Shortman, K., J. C. Cerottini & K. T. Brunner. 1972. Eur. J. Immunol. **2:** 313.
37. Colley, D. G., Wu A. Y. Shih & B. H. Waksman. 1972. J. Exp. Med. **136:** 128.

38. Stobo, J. W. & W. E. Paul. 1972. Cell Immunol. **4:** 367.
39. Yahara, I. & G. M. Edelman. 1972. Proc. Nat. Acad. Sci. U.S. **69:** 608.
40. Gilette, R. W., G. O. McKenzie & M. H. Swanson. 1973. J. Immunol. **111:** 1902.
41. Sharon, N. & H. Lis. 1972. Science **177:** 949.
42. Schlesinger, M. & M. Chaouat. 1973. Transplant. Proc. **5:** 105.
43. Schlesinger, M. & M. Chaouat. 1975. Eur. J. Immunol. In press.
44. Grumet, F. C., G. F. Mitchell & H. O. McDevitt. 1971. Ann. N.Y. Acad. Sci. **190:** 170.

Discussion of the Paper

Dr. Wyburn: Did you try to inhibit the T-rosettes with anti-β 2 microglobulin?

Dr. M. Schlesinger: Not yet.

Dr. A. Wyburn: We tried to inhibit the E-rosettes, which are T-cells, with anti-HLA serum in human systems and we cannot show any type of inhibition.

Dr. M. Schlesinger: I perfectly agree. Now as far as the human system is concerned one can inhibit the E-rosettes with anti-T serum. One can partially inhibit the EAC-rosettes with anti-HLA, not the E-rosettes. The E-rosettes are not inhibitable by anti-HLA serum.

Dr. H. Friedman: Your model system is certainly very intriguing. I believe you also mentioned, as others have suggested, that a macrophage supernatant may replace some factors. Do you believe the supernatants might actually contain some of these membrane receptors?

Dr. M. Schlesinger: No, the active principle in the macrophage supernatant is a very small molecule on the order of less than 10,000 MW in size. It is a very small molecule and has not been identified yet. This may be related to some of the factors that were discussed here, but certainly I do not believe that this is a membrane factor.

NATURE AND BIOLOGICAL ACTIVITIES OF THYMUS HORMONES: PROSPECTS FOR THE FUTURE

Abraham White

Syntex Research
Palo Alto, California 94304

The title designated for this presentation by those individuals who planned this conference provides the opportunity to consider three aspects of thymic hormones: (1) to summarize briefly the origins of some of the present concepts of the nature and role of thymic hormones in immunity; (2) to indicate the present day status of these concepts, as derived from pertinent literature and from the data provided by other participants in this conference; and (3) to project a cautious assessment of prospects for the future.

This presentation is dedicated to the memory of Dr. Thomas F. Dougherty, whose recent untimely death has resulted in the loss of an inspiring teacher, a brilliant investigator, and an irreplaceable friend. Indeed, my own several decades of involvement in studies of the chemistry and metabolism of lymphoid tissue were initiated by Dr. Dougherty who came to Yale in 1942 as a Post-doctoral Fellow, having just completed his Ph.D. training at the University of Minnesota with Dr. Hal Downey. Dr. Downey had transmitted to Tom Dougherty an interest in lymphoid cells, as he had to many students, including some participants in this Conference.

In the course of discussions with Dr. Dougherty about his then current studies with Dr. William Gardner of lymphoid tissue hyperplasia induced by estrogen administration to mice,[1] our attention was directed to the marked involution of lymphoid tissue, notably the thymus, that had been described by Selye[2] as due to a stress stimulus that was mediated by the adrenal glands. Inasmuch as Dr. George Sayers, then a graduate student in our laboratory at Yale, had just isolated highly purified adrenocorticotropic hormone from beef pituitaries,[3] we embarked with Dr. Dougherty on a detailed study of the effects of adrenocorticotropic hormone on lymphoid tissue. A single injection of this hormone in the mouse produced a marked involution of lymphoid tissue,[4] preceded by an acute, dramatic absolute decrease in the numbers of circulating lymphocytes.[5] These results were extended with the then available Upjohn preparation of total adrenal cortical steroids in oil.[6] The synthesis of certain of these hormones, as a result of the brilliant efforts of Kendall, Sarett and their associates, provided us with the opportunity to demonstrate that the effects of adrenal cortical steroids on lymphoid tissue were unique for the 11-hydroxylated compounds. Moreover, the thymus gland, among the lymphoid structures, was the most sensitive to the involutionary effects of the pituitary-adrenal cortical axis.[5] Of particular significance for more recent studies of the role of the thymus as an endocrine gland, the question of cortisol-resistant versus cortisol-sensitive thymocytes, and the probable secretory role of the endodermal reticular cells of the thymus, was the statement by Dougherty and White[5] that due to hormonal treatment, "The disappearance of numerous lymphocytes ordinarily present in the medulla of the thymus left the endodermal reticular cells more exposed, thus giving the impression that an increase in these cells had occurred."

It is fitting also, in a conference devoted to the role of the thymus in immunity, to note an additional contribution in which Dr. Dougherty participated. Using the newly introduced Tiselius moving boundary electrophoretic technique, we demonstrated that normal lymphoid tissue contains a protein with an electrophoretic mobility identical to that of the γ-globulin of the blood[7,8] and that lymphoid cells from the nodes of immunized mice contain demonstrable antibody.[8,9] The continuing synthesis of antibody globulin by lymphoid cells, and their release under the involutionary effects of adrenal steroids, were among early indications of the role of lymphoid tissue in immune phenomena and demonstrated the role of one endocrine system on host immunity. The dissolution of lymphoid tissue by adrenal steroids, which destroy the site of manufacture of antibody globulin, laid the basis for the demonstration by Heilman and Kendall[10] of the effectiveness of cortisone in restraining the growth of a transplantable lymphosarcoma in the mouse and for the subsequent use of adrenal steroids as immunosuppressive agents.[11]

The dramatic involution of lymphoid tissue by adrenal steroids led to our initial interest in thymic extracts and the possible role of the thymus as an endocrine gland. If the adrenal steroids cause involution of lymphoid tissue, did the latter, on dissolution, yield products that might suppress pituitary-adrenal cortical secretory activity in the manner of a feedback mechanism? Pursuing this question with Dr. Sidney Roberts, and utilizing the well-established parameters of lymphoid tissue hypertrophy and lymphocytosis as an index of adrenal insufficiency, we reported in 1949 that specific, partially purified fractions of calf thymus produced lymphoid tissue hypertrophy and a lymphocytosis on injection into rats.[12] The specificity of this response was inferred from the absence of this activity in other protein-containing fractions of calf thymus. This lymphocytopoietic activity of thymic extracts was subsequently confirmed by Gregoire and Duchateau[13] and by Metcalf[14] in 1956, and similar observations are described elsewhere in this volume.[15-17]

The resurgence of interest in the thymus and in thymic extracts and their potential roles in immune phenomena stems, of course, from the almost simultaneous and now classical observations by Miller,[18] and by Archer and Pierce[19] of the deleterious consequences of neonatal thymectomy, observations that were made initially in the mouse and the rabbit, respectively, and subsequently confirmed in a variety of experimental animal species.[20] This basic information, and the recognition that primary and secondary immunodeficiencies in the human were due to thymic aplasia or dysplasias,[20,21] together with subsequent demonstrations that thymic tissue in Millipore® chambers[22] and cell-free extracts of the thymus[23] may function in lieu of the thymus in neonatally thymectomized animals, rekindled our interest, as well as that of many in other laboratories, in the chemical nature of thymic extracts and the possible role of the thymus as an endocrine gland. In addition, stimulus was provided by the arrival in our laboratory of a Postdoctoral Fellow, Dr. Jerome J. Klein, who had completed clinical training in medicine at Mt. Sinai Hospital and had come under the influence of Dr. K. E. Osserman, and the latter's interest in myasthenia gravis. Dr. Klein suggested repetition of Dr. Robert's earlier studies on thymic extracts, and, with Dr. Allan L. Goldstein, who had also joined the program as a Postdoctoral Fellow, developed an assay based upon incorporation of [^{3}H]thymidine into lymph nodes as a means of assessing the activity of potential lymphocytopoietic fractions of calf thymus extracts.[24] This marked the initiation of a most productive collaboration with Dr. Goldstein that, over a 10-year period, has contributed to establishing the thymus as an endocrine gland and confirming its hormonal role in immunity.[25] In 1966, with the help of Mrs. Florence Slater and Miss Norma Robert, we described the preparation of an active, partially purified, thymic lymphocytopoietic fraction, and suggested that this fraction contained a hormone to which was given the name, thymosin.[26]

The early, partially purified preparations of thymosin, albeit not meeting the criteria of physical-chemical homogeneity, were shown to be effective in a number of models accepted as reflecting acceleration of the maturation of cell-mediated immunological competence.[25, 27] In these efforts, particular acknowledgment should be made of the cooperative studies with Dr. Mark Hardy of the Department of Surgery, and Dr. Jack Battisto, of the Department of Microbiology and Immunology, at the Albert Einstein College of Medicine. With Dr. Martin Zisblatt, then a graduate student at the medical school, it was demonstrated that thymosin was also effective in restraining the progressive growth of the sarcoma induced in mice by inoculation with the Moloney Sarcoma Virus.[28] The variety of experimental models, both *in vivo* and *in vitro*, in which thymosin fractions were significantly active led us to propose that thymosin, a lymphocytopoietic factor, acts on a precursor of the immunologically competent T-cell by accelerating the rate at which selected populations of these precursor cells mature to express T-cell characteristics and functions.[29] This hypothesis has been amply supported by several of the presentations at this conference, which appear in this volume.

The later addition of Dr. Arabinda Guha to our research group facilitated achievement of the isolation of thymosin in purified form.[30] No small contribution to our progress was provided by the development in the laboratory of Dr. J-F. Bach in Paris of a modified *in vitro* rosette assay. With Dr. Bach's first demonstration that calf-thymosin-containing fractions we sent him could be quantitatively evaluated by the rosette assay, it became possible for the first time to assay rapidly for thymosin activity the many fractions being prepared by Drs. Goldstein and Guha. Dr. Goldstein and I are indebted to Dr. Bach and his colleagues, Dr. Marie-Ann Bach and Dr. Mirielle Dardenne, for the hospitality of their laboratory extended to us, and later to our associate, Miss Norma Robert, as well as for the numerous rosette assays they have conducted of our fractions.

Thymosin was demonstrated to be a protein with an MW of approximately 12,200, free of carbohydrate, lipid, and polynucleotides. The initial description of the amino acid composition of thymosin was presented at the Federation meetings in April, 1973, and aspects of a new method of isolation and characterization are presented elsewhere in this volume.[31]

Through the courtesy of Dr. Milton Helperin, in charge of the Coroner's office of the City of New York, we succeeded in obtaining human thymus for the preparation of thymosin from the human species. The product isolated appears to have similar biological properties and certain of the chemical properties of calf thymosin. The development of a radioimmunoassay by Mr. Richard Schulof[32] established the presence of circulating thymosin in a variety of species, including *Homo sapiens*. These data, together with those for a circulating thymic humoral factor described by Bach and Dardenne,[33] strongly support the role of the thymus gland as an endocrine gland, influencing several parameters of host immunological competence.

Elsewhere in this volume, Dr. Allan L. Goldstein and his colleagues have presented some of the data derived from the more recent studies of the research group Dr. Goldstein has assembled following his move to Galveston, supplemented with the participation of a number of investigators to whom thymosin preparations have been provided.[31]

In initiating laboratory activities in Palo Alto, we have sought to improve and simplify the initial steps in the isolation of thymosin from calf thymus. This has been achieved through the efforts of Dr. Clarke Brooks, Mrs. Susan Haag, and Mrs. Kathleen Mitchell. Although this methodology has not yet advanced to a final stage of purification, we have succeeded in increasing substantially the total yield of thymosin, both in terms of weight of material and its biological activity.

In preparing the second aspect of this presentation, namely, the nature and activities of thymic extracts, my task has been greatly facilitated by responses to my request, made prior to these sessions to a number of the participants in this conference, who kindly provided me with both published and unpublished information pertinent to the summation task assigned to me. Most of the data sent to me appear elsewhere in this volume. I shall summarize the more significant of these by comparing and contrasting certain of the chemical properties and biological activities of selected products prepared from thymus tissue in the laboratories of other speakers at this conference.

TABLE 1 lists the physical and chemical properties of some of the more extensively studied products obtained from thymus tissue. TABLE 2 lists some of the biological activities reported for these individual preparations. Each of these products is described in other contributions in this volume.

It is apparent from TABLE 1 that there is at present a significant lack of concensus in the area of the physical and chemical properties of the preparations isolated from thymus tissue as well as, by one laboratory, from pig serum. This lack of agreement may reflect the diverse methods of isolation of products or the existence of more than a single hormonal factor, each with single or multiple biological activities, or both. The preparation from thymus of a hypocalcemic factor, albeit one apparently differing in chemical nature from calcitonin, is perhaps not too surprising in view of the common embryological origin of the thymus, and the parathyroid and thyroid glands, all of which contain the characteristic C-cells indicated to be the site of synthesis of calcitonin. Indeed, the latter hormone has been characterized in partially purified extracts of human thymus and thymoma tissue.[34]

With regard to the biological activities of the various described thymus factors, it may be concluded that there is rather good agreement among the several laboratories that lymphoid cells, of primary significance in selected immune phenomena, are influenced in numbers and certain manifestations of immunological function by the diverse thymus products. The molecular basis of this influence, including the elucidation of the nature of the cell types upon which thymic hormones exert their actions, remain to be delineated. Suggestive data regarding a possible basis for the action of thymus factors on lymphoid cells have been presented by both Bach and co-workers and by Trainin and his collaborators at this conference indicating that, as in the case of many other polypeptide hormones, cyclic AMP may be a modulator in the process of T-cell maturation. In addition, the increased intracellular concentration of cyclic AMP produced in lymphoid cells by prostaglandin E_2 and the ability of this latter compound to enhance graft-versus-host reactivity[35] indicate many approaches to the elucidation of the mechanism of action of thymic factors.

Caution is indicated in attempting to dissect further the differences in chemical and biological properties of active thymus preparations that have been only partially characterized from a physical-chemical standpoint. Additional studies are required to ascertain whether more than one of these may be a thymic hormone. Electrostatic and hydrophobic interaction of proteins and polypeptides with other molecules present in tissues from which initial extraction is conducted, as well as in the blood, are not unknown and may lead to erroneous conclusions with regard to the state of purity of a product whose

TABLE 1

PHYSICAL AND CHEMICAL PROPERTIES OF SOME THYMUS PRODUCTS

Product *	Chemical Class	Molecular Weight	Properties
Thymosin [31]	protein	12,000	heat stable no lipid, CHO or polynucleotide
Thymopoietin I [35]	protein	7,000	heat stable N-terminus: glycine C-terminus: lysine
Thymopoietin II [38]	protein	7,000	heat stable N-terminus: glycine C-terminus: lysine
Thymic humoral factor (THF) [39]	polypeptide	$<5{,}000$ >700	heat stable
Serum TA † [40]	polypeptide	$\sim 1{,}000$	heat labile $pH_I \sim 7.5$
Lymphocyte stimulating hormone (LSH_h) [41]	protein	$\sim 17{,}000$	heat labile
Lymphocyte stimulating hormone (LSH_r) [42]	protein	$\sim 80{,}000$	heat stable
Homeostatic thymus hormone (HTH) [43]	glycopeptide	1,800–2,500	heat labile
Thymic hypocalcemic factor (T_1) [44]	protein	68,000 (100,000)	$pH_I = 5.65$ 2.4% CHO
Thymic hypocalcemic factor (T_2) [44]	protein	57,000 (170,000)	$pH_I = 5.40$

* The superscript numbers are to references in this paper.
† Serum TA=Serum "Thymic Activity."

isolation is being sought. Perhaps less than pure preparations of differing properties will, when studied further, prove to resemble one another more closely than presently appears to be the case. In addition, previous experience, for example with insulin and parathyroid hormone, has demonstrated that a biologically active, circulating hormonal agent may be synthesized by its endocrine gland as a molecule with physical, chemical, immunological, and biological properties differing significantly not only from that of the secreted moiety but,

TABLE 2

BIOLOGICAL ACTIVITIES OF SOME THYMUS PRODUCTS

Product	
Thymosin	Lymphocytopoiesis Restoration of immunological competence *in vivo* and *in vitro* Enhancement of expression of T-cell characteristics and functions *in vitro* and *in vivo*
Thymopoietin I	Impairment of neuromuscular transmission *in vivo* Induction of expression of T-cell antigens *in vitro*
Thymopoietin II	Same as Thymopoietin I
Thymic humoral factor (THF)	Restoration of immunological competence *in vivo* and *in vitro* Acceleration of generation of specifically committed lymphocytes Prevention of sensitization against self-antigens
Serum TA (Serum "thymic activity")	Induction of expression of T-cell antigens *in vitro* θ-positive cells in nude mice *in vivo* Retardation of growth of Moloney Virus induced tumors *in vivo*
Lymphocyte stimulating hormone (LSH_h)	Relative lymphocytosis Augmented antibody synthesis in newborn mice
Lymphocyte stimulating hormone (LSH_r)	Leukocytosis; lymphocytosis Augmented antibody synthesis in newborn mice
Homeostatic thymus hormone (HTH)	Antagonism to adrenocorticotropin and thyrotropin in normal resting condition of their target glands, and to thyroxine Antagonism to gonadotropins; delayed puberty Synergistic to growth hormone (lymphocytosis) Chemotactic influence on lymphocytes
Thymic hypocalcemic factor T_1	Hypocalcemia
Thymic hypocalcemic factor T_2	Hypocalcemia Relative lymphocytosis

indeed, from that of the biologically active form responsible for target cell recognition.

Finally, in closing I come to the projection of a cautious assessment of prospects for the future. Acceptance of this last assignment is both a challenging and perhaps unwise decision, since the rate of appearance of new observations relating to the roles of the thymus in immunobiology is so rapid as to make it it possible that such predictions will be out of date by the time the volume of this conference appears in print. Nonetheless, the guidelines and signposts for the direction of continuing developments in the role of thymus factors in immunity appear to be readily discernible. As for any endocrine gland, practical utility may be predicted for thymic factors or hormones in the replacement or augmentation of the functions now delineated for the thymus in immunity. The experimental and clinical evidence clearly establishes at least two roles of the thymus gland in immunity: (1) the export of lymphoid cells of varying types and states of maturity with respect to their capacity to participate in diverse immunological phenomena and (2) the synthesis and secretion of one or more hormonal factors essential for the continuing, and perhaps final, maturation of immunologically competent thymus-derived or T-cells. In this maturation process, thymosin and other active thymus preparations may function in two ways: (a) to induce the appearance of specific types of T-cells, and (b) to influence the reversion of aberrant T-cells to more normal modes of functioning.[36, 37]

The indicated biological functions of the several diverse subpopulations of T-cells permits optimism concerning the possible practical applications of one or more highly purified thymic factors. These applications range from obvious utility in replacement of a lack of a normal functioning thymus gland at birth, to the possible alleviation of primary or secondary immunodeficiencies not restricted to specific age groups, for example, aberrant, unrestrained cellular proliferation, as well as to the later years of aging characterized by declining host immunological competence, including the ability to discern between self and non-self.

References

1. Gardner, W. U., T. F. Dougherty & W. T. Williams. 1944. Cancer Res. **4:** 73.
2. Selye, H. 1940. In The Cyclopedia of Medicine, Surgery and Specialties. Vol. **15:** 15. F. A. Davis Co. Philadelphia, Pa.
3. Sayers, G., A. White & C. N. H. Long. 1943. J. Biol. Chem. **149:** 425.
4. Dougherty, T. F. & A. White. 1943. Proc. Soc. Exp. Biol. Med. **53:** 132.
5. Dougherty, T. F. & A. White. 1944. Endocrinology. **35:** 1.
6. Dougherty, T. F. & A. White. 1945. Am. J. Anat. **77:** 81.
7. White, A. & T. F. Dougherty. 1945. Endocrinology. **36:** 207.
8. White, A. 1947–1948. Harvey Lectures. **43:** 43.
9. Dougherty, T. F., J. H. Chase & A. White. 1944. Proc. Soc. Exp. Biol. Med. **57:** 295.
10. Heilman, F. R. & E. C. Kendall. 1944. Endocrinology. **34:** 416.
11. Schwartz, R. S. 1971. *In* Immunobiology, R. A. Good & D. W. Fisher, Eds. : 240–247. Sinauer Associates, Inc. Stamford, Conn.
12. Roberts, S. & A. White. 1949. J. Biol. Chem. **178:** 151.
13. Gregoire, C. & G. Duchateau. 1956. Arch. Biol. **67:** 269.
14. Metcalf, D. 1956. Brit. J. Cancer **10:** 442.

15. Luckey, T. D. This volume.
16. Robey, W. G. This volume.
17. Comsa, J., H. Leonhardt & J. A. Schwarz. This volume.
18. Miller, J. F. A. P. 1961. Lancet **ii:** 748.
19. Archer, O. K. & J. C. Pierce. 1961. Fed. Proc. Fed. Am. Soc. Exp. Biol. **20:** 26.
20. Good, R. A. & A. E. Gabrielson, eds. 1964. "The Thymus in Immunobiology." Hoeber Division, Harper & Row, Publishers, New York.
21. Goldstein, A. L. & A. White. 1971. Adv. in Metabolic Disorders. **5:** 149.
22. Levey, R. H., N. Trainin & L. W. Law. 1963. J. Nat. Cancer Inst. **31:** 199.
23. Miller, J. F. A. P. & D. Osoba. 1967. Physiol. Rev. **47:** 437.
24. Klein, J. J., A. L. Goldstein & A. White. 1965. Proc. Nat. Acad. Sci. U.S. **53:** 812.
25. White, A. & A. L. Goldstein. 1970. *In* Control Processes in Multicellular Organisms. G. E. W. Wolstenholme & J. Knight, Eds. : 210–237. Churchill. London, England.
26. Goldstein, A. L., F. D. Slater & A. White. 1966. Proc. Nat. Acad. Sci. U.S. **56:** 1010.
27. Goldstein, A. L. & A. White. 1971. Current Topics in Exp. Endocrinol. **1:** 21.
28. Zisblatt, M., A. L. Goldstein, F. Lilly & A. White. 1970. Proc. Nat. Acad. Sci. U.S. **66:** 1170.
29. Goldstein, A. L. & A. White. 1973. Contemporary Topics in Immunobiology **2:** 339.
30. Goldstein, A. L., A. Guha, M. M. Zatz, M. A. Hardy & A. White. 1972. Proc. Nat. Acad. Sci. U.S. **69:** 1800.
31. Hooper, J. A., M. C. McDaniel, G. B. Thurman, G. H. Cohen, R. S. Schulof & A. L. Goldstein. This volume.
32. Schulof, R. S. 1972. Texas Reports Biol. Med. **30:** 195.
33. Bach, J-F. & M. Dardenne. 1972. Transplant. Proc. **4:** 345.
34. Galante, L., T. V. Gudmundsson, E. W. Mathews, A. Tse, E. D. Williams, N. J. Y. Woodhouse & I. MacIntyre. 1968. Lancet **ii:** 537.
35. Kook, A. I. & N. Trainin. 1974. J. Exp. Med. **139:** 193.
36. Dauphinee, M. J., N. Talal, A. L. Goldstein & A. White. 1974. Proc. Nat. Acad. Sci. U.S. **71:** 2637.
37. Talal, N., M. J. Dauphinee, R. Pillarisetty & R. Goldblum. This volume.
38. Goldstein, G. This volume.
39. Trainin, N. This volume.
40. Bach, J-F., M. Dardenne & M-A. Bach. This volume.
41. Luckey, T. D. & B. Venugopal. This volume.
42. Robey, W. G. This volume.
43. Comsa, J. This volume.
44. Mizutani, A., M. Shimizu, I. Suzuki, T. Mizutani & S. Hayase. This volume.

LYMPHOCYTE DIFFERENTIATION FROM PRECURSOR CELLS *IN VITRO* *

M. P. Scheid, G. Goldstein, U. Hammerling, and E. A. Boyse

Memorial Sloan-Kettering Cancer Center
New York, New York 10021

Much of the recent work in our laboratory has centered about an induction assay developed by Komuro and Boyse [1] in which one of the early maturational steps in the T-cell development, the differentiation from prothymocyte to early thymocyte, can be induced *in vitro* within two hours. This assay is based on a decade of work concerned with the characterization of cell-surface markers, especially the cytotypic differentiation alloantigens of murine T-cells. As a result of this work on the cell-surface composition of murine lymphocytes, we can summarize the antigenic phenotype of the cortical thymocyte as shown in FIGURE 1. The maturational step in the pathway of T-cell differentiation that can be induced *in vitro* involves the appearance of this characteristic antigen profile on the surface of the precursor cell; it can be seen that in this differentiation event the products of at least six unlinked genes are expressed.

This rapid *in vitro* T-cell induction assay clearly had potential as a possible bioassay for the identification of the thymic hormone responsible for inducing T-cell differentiation *in vivo*. Our further studies were designed to answer pertinent questions with respect to this possible application of the assay.

Is T-cell Differentiation Induced Only By Thymus Extracts?

Our original experiments with heat-treated extracts of mouse tissues did indeed suggest that T-cell differentiation was induced by thymus extracts and not by extracts of inappropriate tissues.[1] However, when this study was extended to bovine tissue extracts that had been further fractionated we found that extracts of tissues other than thymus could also induce T-cell differentiation.[2] This led us to explore the range of materials that would induce T-cell differentiation *in vitro* and to study their functional characteristics. Clear precedents for nonspecific triggering have already been established in relation to the action of certain polypeptide hormones, which function via cyclic AMP as a second messenger by activating hormone-specific membrane receptors linked to adenylate cyclase. The physiological response to these hormones can be mimicked by substances that elevate intracellular cyclic AMP levels by other mechanisms.

Is Cyclic AMP Involved In T-cell Induction?

We found that cyclic AMP is indeed the intracellular mediator for the differentiation of prothymocytes to thymocytes. This conclusion was reached

* Supported by grants from the National Cancer Institute (CA-08748) and National Institutes of Health (RO-1-08415-01).

from the following experimental observations we made using several different approaches.

First, exogenous cyclic AMP (1 mM) or its analogue dibutyryl cyclic AMP (DBcAMP 0.1 mM) induced T-cell differentiation *in vitro*.[2] Secondly, agents modifying the levels of endogenous cyclic AMP caused appropriate changes in the efficiency of induction.[2] Thus, theophylline (1 mM), which inhibits phosphodiesterase and impairs cyclic AMP hydrolysis, enhanced induction by suboptimal concentrations of thymus extracts; insulin, which lowers endogenous cyclic AMP levels under certain circumstances, prevented induction by thymus extract (TABLE 1).

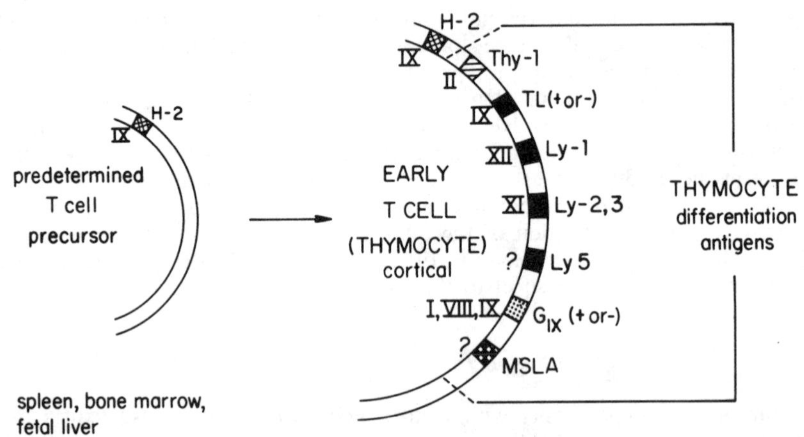

FIGURE 1. Alloantigens of murine prothymocytes and thymocytes showing thymopoietin induced phenotypic conversion *in vitro*. Antigen representation: H-2; on all cell types. Thy-1; on thymocytes, brain, epidermal cells, fibroblasts. G_{IX}; thymocytes, sperm. MSLA; thymocytes, peripheral T-cells, brain, epidermal cells. TL; thymocytes. Ly-1, Ly-2,3, Ly-5; thymocytes, peripheral T-cells.

In addition, epinephrine and β-adrenergic agonists, which are known to elevate cyclic AMP levels in many tissues, were also effective as inducing agents (TABLE 2). Finally, direct measurements of cyclic AMP levels in intact cells during induction showed rapid and appropriate elevations of accumulated cyclic AMP.[3]

The involvement of the adenylate cyclase-cyclic AMP system in the pathway that triggers the prothymocyte to express new surface components explains how a variety of agents can substitute for the physiological inducer. But it raises the question of whether the capacity of these nonthymic agents to initiate cytotypic differentiation is restricted to the triggering of T-precursor cells or whether other precursor cells, for example of the B-line, can be triggered as well.

TABLE 1

SYNERGISTIC EFFECT OF THEOPHYLLINE AND ANTAGONISTIC EFFECT OF INSULIN ON THE INDUCTION OF TL ANTIGEN BY THYMUS EXTRACT *in Vitro*

Treatment		Cells induced (TL^+) (%)
Calf thymus extract		10–15
Calf thymus extract + theophylline	1mM	25
	2mM	23–26
	5mM	21
	10mM	20
Calf thymus extract + insulin	80mU/ml	5
No extract		2
Insulin 80mU/ml		3
Theophylline 2mM		3

TABLE 2

DIFFERENTIATION OF T-PRECURSOR AND IMMATURE B-CELLS BY THYMIC AND NONTHYMIC AGENTS *in Vitro*

Material Tested	Induction of Cytotypic Marker (%) †	
	TL; Thy-1 * T cell	C′3-Receptor B cell
Calf thymus fraction 2	24±4	16±3
DB cAMP (10^{-4}M)	25±5	15±3
Isoproterenol (10^{-4}M)	22±4	20±5
Isoproterenol + propranolol (10^{-4}M)	<2	<2
Epinephrine (10^{-4}M)	18±3	14±4
Endotoxin 25 μg/ml	22±5	20±3
Lipid A 20 μg/ml	25±4	15±5
Poly A:U 10 μg/ml	22±5	18±4

* Results for TL and Thy-1 antigens were always concordant.

These various nonthymic agents and crude thymus extract induce B-cell as well as T-cell differentiation suggesting that they are *not* acting via a hormone-specific receptor restricted to prothymocytes.

† The percentage of cells induced was calculated according to the formula $\frac{a-b}{a} \times 100$.
Where: a=negative cells (percent) after incubation with no inducing agent; b= negative cells (percent) after incubation with inducing agent.

Data summarized above represent means ± SEM from 3–5 experiments with the various inducers under standardized test conditions.

Can B-cell Differentiation Be Induced by Cyclic AMP?

The induction of B-cell differentiation *in vitro* was studied by applying similar principles to those used in the T-cell differentiation assay. In these experiments our cytotypic markers for B-cells were surface immunoglobulin,[4] the Ia alloantigen,[5] Pc,[6] MBLA,[7] MSPCA,[8] and the C′3 receptor.[9] To date we have found the C′3 receptor to be the most useful practical marker. Since a background of C′3-receptor-bearing cells was found in the B layer of the BSA gradient containing inducible cells, these mature cells were removed before the induction; this was done by forming rosettes with sheep erythrocytes coated with antibody and complement (EAC). Using this assay we tested the target cell specificity of various agents known to be active inducers of prothymocyte differentiation by determining their capacity to stimulate early B-cell differentiation. As summarized in TABLE 2, cyclic AMP, or its analogue DBcAMP, catecholamines, endotoxin, and poly A:U were found to be potent inducers of both T-cell and B-cell differentiation. These results suggest that intracellular cyclic AMP elevations may be involved in the inductive signal for both early T-cell and B-cell differentiation. Many polypeptide hormones are known to act via a cyclic AMP second message.

The functional specificity of these polypeptides is determined by the specific hormone receptor in each target tissue; in each of these cyclic AMP produces a response governed by the already established commitment of the cells to a particular differentiative pathway. Because the signals initiating the differentiation of immature lymphocytes along the T as well as B-cell line appear to be mediated in common by cyclic AMP, specificity in the induction of T-cell differentiation must be determined by the interaction of the thymic hormone with receptors expressed only on prothymocytes and not on cells of the B-line. We therefore sought to evaluate this criterion of specificity in studying a putative thymic hormone.

Is Thymopoietin Specific In Inducing T-cell Differentiation?

Thymopoietin is a polypeptide hormone of the thymus isolated by its neuromuscular effects which were first discovered in relation to the human disease myasthenia gravis.[10] Using indirect cytotoxicity assays, we demonstrated that thymopoietin induced T-cell differentiation at putative physiological concentrations ranging down to 20 pg/ml.[11] We studied the specificity of this inducing capacity with respect to T-cell and B-cell differentiation and found that whilst thymopoietin clearly induced T-cell differentiation in the direct cytotoxic test (13% induction of TL^+ cells at 1 ng/ml) no significant induction of B-cell differentiation was obtained even at thymopoietin concentrations as high as 100 ng/ml. We are aware that using this marker combination the T- and B-cell assay are not strictly comparable because TL conversion and acquisition of C′3 receptors (CR) are not strictly comparable events in the sequence of T-cell and B-cell differentiation. Nevertheless the CR^- to CR^+ conversion is a clearly defined step in B-cell maturation as is the TL^- to TL^+ conversion of the prothymocytes.

Ubiquitous Immunopoietic Polypeptide (UBIP)

During the isolation of thymopoietin an additional polypeptide was purified and this was subsequently found to be present in all tissues tested. This polypeptide, termed UBIP, was potent in inducing both T-cell and B-cell differentiation *in vitro* (14% induction of TL^+ cell at 1 ng/ml and 10% induction of cells with complement receptors at the same concentration).

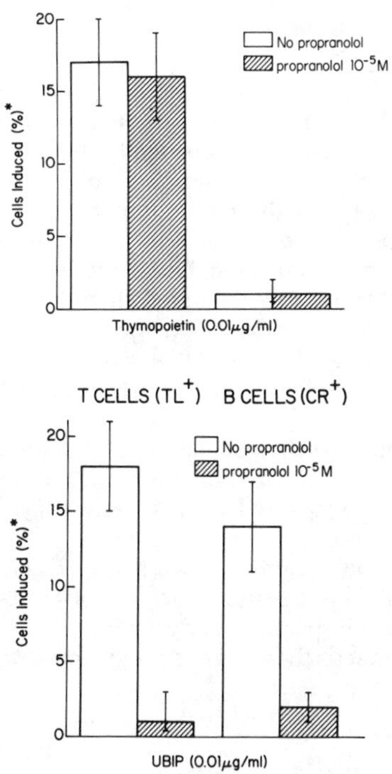

FIGURE 2. Effect of propranolol pretreatment on the induction of T- and B-cell differentiation by thymopoietin (FIGURE 2A, *top*) and UBIP (FIGURE 2B, *bottom*) *in vitro.* The induction of both T-cell and B-cell differentiation by UBIP was inhibited by propranolol whereas thymopoietin induction of T-cell differentiation was unaffected.

Experiments with the β-adrenergic blocking agent propranolol showed that the inductive signals provided by thymopoietin and UBIP are processed by different receptors, which are both linked to the adenylate cyclase complex. Preincubation of the inducible precursor cell with propranolol (10^{-5} M) did not alter T-cell induction by thymopoietin (1 ng/ml, 10 ng/ml) whereas it completely inhibited the induction of T-precursor and immature B-cells by UBIP (10 ng/ml) (FIGURES 2A and 2B). The capacity of thymopoietin to induce the differentiation of T-precursor cells exclusively emphasizes that by virtue of its target-cell specificity thymopoietin is likely to be the physiological inducer of this step in T-cell differentiation.

The physiological function of the widely represented polypeptide UBIP remains unclear at the moment. It seems likely that it does not generally function as an inducer of T-cell differentiation *in vivo,* because it can be isolated from tissues of genetically thymus-deprived mice (nu/nu), which do not differentiate significant numbers of T-cells. On the other hand, UBIP could well be responsible for the capacity of tissue extracts from organs other than thymus to induce the differentiation of immunocytes *in vitro,* and since it is present in far greater amounts than thymopoietin, it clearly complicates the interpretation of inductive effects of thymus extracts.

Are T- and B-precursor Cells Precommitted?

Our studies to date allow no other interpretation than that the cells induced to differentiate to T-cells or B-cells are already predetermined. Inducible cells are found in spleen and bone marrow of normal and genetically thymus-deprived mice; in embryonic liver, cells capable of differentiation to T-cells are found as early as 14 days.[12] This indicates that the commitment of precursor cells to T-cell differentiation develops in the absence of a thymus. Further, our contrasting experiments with thymopoietin and UBIP imply that precommitted T-cell precursors are distinct from precommitted B-cell precursors. One cell has thymopoietin receptors, the other does not. Both execute their predetermined programs in response to elevated intracellular cyclic AMP levels, whether this elevation was caused by stimulation of the thymopoietin receptor or by other means.

Additional evidence for the conclusion that prothymocytes and immature B-cells are two different populations is provided by their different distributions in density gradients, where T-precursor cells are recovered from a denser layer than immature B-cells.

Finally, recent experiments using successive treatments with the T-cell-specific inducer thymopoietin and then UBIP indicate that heterogenous precursor populations can be selectively depleted of prothymocytes with thymopoietin leaving inducible B-cell precursors intact; these can subsequently be stimulated to differentiate by UBIP.

Concept of Early T-cell and B-cell Differentiation

The experiments summarized above imply that separate precommitted prothymocytes and pro-B cells arise in the hemopoietic tissues. These may be characterized as having surface receptors for the respective physiological agents inducing their differentiations. The intracellular effector mechanisms for both cell systems are similar in that both utilize cyclic AMP, which initiates a preprogrammed pattern of differentiation (FIGURE 3) producing in one case T-cells in the other B-cells.

In the case of prothymocyte-to-thymocyte differentiation we infer that thymopoietin is the physiological inducing signal within the thymus. For B-cell differentiation the physiological inducer remains unknown.

In this scheme, differentiation is induced by other agents which elevate cyclic AMP levels. In particular, β-adrenergic receptors, linked to adenylate cyclase, are present on both prothymocytes and pro-B cells, and can be activated by epinephrine, UBIP and other β-adrenergic agonists. Induction of differentiation by agents such as these adequately explains the occasional finding of cells bearing the characteristic T-cell phenotype in genetically athymic mice.

The intracellular mechanism activating the predetermined program of differentiation is of particular interest. Within two hours, and in the absence of cell division, a complex program is executed whereby the products of at least 6 genes are expressed on the cell surface.

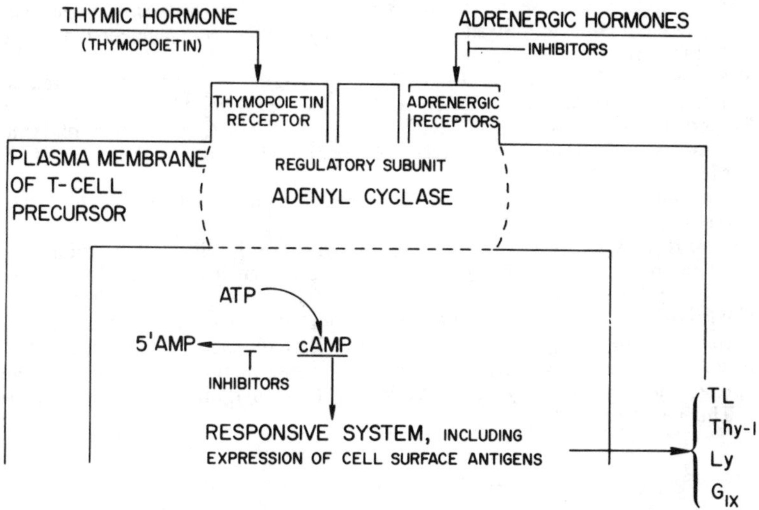

FIGURE 3. Model for reception of the inductive stimulus by prothymocytes. It is implied that thymopoietin interaction with its specific receptor is the physiological mechanism for initiating prothymocyte to thymocyte differentiation. Adenylate cyclase stimulation via the adrenergic receptor, and rise of cellular cAMP levels by other mechanisms, mimic the physiological process. Response of prothymocytes to cAMP elevation depends on preprogrammed commitment. A similar scheme for the cAMP dependent differentiation of B-cells is proposed.

This is accompanied by some functional maturation, as indicated by acquisition of responsiveness to the plant mitogens concanavalin-A and phytohemagglutinin similar to that found in thymocytes;[13] but that is another part of the story.

References

1. KOMURO, K. & E. A. BOYSE. 1973. *In vitro* demonstration of thymic hormone in the mouse by conversion of precursor cells into lymphocytes. Lancet : 740–743.
2. SCHEID, M. P., M. K. HOFFMANN, K. KOMURO, U. HAMMERLING, J. ABBOTT,

E. A. Boyse, G. H. Cohen, J. A. Hooper, R. S. Schulof & A. L. Goldstein. 1973. Differentiation of T cells induced by preparations from thymus and by non-thymic agents. J. Exp. Med. **138:** 1027–1032.
3. Collaborative studies under progress with R. Coffrey and J. Hadden at Sloan-Kettering Institute, New York, N.Y.
4. Takahashi, T., L. J. Old, K. R. McIntire & E. A. Boyse. 1971. Immunoglobulin and other surface antigens of cells of the immune system. J. Exp. Med. **134:** 815–832.
5. Hammerling, G. J., B. D. Deak, G. Mauve, U. Hammerling & H. A. McDevitt. 1974. B lymphocyte alloantigens controlled by the *I* region of the major histocompatibility complex in mice. Immunogenetics **1:** 68–81.
6. Takahashi, T., L. J. Old & E. A. Boyse. 1970. Surface alloantigens of plasma cells. J. Exp. Med. **131:** 1325–1341.
7. Raff, M. C., S. Nase & N. A. Mitchison. 1971. Mouse specific bone marrow derived lymphocyte antigen as a marker for thymus-independent lymphocytes. Nature **230:** 50.
8. Takahashi, T., L. J. Old, C-J. Hsu & E. A. Boyse. 1971. A new differentiation antigen of plasma cells. Europ. J. Immunol. **1:** 478–482.
9. Bianco, C., R. Patrick & V. Nussenzweig. 1970. A population of lymphocytes bearing a membrane receptor for antigen-antibody-complex. J. Exp. Med. **132:** 702.
10. Goldstein, G. 1974. Isolation of bovine thymin, a polypeptide hormone of the thymus. Nature **247:** 11–14.
11. Basch, R. S. & G. Goldstein. 1974. Induction of T-cell differentiation *in vitro* by thymin, a purified polypeptide hormone of the thymus. Proc. Nat. Acad. Sci. U.S. **71:** 1474–1478.
12. Komuro, K. & E. A. Boyse. 1973. Induction of T lymphocytes from precursor cells *in vitro* by a product of the thymus. J. Exp. Med. **138:** 479–482.
13. Basch, R. S. & G. Goldstein. Antigenic and functional evidence for the *in vitro* induction activity of thymopoietin (thymin) on thymocyte precursors. This volume.

Discussion of the Paper

Dr. G. Cohen: Dr. Scheid, I quite agree with you that it would be a bit naive to think that the same substance which would make a T-cell mature would make a B-cell mature. However, I think we have to consider the possibility that triggering a T-cell to mature to a certain state may then result in a signal to a B-cell to make a B-cell mature. Therefore, so long as you have some T-cells or pre-T-cells mixed in with your B-cells when you test for differentiation of B-cell markers, it is hard to exclude that possibility.

Dr. M. Scheid: That is absolutely true; we cannot exclude it. Nevertheless, there is a difference between the activity of the T-cells induced by thymopoietin and those induced by other factors. Thus there must be some difference involved.

Dr. A. Johnson: In your studies with LPS I noticed you were at the 20 microgram per milliliter level. I wonder if you showed any signs of cytotoxicity in lymphocytes at that level?

Dr. M. Scheid: No, not at all. These are concentrations which we use without any difficulty.

Dr. H. Claman: Some of the work that you have done shows the new expression of these surface markers on cells from normal mouse bone marrow. Is that correct?

DR. M. SCHEID: Yes.

DR. H. CLAMAN: You keep calling these cells precursors of T-cells in the normal mouse. What evidence do you have that they might not, in fact, be postthymic cells which have lost their antigen and are reexpressing the same antigen?

DR. M. SCHEID: The evidence is the fact that we find these precursor cells in nu/nu mice and fetal liver.

DR. H. CLAMAN: The nude mouse is a different case, perhaps. But in the normal mouse there is good evidence that the bone marrow contains immunocompetent T-cells which have no θ marker.

DR. M. SCHEID: What is the evidence that this is a mature T-cell if it does not have any markers?

DR. H. CLAMAN: The bone marrow produces GvH reactions, as well as PHA responses, and yet you cannot detect θ-positive cells. It is entirely possible that a cell which has come from the thymic cortex with lots of θ antigen perhaps goes through the medulla with less θ antigen and finally arrives in the bone marrow where you can't find markers; this does not mean it never had the marker.

DR. M. SCHEID: Can you abolish the PHA response with anti-θ sera?

DR. H. CLAMAN: No, and you cannot absorb an anti-θ serum with bone marrow. Dr. Raff has shown that you cannot find θ-positive cells by indirect or direct fluorescent staining. So it is quite clear that the normal bone marrow of a mouse does not have any θ-positive cells; that is clear. It is also clear that the bone marrow has some, although not an awful lot of functions that we attribute to T-cells. Thus this is an interesting dilemma.

DR. M. SCHEID: It is not possible to know the sensitivity of these cells towards induction stimuli, for instance, PHA.

DR. H. CLAMAN: That is the point in question.

DR. M. SCHEID: Yes, that is why I say it is very difficult experimentally to decide between these two possibilities.

DR. H. CLAMAN: One thing that can be done is to ask if these cells in the bone marrow are thymus-dependent and see whether neonatal thymectomy might decrease them. As a matter of fact, neonatal thymectomy at least decreases the PHA response of bone marrow cells by half, which indicates that some of these cells perhaps represent cells that came through the thymus. It is not unequivocal but it points in that direction. It is a difficult question which involves both immunology and perhaps a little semantics.

DR. M. SCHEID: I think the point we would really like to make is that we are looking at T-precursor cells and they are present in nude mice and in fetal liver. Whether or not there are some cells in normal spleen or bone marrow which have the characteristics you were talking about can't be excluded. But we know that our general induction phenomenon is observed in these fetal liver cells and in these nude mouse cells. It is a different question whether or not you can have a cell in a later stage which went through the θ expression and TL expression and is influenced again by thymopoietin.

DR. R. GERSHON: I'd like to go to the opposite tack that Dr. Claman was taking. Were you calling these thymic precursor cells? In my mind that implies this cell is differentiated in the pathway where it now must become a thymic cell or nothing else. And why couldn't this just be any cell that you're inducing? Why do you insist that it is a thymic precursor cell and not just a precursor cell that happens to get turned on by your factors?

DR. M. SCHEID: Are you raising the question whether there is a common precursor which is inducible for both T- and B-cell markers equally well? Our studies of the induction selectivity of thymopoietin and other inducing agents clearly establish that the precursor T-cell is restricted to this differentiation pathway (see text).

Ir GENES AND ANTIGEN RECOGNITION

E. M. Shevach, F. Finkelman, S. Z. Ben-Sasson, I. Green,
and W. E. Paul

Laboratory of Immunology
National Institute of Allergy and Infectious Diseases
National Institutes of Health
Bethesda, Maryland 20014

Over the past decade it has become clear that the capacity of individual animals to mount specific immune responses is regulated by a series of immune response (*Ir*) genes. One important group of *Ir* genes is linked to the major histocompatibility complex of the species; these genes are referred to as histocompatibility (H)-linked *Ir* genes.

The mechanism by which H-linked *Ir* genes and their products control immune responses is still unknown. However, a large body of evidence gained from studies of guinea pig *Ir* genes has indicated that these genes play a critical role in the recognition of carrier functions of antigens. This has suggested that the *Ir* genes and their products are principally expressed within thymus-dependent (T) lymphocytes.[1] Indeed, a major possibility is that Ir gene products function as antigen-recognition units on the surface of T-lymphocytes.[2] More recently, it has been suggested that *Ir* genes may be expressed in other types of lymphoid cells as well. Thus, limiting-dilution cell-transfer studies in mice have raised the possibility that, under certain conditions, *Ir* genes may exert their effect in bone marrow-derived (B) lymphocytes.[3] Moreover, *in vitro* cellular interactions between guinea pig macrophages and T-lymphocytes [4] and between mouse T-lymphocytes and B-lymphocytes [5] have been shown to involve structures controlled by genes closely linked, or perhaps identical, to *Ir* genes. These studies indicate that Ir gene-product function may be quite complex.

We have been interested in the elucidation of the mechanism by which *Ir* genes exert their control of the immune response, and, in particular, in determining whether the genetic linkage between *H* genes and *Ir* genes is reflected phenotypically. To these ends, we have undertaken a series of experiments involving the effect of alloantisera containing antibodies specific for histocompatibility determinants on the capacity of antigens to elicit T-lymphocyte responses controlled by H-linked *Ir* genes.

Our experimental system involves the use of lymphocytes purified from the peritoneal exudate of (strain-2 × strain-13)F_1 guinea pigs. This cell population is highly enriched in T-lymphocytes [6] and is exceptionally antigen-reactive.[7] Peritoneal exudate lymphocytes are obtained from animals that have been immunized 2 to 3 weeks earlier with one or more of a series of antigens, responsiveness to which is controlled by H-linked *Ir* genes. In the initial experiments, we used the 2,4-dinitrophenyl conjugate of the copolymer of L-glutamic acid and L-lysine (DNP-GL) and the copolymer of L-glutamic acid and L-tyrosine (GT). Responsiveness to DNP-GL is controlled by an *Ir* gene linked to strain 2 *H* genes [8] whereas responsiveness to GT is controlled by a 13-linked *Ir* gene.[9]

Lymphocytes from $(2 \times 13)F_1$ guinea pigs primed to DNP-GL and to GT in complete Freund's adjuvant are stimulated to synthesize DNA by both DNP-GL and GT (TABLE 1). This response largely reflects T-lymphocyte function in our system. Responsiveness to both antigens on the part of the F_1 animal is in keeping with the fact that the F_1 possesses *Ir* genes inherited from the strain-2 and from the strain-13 parent. If $(2 \times 13)F_1$ cells from doubly immunized animals are cultured in the presence of heat-inactivated alloantisera raised by immunization of strain-13 guinea pigs with strain-2 lymphoid cells, the response to DNP-GL is completely inhibited whereas the responses to GT, to purified protein derivative of tuberculin (PPD) or to phytohemagglutinin (PHA) are only modestly diminished. On the other hand, when the same cell population is cultured in the presence of heat-inactivated anti-13 serum, raised in an analogous manner to the anti-2 serum, the response to GT is specifically impaired whereas responses to DNP-GL, PPD and PHA are relatively preserved (TABLE 1).

TABLE 1

ALLOANTISERUM INHIBITION OF PROLIFERATIVE RESPONSES OF $(2\times13)F_1$ LYMPHOCYTES *

	DNP-GL	GT	PPD	PHA
NGPS	64,862	13,571	16,550	53,388
Anti-2	0	10,668	9,607	42,802
Anti-13	44,901	286	13,675	26,610

* Peritoneal exudate lymphocytes from $(2\times13)F_1$ guinea pigs were incubated for 30 minutes with DNP-GL (100 μg), GT (100 μg), PPD (100 μg) or PHA (10 μg) and washed. They were cultured for 72 hours in the presence of heat-inactivated anti-2 serum, anti-13 serum or normal guinea pig serum (NGPS) at a final concentration of 10%. The incorporation of tritiated thymodine into acid precipitable material was determined and the results are presented as cpm.

This experiment shows that responses of $(2 \times 13)F_1$ cells that are controlled by 2-linked *Ir* genes are blocked by anti-2 sera whereas responses controlled by 13-linked *Ir* genes are only marginally affected by anti-2 sera. Similarly, anti-13 sera block responses controlled by 13-linked *Ir* genes but have little effect on responses controlled by 2-linked *Ir* genes. These results indicate a phenotypic expression of the genetic linkage between *Ir* genes and histocompatibility (*H*) genes.[10]

Such a linkage might be expressed either at the level of cellular specialization or on the level of an association of gene products on or within the cell. In the former case, one would require that among the population of $(2 \times 13)F_1$ lymphocytes, those responsive to DNP-GL would exclusively (or predominantly) express the strain-2 alloantigens whereas those responsive to GT would show a similar preference in the expression of strain-13 alloantigens. If these relationships held, then alloantiserum-induced blockade could be explained by a general inactivation of the responsive cell. Consequently, we have sought by a variety of means to establish whether or not allelic exclusion (or "allelic preference") exists for the expression of products of guinea pig histocompatibility genes. Thus far, our studies on this point provide no evidence for allelic exclusion. Using indirect immunofluorescence to evaluate $(2 \times 13)F_1$ lymphocytes we find that greater than 95% can be stained by anti-2 serum alone, anti-13 serum alone or anti-2 serum plus anti-13 serum. Similarly, the same degree of complement-mediated lysis of chromated $(2 \times 13)F_1$ lymphocytes is achieved by anti-2 serum, anti-13 serum or a mixture of the two. Finally, if $(2 \times 13)F_1$ peritoneal exudate lymphocytes are treated with limiting amounts of anti-2 serum and complement, the cells remaining alive do not show a preferential diminution in their responsiveness to DNP-GL as compared to their responsiveness to GT. This suggests that the T-lymphocytes richest in strain 2 alloantigens are not more likely to respond to DNP-GL than to GT.

Thus, the explanation for alloantiserum-induced blockade of T-cell activation in this system must involve some type of local relationship on or in the cell between the Ir gene product and the antigen(s) for which the blocking sera are specific. One obvious relationship would be that the blocking antibodies are, in fact, directed at the Ir gene products themselves. First, we must consider whether the Ir gene product may in fact be the histocompatibility antigen against which the principal cytotoxic antibodies in the anti-2 or anti-13 sera are directed. This appears unlikely, principally on genetic grounds. Thus, one encounters, in outbred populations of guinea pigs, individual animals which have associations of alloantigens and *Ir* genes that differ from the association seen in inbred animals. Although some reservation as to the decisiveness of this finding can be raised (see below), it strongly suggests that *Ir* genes and *H* genes, although linked, are distinct from each other. If the H antigens and the Ir gene products are coded for by independent but linked genes, antibodies specific for the Ir gene product and mediating the observed inhibitory activity might nonetheless exist within the alloantisera. Such antibodies might be specific for unique antigenic determinants of the Ir gene product (analogs of anti-idiotype antibodies) or for determinants common to several Ir-gene products of the inbred strain (analogs of antiallotype antibodies). In order to determine whether the blocking antibodies were specific for unique antigenic determinants of a *clonally expressed* Ir gene product, we compared lymph node cells from strain-2 guinea pigs immunized to DNP-GL in Freund's adjuvant to lymph node cells of strain-2 guinea pigs immunized only with adjuvant and saline in their capacity to adsorb the ability of anti-2 sera to block DNP-GL responses of $(2 \times 13)F_1$ cells. If blocking activity were due to "antiidiotype" activity and if clonal expansion occurred upon immunization, one would anticipate that many more cells from DNP-GL-immune animals would bear the relevant idiotype and that such cells would be much more efficient adsorbents of blocking activity than would cells from control animals. In fact, we have observed no difference whatever in the relative adsorptive capacity of the cell populations.[11] Similarly, the use of both DNP-GL-immune cells and control strain-2 cells as immunogens to prepare anti-2 serum in strain-13 guinea pigs did not demonstrate the former to be more efficient in eliciting inhibitory sera. These experiments provide strong evidence against the concept that the inhibitory alloantibodies are directed at unique antigenic determinants of specific Ir gene products that are clonally distributed and that are subject to clonal expansion upon appropriate immunization.

In the determination of whether the inhibitory antibodies are specific for more constant antigens of Ir gene products or for unique antigenic determinants of a nonclonally distributed Ir gene product, an analysis of genetic recombinant animals would be decisive. For example, in strain-2 guinea pigs a close association between the *Ir* gene controlling responsiveness to the copolymer of glutamic acid and alanine (GA) and the strain-2 *H* gene(s) exists.[9] Anti-2 serum blocks the response of lymphocytes from $(2 \times 13)F_1$ guinea pigs to GA.[2] An ideal test of the specificity of the blocking antibodies would involve the capacity of anti-2 serum to block responsiveness to GA of cells from guinea pigs whose histocompatibility regions derived from recombination between 2^-GA^- and 2^+GA^+ chromosomes leading to a 2^-GA^+ chromosome. If anti-2 serum blocked the response to GA of such 2^-GA^+ cells, it would strongly suggest that the blocking antibodies were specific for the GA-Ir gene product rather than for the strain-2 H-antigen. Similarly, if the anti-2 serum failed to block responses of such cells, it would lead to the suggestion that the blocking activity depended upon the interaction of anti-2 antibody with strain-2 histocompatibility antigens. The latter would imply an indirect blockade of Ir-gene product function.

Unfortunately, no genetically documented recombinant chromosomes of the type required exist in progeny of inbred animals. However, a substantial fraction of outbred guinea pigs are 2^-GA^+. These animals may provide the desired genetic situation. We have compared the capacity of anti-2 serum to block the response to GA of cells from 2^+GA^+ and from 2^-GA^+ animals. We find that in the great majority of individual cases, anti-2 serum blocks responses to GA of cells from 2^+GA^+ animals but has little or no effect on the response to GA of cells from 2^-GA^+ animals.[2] This strongly suggests that the blocking activity is mediated by antibodies specific for the linked strain 2 alloantigen rather than for the Ir gene product itself. One reservation concerning this conclusion must be expressed. That is, it is possible that the GA-Ir gene product of 2^-GA^+ cells is different from the GA-Ir gene product of 2^+GA^+ cells. Thus, antibodies specific for the GA-Ir gene products of 2^+GA^+ animals might fail to block the response to GA of 2^-GA^+ cells not because the latter lacked the 2 histocompatibility antigen but rather because the GA-Ir gene product they possessed failed to cross react with the GA-Ir gene product against which the inhibitory antibodies were directed. Although we believe this possibility to be somewhat unlikely, we attempted to produce antibodies against the GA-Ir gene product of 2^- guinea pigs by immunizing strain-13 guinea pigs with cells from 2^-GA^+ animals. We found that these sera failed to block responses to GA of 2^-GA^+ cells, further supporting the contention that the blocking antibodies are specific for "histocompatibility" antigens rather than Ir gene products.

Our experiments thus lead us to conclude that the function of a given Ir gene product is blocked by alloantisera but that this blockade is indirect in that it involves the interaction of the alloantisera with the product of a gene linked to but distinct from the *Ir* gene. This finding suggests that the 2 alloantigen and the GA-Ir gene product must be closely related. Indeed, current views of the fluidity of lymphocyte surfaces and of the apparent capacity of individual molecules to diffuse freely in the plane of the membrane lead us to propose that the 2 alloantigen and the GA-Ir gene product exist as a molecular complex. If the molecules were entirely independent, one would anticipate that any associations between them would be random. In such a case, it would seem unlikely that anti-2 antibody could specifically block unresponsiveness to GA or GL. One could, of course, argue that the molecules normally exist independently but form a transitory complex as a requisite for specific activation. This is clearly a possible alternative to the notion that the histocompatibility antigen and the Ir gene product exist as a stable molecular complex.

Because of the potential importance of such an alloantigen-Ir gene product complex, we have turned our attention to an examination of the alloantigens controlled at the 2/13 locus, both in terms of chemical structure and tissue distribution of these antigens.

As a control for studies of the 2/13 alloantigens, we have also studied a group of histocompatibility antigens recently described by Sato and deWeck.[12] These antigens include the specificities B, C, and D, and appear to be coded for at a single locus or at closely linked loci. In our laboratory at least one additional specificity controlled at the *"B,C,D"* locus has been identified. In limited studies of responsiveness of strain-2 and strain-13 lymphocytes to antigen, anti-B serum produced a generalized depression of T-lymphocyte proliferation, in contrast to the specific blockade produced by anti-2 and anti-13 sera. This suggests important biological differences between the relationship of Ir gene products to 2/13 antigens and to the B,C,D antigens. In addition, the B antigen has been demonstrated to be present on several nonlymphoid tumors and appears to have a wide tissue distribution. The strain-2 and -13 antigens, on the other hand, have a much more limited tissue distribution and are principally expressed on lymphoid cells; they occur in larger amounts on bone-marrow-derived lymphocytes than on thymocytes, but they may be identified on both cell types.

Surface labeling studies using lactoperoxidase-catalyzed iodination and analysis by specific immunoprecipitation followed by electrophoresis in sodium dodecyl sulfate (SDS)-polyacrylamide gels indicate a molecular weight for B of ~45,000 Daltons with an associated low molecular weight chain of ~11,000 Daltons. The 2 and 13 antigens have apparent molecular weights of ~25,000 Daltons and no linked low molecular weight chain has yet been demonstrated.

These studies thus suggest that the B,C,D series of antigens are analogs of the D and K series of antigens of mice and of the LA and Four series of antigens of humans. The 2/13 antigens appear analogous to the recently described Ia antigens of mice,[13-16] which are controlled by genes located in the same portion of the mouse H-2 region as are all the mouse *Ir* genes thus far mapped. Intensive studies of the structure of the 2 and 13 antigens promises to yield important insights into the functional role of Ir gene products.

In closing this discussion of guinea pig H-linked *Ir* genes, a consideration of the major possible roles of *Ir* genes and their products may be illuminating. The finding that possession of a given *Ir* gene endows an animal with the capacity to respond to a single antigen or to a group of closely related antigens implies some specific role for *Ir* genes rather than a general role in cell activation. Although the possibility has been considered that *Ir* genes function only during development to control the emergence of cells with specific receptors,[17] our findings that activation of $(2 \times 13)F_1$ cells can be specifically blocked by alloantisera at the time of antigenic challenge, strongly suggests that such a role for *Ir* genes is unlikely.

Rather, it appears that Ir gene products function in the actual recognition of, or activation of the cell by, antigen. We have previously suggested that one obvious mechanism for the control exerted by Ir genes would be that they are structural genes for variable portions of T-lymphocyte receptors.[2] This model has certain appealing features. It provides an obvious explanation for alloantisera-mediated inhibition of T-lymphocyte activation. In such a case, one envisages the 2/13 alloantigens to be an analog of immunoglobulin H chain constant regions and the Ir gene products to be analogs of immunoglobulin H chain variable regions. Indeed, it would seem logical to propose that both the IgC_H and the IgV_H genes of immunoglobulin and the *Ir* genes and genes controlling alloantigens such as 2 and 13 are derived from a common primordial "recognition" gene. Furthermore, the increased efficiency of cellular interactions between syngeneic or semisyngeneic macrophages and T-lymphocytes[4] and T-lymphocytes and B-lymphocytes[5] might reflect a recognition function exerted by the so-called constant portion of the postulated alloantigen-Ir gene product complex. That is, the 2 alloantigen on the T-lymphocyte might interact with 2 alloantigen on either macrophages or B-lymphocytes to allow intimate cell contact and/or efficient cellular interaction.

Although the specific aspects of Ir gene product function are easiest to explain by postulating that the Ir gene product is the prime antigen-binding receptor of the T-lymphocytes, other roles for these genes must be carefully considered. This is especially true in view of some recent work on antigen-recognition by T-lymphocytes. Some,[18, 19] but not all,[20-22] investigators report the presence of surface immunoglobulin on T-lymphocytes and experiments indicating a crucial role for "T-lymphocyte immunoglobulin (IgT)" have been presented.[23] In addition, in mouse systems involving Ir-gene-controlled responses to multichain polymers, it has been reported that some aspects of T-lymphocyte functions are normal in "unresponsive" strains, but that B-lymphocyte activation is defective in such animals.[3] Although these studies are still not definitive, they suggest that considerable attention should be given to the concept that Ir gene products function principally to regulate interaction between cells or to determine whether an antigen that has been specifically bound to a cell by its "prime" antigen-binding receptor will activate that cell. In both these cases, the specificity envisaged for the Ir gene product is of a relatively low order. It would be unlikely that, for such functions, a specific recognition resembling that of antibody and antigen would be feasible or desirable. Rather, the identification of "general" molecular characteristics such as charge or hydrophobicity would be more reasonable. The evidence regarding specificity in *Ir* gene controlled systems is not decisive on this point. On the one hand, there are findings that the guinea pig *Ir* genes controlling responses to low doses of DNP-bovine serum albumin[24] are different from those controlling responses to low doses of DNP-guinea pig albumin[25] and the findings that mouse *Ir* genes controlling responses to IgG and IgA myeloma proteins are different.[26] These observations suggest a rather sophisticated system of molecular interaction capable of distinguishing rather similar molecules. On the other hand, it has been shown that responsiveness of guinea pigs to a series of antigens with concentrations of positive charges (poly-L-lysine, poly-L-arginine, poly-L-ornithine, protamine and the copolymer of L-glutamic acid and L-lysine) are all controlled by 2-linked *Ir* genes.[27] It is possible that this linkage reflects the fact that the same Ir gene product recognizes each of these antigens despite the fact that T-cell responses distinguish these antigens. This would imply a clear difference between the specificity of Ir gene products and that of T-cell receptors. Alternatively, the genes controlling these responses may be either a linked series of *Ir* genes that arose by duplication and mutation from a single gene or a group of genes derived by somatic mutation from a single germ line *Ir* gene. In the latter two cases, it would be possible for *Ir* genes to code for specific T-cell receptors and still explain the apparent specificity difference between genetic control and T-lymphocyte recognition of antigen.

To reach a definitive conclusion on the mode of function of Ir gene products and their role in antigen recognition will clearly require both the isolation and characterization of Ir gene products on the one hand and a definitive solution to the nature of the T-lymphocyte receptors on the other. This area of modern immunology promises to be an exciting and fruitful avenue of current research.

References

1. Benacerraf, B. & H. O. McDevitt. 1972. Science **175:** 273.
2. Shevach, E. M., W. E. Paul & I. Green. 1974. J. Exp. Med. **139:** 679.
3. Shearer, G. M., E. Mozes & M. Sela. 1972. J. Exp. Med. **135:** 1009.
4. Shevach, E. M. & A. S. Rosenthal. 1973. J. Exp. Med. **138:** 1213.
5. Katz, D. H., T. Hamaoka, M. E. Dorf, P. H. Maurer & B. Benacerraf. 1973. J. Exp. Med. **138:** 734.
6. Rosenthal, A. S., D. L. Rosenstreich, J. M. Davie & J. T. Blake. 1972. Proc. of the Sixth Leucocyte Culture Conf. : 433. Academic Press. New York, N.Y.
7. Rosenstreich, D. L., J. T. Blake & A. S. Rosenthal. 1971. J. Exp. Med. **134:** 1170.
8. Ellman, L., I. Green, W. J. Martin & B. Benacerraf. 1970. Proc. Nat. Acad. Sci. U.S. **66:** 322.
9. Bluestein, H. G., I. Green & B. Benacerraf. 1971. J. Exp. Med. **134:** 458.
10. Shevach, E. M., W. E. Paul & I. Green. 1972. J. Exp. Med. **136:** 1207.
11. Shevach, E. M., W. E. Paul & I. Green. 1974. J. Exp. Med. **139:** 661.
12. Sato, W. & A. L. deWeck. 1972. Z. Immunitaetsforsch. Allerg. Klin. Immunol. **144:** S. 49.
13. Hauptfeld, V., D. Klein & J. Klein. 1973. Science **181:** 167.
14. David, C. S., D. C. Shreffler & J. A. Frelinger. 1973. Proc. Nat. Acad. Sci. U.S. **70:** 2509.
15. Sachs, D. H. & J. L. Cone. 1973. J. Exp. Med. **138:** 1289.
16. Hammerling, G. J., B. D. Deak, G. Mauve, U. Hammerling & H. O. McDevitt. 1974. Immunogenetics **1:** 68.
17. Jerne, N. K. 1971. Eur. J. Immunol. **1:** 1.
18. Marchalonis, J. J., R. E. Cone & J. L. Atwell. 1972. J. Exp. Med. **135:** 956.
19. Moroz, C. & Y. Hahn. 1973. Proc. Nat. Acad. Sci. U.S. **70:** 3716.
20. Vitetta, E. X., C. Bianco, V. Nussenzweig & J. W. Uhr. 1972. J. Exp. Med. **136:** 81.
21. Grey, H. M., R. T. Kubo & J. C. Cerottini. 1972. J. Exp. Med. **136:** 1323.
22. Lisowska-Bernstein, B., A. Rinuy & P. Vassalli. 1973. Proc. Nat. Acad. Sci. U.S. **70:** 2879.
23. Feldman, M. 1972. J. Exp. Med. **136:** 737.
24. Green, I. & B. Benacerraf. 1971. J. Immunol. **107:** 374.
25. Green, I., W. E. Paul & B. Benacerraf. 1972. J. Immunol. **109:** 457.
26. Lieberman, R., W. E. Paul, W. Humphrey, Jr. & J. H. Stimpfling. 1972. J. Exp. Med. **136:** 1231.
27. Green, I., W. E. Paul & B. Benacerraf. 1969. Proc. Nat. Acad. Sci. U.S. **64:** 1095.